P9-DUP-364

THE PRINCIPLES AND PRACTICE OF BLOOD GROUPING

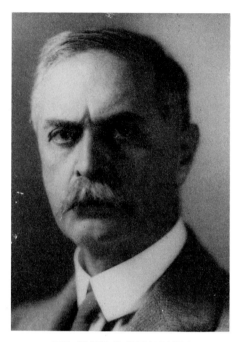

DR. KARL LANDSTEINER

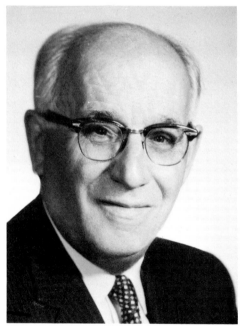

DR. PHILIP LEVINE

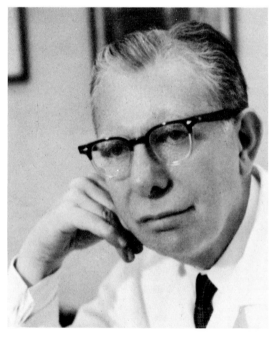

DR. ALEXANDER S. WIENER

THE PRINCIPLES AND PRACTICE OF
BLOOD GROUPING

ADDINE G. ERSKINE, D.Sc., Litt.D.(Hon.)

Chairman, Board of Directors, The Gradwohl School
of Laboratory Technique, St. Louis, Mo.; Editor of The
Quarterly Bulletin of the Missouri Branch, American
Society for Microbiology; formerly Consultant to
the Medical Division of the United States Department
of State, Washington, D.C.

WLADYSLAW W. SOCHA, M.D., Habil. Dozent

Research Professor of Forensic Medicine, Department
of Forensic Medicine, New York University School of Medicine;
Associate Director, Primate Blood Group Reference Laboratory
and World Health Organization Collaborating Centre for
Haematology of Primate Animals; Chief Pathologist, Laboratory
for Experimental Medicine and Surgery in Primates (LEMSIP)
of the New York University Medical Center, New York, N.Y.

SECOND EDITION

with 105 *illustrations*

THE C. V. MOSBY COMPANY

Saint Louis   1978

SECOND EDITION

Previous edition copyrighted 1973

Printed in the United States of America

Distributed in Great Britain by Henry Kimpton, London

The C. V. Mosby Company
11830 Westline Industrial Drive, St. Louis, Missouri 63141

Library of Congress Cataloging in Publication Data

Erskine, Addine G   1904-
 The principles and practice of blood grouping.

 Bibliography: p.
 Includes index.
 1. Compatibility testing (Hematology).   2.   Blood
groups. 3. Blood groups in animals. I. Socha,
Wladyslaw W., 1926-   joint author. II.   Title.
[DNLM: 1. Blood groups.   QY415 E73p]
RB45.5.E77 1978   612′.11825   77-13042
ISBN 0-8016-1531-3

CB/CB/B   9 8 7 6 5 4 3 2 1

TO

DR. LESTER SAWYER

CLINICAL DIRECTOR, MEDICAL DIVISION (RET.)
UNITED STATES DEPARTMENT OF STATE
WASHINGTON, D.C.

Foreword to first edition

The science of blood grouping, with its manifold applications in clinical and legal medicine, anthropology, and genetics, has greatly advanced and expanded in scope since I entered the field about forty-five years ago. There has been a great need for an up-to-date general textbook such as I visualized when I prepared the first edition of *Blood Groups and Transfusion* some forty years ago. This text was suitable for beginners and teachers because of its emphasis on basic principles, yet comprehensive enough in scope to be useful also for active advanced investigators in the field. The third and last edition of *Blood Groups and Transfusion* is now almost thirty years old and therefore does not include all the important developments initiated and stimulated largely by the discovery of the Rh factor in 1937. In this discovery I was fortunate to be associated with my mentor, Karl Landsteiner, the father of blood grouping immunochemistry, who received the Nobel Prize for his discovery of the A-B-O blood groups.

Since 1943 there has been no dearth of books on blood groups, which have attempted to include these newer advances in the field. The most important one is the deservedly popular book of Robert R. Race and Ruth Sanger, *Blood Groups in Man.* However, this book, as an up-to-date reference source, although indispensable for advanced investigators in the field, is unsuitable as a teaching text. A general text must explain basic principles, describe testing technics, outline methods of avoiding common pitfalls, and include all the details important for blood bank technicians.

Most of the available books on blood grouping have been far too limited in scope for use as a general textbook. Some have been restricted solely to description of technics with little or no explanation of the principles underlying the tests or theories proposed to explain the reactions, whereas others have been limited to such specific subjects as the use of blood grouping for blood transfusion, the applications of blood grouping to anthropology, or the exclusion of parentage in forensic cases of disputed parentage. There have even been monographs restricted simply to the use of proteolytic enzymes in the tests, books on the use of extracts of seeds as reagents, monographs limited to the antiglobulin tests, or to erythroblastosis fetalis in which tests for the Rh factor, Rh sensitization, and A-B-O sensitization play such a prominent role.

Aside from the important book by Race and Sanger, the only other comprehensive volume is the important work of O. Prokop and G. Uhlenbruck, *Human Blood and Serum Groups,* which after two German editions finally became available in English a few years ago. This ponderous volume is more ambitious than *Blood Groups in Man.* It contains an extensive bibliography, even including an elaborate list of the names and addresses of the leading workers in the field. Again, this book, although it does constitute an outstanding reference source for advanced investigators, cannot be used as a general textbook because of its uncritical and excessively detailed citations of the literature.

From time to time I have planned to prepare a new edition of *Blood Groups and Transfusion* or to prepare a new similar book incorporating the advances of the past thirty years. The pace of the investigative work of our research team has been such, however, that the need to prepare our findings for publication has forced me to restrict my own efforts to monographs of more limited scope and to several volumes of collected reprints. However, during the past few decades I have been fortunate enough to become aware of the outstanding contributions of the distinguished teacher, Addine G. Erskine, to the advancement of the field of blood groups in her capacity as both instructor and principal of the Gradwohl School of Laboratory Technique at St. Louis and as author of the outstanding section on blood groups in the widely used *Gradwohl's Clinical Laboratory Methods and Diagnosis*. While her famous uncle, R. B. H. Gradwohl, was still alive, I valued my relationship with him as colleague and friend. Since I was aware of her extensive familiarity with the field of blood grouping and her outstand-

ing abilities as author and teacher, it was natural for me to induce her to undertake the preparation of the greatly needed, modern textbook on blood grouping. Fortunately, she agreed to undertake this difficult task, with the present book the result of her efforts.

This book entirely fulfills my expectations. Because I have been partly responsible for the author's having undertaken this difficult assignment, I have closely watched its development and acted as advisor from the onset, carefully reading and editing the manuscript from beginning to end; therefore I share with the author responsibility for any errors of commission or omission. I feel grateful to her for having undertaken this task. I am convinced this useful result will do much to advance the subject of blood grouping. I recommend the book highly to the general reader, and especially to teachers, students, and to seasoned workers in the field. I trust that the book will find its proper place on the work bench of technicians in blood banks, where it will contribute to the safety of blood transfusion by stimulating in technicians greater interest in their work.

Alexander S. Wiener
1972

Preface

It has now been five years since the first edition of this book was conceived and written and four years since its publication. During that time many changes have taken place in blood grouping.

In the preface to the first edition it was stated that although there is a vast literature on blood grouping, it is difficult if not impossible to find a single book that encompasses all aspects of the subject and at the same time is suitable for both beginners and advanced workers in the field. The first edition was written to fill that void; the second edition continues with that goal in mind.

The subject matter is still presented from the point of view of the teacher so that the book is useful as a classroom text, as well as a laboratory manual and reference source in colleges, junior colleges, schools of medical laboratory technology, hospitals, and medical schools.

The text is divided into three parts and a Glossary. Part One presents the fundamental principles of blood grouping, the genetics of the blood groups, and a summary of every known blood group system as well as "private" and "public" antigens. Part Two contains two new chapters on the blood groups of nonhuman primates. Part Three is the section on methodology and can be used as a laboratory manual. Along with detailed instructions in general methods for all the blood group systems and tests made before a transfusion and in pregnancy, Part Three also contains methods helpful in medicolegal examinations,

such as identification of dried blood stains, paternity and maternity tests, the mathematics involved in blood grouping and population genetics, and all the necessary controls. It includes, also, methods used in studying the blood groups of nonhuman primates.

With the steadily accelerating progress in immunohematology and immunogenetics, it has become imperative to update the book to include the most important and latest contributions and discoveries in these fields. The scope of the various disciplines involved in the modern science of blood grouping is now so broad that the knowledge and experience of more than one person are required to cover the subject adequately. Again the advice of one of the greatest serologists of all time, Dr. Alexander S. Wiener, was sought. His last illness and untimely death, however, prevented his taking part in the actual preparation of the second edition, but he had made many suggestions as to the choice of revisions and subject matter to be added. Knowing the nature of his illness and the probable prognosis, he suggested that Dr. Socha, his closest collaborator, become the coauthor of this book.

It seemed mandatory to us, with the passing of one of the last persons who had participated in the fundamental discoveries in blood grouping, to recall the undistorted historical facts of these discoveries. This is especially advisable because of the many misrepresentations of these basic facts that have infiltrated the literature and have been indiscriminately repeated from text to text and from journal article to journal article. What had been published as the Appendix in the first edition now constitutes an integral part of the chapter on history.

We are not producing a textbook of immunology per se, but it was considered necessary to include some of the new findings in immunology, particularly the classification and role of lymphocytes in the immune response, and the nature and nomenclature of antibodies.

The discussions on chimerism and polyagglutinability have been greatly elaborated.

The complexity of the Lewis system is reflected in the revision of the chapter dealing with this subject. The important findings in the Duffy system that have stimulated the mapping of human chromosomes have been added, together with the recent discovery of the relationship between the Duffy phenotype and susceptibility to *Plasmodium vivax* malarial infection. This last problem is also discussed in the new chapter on blood groups and disease.

Considerable revision and expansion of the chapters on the high- and low-frequency antigens (private and public blood groups) have been made because of the increasing numbers of reports of incompatible transfusion reactions and transplacental immunization due to these antigens. Special attention is also paid to the so-called "null" blood group factors. These are covered in the discussion on the various blood group systems and are also recapitulated later in tabular form.

The chapter on heredity of blood groups has been enriched by discussion of linkage, mapping of chromosomes, and determination of zygosity of twins, as well as the problem of identity.

The first edition of this book included a short chapter on blood groups of nonhuman primates, unique in textbooks of this kind. Because of the increasing use of simian primates in medical experimenta-

tion and research, primarily in the fields of virology, transplantation, and cardiac and vascular surgery involving tissue and organ rejection, knowledge of the blood groups of these close relatives of man is now required. Although the necessary information is available, it is spread over many articles published in many languages, often in narrowly specialized periodicals. This second edition is the first textbook on blood grouping to include not only the general principles and most recent findings in the field of blood groups of simian primates but also the methodology involved.

Part Three on methods has been enlarged to include quality controls; these are described with each subject as it is discussed. The important substitutes for blood grouping reagents of human origin are extracts of seeds and snails, known as lectins. These are included in an entirely new section. Blood grouping laboratories more and more frequently use physical methods to detect and identify antibodies or antigens. Among such methods, counterelectrophoresis seems of prime importance, especially in screening blood donors and examining blood stains. This method is given in its entirety in the new edition.

The extensive use of blood transfusion therapy has required improvement of methods of storage of blood and blood products and has given birth to a new discipline—cryobiology. Some of the methods devised by cryobiology—those used for long-term storage of small quantities of blood cells containing selected antigens—are also included in methodology.

Rudiments of statistics must be a part of every laboratory armamentarium; therefore the short discussion that appeared in the first edition has been considerably extended. The amount of information contained in the revised chapter now seems sufficient to cover the everyday needs of a worker in the field of blood grouping.

Although blood grouping tests may appear on the surface to be simple to perform, by comparison with some of the more elaborate chemical and microbiologic tests, the possibility for error due to over-confidence is great, and strict adherence to detail and the use of sufficient controls are mandatory. This is stressed throughout Part Three.

The Glossary had to be extended to accommodate the new material, facts, and problems included in the text. It now has been moved to the end of the book.

As in the first edition, we have attempted to give credit to those who have contributed, by their research and study, to the increasing knowledge in this field. Not every article, however, could be cited, or the list of references would have been longer than the text. A list of recommended readings has been included in most chapters. Not included, however, is the typing of leukocytes and platelets. These are specialty subjects that are still in the experimental stage.

It is our hope that this second edition will continue to contribute to the safety of procedures that depend on accurate examination of blood, their groups, antigens, and antibodies.

Addine G. Erskine
Wladyslaw W. Socha

Contents

PART ONE □ **Principles**

1 □ History of blood transfusion and basic principles of the blood groups

HISTORY OF BLOOD TRANSFUSION

For at least as long as recorded history, man has been interested in and mystified by blood. He has assigned to blood both natural and supernatural qualities. The ancients surmised the curative capabilities of blood, although they could neither prove nor utilize these properties. Blood was used for baths by ancient Egyptians to resuscitate the sick. Many individuals believed, as some still do, that the sick could be helped or even cured by drinking the blood of healthy animals.

The first reference to an attempted transfusion of blood is in a story by Ovid in which he refers to the efforts of Medea to rejuvenate Old Anchises and to restore his youthful vigor by removing blood from his cervical vessels and replacing it with blood from a healthy youth.

It has been said that during the days of the gladiators, spectators would rush into the arena after the fight to drink the blood of the dying man. It has also been told that during the French Revolution the blood of the beheaded aristocrats was offered as a special drink to a favored few of the poor. Drinking blood has been advocated over the years as a tonic and a treatment for disease. In Africa some of the tribes are said to drink the blood of the first animal killed by the young male hunter who has just become a man.

Legend has it that Genghis Khan was able to restore the health of and feed his men by the ingenious method of bleeding his horses, then letting the horses graze until their blood supply was restored; meanwhile, the soldiers who drank the horses' blood had received enough sustenance to enable them to continue their exploits.

Blood has traditionally been considered the seat of emotion, as in expressions like "it stirs one's blood," "it makes one's blood boil," an act is committed in "cold blood," or "my heart bleeds for him." The Bible mentions blood "shed as a sacrifice." A common expression is "blood kin," or "related by blood." "Fresh blood" means introduction of new stock, and some people also use such expressions as "good blood," "bad blood," "blue blood," and "royal blood." "Flesh and blood" usually refers to humanity as opposed to animal life. To be "in blood" once meant to be alive, and to be "out of blood" meant not vigorous. Even now the expression "blood money" is used.

The idea of removing blood from a healthy animal or human and placing it into the system of a sick individual seems to have intrigued man for centuries. In 1492 blood was taken from three young men and given to Pope Innocent VIII to drink, with the hope of reviving him. The Pope and all three young men died.

No real transfusion of blood was performed, however, until something had been learned of the circulatory system. In 1616, after painstaking investigations, Sir Wil-

3

liam Harvey described the circulation of blood, claiming that he had pumped water through the blood vessels of a dead man. His classic monograph was not published, however, until 1628. Andreas Libavius, in 1615, had suggested transferring blood from one human to another. Johannes Colle, of Padua, had also mentioned blood transfusion as a possible means of prolonging life.

Although Sir Christopher Wren is best known for his great architecture, he was primarily a doctor of medicine. Sir Christopher invented an instrument for intravenous therapy and was successful in injecting medications into the veins of dogs. The instrument consisted of a cannula made from a slender quill, which in turn was attached to a bladder. The quill worked like an eyedropper, with a pointed tip enabling it to penetrate the skin and enter the vein. His work was reported around 1657. Robert Boyle, in 1663, described and published Wren's experiments. Boyle was the first person to give intravenous infusions to humans, using inmates of a London prison as his subjects.

According to the Journal Book of the Royal Society, Birch's *History of the Royal Society* (1756) states that between 1665 and 1666 there was some discussion by Dr. Wilkins, Dr. Coxe, and others of the possibility of experimentally injecting the blood of one animal into the vein of another. However, Richard Lower was evidently the first to succeed in carrying out the actual experiment as described vividly by Samuel Pepys[1] in his diary on November 14, 1666:

Here [at the Pope's Head] Dr. Croone told me, that, at the meeting at Gresham College tonight . . . there was a pretty experiment of the blood of one dog let out, till he died, into the body of another on one side while all his own run out on the other side. The first died upon the place, and the other very well, and likely to do well. This did give occasion to many pretty wishes, as of the blood of a Quaker to be let into an Archbishop, and such like; but, as Dr. Croone says, may, if it takes, be of mighty use to man's health, for the amending of bad blood by borrowing from a better body.

An earlier date, May 31, 1665, cited in Pepys' diary, actually marks the first mention of a direct blood transfusion. The entry credits Lower with this experiment, too. Using a tube, Lower injected blood from the carotid artery of one dog into the jugular vein of another dog. His first apparatus was a quill. Later he used silver tubes with flanges to transfer the blood. The flanges enabled him to tie the tubes securely into the blood vessels. In his report, Lower carefully established the dates of the experiment because he complained that a "certain Denis" was trying to deprive him of his priority. Actually, Jean Denys, who was Professor of Philosophy and Mathematics at Montpellier, wrote a long letter from Paris in June, 1667, describing his own work.

In his experiments, Denys used animal blood, usually from lambs, to transfuse humans. In one experiment he bled a 15-year-old youth, ill with a fever, removing about 3 ounces of blood, and then injected 9 ounces of blood that he had procured from the carotid artery of a lamb. Because the boy felt well and had no ill effects, Denys continued his experiments on other patients. His next transfusion was of about 20 ounces of lamb's blood into an older man, and this, too, was successful. Denys claimed that he had cured another patient suffering from "an inveterate phrensy" by transfusion of calf's blood. Unfortunately this patient developed all the symptoms presently regarded as signs of an incompatible transfusion reaction—pain in the arm, rapid and irregular pulse, sweating, pain in the back, vomiting, diarrhea, and later black urine. This patient recovered. One of his patients died in 1668 after having received the third of a series of transfusions, and, after an investigation into the death, a verdict was directed against Denys. No further work was published on such transfusions after this, and transfusion of animal blood into man fell into disrepute.

After the verdict against Denys, nothing of importance was reported in this field throughout the eighteenth century, except that Anthony Wood stated in 1721 that the Reverend Francis Potter had tried to transfuse blood from a hen to a man but was unsuccessful because he was unable to obtain enough blood.

The first transfusion in the modern sense may be said to have been performed in the nineteenth century. James Blundell studied the possibilities of blood transfusion from 1814 to 1816 and used only human donors because he was convinced that the blood of animals would be harmful if injected into humans. Blundell found that a dog bled almost to the point of exsanguination could be restored to health if transfused with the blood of another dog, but when blood from a sheep was used, the transfused dog invariably died. This might be considered the first indication of possible incompatibility of bloods. This effect was explained later in the same century by the in vitro experiments of Landois, who showed the serum of one animal would agglutinate or hemolyze* red cells of other animals of a different species.

The first transfusion of human blood was performed by Blundell on December 22, 1818. Using a syringe, he injected 12 to 14 ounces of blood from several donors into his patient, continuing the injections over a period of 30 to 40 minutes. The subject, an incurably ill patient, improved temporarily but relapsed and died 56 hours after the transfusion. Blundell continued his experiments, however, performing more transfusions (six in 1824) but having no uniformity of success. Two of his patients were probably already dead when he be-

gan the transfusion, and the others were too ill to have recovered under any circumstances. In 1829 he successfully transfused 8 ounces of blood from the arm of his assistant into a postpartum patient over a 3-hour period of time. The patient made a good recovery. Unfortunately, out of twenty transfusions only four were successful. Blundell also appears to have been the first to realize that a few bubbles of air in the circulation are not necessarily dangerous.

Further experiments in blood transfusion followed in rapid succession: Charles Waller, in 1825 and 1826, transfused women having hemorrhages in childbirth, giving 4 to 8½ ounces of blood, using a syringe for the injections. Doubleday gave as much as 14 ounces of blood in 1825. J. H. Aveling, in 1863, devised direct blood transfusion from the arm of one human to the arm of another; he performed seven such transfusions, claiming that the blood that passed from the tube of the donor into the vein of the recipient was virtually unchanged.

The tendency of blood to clot was the principal obstacle to transfusions. Attempts to find a nontoxic anticoagulant began during the nineteenth century when Braxton Hicks, in 1869, recommended the use of sodium phosphate. Unfortunately, all his patients succumbed because of the toxicity of the anticoagulant. Provost and Dumas, in 1821, and later Sir Thomas Smith used defibrinated blood. Smith's apparatus was a wire eggbeater with a hair sieve to remove the clot, but unfortunately in removing the clot he also removed a large portion of the blood and protein. The defibrinated blood proved toxic (probably because it contained thrombin).

Higginson, in 1857, applied the principle of a rubber syringe with ball valves for transferring blood from one individual to another; he performed seven transfusions with this device, five of which he claimed were successful. Roussel, in 1865, used a direct transfusion from arm to arm to treat a patient with puerperal hemorrhage and

---

*Agglutination of red cells of an animal by serum of an animal of a different species is called heteroagglutination. Agglutination of red cells of an individual by his own serum is called autoagglutination. Agglutination of red cells of an individual by serum of a different animal of the same species is called isoagglutination. The prefix "allo-" often used by modern investigators in place of "iso-" will not be used in this book. Obviously, the prefixes have a similar meaning in words such as isohemolysis, isoimmunization, and isoantibodies.

emphasized the importance of using only human blood. His book *Transfusion of Human Blood*, written in 1877 in French, was translated into English and published in London. He reported sixty transfusions since 1865 in Switzerland, Austria, Russia, Belgium, England, and France. The French Army adopted his apparatus and used it in the Franco-German War—the first time that blood transfusion on the battlefield was attempted. Despite all this, transfusions were considered too dangerous for general use, and they were to be employed only as a last resort, especially because many severe reactions and even deaths followed the procedure.

The first major contribution to blood transfusion was that of Karl Landsteiner, who, in 1901, discovered the A-B-O blood groups and pointed out that blood group differences could explain the serious reactions to blood transfusions that occurred even when human instead of animal donors were used. Landsteiner, the "Father of Blood Grouping," was born in Vienna, Austria, on June 14, 1868, and died in New York on June 25, 1943. He had devoted his entire life to research. His book *The Specificity of Serological Reactions* forms the basis of present-day knowledge and methods in immunochemistry and contains fundamental information still not fully appreciated or used by scientific workers. However, of all his pathfinding discoveries, the one that has the greatest application in medicine is that of the A-B-O blood types. Next in importance is the Rh blood factor, which he and Dr. Alexander S. Wiener, his eminent pupil, reported in 1940, although the work had been performed and completed in 1937. Application of the A-B-O blood grouping results for selection of blood donors in transfusions, suggested by Landsteiner in his first paper on the subject, has made blood transfusion a safe procedure and has saved the lives of millions of persons, many of whom have never even heard his name. Landsteiner was awarded the Nobel Prize in medicine in 1930 in recognition of his discovery of the

blood groups in 1901. More information on this is presented later in this book.

Although Landsteiner discovered the blood groups in 1900 to 1901, the discovery did not find practical application until 1907 to 1910, since at the turn of the century blood transfusion was still a rare procedure because of the difficulty caused by coagulation. Crile, in 1908, devised a cannula that he used to connect the radial artery of the donor to the vein of the recipient. This was a difficult operative procedure that few surgeons could master, and there was no way of gauging the amount of blood transfused until the patient's color improved and the donor fainted. Other workers devised other cannulas or used paraffinized containers and similar devices without significant success.

Lindemann was the first to really succeed with vein-to-vein transfusion of unmodified blood by using multiple syringes and a special cannula for puncturing the vein through the skin, but this required a skilled team of assistants. Unger's syringe-valve apparatus was the first practical device that made it possible for an unassisted operator to transfuse the required amount of unmodified blood from donor to patient. The apparatus consisted essentially of a syringe with a two-way stopcock connected by rubber tubing to two needles inserted in the antecubital veins of the donor and patient. Other physicians soon modified Unger's apparatus but did not introduce any new principles. His method, although quite practicable, still required a certain amount of skill and training on the part of the operator.

Another milestone was reached in 1914 when A. Hustin in Belgium, L. Agote in Buenos Aires, and Richard Lewisohn in New York, independently of one another, introduced the use of sodium citrate as an anticoagulant and demonstrated that it is effective and not toxic in concentrations of 0.2%, provided that the amount administered does not exceed 5 gm. The results of their studies were published in 1915. The first transfusion of human citrated blood was given by Agote on November 14, 1914. In 1917 the use of sodium citrate as an anticoagulant for blood transfusions was introduced for military use in France. This method made transfusions more practicable and better for the operator, as well as for the patient, because the transfusions did not have to be rushed.

For a long time the relative advantages of the syringe-valve method and the use of citrate in transfusions were debated. Febrile reactions that frequently accompanied transfusions were ascribed to the citrate solution. The problem was resolved when Florence Seibert showed that the fever was due to bodies of dead bacteria (pyrogens) in tap water and not to the citrate. Such pyrogens could be eliminated by using special stills, and the more practicable citrate method of transfusion was then universally adopted. The natural sequel was the development of preservative solutions containing glucose, notably acid-citrate-dextrose (ACD), and the manufacture by commercial firms of disposable plastic transfusion apparatus and disposable needles and syringes. Blood transfusion is no longer the formidable operation it used to be and is often carried out by technical personnel under direct or indirect supervision by a physician.

Perfection of preservative solutions for blood, including citrate, made storage of blood and after that the development of blood banks inevitable. The initial work on blood storage must be credited to the Russians, who established the first blood bank. They removed blood from healthy individuals who had met accidental death and stored it under refrigeration until it was needed. In the United States, storage of blood began later, based on the experiments of Fantus in Chicago in 1937. In 1904, however, shortly after the announcement by Landsteiner of the discovery of the A-B-O blood groups, Dr. R. B. H. Gradwohl[2] of St. Louis, working at the Pasteur Institute in Paris, was performing experiments to determine how soon after death the natural bacteria in the body invade the bloodstream. He explained that he believed it might be practical to drain the blood from the body of a healthy individual who had died accidentally and to preserve this blood for later transfusion. Gradwohl discovered, however, that during life the blood vessels act as a barrier against bacterial invasion, but at death the organisms from the intestines and other portions of the body can cross the natural barrier to invade the bloodstream and organs and are recoverable in the heart's blood. He therefore abandoned his idea of using cadaver blood for transfusion purposes.

As a result of these many developments, blood transfusion, at one time a rare and hazardous procedure to both donor and patient, as well as a trying experience for the surgeon, has now become commonplace. In the United States alone some eight million transfusions are given each year, and the blood bank has become one of the most important departments in the hospital. The massive use of blood in open heart surgery, vascular therapy, and organ transplantation is the natural outcome of the many painful and painstaking experiments described.

Discovery of other blood group systems has opened up an entirely new field, with which this text is concerned—immunohematology and immunogenetics. The mechanism of inheritance of the A-B-O blood groups by multiple allelic genes was established in 1924 by Bernstein. In 1927 to 1928 Landsteiner and Levine discovered the M-N types and the P factor.

For a long time Unger had been insisting that it was not sufficient that donor and patient be matched merely for the A-B-O groups. He described so-called "minor" agglutinins in addition to the "major" isoagglutinins that determine the four blood groups. A number of physicians had encountered hemolytic transfusion reactions despite the use of blood of the correct A-B-O type. The solution to this problem came with the discovery of the Rh factor by Landsteiner and Wiener in 1937 and the demonstration by Wiener and Peters in 1940 of the predominant role of Rh sensitization in intragroup hemolytic transfusion reactions. Shortly thereafter, in 1941, Levine, Burnham, et al. demonstrated the role of maternofetal incompatibility with respect to the Rh factor in the pathogenesis of erythroblastosis fetalis. Wiener's work led to the routine Rh typing of patient and donors in addition to the A-B-O grouping when selecting donors for transfusion.

The puzzling inability to demonstrate the expected Rh antibodies in many clinical cases was solved when Wiener showed the existence of two major forms of antibodies—agglutinating, presently called gamma M (19S, IgM), and blocking, now designated gamma G (7S, IgG). New testing methods were the result of this discovery, especially the antiglobulin test of Coombs et al. and the proteolytic enzyme test of Pickles, as well as the conglutination test of Wiener. With these newer methods, studies on posttransfusion sera and on sera from mothers of erythroblastotic babies led to the discovery in rapid succession of new blood factors and new blood systems. At present more than 100 blood group factors belonging to fifteen blood group systems are known to exist.

A more recent advance has been an effective and safe method of treating erythroblastosis fetalis by exchange transfusion, devised by Wiener and Wexler in 1944 and followed by Diamond and Allen's simple method in 1949, utilizing an umbilical catheter. The availability of disposable apparatus has made this the method most used at present. More recently a method has been perfected by two teams of investigators working independently of one another —R. Finn, E. A. Clarke, et al. in England and V. J. Freda, J. Gorman, et al. in the United States—to prevent the occurrence of Rh sensitization. It entails injection of high titered purified Rh_0 IgG into Rh-negative mothers of Rh-positive babies at the time of birth.

Whereas the great advances in knowledge of the blood groups and the perfection of methods of cross matching blood that resulted from the introduction especially of the antiglobulin test virtually eliminated the possibility of hemolytic reactions, there still remained rare instances in which transfusions of blood were followed by severe chills and fever or other adverse manifestations. Some of these reactions have been attributed to individual differences of other blood components besides red cells. Intensive studies of this problem have led to discovery of the so-called serum groups, isozyme groups, and leukocyte groups. The last have found their principal application in the field of transplantation of organs and tissues. Serum, isozyme, and leukocyte groups have been shown to be genetically transmitted, and this has found extensive application, especially in forensic medicine in problems of disputed parentage. Because of significant differences in distribution of blood and serum groups and isozyme types in the different human populations, those tests are now routinely applied in physical anthropology. The technics of serum grouping differ from those of blood grouping, and since the field has grown greatly in complexity, it will not be included in the present book, so as to keep the book within reasonable limits of size.

Chromosome mapping is another subject that has come into the foreground in the last decade. It utilizes red cell antigens, white cell antigens, and serum groups in studies of linkage. Up to 1966, blood group markers supplied all the autosomal linkages known to that date. Evidence was thus established of linkage between the *Lu* and the *Se* genes, at the same time proving that the *Lewis* genes are *not* linked to the *Lu* or *Se* genes. The number of known markers has increased in the last 15 years as the extent of the genetic diversity of man has been demonstrated by biochemical and immunologic means. More than fifty useful polymorphic marker traits are now available for linkage studies in families.

With the perfection of blood typing and

cross-matching technics, blood transfusion is now not only a simple but also a safe procedure, barring human clerical errors. The tests have been simplified by the commercial availability of sterile potent blood grouping sera in convenient dropper bottles. The Division of Biological Standards (DBS) of the National Institutes of Health (NIH) has played a dominant role in regulating these products.

Preparation of commercial typing sera was facilitated by Witebsky's introduction in 1944 of a method of producing high-titered anti-**A** and anti-**B** blood grouping sera by injecting volunteer donors with purified solutions of A and B blood group–specific substances. In 1945 Wiener devised a practicable method of producing high-titered anti-**Rh** serum by injecting Rh-negative volunteer donors with small amounts of Rh-positive blood.

The most recent advances in blood grouping and blood transfusion entail still further refinement in technic. First, in present practice the use of disposable equipment ensures sterility—not only for collecting blood from donors but also for collecting small samples for blood typing and other tests—with disposable needles and syringes. Although this may seem wasteful, elimination of the danger of infection and the saving of time formerly required for cleaning and sterilizing used equipment, sharpening needles, etc. has proved economical because it eliminates the need for specially trained personnel formerly required to carry out such chores.

Another recent development has been to discontinue the former practice of the routine use for transfusion of only whole blood as collected with the anticoagulant, and the frequent use instead of fractions of the blood to meet individual patients' requirements. For example, packed red cells are used in chronic anemias and leukemias or other conditions characterized by chronic anemias without active bleeding that would require restoration of blood volume. The plasma that remains after removal of the red cells can then be used for other patients with reduced blood volume but without anemia. Another useful fraction separated at the same time contains almost entirely only platelets useful for treating patients with purpuras, such as patients receiving chemotherapy in leukemias, and to protect the patient being subjected to splenectomy for thrombocytopenia, thus rendering this formerly dangerous operation safe to perform. Similarly, leukocyte fractions separated from blood are being used for treatment of agranulocytosis and aplastic anemias. A further advance has been to fractionate blood plasma into its various components—principally albumins, globulins, and fibrinogen—each of which has found its place as a therapeutic agent in medical, obstetric, and surgical practice. A useful fraction has proved to be the cryoglobulins that separate when plasma is frozen and thawed; it contains the antihemophilic globulin (AHG) used for the treatment of hemophilia.

Fractionation of blood into its components has been facilitated by the introduction of plastic disposable transfusion units in place of bottles for collecting and storing blood for transfusion. With this closed technic it is easy to divide a unit of blood into several small subunits convenient for use in pediatric practice or for fractionation of blood components.

Blood that has been collected in ACD or an equivalent anticoagulant-preservative is considered to have an expiration date of 28 days after withdrawal when used for transfusion in adults. To extend the useful life of blood for transfusion, methods of freezing have been devised that protect the red cells from the damage inherent in the process of freezing and make possible the reconstitution, after thawing, of red cells which can safely be used for transfusion even after years of storage. This has given a boost to autotransfusion, the safest of all transfusions, in which the patient acts as his own donor, thus raising the possibility of storing blood collected from individuals when they are well for possible future use when the need arises.

One of the most serious problems associated with the increased use of blood transfusion has been the transmission of disease from donor to recipient. The most important of such diseases is serum hepatitis. The discovery of a practicable, simple method of screening blood, such as immunocounterelectrophoresis, for the presence of hepatitis B virus, has been an important advance, even though the method can detect only about one fifth of hepatitis carriers.

Considering the intensive work going on in this field, further important advances are to be expected that will render transfusion even safer.

HIGHLIGHTS IN THE HISTORY OF THE BLOOD GROUPS

It is a well-known fact that errors which inadvertently creep into some textbooks and journal articles are often repeated by authors who do not challenge the truth of certain statements. As an example, it was believed for at least half a century that the precipitin test for the identification of human blood was specific for the human species until this belief was challenged and proved to be erroneous. Cross reactions do occur between the bloods of humans and nonhuman primates in some cases. Perhaps nowhere have the historical facts been more misquoted or misunderstood than in the field of immunohematology and immunogenetics. For this reason the following quotations from the literature are included as history.

Discovery of the A-B-O blood groups

The reasoning that led Karl Landsteiner to the discovery of the A-B-O blood groups is best explained by citing from his Nobel lecture in Stockholm in 1930.[3]

The discovery of biochemical species specificity prompted the question which formed the basis of the investigations about to be discussed, as to whether the species differentiation goes beyond the limits of species, and whether also the individuals within a species show similar, though presumably slighter, differences. As no observations whatever were available pointing to such behavior, I chose the simplest among the possible plans of investigation, and that material which gave promise of useful application. Accordingly, the investigations consisted of allowing blood serum and red corpuscles of different human individuals to interact.

The results were only partially those which had been expected. In many tests, just as if the red cells had been mixed with their own serum, no changes were observed. Frequently, however, a phenomenon described as agglutination occurred, the serum causing a clumping of the cells of the other individual.

The unexpected feature was that the agglutination, when it did occur, was as marked as the well-known reactions in which the serum and cells of different animal species interact, whereas in other cases there seemed to be no difference in the blood of various individuals. At this point it was still to be considered that the phenomenon observed did not signify the individual differences sought for and that the reaction, though obtained with the blood of healthy individuals, might have been due to a past history of disease. It soon became evident, however, that the reactions follow a law which holds for the blood of all human beings, and that the properties observed are as characteristic for single individuals as are the serological properties distinguishing species. There are in the main four different kinds of human blood, constituting so-called blood groups. The number of groups depends on the existence in the erythrocytes of substances (isoagglutinogens) having two different structures, either or both of which may be present or absent in the erythrocytes of a given person. This alone would not be sufficient to explain the reactions; the active substances of sera, the isoagglutinins, must also occur in a definite distribution. Such is indeed the case, for every serum contains those agglutinins which act upon the agglutinogens not present in the cells, a remarkable phenomenon, the cause of which has not yet been definitely established. From these facts there follow definite relationships shown in the table [Table 1-1], between the various blood groups, which makes the task of their determination a simple one. The groups are designated according to the agglutinogens contained in the cells. (In the table the sign + indicates agglutination.)

In his original report in 1901, Landsteiner[4] presented three tables in which sera from each of five or six different individuals were cross matched with one another's red cells.

Table 1-2 shows the first of the three tables, which includes the blood of Dr. Landsteiner and of one of his students, Dr. Sturli. As can be seen, in some combinations agglutination was observed, indicated by plus signs, whereas in other combinations there was no apparent reaction, indicated by minus signs. In Landsteiner's words (translated):

In a number of cases (group A), the serum reacts with cells of another group (group B), but not with those of group A; those A cells are acted upon in the same manner by serum B. In the third group (C), the serum agglutinates the corpuscles of A and B, while the red cells of group C are not acted upon by the serum from A and B. According to customary terminology, one can say that in these cases there must be at least two kinds of agglutinins present, the one in A, the other in B, and both together in C. Naturally, the corpuscles must be considered insensitive to the agglutinins which are present in the same serum.

It is evident from this quotation that Landsteiner, in his original investigation, described the three blood groups, O, A, and B; even the terminology is modern except that group O was called group C in that first report. The fourth and rarest group, AB, was described the next year by Decastello and Sturli, the latter a pupil of Landsteiner who continued the work at Landsteiner's suggestion. Decastello and Sturli[20] extended the studies to a much larger series of individuals and encountered several whose blood gave reactions that did not fit into the scheme of only three blood groups. To cite them (translated):

A total of 155 persons over 6 months old, with the exception of 4 cases, showed the presence of agglutinating substances in the serum as well as a strict division into three groups. . . . The four exceptions to this rule behave in the following manner: the serum reacted with none of the blood samples and thus did not contain any agglutinins, whereas the erythrocytes were agglutinated by all the other sera.

By 1902 therefore Landsteiner, with his pupils, had fully described the four A-B-O groups, O(C), A, B, and AB. Moreover, Landsteiner's explanation of the reactions, postulating two agglutinogens and two corresponding agglutinins, was supported by

Table 1-1. Composition of the four A-B-O blood groups, as shown by cross matching of red cells and sera*

Serum of group	Agglutinins in serum	Erythrocytes of group			
		O	A	B	AB
O	$\alpha\beta$	−	+	+	+
A	β	−	−	+	+
B	α	−	+	−	+
AB	−	−	−	−	−

*From Landsteiner, K., Nobel lecture, Stockholm, 1930, Science 73:403, 1931.

Table 1-2. Results of Landsteiner's original experiment that led to the discovery of the A-B-O blood groups*

Serum from	Blood cells from					
	Dr. St.	Dr. Plecn.	Dr. Sturl.	Dr. Erdh.	Zar.	Landst.
Dr. St.	−	+	+	+	+	−
Dr. Plecn.	−	−	+	+	−	−
Dr. Sturl.	−	+	−	−	+	−
Dr. Erdh.	−	+	−	−	+	−
Zar.	−	−	+	+	−	−
Landst.	−	+	+	+	+	−

*From Landsteiner, K.: Wien. Klin. Wochenschr. 14:1132, 1901.

absorption experiments fully described in the early article of Decastello and Sturli, as follows:

> If a serum of group A is mixed with a sufficient quantity of group B blood cells and the mixture centrifuged, serum A not only loses the ability to agglutinate fresh blood from the same person of group B but also to agglutinate any blood of this group. Conversely, the same is true for a group B serum and an A blood. However, if a C serum is mixed with an A blood, the agglutinating power is lost only for this group, and not for group B (the same is true for B). If serum A and serum B are mixed, the mixture agglutinates the blood cells of A and B.

It is of interest that Hektoen[5] in 1907, although familiar with the prior work of Landsteiner and his students, incorrectly believed that there were only three blood groups. To cite from his article:

> Landsteiner, and following him, Descatello [sic] and Sturli, point out that individuals may be divided into three main groups.

When Hektoen encountered individuals of group AB, he thought they were merely exceptions to Landsteiner's classification of three (sic) blood groups and remarked:

> The exceptions to Landsteiner's typing are given in heavy type. . . . The absence of agglutinins in the sera of persons whose corpuscles fall into group III is not at all unusual.

In addition to citing the literature incorrectly, a common fault of some modern books and articles on blood grouping, Hektoen carried out no absorption tests and therefore was in no position to discover the third kind of agglutinin, anti-C of group O serum, for which the book *Blood Groups*

in Man by Race and Sanger incorrectly credits him.

Although the designation of the four blood groups by letters, as O, A, B, and AB, is simple and instructive, Jansky[6] suggested instead that they be numbered as I, II, III, and IV, respectively, and Moss[7] introduced further confusion by numbering the blood groups differently, as IV, II, III, and I. For their contributions to confusion of the subject of blood grouping, Jansky and Moss were awarded by many authors the credit for the discovery of the A-B-O blood groups, even after Landsteiner had received the Nobel prize for that discovery. Moss did attempt to give an interpretation different from that of Landsteiner for the isoagglutination reactions, which were tabulated according to his numberings (Table 1-3). Instead of Landsteiner's simple explanation of the reactions, postulating two agglutinogens and two corresponding agglutinins, Moss suggested three agglutinogens and three corresponding agglutinins. Not satisfied with a single scheme, he suggested two possible schemes, which, translated into modern terminology, are as given in Table 1-4.

Both of these schemes are obviously incorrect, as was pointed out by Landsteiner. Even though they both could explain the reactions in Table 1-3, they are refuted by the results of the absorption experiments. According to the first scheme, group AB blood could not absorb all the agglutinins out of the sera of the other three groups, which is obviously incorrect; and according to the second scheme, the agglutinins

Table 1-3. Moss' designation of the four A-B-O blood groups compared with that of Landsteiner

		Reactions with red cells of groups			
		O	A	B	AB
Serum of group		IV	II	III	I
O	IV	−	+	+	+
A	II	−	−	+	+
B	III	−	+	−	+
AB	I	−	−	−	−

of group O serum could not be fractionated by separate absorption with A or B cells. Despite his faulty ideas, again, Moss has been credited in the Race and Sanger book with having made the first observation on the antibody anti-C of group O serum, even though he made no absorption experiments. The coincidental use of the letter C by Moss obviously bears no relation to the problem of the third antibody in group O serum. (See pp. 57 and 58.)

Discovery of the Rh-Hr blood types

Landsteiner and Wiener[8,9] were led to their discovery of the Rh factor in blood by studies on homologues of the M-N agglutinogens in apes and monkeys. The original report of the discovery of the Rh factor has proved to be so important that it is cited here in its entirety.[10]

The capacity possessed by some rabbit sera, produced with the blood of Rhesus monkeys, of reacting with human blood that contains the agglutinogen M, has been reported previously. Subsequently, it has been found that another individual property of human blood (which may be designated as Rh) can be detected by certain of these sera.

Upon exhaustion of such a serum with selected bloods, for instance OM, the absorbed serum still agglutinated the majority (39 of 45) of other human bloods, independently of the group or the M-N types; moreover, reactions took place with bloods lacking the property P. An example of the reactions is given in Table 1 [Table 1-5].

The results are of some interest in that they suggest a way of finding individual properties of human blood, namely, with the aid of immune sera against the blood of animals. As an analogy may be cited the demonstration of differences in sheep erythrocytes with immune sera for human A blood.

The reactions observed, although of moderate intensity only, were obtained with immune sera produced at different times. Whether the observations may possibly lead to a method suitable for routine work is still under investigation.

The observations described in this report were a sequel to the production of anti-M sera by Landsteiner and Wiener, who immunized rabbits with rhesus monkey blood. Landsteiner and Wiener delayed the report of their 1937 discovery of the Rh factor until 1940, at which time its importance became evident when Wiener and Peters[11] demonstrated the role of the Rh factor in isosensitization to the Rh factor in man in hemolytic reactions to transfu-

Table 1-4. Moss' schemes of serology of the four A-B-O blood groups

Blood groups	Moss' first scheme		Moss' second scheme	
	Red cells (agglutinogens)	Serum (agglutinins)	Red cells (agglutinogens)	Serum (agglutinins)
O	None	Anti-A, anti-B, anti-C	None	Anti-C
A	A	Anti-B and anti-C	A and C	Anti-B
B	B	Anti-A and anti-C	B and C	Anti-A
AB	C	None	A, B, and C	None

Table 1-5. Reactions of absorbed anti-rhesus rabbit serum with various human red cells, all lacking the property P°

	Bloods (all group O)									
	Type M				Type N			Type MN		
	1	2	3	4	5	6	7	8	9	10
Absorbed immune serum	+	+	+	0	0	+	+	+	0	+

°From Landsteiner, K., and Wiener, A. S.: Proc. Soc. Exp. Biol. Med. 43:223, 1940.

sions of blood of the homologous A-B-O blood group. Wiener and Peters described three such cases in which the same agglutinogen, Rh, was responsible, summarizing their findings as follows:

Three cases are reported in which transfusion of blood of the proper blood group gave rise to hemolytic reactions, two of the three reactions resulting in the death of the patient.

In two cases there was noted the appearance in the patient's serum of an isoagglutinin designated as anti-Rh. This is explained by the immune response to the injection of Rh+ blood into Rh− individuals, the group playing no role. Following the appearance of anti-Rh agglutinins the transfusion of Rh+ blood gave rise to hemolytic reactions. Remarkably the reactions of the anti-Rh sera corresponded with those of immune rabbit sera prepared by Landsteiner and Wiener by the injection of rhesus blood. The frequency distribution of agglutinogen Rh in the general population is approximately 85% Rh+ and 15% Rh−.

Our cases were compared with others reported in the literature and various similarities and differences pointed out. A hypothesis is offered to explain the occurrence of hemolytic intragroup reactions in certain individuals who had not received previous blood transfusions. The role played by the properties A_1, A_2, M, N, and P in transfusion reactions is discussed. Methods are suggested for the prevention of occurrence of intragroup hemolytic reactions.

The report of Wiener and Peters of the role of Rh sensitization as the prime cause of intragroup hemolytic transfusion reactions was quickly confirmed and additional cases reported.[12] The heredity of the Rh factor was then established by Landsteiner and Wiener, who improved the preparation of anti-Rh sera by using guinea pigs instead of rabbits for producing the anti-rhesus sera. At the same time, limited amounts of human anti-Rh sera became available from clinical cases of Rh sensitization. Landsteiner and Wiener[13] summarized these additional findings as follows:

A method for the determination of the presence or absence of the new blood factor Rh is described, which can be used for typing patients and prospective donors.

Examination of families showed that the agglutinogen is inherited as a simple Mendelian dominant. The distribution of the Rh factor among

white individuals and Negroes may indicate racial differences. The property is probably genetically independent of the blood groups and the factors M and N.

Whereas Wiener later devised a method of producing potent anti-Rh sera in human volunteers by deliberate isoimmunization, human anti-Rh sera were not readily available at first, especially since the existence of "blocking" antibodies was still unknown, and the early work had to be done mainly with the anti-rhesus sera of Landsteiner and Wiener made in guinea pigs. This is illustrated by consulting contemporary (at that time) laboratory textbooks, for example, Todd and Sanford's *Clinical Diagnosis by Laboratory Methods.*[*]

The assertion made in some recent textbooks that the designation Rh factor is a misnomer is obviously scientifically and historically erroneous, as is the artificial distinction sometimes made between a so-called "animal" Rh agglutinogen (demonstrable with guinea pig anti-rhesus serum) and a so-called "human" Rh agglutinogen (demonstrable with isoimmune human anti-Rh serum). Actually these two kinds of reagents, although different in *specificity,*[†] identify *the same agglutinogen Rh,* just as two portraits, one a profile view and the other a full-face view, although different in appearance, identify one and the same individual. At any rate this point, which has been raised, only serves to fortify Wiener's priority and predominant role in the discovery of the Rh factor, since he was the first to describe *both* kinds of reagents—animal (with Landsteiner) and human (with Peters).

Shortly after Wiener and Peters had demonstrated the role of Rh sensitization in intragroup hemolytic transfusion reactions, Burnham[14] and Levine et al.[15,16] dem-

---

*Todd, J. C., and Sanford, A. H.: Clinical diagnosis by laboratory methods, ed. 11, Philadelphia, 1948, W. B. Saunders Co.

†Wiener also pointed out that potent human anti-Rh sera, contrary to expectation, do not agglutinate rhesus monkey red cells—a phenomenon that has been designated as a nonreciprocal reaction.

onstrated its role also in the pathogenesis of erythroblastosis fetalis. In Burnham's report, before the *Case Reports,* the following appears:

> The association of erythroblastosis and transfusion accidents was first suggested by the following case which was observed in June, 1940.

It should be noted that the date, June, 1940, was *after* publication of the reports of Landsteiner and Wiener, and of Wiener and Peters. Levine et al.,[16] whose work was published in 1941, state:

> The data to be presented indicate that erythroblastosis fetalis results from isoimmunization of the mother by dominant hereditary blood factors in the fetus. . . . In the majority of the cases the blood factor involved has been shown to be either identical with or related to the Rh (Rhesus) agglutinogen first described by Landsteiner and Wiener with the aid of rabbit sera prepared by the injection of rhesus blood. . . . Accordingly, a pregnant woman whose blood does not contain the factor (Rh-, occurring in about 15 percent of the general population) if married to an Rh+ husband (85 percent of the random population) may produce anti-Rh agglutinins as a result of immunization with the Rh+ fetal blood. Should these agglutinins penetrate the placenta in suitable concentration they may serve as a source of the intrauterine hemolysis of fetal blood, the characteristic feature of which is erythroblastosis fetalis.

In this connection, it is necessary also to cite the earlier article of Levine and Stetson,[17] which is cited by Race and Sanger in their book as the first description of the Rh factor and by other authors as the first demonstration of the role of Rh sensitization in the pathogenesis of erythroblastosis fetalis. As Wiener[18] pointed out in his history of the Rh factor, this was merely a case report of another unexplained intragroup hemolytic transfusion reaction, comparable to others reported about the same time by Unger, Zacho, Neter, Landsteiner, Levine and Janes, Culbertson and Ratcliffe, and others. To quote from the article by Levine and Stetson:

> Another specimen drawn two months later still exhibited the agglutinin, which, however, gave far weaker reactions. Here again the reactions at 37° C were quite as intense as those at room temperature or lower. It was not possible to examine the serum of this patient until a year later, when all traces of reactions had disappeared.

> In several respects this iso-agglutinin, as already mentioned, resembles the iso-agglutinins described by Landsteiner, Levine and Janes, and that of Neter, namely (1) reactions with the same group equally active at room temperature and at 37° C and (2) temporary character of the agglutinin. . . . Consequently attempts were made to produce a hetero-immune agglutinin of identical or similar specificity by repeated injections of a positive blood into a series of rabbits.

There were early case reports, before the discovery of Rh, of intragroup transfusion reactions, and of intragroup incompatibility, independent of the A-B-O blood groups, in which, as in the Levine and Stetson case, the antibodies responsible were never clearly identified.

As can be seen, the case of Levine and Stetson differed in no important respect from other cases reported at about the same time, and the fact that the patient's serum lost its activity (blocking antibodies were not yet known) precluded any further work with it. The claim sometimes made that the Levine-Stetson antibody was shown to be the same as anti-Rh therefore obviously has no basis.

With respect to the claim that the Levine and Stetson article is the first description of the role of Rh in erythroblastosis fetalis, the disease is not even mentioned in the article. The only statement is as follows:

> In view of the fact that this patient harbored a dead fetus for a period of several months, one may assume that the products of the disintegrating fetus were responsible not only for the toxic symptoms of the patient but also for the iso-immunization.

Thus it can be seen that no mention was made that the source of the maternal iso-sensitization might have been the *intact red cells* of a *live fetus* that had traversed the placental barrier into her circulation, nor was the fetal death in any way suspected to be the end result of the maternal isosensitization.

In his article describing further cases of

hemolytic transfusion reactions due to Rh sensitization, Wiener[19] detailed a case in which the patient had produced an immune isoantibody giving only 70% positive reactions (at present known as anti-**rh'**) as compared with the 85% positive reactions given by the other sera (presently called anti-**Rh**$_o$). The two antisera together defined four types of blood, and the close association between the newly found **rh'** factor and the **Rh**$_o$ factor indicated that they were both part of the same blood group system, the Rh-Hr types. Analyzing data on the distribution of the four types in the general population to deduce a reasonable genetic theory, Wiener, in the third edition of *Blood Groups and Transfusion* (1943), wrote as follows (in this analysis the serum now designated anti-**Rh**$_o$ was then called anti-Rh$_1$, and the serum now designated anti-**rh'** was then called anti-Rh$_2$):

> The reactions could be explained most simply by assuming the existence of two qualitatively different agglutinogens, Rh$_1$ and Rh$_2$, in the blood cells, corresponding to the agglutinins anti-Rh$_1$ and anti-Rh$_2$. The four types of blood would then have the composition, Rh$_1$Rh$_2$, Rh$_1$, Rh$_2$, Rh-negative, respectively. This assumption would imply the existence, however, of two corresponding genes, *Rh$_1$* and *Rh$_2$*, which would have to be either independent, linked, or allelic. The first two possibilities are excluded since the product of the frequencies Rh$_1$Rh$_2$ × Rh-negative is much greater than Rh$_1$ × Rh$_2$. Moreover, the existence of allelic genes *Rh$_1$* and *Rh$_2$* in individuals whose blood reacts with both anti-Rh$_1$ and anti-Rh$_2$ would necessitate that this class not exceed 50 percent, while the actual frequency is 70 percent. Accordingly, the observations are best explained by assuming the existence of 3 qualitatively different Rh agglutinogens instead of only 2, one type reacting with anti-Rh$_1$ serum but not anti-Rh$_2$, a second reacting with anti-Rh$_2$ but not anti-Rh$_1$, and a third reacting with both sorts of anti-Rh sera.

This basic summary of the possibilities led Wiener to develop his theory of multiple allelic genes and his nomenclature for the Rh-Hr blood types as described in this book. Two years later, Fisher revived the theory of linkage, which had been disproved and discarded by Wiener, and extended it to include triple linked genes in place of double linked genes. At the same time, he introduced the C-D-E notations for the Rh-Hr types, with its attendant errors and confusion. In a way, Fisher's contribution is comparable to that of Moss. Moss tried to introduce a theory of three agglutinogens and corresponding agglutinins in place of Landsteiner's concept of two agglutinogens and corresponding agglutinins. As has been shown here, Moss' ideas were entirely incorrect. Similarly, Fisher extended to triple linked genes the theory of double linked genes previously disproved and discarded by Wiener. Again, Fisher's ideas have been proved to be entirely incorrect. Moss and Fisher both introduced new and unnecessary notations to replace the rational nomenclature of the discoverers of the A-B-O blood groups and Rh-Hr blood types, respectively, and in both cases Race and Sanger in their book credit Moss and Fisher for contributions they did not make.

SCIENTIFIC SYMBOLS—THEIR APPLICATION TO BLOOD GROUPS

The complex developments in the field of blood grouping have created the problem of communication and storage of information that can be done satisfactorily only with the help of appropriate scientific nomenclature.

Scientific symbols should be simple enough to be easy to use, and they should give some clue as to what they represent. They must not alter, distort, or misrepresent facts. They should be international. As an example, the same chemical symbols for the elements are used by scientists throughout the world. Blood grouping symbols should also be adaptable for international usage. The nomenclature in this field must consider not only the agglutinogens but also the **genes** and the **serologic specificities** (**factors**) by which the agglutinogens are identified. Wiener suggested that symbols for genes and genotypes be printed in *italics,* symbols for the blood factors (specificities) and their corresponding antibodies in **boldface** or black type, and symbols for agglutinogens and phenotypes in regular lightface type. This convention will be followed in this book.

The order of discovery of the various blood group systems was as follows: A-B-O, M-N, P, Rh-Hr, K-k (Kell), Lu (Lutheran), Le (Lewis), Fy (Duffy), Jk (Kidd), Di (Diego), Yt, Do (Dombrock), Au (Auberger), the high- and low-frequency systems, I-i, Xg (sex-linked), and others. New blood group systems are often discovered when antibodies are formed by a patient as a result of a blood transfusion or pregnancy or by experimental means using animals. A new antibody must be shown to be different from any of those already discovered or known, the antigen it identifies must be detectable, and allelic genes must be identified. It is usually demonstrated, also, that the antibodies within systems react in like media in the laboratory or that they fail to react in certain media. As an example, some antibodies will not react with red cells that have been treated with a proteolytic enzyme, whereas in some of the systems enzymes are required for a reaction. This is explained when the various blood group systems are discussed in their respective chapters.

Of all the blood group systems, the most complex and the one around which the most controversy has revolved is the Rh-Hr system. The A-B-O and Rh-Hr systems are the most important, especially in transfusion and in maternofetal incompatibility. The M-N-S system, along with the A-B-O and Rh-Hr, is important in investigations of paternity suits and in the identification of blood stains (although the M-N-S and Rh-Hr systems cannot be used at present to identify dried blood stains). Some of the other blood group systems have also been used in disputed parentage cases.

Most of the laboratory tests done as a routine are directed toward the three systems, A-B-O, M-N-S, and Rh-Hr, although the M-N-S system is not usually involved in transfusions and the remaining twelve or so blood group systems are of concern in only rare incompatible reactions.

The order of arrangements of the various blood groups in their respective systems, especially those of the A-B-O and Rh-Hr systems, is important in preparing the laboratory results for computerization. A uniform system of arrangement and nomenclature throughout the world would enable the results obtained in one laboratory to be transferred to another laboratory, as well as from country to country. If such an order is adopted, there can be a uniform code for computers, as discussed later in this text.

REFERENCES

1. Pepys, S.: Diary, 1666, edited by Wheatley, London, 1924.
2. Gradwohl, R. B. H.: Ann. Inst. Pasteur **18:** 766, 1904.
3. Landsteiner, K.: Nobel lecture, Stockholm, 1930, Science **73:**403, 1931.
4. Landsteiner, K.: Wien. Klin. Wochenschr. **14:** 1132, 1901. English translation in Selected contributions to the literature of the blood groups and immunology, vol. 1, Fort Knox, Ky., 1966, Blood Transfusion Division, U.S. Army Medical Research Laboratory.
5. Hektoen, L.: J. Infect. Dis. **4:**297, 1907.
6. Jansky, J.: Jahresbericht Neurol. Psychiatrie, p. 1028, 1907.
7. Moss, W. L.: Bull. Johns Hopkins Hosp. **21:** 67, 1910.
8. Wiener, A. S.: J. Immunol. **34:**11, 1938.
9. Landsteiner, K., and Wiener, A. S.: J. Immunol. **33:**19, 1937.
10. Landsteiner, K., and Wiener, A. S.: Proc. Soc. Exp. Biol. Med. **43:**223, 1940.
11. Wiener, A. S., and Peters, H. R.: Ann. Intern. Med. **13:**2306, 1940.
12. Wiener, A. S.: Arch. Pathol. **32:**227, 1941.
13. Landsteiner, K., and Wiener, A. S.: J. Exp. Med. **74:**309, 1940.
14. Burnham, L.: Am. J. Obstet. Gynecol. **42:** 389, 1941.
15. Levine, P., Katzin, B. M., and Burnham, L.: J.A.M.A. **116:**825, 1941.
16. Levine, P., Burnham, K., Katzin, B. M., and Vogel, P.: Am. J. Obstet. Gynecol. **42:**925, 1941.
17. Levine, P., and Stetson, R. E.: J.A.M.A. **113:** 126, 1939.
18. Wiener, A. S.: N.Y. State J. Med. **69:**2915, 1969.
19. Wiener, A. S.: Arch. Pathol. **32:**227, 1941.
20. vonDecastello, A., and Sturli, A.: Münch. Med. Wochenschr. **49:**1090, 1902.

RECOMMENDED READINGS

Erskine, A. G.: What you should know about blood types, transfusion, Rh, and heredity, Berkeley, Calif., 1970, Altamont Press.

Giblett, E. R.: Genetic markers in human blood, Philadelphia, 1969, F. A. Davis Co.

Hollán, S. R., editor: Current topics in immunohematology and immunogenetics, Alexander S. Wiener Festschrift, Budapest, 1972, Akadémiai Kiadó.

Keynes, G. L., editor: Blood transfusion, Bristol, England, 1949, John Wright & Sons, Ltd., and London, 1949; Simpkin Marchall, Ltd. (1941).

Prokop, O., and Uhlenbruck, G.: Human blood and serum groups (translated by J. L. Raven), New York, 1969, John Wiley & Sons, Inc.

Ranganathan, R. S.: Essentials of blood grouping and clinical applications, New York, 1968, Grune & Stratton, Inc.

Speiser, P.: Karl Landsteiner, Entdecker der Blutgruppen, Vienna, 1961, Brüder Hollinek.

White, C. S., and Weinstein, J. J.: Blood derivatives and substitutes, Baltimore, 1947, The Williams & Wilkins Co.

Wiener, A. S.: Blood groups and transfusion, ed. 3, Springfield, Ill., 1943, Charles C Thomas, Publisher; reprinted New York, 1962, Hafner Publishing Co.

Wiener, A. S.: J. Hist. Med. 7:369, 1952.

Wiener, A. S.: Advances in blood grouping, vol. 3, New York, 1970, Grune & Stratton, Inc.

Wiener, A. S., and Socha, W. W.: A-B-O blood groups and Lewis types, New York, 1976, Stratton Intercontinental Medical Book Corporation.

2 □ Immunologic basis of the blood groups

Blood grouping serology constitutes a portion of the broad field of immunology. **Immunology** is that aspect of science that deals with immunity, that is, the reaction of the living organism to the introduction of foreign substances, usually by parenteral route, which have the capacity to stimulate the body to produce reactive substances specific for the introduced foreign substance. The introduced foreign substance may be particulate or soluble, most commonly protein in nature, and of a substantial molecular weight. Such substances are called **antigens.** The reacting substances elicited by their introduction into the body are called **antibodies.** In the earliest stages of immunology, medical scientists were concerned mainly with antibodies produced in response to infection with bacteria, toxins, molds, or viruses; because individuals with such bacterial and other antibodies are resistant, or immune, to the specific disease in question, the science acquired its name of immunology. However, antibodies can also be produced against innocuous foreign materials such as red cells, as the antibodies used in blood grouping. Moreover, instead of being beneficial, the antigen-antibody reaction may be harmful, as in erythroblastosis fetalis and anaphylaxis in allergy, and in autoimmune diseases such as systemic lupus erythematosus, Hashimoto's thyroiditis, and autohemolytic anemias—phenomena that constitute a branch of immunology known as **immunopathology.**

TERMINOLOGY

The term **serology** is applied to that field of immunology in which laboratory tests using antisera are under consideration. Blood grouping is a branch of serology for which the terms **immunohematology, serohematology,** or **immunogenetics** are also used, depending on the aspect being discussed. Two basic laboratory materials are involved in serology: (1) **serum,** the fluid that separates when blood clots and the clot retracts, and (2) **cells**—in the broader sense, cellular elements—which constitute the bulk of the remaining portion of the blood. When the term **blood cells** is used in this book, it generally refers to the **erythrocytes,** or red blood cells. The terms **leukocytes,** for the white blood cells, and **platelets** are also employed.

Antibodies are found in the serum, and antigens are on or in the cells or in solution in secretions such as saliva. Antibodies bring about a reaction; the cells react (or are acted on) either by clumping together or by dissolving, whereas **blood group substances** in solution may be precipitated. However, red cells may become coated with antibodies without visible reaction. When the specificity of the antibody in the serum is known, the antigen in or on the cells can be identified. This is true because antigen and antibody are specific for one another, even though there is not a 1:1 correspondence between antibodies and antigens, as explained more fully on the following pages.

In human blood grouping, in which the reading of tests is based usually on clumping (agglutination) of red cells, the antigens on the red cells have been called **agglutinogens**. However, in cattle blood grouping, in which the tests are based on hemolysis, the term would seem to be inappropriate, and **hemolysinogen** could be used. As neutral terms, Wiener suggested **erythrogens** for red cell antigens and **leukogens** for white cell antigens, with **thrombogens** being used for platelet antigens; however, these three terms have not found favor and will not be used in this book.

The agglutinogens on the red cells are identified with the aid of the antisera, each one being "monospecific" for a particular **blood factor**. The term blood factor has been used inconsistently in the past, and its meaning is often poorly defined. As used more recently, it refers to **serologic specificities** of red cells, and where possible the term **specificity** should be used in preference to blood factor. The relationship of antibodies to antigens is not necessarily 1:1, but rather it is analogous to the relationship of photographs to the object visualized. Unlimited numbers of different photographs can be made of a single object, and theoretically an unlimited variety of antibodies can correspond to each antigen, as Wiener emphasized. Knowledge of the multiplicity of antibodies corresponding to a single antigen dates back to the work of Landsteiner. **Each separate antibody that reacts with an antigen defines a separate specificity,** just as each photograph discloses a different aspect of the object. Each agglutinogen therefore has multiple serologic specificities, or blood factors. Although the outstanding characteristic of antigen-antibody reactions is their specificity, evidently this specificity is not absolute, and an antibody produced to one antigen may react with other apparently unrelated antigens. Specific examples of this are the ability of antisera to guinea pig kidney to hemolyze sheep red blood cells (the so-called Forssman anti-sera), the ability of anti-**A** human blood grouping sera to hemolyze sheep cells, and the ability of anti-**B** human sera to react preferentially with rabbit red cells.

The difference between **agglutinogens** (**intrinsic** attributes of red cells) and **blood factors,** or **serologic specificities** (the corresponding multiple **extrinsic** attributes of each agglutinogen) has been difficult not only for beginners but even for seasoned workers to understand. The reason appears to be that when the scope of the work is limited, a single antiserum may serve to identify each agglutinogen, just as a single photograph usually suffices to identify a person. In routine blood banking, for example, the three reagents anti-**A**, anti-**B**, and anti-**Rh** serve to identify the three blood antigens A, B, and Rh, respectively. In this case, for practical purposes a 1:1 correspondence between antigen and antibody does hold and has led to the tacit assumption that every antigen has its one unique corresponding antibody, even in more complex situations where such a 1:1 correspondence is manifestly invalid.

ANTIBODY BEHAVIOR

The antibodies in the different blood group systems, in general, behave differently from one another. Rh-Hr antibodies can be recognized by the sharp reaction given by most of the known technics, including conglutination, antiglobulin, and especially the proteolytic enzyme methods. On the other hand, proteolytic enzymes destroy antigens of the M-N-S system, which therefore cannot be tested for by that method.

Fy (**Duffy**) and **Jk** (**Kidd**) antibodies generally react best by the antiglobulin method. Cells maximally coated with such antibodies generally react with antiglobulin sera to about one tenth of the titer of cells maximally coated with Rh antibodies. **Kidd** antibodies react best in serum from freshly drawn blood because **complement,** which is ordinarily present in fresh blood, is essential in such reactions. Antibodies of the A-B-O, Lewis, and Vel systems can, together with complement, hemolyze red cells, whereas antibodies of the Rh-Hr system never cause hemolysis in vitro.

K-k (Kell-Cellano) antibodies have properties intermediate between those of the Rh-Hr and the **Fy** antibodies.

Because the antibody in the serum causes such effects as clumping and dissolving of the cells, the serum containing the antibody is referred to as **antiserum,** meaning a serum that reacts against something. Antiserum may often be produced artificially by injecting cells or other body products containing the antigen into a susceptible animal or human. The organism then forms the antibodies (**immune antibodies**) against the kind of cell or fluid that was injected. Antibodies may be a result of natural phenomena, and in such cases they are called **natural antibodies** in contrast to immune antibodies. Warm and cold antibodies and autoantibodies are discussed on p. 44.

When new blood group specificities or systems are discovered and the antibody is shown to be different from all other known antibodies, as a general rule, it is named for the person in whom it was found. Each antibody symbol contains the prefix "anti-," followed by the name of the antigen for which it is specific. If an antibody were to be found, for example, in the blood of an individual named Johnson, the antibody would be called anti-Johnson and the specificity or antigen it defines would be assigned the name "Johnson," or "Jo." When an antiserum contains antibodies of known specificity, an unknown antigen can be identified. Similarly, cells with known antigens are used to identify unknown antibodies.

ANTIGENS

An antigen is generally defined as a substance, present in or on a cell or in body fluid, that is capable of stimulating production of an antibody more or less specific

in its action against that cell and others like it. The serum containing the antibody is the diagnostic reagent used in the laboratory. It is produced by an animal or human in response to stimulation by the presence of a foreign antigen. Not all substances present in a cell are antigenic, and not all of them therefore can stimulate formation of antibodies.

An antigen contains structural groupings, or **antigenic determinants,** that are absent from or "foreign to" the immunized organism. When an antigen is present on the cell surface, as in the blood cells, it can be identified by agglutination tests; that is, if the cells are mixed with a specific antiserum and come together in clusters, or clumps, the antigen is then identified by the specificity of the antiserum used. The cells are said to have **agglutinated.** The clumps of cells are more or less permanent; it is difficult and at times impossible to separate the individual cells once they have undergone agglutination. The antibodies that cause this type of clumping are called **agglutinating antibodies,** and the clumps of cells are **agglutinates.** There are also **precipitating antibodies, hemolyzing antibodies, coating antibodies,** etc. Precipitating antibodies cause a precipitate to form when mixed with solutions of blood group substances, such as in saliva. Hemolyzing antibodies, with complement—a third substance needed in the reaction of hemolysis—cause the cells to break up, or lyse.

CLASSES OF ANTIBODIES

Antibodies belong to a large group of substances called **immunoglobulins.** Immunoglobulins (Ig) are serum globulins that, when suitably modified, act as antibodies. They are an end product of the immune responses. Five major classes have so far been identified and have been designated IgG, IgM, IgA, IgD, and IgE. Greek letters are also used, and because all the immunoglobulins are gamma globulins, the Greek letter gamma (γ) precedes the iden-

Table 2-1. Some characteristics of the immunoglobulins[*]

	IgG	IgA	IgM	IgD	IgE
Synonyms	Gamma G, γG, 7S, 7Sγ, γ_2, γss, 6.6S, 7Sγ_2	Gamma A, γA, β_2A, γ_1A, 7S-13S, 7S-14Sγ_1, $\beta_\mathbf{x}$	Gamma M, γM, β_2M, 18S, 19S, β_2-C, iota-globulin, macro-globulin	Gamma D, γD, γ_2D	Gamma E, γE
Molecular weight	160,000	170,000 + polymers	900,000; 1 million; + polymers	160,000	200,000 + polymers
Sedimentation coefficient	7S	17S (9, 11, 13, 15S)	19S	7S	8S
Normal serum immunoglobulins (%)	75 (60-70)	15 (15-20)	7 (5-10)	0.2	?
Normal serum proteins (%)	15 to 20	?	1 to 2	?	?
Normal immunoglobulin in serum mg/100 ml	1240 ± 224	250	120 ± 35	3	0.05
Half-life (days)	30	5.8	5.1	2.8	2.3
Daily turnover	6.7%	25%	18%	37%	Rapid
Electrophoretic mobility	γ_2 to α_2; γ	γ_1 to α_2 fast; slow β	Fast γ; slow β_2	γ to β; γ and β	γ_2 to α_2; γ and β
Chromatographic peaks	4, 5, 6, 7 ± + + +++ ++	4, 5, 6 + + ±	1, 2, 3 ± + ±	?	?
Solubility	Euglobulin	Pseudoglobulin	Euglobulin	Unknown	Pseudoglobulin
Carbohydrate (%)	2.9	7.5	11.8	—	10.7
Antibodies	Major antibacterial, antiviral, and antitoxic; sensitizing to Rh; warm, incomplete, blocking; IgG$_1$ and IgG$_3$ fix complement well, IgG$_2$ weakly, IgG$_4$ not at all, antinuclear	Bacterial agglutinins, skin sensitizing, cold agglutinins, isoagglutinins, anti-insulin, antinuclear (?)	Natural heterophil; ABO isoantibodies; rheumatoid factor; antinuclear; cold agglutinins; certain Rh complete saline; typhoid antisomatic O; binds complement; Waldenström's macroglobulinemia abnormal monoclonal; first antibody formed in primary immune response; IgM autoantibody to IgG	?	Neutralizes allergens; fixes to skin; human skin sensitizing; myeloma protein
Cross placenta (?)	Yes	No	No	?	?
Increased in	Dysproteinemias, severe malnutrition, infectious hepatitis, lupus erythematosus, chronic infections, infectious mononucleosis, cystic fibrosis, monocytic leukemia	Cystic fibrosis, "A" myeloma, Laennec's cirrhosis, monocytic leukemia, at times in infectious hepatitis, infectious mononucleosis, sarcoidosis, Hodgkin's disease; high in tears, saliva, colostrum,	Malaria, actinomycosis, trypanosomiasis, Waldenström's macroglobulinemia, Laennec's cirrhosis, biliary cirrhosis, rheumatoid arthritis, infectious mononucleosis, monocytic leukemia; at	?	Allergy

[*]From Erskine, A. G.: Lab. Digest 33:(2):6, 1971.

Table 2-1. Some characteristics of the immunoglobulins—cont'd

	IgG	IgA	IgM	IgD	IgE
		nasopharyngeal, trache- obronchial, and gastro- intestinal secretions	times in infectious hep- atitis, lupus erythema- tosus, chronic infec- tions, sarcoidosis, cystic fibrosis, Hodg- kin's disease		
Decreased in	Congenital hypogam- maglobulinemia or agammaglobulinemia	Ataxia telangiectasia	Lymphoid aplasia, G and A myeloma, agamma- globulinemia, dys- gammaglobulinemia		

tifying initial, such as γG, γM, γA, γD, and γE. The letters refer to their distintive electrophoretic behaviors, or mobilities, as given in Table 2-1.

Simple **gel diffusion** is used, as well as **immunoelectrophoresis,** to identify the various immunoglobulins. In gel diffusion (Fig. 2-1) the antigen and its corresponding antibody diffuse through the gel directly into one another. In **double diffusion** of Ouchterlony (Fig. 2-2) a blank volume of gel is interposed between the antigen and antibody. The test is often performed on plates. The antigen and antibody, placed in separate holes in the gel, diffuse toward one another in the thin layer of gel. **Lines of precipitation** are formed in the gel; these lines can then be stained with any of a variety of dyes such as Ponceau red, azocarmine, chlorazol black, and wool black, and these records may be kept permanently after drying. This double diffusion method enables one to identify either an unknown antibody or an unknown antigen.

In **immunoelectrophoresis,** on the other hand, the components are first separated by electrophoresis (Fig. 2-3). The antiserum is then allowed to diffuse toward these components from a parallel trough cut in the agar. Arcs of precipitate form when the diffusing antibody meets the separated antigens.

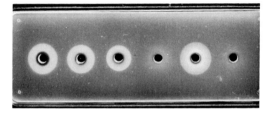

Fig. 2-1. Gel diffusion. The three tests at the left side show the rings of precipitation formed by immunoglobulins IgM, IgG, and IgA of a normal serum; those at the right were formed by a serum with a high IgG concentration. The serum being tested for immunoglobulin content is placed in the well and allowed to diffuse into the surrounding agar, which contains the known antibodies. The size of the halo that results is proportional to the concentration of the antigen in question. (Courtesy Dr. J. D. Bauer, DePaul Hospital Division, St. Louis, Mo.)

IMMUNOGLOBULINS[1-3]

The likely site for production of serum globulins is either the small lymphocyte or the plasma cell, or both, possibly within the lymph node. The spleen seems also to have some function with respect to the immunoglobulins. Production of gamma globulin also appears to be part of the normal function of small lymphocytes and plasma cells. When a foreign antigen is introduced into the body, an **immune response** occurs, and the antibody-containing gamma globulin is produced. If an immune response

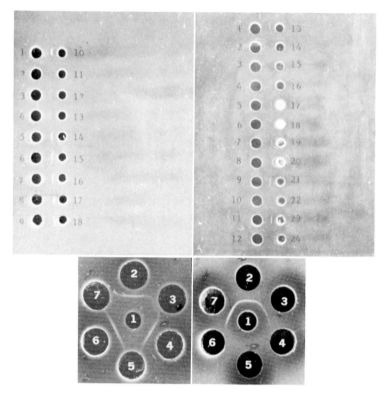

Fig. 2-2. Immunoelectrophoresis (top) and Ouchterlony agar double diffusion (bottom) test showing precipitation bands. Although these procedures were actually made for the hepatitis-associated antigen (HAA) test, the method is the same in the identification of the various immunoglobulins. (Courtesy Dr. A. H. Cioffi, Eastern Biologicals, Inc., New York, N.Y.)

takes place simultaneously with a number of different antigens, then other sets of lymphocytes or plasma cells react and produce different antibodies. The lymphocytes appear to develop in **clones.** A clone, or colony, of lymphocytes is composed of related cells that were derived from one precursor cell, and all the lymphocytes in a single clone seem to have identical functions and reaction behavior patterns.

The **biological activity** of the various immunoglobulins can be classified into two general categories. The first is antibody activity (Table 2-1), and the second is a group of others, including (1) reaction with rheumatoid factors, (2) fixation of complement, (3) sensitization of skin, (4) active transport across placental and possibly other membranes, and (5) regulation of immunoglobulin molecular catabolism. Antibody activity has been demonstrated in IgG, IgM, and IgA proteins.

The various immunoglobulins differ from one another chemically, and since IgG, IgM, and IgA seem to be components of the blood group antibodies in different quantities and mixtures, the blood group antibodies also differ from one another. Because of a difference in molecular structure and probably also because of the small size of the molecule as first postulated, IgG antibodies can be transported across the placenta. IgM, a large-molecule antibody, does not cross the placenta, but even some of the smaller molecular size antibodies like IgA do not have the ability of transplacental transport (Fig. 2-4).

Differentiation of IgG, IgM, and IgA from one another is accomplished by (1) fractionation on DEAE-cellulose or cross-linked dextran (Sephadex) columns, (2) ultracentrifugation, (3) electrophoresis,

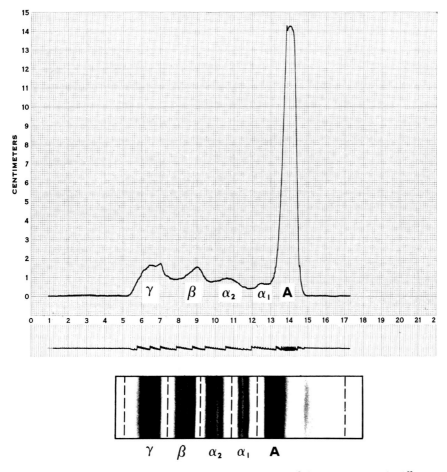

Fig. 2-3. Cellulose acetate electrophoretic pattern of normal human serum. A, Albumin; α_1 and α_2, alpha globulins; β, beta globulins; and γ, gamma globulins. (From Bauer, J. D., Ackermann, P. G., and Toro, G.: Clinical laboratory methods, ed. 8, St. Louis, 1974, The C. V. Mosby Co.)

(4) treatment with sulfhydryl compounds, or (5) sensitivity to heat.

The **immunoglobulin molecule**[4-6] is composed of a four-unit structure that consists of two light- and two heavy-chain polypeptides connected by disulfide linkages. The heavy chains are characteristic in their amino acid sequence and biological function, and they are represented by the small Greek letter corresponding to their respective class. The light chains are of two types common to all classes and are designated as kappa (κ) or lambda (λ), but only one of these types is associated with any individual antibody. Each light chain is co-

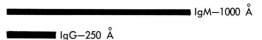

Fig. 2-4. Relative lengths of IgM and IgG molecules. The longer IgM molecule can bridge the gap more easily between red cells suspended in saline media than can the shorter IgG molecule, causing the red cells to agglutinate without the addition of a third substance such as antiglobulin.

valently bound to one heavy chain by a disulfide bond. The two heavy chains are joined together by at least one and possibly two or three disulfide bonds. This basic molecular unit of two heavy and two light polypeptide chains characterizes the immunoglobulin molecules and is found in IgG, IgM, IgA, and IgD. Antibody-specific activity is believed to be located in the Fab fragments of the immunoglobulin molecule (Fig. 2-5).

In Fig. 2-5 the left-hand extremes of the chains are known as the N terminals because of the amino groups present there, and the right-hand ends are known as the C terminals because of the carboxyl groups located there. As has been shown by amino acid sequencing, each chain can be subdivided into constant, or C, segments (at the right hand side) and variable, or V, segments, at the Fab location. The C portions are genetically determined and are responsible for the so-called Gm groups, of which by now at least twenty varieties are known, whereas the V segments are responsible for the specificities of the antibody activity of immunoglobulin molecules.

The intact **IgG antibody molecule is bivalent;** that is, it has two antibody-combining sites and can therefore combine with two antigen molecules. However, the IgG molecules can be split into **fragments** by cleavage of peptide bonds by proteolytic enzyme. When papain is used, three fragments are formed—two Fab, and a third, Fc, containing half of each of the two

heavy chains (Fig. 2-5).* When the IgG molecule is digested with pepsin, different fragments are produced. The IgG heavy chains are antigenically different from the IgG light chains. There are subvarieties of the IgG heavy chains, and similar subclasses have also been described for IgM and IgA. In fact, at least twenty types of immunoglobulins are definable by antigenic and functional criteria. The IgG molecule contains carbohydrate to the extent of 2% of its molecular weight. For other characteristics of IgG, consult Table 2-1.

The **IgM molecule** is larger and consists of five subunits; each subunit also has two heavy chains and two light chains linked by disulfide bridges. The IgM light chains are like those of IgG and IgA. About 10% of the molecular weight of IgM is carbohydrate. It exists as a five-subunit molecule with a sedimentation constant of 18S, whereas IgA seems to occur naturally as a series of polymers. The basic unit of IgA is a molecule composed of two light and

---

*Fab refers to fragment, antigen binding; Fc refers to fragment, crystalline. Each light chain has two globular regions or domains, one constant (C_1) and one variable (V_1), and each consisting of about 110 amino acids.

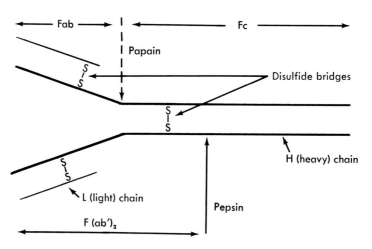

Fig. 2-5. Diagram showing four-chain structure of an IgG molecule and fragments produced by splitting the molecule with enzymes papain and pepsin. (Modified from Fudenberg, H. H., et al.: Basic immunogenetics, Oxford, 1972, Oxford University Press.)

two heavy chains. Some **IgA molecules** form polymers with sedimentation coefficients of 9S, 11S, or 13S, but the ultracentrifugal sedimentation coefficient is most often 7S. Some secretions like saliva and colostrum contain relatively high concentrations of IgA with a sedimentation constant of 11S. About 10% of the molecular weight of IgA is carbohydrate.

The molecular structure and function of **IgD** are not well understood, and antibody activity has not been demonstrated; again, there are two light and two heavy polypeptide chains.

The term **IgE** has been proposed for reaginic antibodies, that is, antibodies that have the ability to passively sensitize human skin for allergic reactions.

19S AND 7S GAMMA GLOBULINS

In describing the differences between 19S and 7S gamma globulins and the manner in which they react in vitro, Campbell et al.[7] in 1955 fractionated anti-**Rh** antibodies—both the agglutinating and the blocking, or incomplete,[*] types—by ultracentrifugation, which separated them into 19S and 7S gamma globulins. Agglutinating antibodies, which are those capable of clumping red cells suspended in saline, appear to be of the 19S type, whereas incomplete antibodies are 7S. Anti-**M,** anti-**N,** anti-**P**$_1$, anti-**Rh** agglutinating antibodies, and naturally occurring anti-**A,** anti-**B,** and anti-**Le**^{a} are usually 19S globulins (see below). The serologic activity of anti-**A**$_1$, anti-**B,** and anti-**Rh** saline agglutinating antibodies and the so-called nonspecific cold agglutinins are destroyed by treatment with 2-mercaptoethanol according to Grubb and Swahn[8]; most immune, so-called incomplete, antibodies such as anti-**Rh** univalent, anti-**K,** and anti- **Fy**^{a} behave as 7S globulin. The serologic activity of incomplete anti-**Rh,** as well as other IgG antibodies, is not destroyed by treatment with 2-mercaptoethanol.

The **newborn infant** usually has about the same content of 7S globulin as the mother, but this declines after birth,[9] with a "half-life" of 30 days. IgG (immunoglobulin G, or gamma globulin) is not normally produced by the infant until he is 2 or 3 months old (Fig. 2-6), and those present in the newborn are of maternal origin, passively acquired by the fetus by transplacental transfer, thus accounting for the equality of titers in mother and newborn. The 19S gamma globulin in the cord serum, however, is only about one tenth to one twentieth of that of a normal adult.[10] **Gamma globulin synthesis** occurs normally after the first few weeks of life, but antibody formation capacity develops only during the second month after birth. However, antibodies may be produced if an appropriate antigenic stimulus is given, even in the newborn.

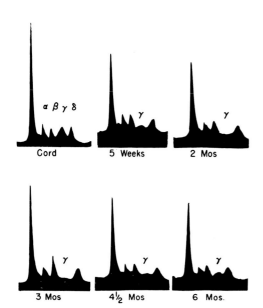

α β γ δ

Cord   5 Weeks   2 Mos

γ   γ

3 Mos   4½ Mos   6 Mos.

Fig. 2-6. Serum gamma globulin in babies. (From Wiener, A. S.: The Rh-Hr blood types, New York, 1954, with permission of Grune & Stratton, Inc.)

---

*The term "IgG (7S)" antibodies has replaced the terms blocking antibodies, incomplete antibodies, and univalent antibodies. Similarly, "IgM" has replaced complete antibodies and bivalent antibodies, but "agglutinating" antibodies is still in good usage.

COMPLEMENT

Complement is a thermolabile substance present in all normal human sera and is a necessary component for a biological hemolytic reaction. Apparently it is adsorbed onto erythrocytes that have been sensitized by a **hemolysin (amboceptor)** and aids in or brings about dissolution of the cells. Complement has four principal components and at least nine globulins, as well as many subcomponents. It is **inactivated** at a temperature of 56° C in from 15 to 30 minutes. Blood taken in heparin may show considerable impairment of complement activity. In blood grouping reactions, complement is important only in hemolytic reactions and for identification of some of the blood group factors, for example, **Kidd.** Use of fresh serum is important because storage of typing serum or simply time will remove or inactivate the natural complement of serum that is necessary for the reaction. To prevent isohemolysis during in vitro reactions when testing serum against cells in the A-B-O system, it may be necessary to inactivate the serum prior to testing. In many cases, using fresh serum results in hemolysis of the opposing red cells, but after the serum has been inactivated, the cells can be and are acted on by the agglutinating antibodies in the serum, and then they will clump. The hemolysins and agglutinins in such a case are of the same specificity.

ISOAGGLUTININS

The blood group antibodies in the A-B-O system are usually called isoagglutinins because they cause blood cells of individuals of the same species to clump. ("Iso-" refers to the intraspecies reaction; "agglutinin" refers to the clumping antibody.) The two isoagglutinins are designated anti-**A** and anti-**B,** and these are said to be naturally occurring in humans. Anti-**A** reacts against cells having the A agglutinogen, as in blood groups A and AB but not B or O; anti-**B** reacts with cells having the B agglutinogen, as in groups B and AB but not A or O.

The composition of the four A-B-O blood groups with respect to agglutinogens and agglutinins is as follows:

Group O—No agglutinogens; anti-**A** and anti-**B** agglutinins
Group A—Agglutinogen A; anti-**B** agglutinin
Group B—Agglutinogen B; anti-**A** agglutinin
Group AB—Agglutinogens A and B; no agglutinins

For a continuation of this discussion, refer to Chapters 3 and 5.

Anti-**A** and anti-**B** appear to be both 7S and 19S globulin antibodies.

ANTIGEN-ANTIBODY REACTIONS

Blood grouping tests belong to the broad category of antigen-antibody reactions. In the laboratory an observable change takes place when an antigen combines with an antibody. The reaction is believed to be caused by the combination of the terminal nonreducing sugar units of the antigen with the gamma globulin antibody molecule. Antigen-antibody reactions are **specific;** that is, anti-**A** antibody molecules will attach to the terminal sugar units on the A antigen polysaccharide chain but will not attach to terminal units on the B antigen chain. For this reason, anti-**A** will clump cells having the A but not the B antigen, or, to be more explicit, this antibody will cause agglutination of A and AB cells but not of B or O cells.

There are different types of antigen-antibody reactions, as well as different types of antibodies. In blood grouping the usual reaction is agglutination, and hemolysis can also occur. Sensitization, neutralization, and complement fixation are other types of antigen-antibody reactions.

LYMPHOCYTES AND THE IMMUNE RESPONSE

There are two populations of lymphocytes in the mammalian body; one survives in the circulation for only 2 to 5 days, and the other survives for 3 or 4 years or even for as long as 20 years. Lymphocytes can leave the circulation and accumulate at sites of inflammation and in such organs as the spleen, bone marrow, and lymph nodes, where they are stored. They return to the bloodstream by way of the thoracic duct and lymphatics.

In fetal life, lymphocyte precursors of the specifically sensitized lymphocytes of cell-mediated immune response (CMIR) and of plasma cells that synthesize immunoglobulins are found in the liver and later in the developing bone marrow. Certain lymphocytes are under the influence of the thymus in late fetal or early neonatal life and are therefore called **T-lymphocytes** (for thymus). The lymphocytes that become plasma cell precursors do not depend on the thymus. These are responsible for cellular immunity and are the cells involved in graft rejection in mammals, including man. In birds they are influenced by the bursa of Fabricius. In humans and mammals the bursal equivalent is provided by the lymphoid tissue that lines the intestinal tract, such as Peyer's patches and the appendix. Lympho-

cytes from such sources are referred to as **B-lymphocytes** (from bursa). These are the cells involved in humoral antibody production. T-lymphocytes are usually long lived and mobile. B-lymphocytes are usually short lived and far less mobile than T-lymphocytes.

The two forms of lymphocytes can be explained as in Fig. 2-7.

The immune response begins when the antigen reacts with the lymphoid tissues of the host. Antigen recognition seems to be brought about by specific receptors that are present in patches on the surface of the lymphocytes, but it can also be associated with active cell proliferation and the interaction of different cell types. Such actions lead to antibody formation, to immunologic memory, or even to cellular immunity. The immunogenic capacity of the antigen, the quantity of the antigen, the route of administration or access to the tissues, the susceptibility of the host, and the

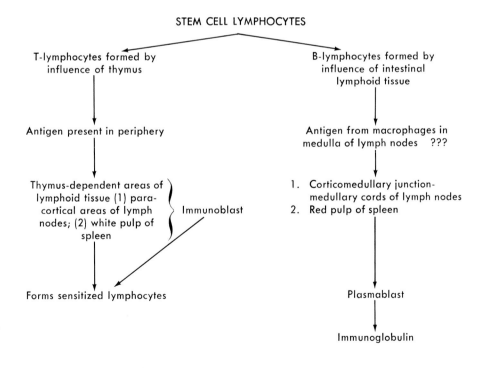

Fig. 2-7. Two forms of lymphocytes. (Modified from Turk, J. L.: Immunology in clinical medicine, ed. 2, New York, 1972, Appleton-Century-Crofts.)

physiologic condition of the host all influence antibody production.

NATURE OF ANTIBODIES

At one time, a sharp distinction was made between immune antibodies and so-called "natural" antibodies. It is presently accepted that this distinction is an artificial one and that so-called natural antibodies are also of immune origin, with the difference that the antigen eliciting their pro-duction is unknown or inapparent. Presumably, naturally occurring antibodies result from inapparent infections during early life or, in the case of blood group antibodies, from exposure to substances that are antigenically similar to the human blood group substances but are not blood group substances themselves. As Springer et al.[12] have demonstrated by experiments with germfree chickens, some of these antibodies come from stimulation by certain

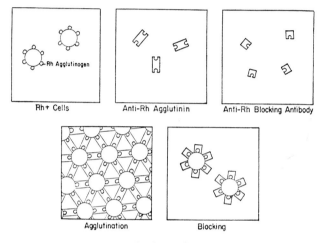

Fig. 2-8. Diagrammatic representation of Rh agglutination and blocking reactions. (From Wiener, A. S.: Am. J. Clin. Pathol. **15**:106, 1945.)

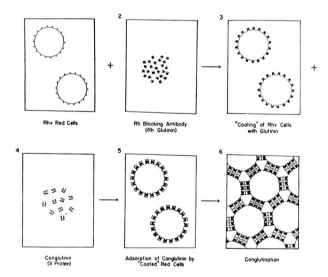

Fig. 2-9. Diagrammatic representation of Rh conglutination reaction (test in plasma or serum media). (From Wiener, A. S.: Lab. Digest **14**[6], 1950.)

bacteria in the bowel, such as *Escherichia coli*, whereas others come from food.

There are two principal forms of antibodies: (1) IgM (agglutinating, complete, precipitating, or 19S, formerly referred to as "bivalent"), and (2) IgG (conglutinating, blocking, 7S, incomplete, or coating, formerly referred to as "univalent"). **Univalent** and **bivalent** must not be confused with chemical valence. These terms were coined by Wiener to give a visual concept of in vitro reactions, as in Figs. 2-8 to 2-11, but the terms must not be taken literally.

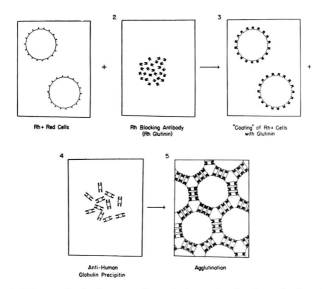

Fig. 2-10. Antiglobulin method of testing for IgG (univalent) Rh antibodies. (From Wiener, A. S.: Lab. Digest **14**[6], 1950.)

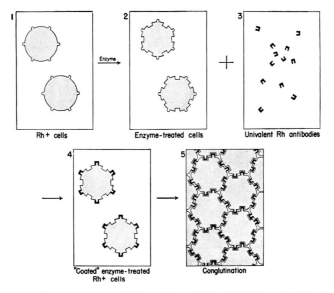

Fig. 2-11. Clumping of enzyme-treated Rh-positive cells by IgG Rh antibodies. (From Wiener, A. S.: Lab. Digest **14**[6], 1950.)

Antibodies in intragroup transfusion reactions

As early as 1921 Unger[11] noted that occasionally a patient's serum would clump the cells of a donor, even though both belonged to the same A-B-O blood group, and that transfusion of such blood resulted in chills and fever, which he attributed to incompatibility. This was apparently the first report of an intragroup transfusion reaction. Unger called the antibodies responsible for the incompatibility **minor agglutinins** to distinguish them from the **major** anti-**A** and anti-**B** agglutinins. He had used a 2% suspension of the cells in the individual's own plasma for the cross-matching tests, even though at that time it was customary to use only saline-suspended cells. Without realizing it, he had observed the reactions produced by IgG, 7S antibodies, as they are presently known.

IgM ANTIBODIES

IgM antibodies react with cells suspended in saline as well as with cells suspended in high molecular colloid media, and were formerly designated as "bivalent," or "complete," antibodies. As a matter of fact, IgM antibodies are now known to be pentavalent and are no more complete than are other antibodies. The ability of IgM antibodies to agglutinate red cells in saline media is now believed to be due to their large molecular size—about 1,000 Å in length; thus they are able to bridge the gap between the red cells and link them together, causing agglutination despite the net negative charge that tends to keep the red cells apart. Antibodies of smaller molecular size could not act in this manner without the intervention of a third accessory substance (Fig. 2-4).

IgM antibodies cannot traverse the placenta. Such antibodies usually occur in the earlier stages of immunization and are relatively thermolabile; that is, they are damaged or destroyed by heating above 65° C. IgG antibodies, in contrast, tend to appear later in the course of immunization, can traverse the placenta, and are relatively

thermostabile. The IgM antibody produced in syphilis is a **flocculating** antibody, whereas the IgG antibody is a **complement-fixing** one. **Antisheep hemolysin** used in complement fixation tests is an IgG antibody that requires complement to complete its reaction with sheep cells.

Anti-**A** and anti-**B** agglutinins are usually IgM antibodies, but anti-**C** (of the A-B-O system) is more often IgG. Rh antibodies can be IgM or IgG, or both types can be present at the same time in the same blood serum. It is for this last reason that laboratory tests for antibodies are directed toward identifying both IgG and IgM antibodies in a single specimen of serum.

IgG ANTIBODIES

In 1944 Wiener[13] and Race,[14] independent of one another, discovered the blocking, or incomplete, Rh antibody; Wiener designated it a blocking antibody, and Race called it incomplete. Wiener originally explained the in vitro reactions of the blocking antibody by representing it diagrammatically as univalent, and he pointed out its ability to pass the placental barrier and its consequent greater than realized role in the pathogenesis of erythroblastosis fetalis. A number of different authors suggested various tests to detect the blocking antibody. In 1945 a new technic was announced, primarily by Coombs et al.[15] The original test has become known as the **Coombs test,** but at present it is preferably designated as the **antiglobulin test.** The antiglobulin serum was prepared by immunizing rabbits with human whole serum or preferably purified human gamma globulin, so that the resulting antiserum contained an anti–human gamma globulin, presently called antiglobulin. When red cells that have been sensitized (coated) by incomplete anti-Rh antibodies are washed free of detectable amounts of serum and mixed with antiglobulin serum, the cells agglutinate.

Blocking antibody (7S, IgG) cannot cause agglutination of red cells suspended in a saline medium, but it can combine with the antigen to bring about clumping of the cells when another substance is added. These incomplete antibodies are usually of the IgG variety with a length of only 250 Å.

IgG antibodies fail to agglutinate red cells in saline media not because they are univalent (they are actually bivalent), but because they are so short that they cannot bridge the gap between the red cells, which are kept apart by their net negative surface charge (Fig. 2-4).

The suggestion to use centrifugation as a mechanical means to reduce the gap be-tween the cells coated with IgG antibodies has the difficulty that a centrifugal force of 8,000 g is required, which could cause the red cells to disintegrate. A better method is to suspend the red cells in colloid media that, by reducing the zeta potential, makes it possible for the red cells to approach one another closely enough to be linked to-gether by the smaller IgG antibodies. An-other method is based on the fact that the antibodies are gamma globulins so that the coating can be detected by adding an anti-gamma globulin serum to the coated cells; the antiglobulin then reacts with the glob-ulin on the coated cells, and the cells clump.

Table 2-2. Properties of agglutinating (IgM) and blocking (IgG) antibodies*

Characteristic	IgM (19S) antibodies	IgG (7S) antibodies
Common name	Agglutinin, precipitin, agglutinat-ing antibody, complete antibody, IgM, γM	Glutinin, blocking antibody, con-glutinating antibody, incomplete antibody, IgG, γG
Usual time of appearance in course of immunization	Early	Late
Resistance to heating	Relatively thermolabile	Relatively thermostable
Reaction of **Rh**o antibodies† in saline medium	Clumps cells by agglutination	Coats cells without clumping them — blocking reaction
Reactions of **Rh**o antibodies in colloid medium	Clumps cells by agglutination	Clumps cells by conglutination
Behavior in mixed agglutination tests	Specific clumps are formed	Clumps contain more than 1 kind of cell
Opsonic effect	None	Positive in presence of complement
Chemical nature	Euglobulin; precipitated by so-dium sulfate solutions of con-centrations 13.5% to 17.4%	Pseudoglobulin; precipitated by sodium sulfate solutions of con-centrations 17.4% to 21.5%
Electrophoretic behavior	Alpha and beta globulins	Gamma globulins
Sedimentation constant	19S	7S
Probable molecular weight	900,000	150,000
Diffusibility	Poor	Good
Behavior relative to placenta	Held back by intact placenta	Passes through placenta readily
Half-life	Probably 2 wk or less	30 to 35 days
Role in syphilis	Flocculating antibody	Complement-fixing antibody
Role in disease	Precipitating and agglutinating antibody	Protective antibody; antitoxin
Role in allergy	Sensitizing antibody (reagin)	Blocking antibody
Role in erythroblastosis	Not significant	Major

*Modified from Wiener, A. S., and Wexler, J. B.: An Rh-Hr syllabus, the types and their applications, ed. 2, New York, 1963, Grune & Stratton, Inc.
†The in vitro reactions are somewhat different, depending on the antigen-antibody system.

Because later evidence indicated that both forms of antibodies are actually bivalent or multivalent, Wiener modified his ideas concerning in vitro reactions. He likened IgG antibody to an adapter on a syringe—it fits the antiglobulin antibody and then links the cells together. He concluded that red cells have negative charges all around the surface and that the surface potential keeps the cells apart. The IgM antibodies are longer molecules and also cover more of the ionic polarities of the red cell than can the small-molecule 7S antibody, and so when IgM antibody attaches itself to the red cells containing the proper antigen, agglutination takes place. When the shorter IgG antibody combines with red cells, there can be no agglutination because it cannot cover up enough of the ionic polarities. There is a critical potential below which clumping can occur. When the combining sites are coated with antibody and the potential that keeps the red cells apart is sufficiently lowered, the cells clump. If the red cells are suspended in a surface colloid like **acacia,** some of the medium is adsorbed onto the red cell surface, and the electric surface charge is reduced. The appropriate antibody—even the small, 7S variety—can then bring them together, and clumping occurs.

Table 2-2 gives a detailed outline of the differences between IgM (19S) and IgG (7S) antibodies. The difference between the reactions of Rh IgM and Rh IgG antibodies are explained as follows:

1. Anti-**Rh** IgM antibodies + Rh-positive cells = Rh agglutination
2a. Anti-**Rh** IgG antibodies + Rh-positive cells suspended in saline = coating of the cells but no agglutination
2b. Antiglobulin serum added now = clumping of coated cells

There is in serum a normal component, called **X protein,** that is adsorbed onto specifically sensitized red cells, causing them to stick together. It is a colloidal constituent or **conglutinin,** a large molecular complex of albumin, globulin, fibrinogen, and phospholipid. Although it is heat resistant, it dissociates readily into its constituent, smaller molecules of albumin and globulin when diluted with water. The use of saline to suspend cells or to dilute serum may either partially or completely dissociate the X protein of serum. Crystalline solutions are therefore avoided when attempting to identify or detect the presence of IgG antibodies.

ZETA POTENTIAL

Pollack et al.[16-18] explained the reactions of IgM and IgG antibodies as follows. For red cells to agglutinate, they must first approach each other closely enough to be spanned by the antibody molecules. The IgM molecules are long enough to span this distance, but the 7S, or IgG, molecules are not. The distance between the cells must be three or four times shorter for the IgG molecules than for the IgM varieties to cause linkage of the cells in an agglutination reaction. The position of the antigen on the cells is important because if it protrudes several hundred angstroms beyond the outer portion of the cell, agglutination is more likely to occur in a saline medium, as with anti-**A** or anti-**B** of the A-B-O system. If the antigen, on the other hand, is buried beneath the red cell surface, then even the 19S molecule may not be long enough to combine with the antigens on adjacent cells to link them together.

All similar particles, including red cells, in suspension have a general tendency to come together in a single whole, or cohesion, reaction. The forces of attraction are between the red cells and arise from the free energy either contained in or trapped on the surfaces. The cohesion of two particles results in the loss of the two surfaces that come in contact with one another. The lost surface area consists of one side from each of the joining objects and is equal to twice the area of contact. The energy that had been trapped by these two joining surfaces is liberated and seems to force the particles together. This is called the **cohesive force.** Forces that oppose the attraction forces are also present; otherwise, red cells would not exist as separated individual units. Suspension stability is thus maintained by these repelling forces.

Red blood cells carry on their surfaces an excess of negative polar groups. These are believed to arise mostly as a result of ionization of the carboxyl groups of sialic acid residues. The red cell can be thought of as analogous to one pole of a magnet that repels the like pole of another magnet when brought within its sphere of influence.

The considerable force between the red cells is sufficiently strong to prevent agglutination by the shorter IgG agglutinins if the cells are suspended in a saline medium. The relative strengths of the two opposing forces control agglutination or lack of it under these circumstances. The repulsive forces can be overcome by high speed centrifugation. The repulsive forces, moreover, can be decreased by a number of methods, for example, treatment of the red cells with proteolytic enzymes.

When red cells are suspended in a saline medium, the strongly negative-charged cells attract positive-charged sodium ions. A cloud is formed that decreases in density as the distance from the surface of the erythrocytes increases. Since the force with which one red cell repels another is proportional to the charge on its surface, the force between these charges is reduced in an atmosphere of sodium ions. The sodium ions within the boundary of the double layer always move as if they were part of the red cell, and they form part of its kinetic unit. Outside this plane they do not. Pollack has termed this the **slipping plane,** or the **shear boundary.** Sodium ions outside this boundary do not move as if they were part of the erythrocyte. The force between the shear boundaries of erythrocytes is related to the voltage, or potential, at this point. Voltage, or potential, is defined as the charge per unit of distance.

The potential at the shear boundary is termed the **zeta potential.** Its magnitude is proportional to the force and thickness of the double layer. If the electrolyte concentration is raised, that is, if the ionic strength is increased, more cations are packed around the red cell, and the zeta potential is reduced, even though the charge on the red cell surface itself may not be affected. The presence of electrolytes in isotonic solutions therefore permits agglutination by the 19S antibody molecules but not by the 7S molecules. Were the sodium content of the saline increased sufficiently to reduce the zeta potential, 7S antibody molecules still could not cause agglutination because the concentration of sodium chloride required to lower the zeta to levels to bring this about would completely elute the antibody. Pollack and his associates have calculated that 0.87M sodium chloride would be required to lower zeta sufficiently, and at only half that concentration 7S univalent antibodies are almost completely eluted from the red cells.

There are some **natural** and **synthetic polymers** that can bring about agglutination with IgG antibodies. The water-soluble polymers—albumin, PVP, dextran, etc. —all raise the dielectric constant of water by an amount dependent on the degree to which they become polarized, or oriented in an electric field. Parts of the molecule of substances that raise the dielectric constant become attracted to the charges on the red cell, but these substances also have other parts that are repelled by the red cell charges and are therefore forced to orient, or rotate, in such a way that they are less randomly distributed in the medium. This activity consumes much of the electric energy of the red cells, thereby reducing the zeta potential. It is possible to prepare solutions of polymers that are similar to serum in serologic reactions.

Agglutination of the red cells occurs when the strengths of forces are such that the cells can approach closely enough to each other for antibody molecules to span the intercellular gap. The two major **competing forces** are the surface free energy that tends to cause aggregation and the electrostatic force of repulsion that depends on the zeta potential. If the zeta potential is less than 19 mv, agglutination occurs with saline IgM agglutinins. Agglutination will occur with albumin IgG agglutinins only when zeta potential is below 10 mv.

Actions that reduce the zeta potential of erythrocytes are those in which reduction of surface charge takes place, such as absorption of antibody and treatment with blood group enzymes. Those that cause changes in a reaction medium do so by increasing either the ionic strength or the dielectric constant.

Proteolytic enzymes act differently. They split off polar groups and thus reduce the surface charge on the red cells, enabling IgG antibodies to bring about agglutination. However, treatment of red cells with proteolytic enzymes, in the M-N-S system especially, modifies the antigens so that the cells will no longer react with their corresponding antibodies. In using such enzymes as ficin in tests, one must be careful not to treat the cells for too long a time; otherwise, the cells tend to stick together and cannot be separated.

ANTIGLOBULIN TESTS

Antiglobulin tests are described in Chapter 15.

As previously stated, certain antibodies can combine with red cells but cannot bring about agglutination because they are too short to link adjacent cells together. Since the combining antibodies are serum gamma globulins, addition of antibodies artifically produced in rabbits against human serum globulin (called anti–human globulin or antiglobulin) can link the coated human red cells and cause them to agglutinate, with the antibodies acting as adapters.

There are two types of antiglobulin tests: (1) direct, applied to red cells already coated in vivo with antibody, and (2) indirect, applied to serum to detect the presence of antibody. There are also two types of antiglobulin reagents: (1) anti–gamma globulin for antibodies that react without the aid of complement and (2) anti–nongamma globulin applied to antibodies that clump red cells only in the presence of complement. Anti–human globulin reagent for the antiglobulin test (also called the Coombs test) can be produced artificially in animals by injecting them with human serum or its globulin fraction and then absorbing out the species-specific hemagglutinins. An antibody specific for human globulin remains in the animal serum, which, subsequently, can be standardized for its ability to react with gamma globulin as well as with complement. This, in turn, determines the capability of the serum to detect different types of antibodies.

If the antiglobulin serum is to be used only with IgG globulin, antibodies of this type only will be detected. Most complement-dependent antibodies require anti–nongamma globulin activity to be detectable by the antiglobulin reaction. Some of the antibodies that do not react with anti–gamma globulin serum are anti-**H**, anti-**Lewis**, anti-**Jk**^{a}, and anti-**Fy**^{a}, which apparently require the presence of human complement in order to react.

If human gamma globulin is added to or is present in excess in a test, the direct antiglobulin test will be inhibited. Addition of gamma globulin does not inhibit a positive nongamma globulin antiglobulin test in which complement is involved, but this reaction is inhibited by addition of human α and β globulins.

The **direct antiglobulin test** is used mostly in the diagnosis of hemolytic disease of the newborn, in autoimmune hemolytic anemias, and in the investigation of transfusion reactions. Direct antiglobulin tests may at times give false positive results, due to high reticulocyte counts or due to adsorption onto the red cells of serum globulins that are not antibodies, which occurs in lead poisoning, drug-induced hemolysis, and some viral diseases.

The **indirect antiglobulin test** is used in determining compatibility, in cross-matching tests, in finding and identifying irregular antibodies, in detecting antibodies not identified by other means, or in investigative studies.

The antiglobulin tests are critically affected by variations in timing and temperature, and it is therefore important that in testing with these reagents the manufacturers instructions for their specific products be followed to the letter. Enzyme treatment of cells, as for the Jk factors, increases the sensitivity of the tests, but in some instances, as already pointed out, enzymes cannot be used.

When the antiglobulin test is performed, the cells must be washed four times in saline after sensitization with the coating antibody. If the washing is not done thoroughly and rapidly and if all the saline is not completely removed between and after the washings, the tests could give false negative results. Under no circumstances must the finger of the operator be placed over the tubes when they are inverted to mix after each washing because the small amount of protein present on the finger could inactivate the antiglobulin reagent. Time and speed of centrifugation after the addition of antiglobulin serum are critical.

Cells that give a direct positive antiglobulin test cannot be used for indirect tests because antibody has already coated the cells. If the test cells are contaminated with bacteria, they may agglutinate even in the absence of specific antibodies. The same is true of cells derived from a patient with bacteremia. Umbilical cord specimens contaminated with Wharton's jelly must be washed at least four times (or more) with saline before testing, or hyaluronidase may be added to the test cells to keep them from sticking together.

Saline should not be stored too long in glass containers because the colloidal silica that may dissolve into the solution from the glass can interfere in antigen-antibody reactions. Contact of the reagents with metal parts must also be avoided because the metallic ions can cause protein coating or direct agglutination of red cells. Whenever antiglobulin tests are only weakly positive, it is good practice to check the glassware and to repeat the tests with new glassware before reporting the results.

Broad-spectrum antiglobulin sera that contain both anti–gamma and anti–non-gamma globulin antibodies are available commercially.

REFERENCES

1. Kochwa, S., Rosenfield, R. E., Tallal, L., and Wassermann, L. R.: J. Chem. Invest. **40**:874, 1961, and Rosenfield, R. E., cited by Freda.[2]
2. Freda, V. J.: Am. J. Obstet. Gynecol. **84**:1756, 1961.
3. Wiener, A. S., and Sonn, E. B.: J. Lab. Clin. Med. **31**:1020, 1946.
4. Issitt, P. D.: Applied blood group serology, 1970, Spectra Biologicals, Becton-Dickinson & Co.
5. Barrett, J. T.: Textbook of immunology, St. Louis, 1970, The C. V. Mosby Co.
6. Erskine, A. G.: In Frankel, S., Reitman, S., and Sonnenwirth, A. C., editors: Gradwohl's clinical laboratory methods and diagnosis, ed. 7, St. Louis, 1970, The C. V. Mosby Co.
7. Campbell, D. H., Sturgeon, P., and Vinograd, J. R.: Science **122**:1091, 1955.
8. Grubb, R., and Swahn, B.: Acta Pathol. Microbiol. Scand. **43**:305, 1958.
9. Wiener, A. S.: J. Exp. Med. **94**:213, 1951.
10. Wiener, A. S.: Ann. Allergy **10**:535, 1952.
11. Unger, L. J.: J.A.M.A. **76**:9, 1921.
12. Springer, G. F., Horton, R. S., and Forbes, M.: J. Exp. Med. **110**:221, 1959.
13. Wiener, A. S.: Proc. Soc. Exp. Biol. Med. **56**:173, 1944.
14. Race, R. R.: Nature (Lond.) **153**:771, 1944.
15. Coombs, R. R. A., Mourant, A. E., and Race, R. R.: Lancet **2**:15, 1945; **1**:264, 1946.
16. Pollack, W.: From a lecture, Nov., 1965, Kansas University School of Medicine.
17. Pollack, W., Hager, H. J., Reckel, R., Toren, D. A., and Singher, H. A.: Transfusion **5**:158, 1965.
18. Pollack, W.: Ann. N.Y. Acad. Sci. **127**:892, 1966.

RECOMMENDED READINGS

Day, E. D.: Advanced immunochemistry, Baltimore, 1972, The Williams & Wilkins Co.

Fudenberg, H. H., Pink, I. R. L., Stites, D. P., and Wong, A. C.: Basic immunogenetics, New York, 1972, Oxford University Press.

Gell, P. G. H., and Coombs, R. R. A.: Clinical aspects of immunology, ed. 2, Philadelphia, 1968, F. A. Davis Co.

Hollán, S. R., editor: Current topics in immunohematology and immunogenetics: Alexander S. Wiener Festschrift, Budapest, 1972, Akadémiai Kiadó.

Wiener, A. S.: Rh-Hh blood types, New York, 1954, Grune & Stratton, Inc.

Wiener, A. S., and Socha, W. W.: A-B-O blood groups and Lewis types, New York, 1976, Stratton Intercontinental Medical Book Corporation.

3 □ Blood group antigens and antibodies

THE NATURE OF BLOOD GROUP ANTIGENS, AGGLUTINOGENS, AND FACTORS

The term **antigen** (anti = against; -gen = a thing produced, or generated) refers to any substance that when injected into humans or animals stimulates the production of antibodies. **Antibodies** are immune bodies capable of reacting with or destroying the antigen that called them into being. Antigens are often proteins, but they may be polysaccharides, polypeptides, or polynucleotides. The antibodies are specific in nature; that is, they react with the antigen that caused their formation and, except for particular cross-reactions, do not react with other antigens. In the case of the A-B-O blood groups, the antigen is found usually on the red blood cells and is also recoverable in solution in certain body fluids and secretions of individuals known as **secretors**. Thus in secretors it is often possible to identify the particular A-B-O blood group not only by testing the red cells for antigen or the blood serum for antibody (agglutinin) but also by testing the saliva, semen, vaginal secretions, gastric contents, and other fluids for **blood group substances**.

Agglutinogens and factors (serologic specificities)

The red blood cells have agglutinogens that render them capable of being clumped, or agglutinated, by antibodies. They react because of the serologic speci-ficities (blood factors) that characterize them. The number of serologic specificities that an agglutinogen might have is theoretically unlimited. However, when the methods of testing for such factors are more or less limited, as in A-B-O tests, there may appear to be a 1:1 correspondence between agglutinogen and blood factors, although at present agglutinogen A, for example, is known to have blood factor C in addition to specificity **A,** and so on. A **blood factor** is a serologic specificity of red cell agglutinogens. Antibodies of different specificities are arbitrarily designated by symbols, using the prefix "anti-," followed by the identifying term of the blood factor. Thus there are anti-Rh_o, anti-**rh'**, anti-**hr**, etc. in which the Rh_o, **rh'**, and **hr**, respectively, represent specificities of one or various agglutinogens. When dealing with the subgroups in the A-B-O, M-N-S, Rh-Hr, and other systems, it is imperative that a differentiation be made between agglutinogens and their specificities, or blood factors; otherwise, understanding the numerous antibodies with which each agglutinogen can react would be difficult, if not impossible. It is also important, in studying the genetics of blood grouping, that blood factors and agglutinogens be clearly differentiated in one's mind for maximum comprehension. As an example of the multiplicity of specificities that characterized a single agglutinogen, agglutinogen Rh_1 has factors Rh_o, Rh^A, Rh^B, Rh^C, Rh^D, **rh'**, **hr''**, and others.

Blood group systems

Blood group antigens fall naturally into groups, or systems, depending on their relationship to each other and to the other blood groups. The blood group systems that have been identified to date are A-B-O, M-N-S, Rh-Hr, P-p, Lu, K-k, Lewis, Fy, Jk, Yt, Vel, Xg, Di, I-i, Do, and others, for example, Au, Sm, and Bu. In addition there are certain agglutinogens that are characterized either by their extremely high or low frequencies in the population. **Xg** is the only sex-linked factor known to date.

The agglutinogens in each system are hereditarily determined by **allelic genes** occurring at specific loci on the chromosomes. Each system of antigens is inherited separately from the antigens in other blood group systems (Table 3-1).

Agglutinogens and genes

When genes are situated on the same chromosome, they tend to be inherited together, depending on the distance between them, and are said to be **linked**; that is, the two genes remain on the same piece of chromosome when the chromosome material separates, unless there is **crossing over**. The concept of *complete* linkage has been invoked in an attempt to explain the tendency of blood factors of one and the same system to be inherited in sets, or blocks, as in the Fisher-Race C-D-E hypothesis. Wiener, however, has demonstrated that the various Rh-Hr agglutinogens are actually inherited by corresponding multiple allelic genes and that the blocks of so-called antigens are really sets of multiple **serologic specificities,** or blood **factors,** that is, the extrinsic attributes of unit antigens

Table 3-1. Blood group systems in man

Blood group system	Specificities identified
A-B-O	**A, A₁, B, C, H***
M-N-S	**M, N, Nᵛ, S, s, U, Hu, He, Me, Hil, Mᶜ, Mᵍ, Mᵛ, Mᴬ, M₁, M′, Miᵃ, Mtᵃ, Mur, Hut, Nyᵃ, Clᵃ, Stᵃ, Sul, Far, Vr, Riᵃ, Tm, Sj, Sᴮ, Mᵏ, Uᴮ, Mᶻ, Mᵃ, Nᵃ, Mʳ**
P	**P₁, P, Luke**
Rh-Hr	**Rh₀, rh′, rh″, hr′, hr″, hr, Rhᴬ, Rhᴮ, Rhᶜ, Rhᴰ, hrˢ, hrᵛ, hrᴴ, hrᴮ, rh₁, rh₁₁, rh, rhᵀ, Goᵃ, Rhᵂ**
Kell	**K, k, Kpᵃ, Kpᵇ, Ku, Jsᵃ, Jsᵇ, Ulᵃ, Wkᵃ, KL, K11, K12-16**
Kidd	**Jkᵃ, Jkᵇ, Jk**
I	**I, i, Iꟳ, Iᴰ, IH, IA, IB, iH, Iᵀ**
Lewis	**Leᵃ, Leᵇ, Leᶜ, Leᵈ, Leˣ, Mag., A₁Leᵇ (Siedler)**
Lutheran	**Luᵃ, Luᵇ, Lu (Lu3), Lu4-9, Lu10-17**
Duffy	**Fyᵃ, Fyᵇ, Fy (Fy3), Fy4**
Diego	**Diᵃ, Diᵇ**
Dombrock	**Doᵃ, Doᵇ**
Cartwright	**Ytᵃ, Ytᵇ**
Colton	**Coᵃ, Coᵇ, Co**
Sm-Burrell	**Sm, Buᵃ**
Sid	**Sdᵃ**
Scianna	**Sc1, Sc2**
Xg	**Xgᵃ**
High-frequency groups	**Atᵃ, Dp, Enᵃ, El, Ge, Gyᵃ, Joᵃ, Jrᵃ, Knᵃ, Hᴛ, Lan, Vel, Wrᵇ, Yk-a, Sp₁, Soᵃ,** and many other unpublished
Low-frequency groups	**Anᵃ, Beᵃ, Bi, Bpᵃ, Br, Bxᵃ, By, Chrᵃ, Cross, Donavieski, Dropik, Evans, Far, Finlay, French, Good, Gfᵃ, Gladding, Gon, Hartle, Heibel, Hey, Hov, Hollister, Htᵃ (Hunt), Jeᵃ, Jnᵃ, Job, Kamhuber, Levay, Lsᵃ, Mansfield, Marriot, Nijhuis, Noble, Peacock, Prᵃ, Wrᵃ (Ca),** and many other unpublished

*A genetically independent antigen closely associated with the A-B-O system.

(agglutinogens). Recently, C-D-E workers have modified their hypothesis and in place of sets of linked genes speak of **cistrons,** or regions containing multiple **gene subloci.** However, family studies by Wiener and others have failed to reveal any examples of crossing over among the so-called subloci so that the "cistrons" are functional genes that act as units in conformity with the Wiener theory.

Leukocyte antigens

Claims have been made that blood group antigens have been demonstrated on the leukocytes as well as on the red cells in the A-B-O, M-N-S, and P systems but not in the Rh-Hr system. Leukocytes do, as a matter of fact, have other antigens not present on the red blood cells. For homografts especially, the role of leukoagglutinins has been extensively studied. The subject of leukoagglutinins and incompatibility of platelets will not be included in this book, since this is a speciality of its own.

Antigenicity of the blood factors

Of all the blood group antigens, those in the A-B-O and Rh-Hr systems are the most antigenic and therefore the most important clinically. In the Rh-Hr system the most antigenic factor is Rh_o, found in agglutinogens and types Rh_o, Rh_1, Rh_2, and Rh_z, for which reason the Wiener nomenclature utilizes the capital "R" in writing the symbols for these types. Agglutinogens that lack Rh_o and its cognates, such as rh′, rh″, rh_y, hr′, hr″, and hr, are written with the small "r" or "h" to show their relatively lesser antigenicity.

Today more than 200 blood group factors are known to exist, determining individual serologic differences among humans. The three most important are **A, B,** and Rh_o, and these form the basis for the bulk of the clinical problems. There are many opportunities for sensitization to the other blood factors, both through transfusion and pregnancy, but sensitization is relatively uncommon. Such factors as **M, N, S, s, U, P, rh′, rh″, hr′, hr″, K, Fy, Vel, Tjᵃ, I,**

Rh^A, Rh^B, Rh^C, Rh^D, and the rest of the specificities are much less antigenic than **A, B,** or Rh_o. Some individuals such as those with disseminated lupus erythematosus have a greater propensity to form antibodies than do others, and such people may form multiple antibodies and become multiply sensitized. These people often produce **autoantibodies** as well as group-specific antibodies. Wiener and his co-workers[1] have found autoantibodies in the serum of many individuals sensitized to the less antigenic factors **hr′** and **hr″.**

In addition to group-specific antigens, there are individual antigens, that is, those that seem to occur in only a few persons and in their siblings. There are also antigens that are almost universally shared.

The agglutinogens are formed in prenatal life, as contrasted to the antibodies, which develop after birth.

Distribution of the blood groups[2]

Family studies have demonstrated that there is no linkage between any of the major blood group systems, and there is apparently no relationship to sex except for the Xg characteristic. Different racial groups seem to have different distributions of blood groups. Blood group systems that are homologous to those in humans have been found in nonhuman primates and in other animals. This is discussed in Part Two. The science of blood grouping has become a part of serology, anthropology, and genetics, as well as biochemistry.

Blood group frequencies and blood group gene frequencies must not be confused. For example, a person of blood group A might carry genes *A* and *O* so that the gene frequency would be different from the blood group frequency. Blood group O is found in about 45% of all white people in the United States (in this case the frequency of gene *O* is about 67%), but in the Indians of South and Central America the frequency of group O is almost 100% and so is the gene frequency.

In Scandinavia and the mountain chain of the Pyrenees, Alps, and Carpathians, the frequency of group A is higher than in other countries like the United States and England, where it is only 42% of the population. The highest group A frequencies occur in certain American Indian tribes in the western regions of North America, but the North American Indian tribes are in many cases composed almost entirely of group O individuals. Subgroup A_2 shows many variations, being somewhat higher in England than in the United States; it has its highest frequency in Finland. An intermediate subgroup $A_{1,2}$ is found especially in Negroids, whereas A_2 is absent among people of Mongoloid extraction.

The B antigen is almost completely absent from the American Indians and the Australian aborigines, with a maximum frequency found in central Asia and northern India. In the United States it is present in 13% of the population. In some portions of the Netherlands, France, Spain, and Portugal the B frequency is about 5%. The Basques have the lowest B gene frequency among Europeans—below 3% and down to zero in some 400 individuals tested in southern France. The A-B-O frequencies have a greater tendency to vary in some localities in small countries, compared with the frequencies of Rh and M-N.

The frequencies in the Rh-Hr blood groups have been well documented by Wiener. These are presented in Table 8-3.

The frequency of gene M is between 50% and 60% in most populations in Europe, Africa, and eastern Asia, as well as in the United States. It is higher in the east Baltic countries through European Russia and most of southern Asia and Java. American Indians and Eskimos have high M frequencies.

High N frequencies are found throughout the Pacific area, including Australia, the highest known being in New Guinea. The highest N frequencies are among the Lapps in Europe and the Berbers in North Africa.

Blood factor S is almost completely absent from Australian aborigines, but it is present in 23% of the population of New

Guinea. In Europe about half the M genes carry S and half carry s. Only one sixth of the N genes carry S and the rest s. M is more commonly found in India, and S is mainly associated with M there. S is rarer in Africa, almost equally divided between M and N.

The population statistics of the various blood group systems are included in the respective chapters on those systems and will not be repeated here.

For further information with respect to gene frequency distribution, refer to Mourant.[2]

GENERALITIES IN IDENTIFICATION OF ANTIBODIES, ANTIGENS, AND THE BLOOD GROUPS

The most frequent method of identifying antigens on the blood cells is to suspend the cells in saline, in their own plasma, or in a colloid medium and then to mix them with serum containing a specific, known antibody. If the cells then clump, or agglutinate, they have the antigen specific for the antiserum used in the test. For example, if the unknown cells react with or are clumped by serum that has anti-**B**, the cells have the **B** specificity and therefore have the B agglutinogen. If they are not clumped by serum containing anti-**A**, they do not have the **A** specificity. If both anti-**A** and anti-**B** cause the cells to clump, the cells have both **A** and **B** specificities and are therefore group AB. Similarly, if neither the anti-**A** nor anti-**B** sera cause clumping, the cells obviously have neither **A** nor **B** specificity. These reactions form the basis for the identification of the four principal A-B-O blood groups. (See Table 3-2.)

If the group A or AB red cells are further tested using an anti-A_1 reagent and they agglutinate, the A agglutinogen present is said to be A_1. If they fail to clump, the A agglutinogen is designated as A_2.

If anti-**Rh**$_o$ serum causes cells to clump, the cells have the specificity (blood factor) **Rh**$_o$. If anti-**rh'** likewise causes clumping of the cells, they also have the specificity **rh'**. If anti-**rh''** serum does not cause

Table 3-2. Identification of the four principal A-B-O blood groups

Blood group	Reactions of red cells with serum		Specificities (blood factors) detected	Agglutinogen(s) present
	Anti-A	Anti-B		
O	−	−	None	Neither A nor B
A	+	−	**A**	A
B	−	+	**B**	B
AB	+	+	**A** and **B**	A and B

+ = agglutination; − = no agglutination.

clumping of the cells, they lack specificity **rh″**. Cells having specificities **Rh₀** and **rh′** but lacking **rh″** are designated as type Rh_1. In this case an agglutinogen Rh_1 is postulated as having the two designated specificities **Rh₀** and **rh′** but not **rh″**.

If an anti-**M** serum causes clumping, the cells have specificity **M** and therefore agglutinogen M. If anti-**N** also causes these same cells to clump, they have specificity **N** in addition to **M** and are therefore type MN.

In general, if an antiserum anti-**X** is available to test cells and if the cells are induced to clump by the action of this antiserum, the red cells are said to have the corresponding specificity, or blood factor, **X**. As stated previously, antisera are designated as "anti-," followed by the symbol for the particular specificity they detect.

As previously noted in the discussion of direct and indirect antiglobulin tests, at times it is necessary to perform more than simple agglutination tests with cells suspended in saline. Sometimes it is necessary to coat the cells first with an IgG antibody and then test them by the antiglobulin method. If they form clumps after this, they were, in fact, coated, and because the identity of the antiserum used to coat the cells is known, naming the specificity on the cells is an easy matter. At times the cells are already coated with antibody in vivo. Such is the case when testing **infants' cells** or cells from **cord blood** in suspected erythroblastosis fetalis. In such cases the only procedure necessary to show the presence of an IgG, or 7S, antibody coating the red cells is to wash the cells and then mix them with antiglobulin serum. If they clump, the cells are definitely shown to be coated with antibody, but the specificity of the antibody cannot be identified in this way.

Antibodies can be identified by mixing serum containing the antibody in question with red cells of known antigen content. For example, if only red cells of group **A** are agglutinated, but those of group **B** are not, obviously that serum contains anti-**A** but not anti-**B**.

At times antisera fail to agglutinate red cells when the sera are used undiluted but give strong agglutination reactions when the sera are diluted. When such sera are titrated, a **prozone** will be seen, in that the initial dilutions give little or no reactions, and higher dilutions produce reactions that become progressively stronger, reach a maximum, and then gradually diminish. This phenomenon has often been attributed to the lack of optimal proportions between antigen and antibody, but according to Wiener,[3] it may actually occur in one or two ways. In some cases the prozone is due to the use of fresh sera containing complement, as is sometimes evident from the presence of hemolysis initially in the tubes used for the titration. This can be readily proved by inactivating the serum and retitrating, whereupon the prozone disappears. In other cases the prozone is due to the presence in the same serum of both IgG and IgM antibodies[4] (Table 3-3), and the prozone disappears if the tests are carried out in a high-viscosity medium such as human AB serum, bovine albumin, dextran, or polyvinylpyrrolidone (PVP) in place of saline.

Table 3-3. Titration of IgM (agglutinating) and IgG (blocking) antibodies*

Day of tests	Type of tests	Test cells (group O)	Dilutions of serum§								
			1:1	1:2	1:4	1:8	1:16	1:32	1:64	1:128	1:256
6 days after delivery	Direct titration†	Rh₁	−	−	tr.	+	+±	+±	tr.	−	−
		Rh₂	±	+±	++	++	++	++	++	+±	tr.
1 month after delivery	Direct titration†	Rh₁	−	−	−	tr.	+	−	−	−	−
		Rh₂	−	−	−	−	−	−	−	−	−
	Blocking‡	Rh₁	−	−	tr.	+±	++	++±	++±	++±	
		Rh₂	−	−	−	++	++±	++±	++±	++±	

*Modified from Wiener, A. S.: Rh-Hr blood types, New York, 1954, Grune & Stratton, Inc.
†Direct titrations incubated 45 minutes in a 38° C water bath.
‡Blocking tests: in tests with Rh₂ cells, the supernates were removed before adding the anti-Rh₀ serum; with Rh₁ cells, the supernates were not removed.
§The serum was that of a patient with an erythroblastotic infant. Both IgG and IgM antibodies were present.

As previously mentioned, at times the cells must be treated with certain enzymes to render them agglutinable, and in other cases the cells will not react if treated with enzymes. The enzymes employed for this purpose are papain, trypsin, ficin, and bromelin, all of which are proteolytic. These enzymes apparently act by dehydrolysing mucopeptides on the cell membrane and releasing glycopeptides into the medium; that is, they remove polar groups and thus reduce the zeta potential. This then brings about the close apposition necessary before cells will clump when the small IgG, or 7S, molecule antibodies are present.

Antibodies have been conjugated with fluorescent dyes, but these methods adapt themselves better to microbiology, parasitology, and virology than to blood grouping. The fluorescent dye antibody method is useful to demonstrate the corresponding antigens present in tissue, to detect pathogenic bacteria and identify them, and to localize viruses. At times antiglobulin serum tagged with a fluorescent dye is used, which obviates tagging each antiserum separately.

Radioactive labeling is used to measure very small amounts of antigen and antibody, but, again, such methods have mostly been employed in fields other than blood grouping.

Although the blood group antigens are usually limited to the blood cells, the blood group substance, for example, H substance, is also found in solution in individuals called **secretors** in such body fluids as saliva and nasal secretions. It is necessary in some cases to perform an inhibition (absorption) test when dealing with soluble substances, since no visible reaction occurs when secretions are mixed with antisera unless the titers of the sera are high enough that a precipitate is produced.

Agglutinin absorption

In the **agglutinin absorption** methods the unknown material is mixed with serum or lectin containing known antibodies, and the mixture is allowed to remain long enough for the antibody to be removed by absorption or neutralization. The resulting absorbed fluid is then tested to determine whether the antibody has in fact been removed; if it has, the material used to remove the antibody from the serum must have contained an antigen corresponding to the antibody in the serum. As an example, a blood stain is mixed with anti-A serum and also in a separate container with anti-B serum. Later, after centrifugation to remove any solid particles, the absorbed serum solutions are mixed with known A and known B cells, respectively. If the absorbed anti-A serum still clumps A cells, obviously it still has its anti-A agglutinin, and the blood stain did not contain A substances. If, however, it now does *not* clump A cells, the anti-**A** has been removed, and the blood stain that removed it contained the A antigen.

When antisera are artificially produced by injecting animals with cells or extracts of cells or tissue, etc., the serum from the blood of the injected animals usually contains more than one antibody. For example, in producing anti-**M** serum, group O type M cells that do not contain either A or B agglutinogen but do have M, are used to inoculate a rabbit. After a number of injections, the rabbit produces antibodies against the M agglutinogen, but the serum of the rabbit also has human species-specific agglutinins that must be removed. The rabbit's serum must therefore be absorbed with human red cells of type N to remove these species-specific antibodies, leaving the anti-**M** in the absorbed serum that can then be used for testing purposes.

Elution

When cells have adsorbed antibody— that is, when the antibody is on the surface of the cells—it is possible to remove that antibody by a process of **elution.** The eluted antibody then is specific for whatever antigen it had combined with on the cells. This method is useful at times to demonstrate and identify weak subgroups or variants within a blood group system, for example, in the A-B-O system. It is also useful in demonstrating and identifying the antibody on the red cells of infant or cord blood, as in hemolytic disease of the newborn. This **eluate** can be used for compatibility tests when the mother's serum is not available in cases of erythroblastosis fetalis. **Elution experiments** are also made to demonstrate and identify antibody on the red cells of patients with acquired hemolytic anemia or to determine coating of red cells in suspected transfusion reactions. They can be used to separate and identify antibodies in a serum containing a mixture of antibodies.

Any antibodies adsorbed onto the red cell surface not because of combination with the antigen have to be completely removed before elution experiments are made, which means that the coated cells have to be washed many times.

The eluate usually contains hemoglobin, but this is not an interfering substance. Eluates should be tested on the day they are prepared because they are unstable, although they may be stored in a deep freeze at $-20°$ C or lower.

Elution methods may involve heat, alcohol precipitation, or the use of either. For details see Part Three.

Effect of temperature

It is important in blood grouping tests that the temperature of reaction be properly maintained. Agglutination tests are adversely affected by improper temperature, as well as by improper centrifugation and improper timing. The anti-**A** and anti-**B** antibodies, for example, react best at room temperature or between $4°$ and $18°$ C and may be adversely affected by overheating. **Rh** antibodies, on the other hand, react optimally at $37°$ C. There are cold as well as warm agglutinins. Cold agglutinins react in vitro best at refrigerator temperature, and in many cases the reaction must be read before the tests warm to room temperature and cause the reaction to reverse.

Miscellaneous

As previously stated, the IgM molecule antibodies are agglutinating antibodies and will react with cells suspended in a saline medium. The IgG type antibodies usually react only in a high colloid medium.

Theoretically, antibodies could be produced against almost any antigen not possessed by an individual, but the individual would have to be susceptible to that antigen, and there would have to be sufficient antigenic stimulus to cause the subject to produce antibodies. The antibodies are usually formed within 10 to 14 days after injection of an antigen and reach a peak in titer in about 20 days or 3 weeks, after which a gradual diminution in titer occurs.

Once a person has been sensitized to an antigen, he generally remains so for life, even though the antibodies may have declined in titer to such a degree that they are no longer demonstrable in the in vitro test. When such a person is reinjected with the same antigen, the response (**secondary response**) to the injection is much more prompt so that the antibodies appear more rapidly and reach a higher titer within a shorter time. This is generally called the **anamnestic reaction.**

In the A-B-O blood group system, the only antibodies regularly found in the serum are those for which the corresponding agglutinogens are absent from the red blood cells (**Landsteiner's rule**), except during the neonatal period. For example, group A blood cells have A but not B agglutinogen, and therefore the serum has anti-**B** and not anti-**A.**

Antibody production hardly ever occurs in cases of agammaglobulinemia, and therefore the expected isoagglutinins are absent as one more manifestation of this disease, which affects all antibody production.

Isosensitization (isoimmunization)

Production of antibodies against an antigen present in the same species of animal was first induced by Ehrlich and Morgenroth in goats in 1900. This type of immunization is called **isoimmunization,** or **isosensitization,*** as contrasted to **heteroimmunization,** in which antibodies are produced by a species against an antigen from a member of a different species. Ehrlich first introduced the term "horror autotoxicus" to indicate that the organism "fears" to form antibodies harmful to its own tissues. Such antibodies, if formed, would be termed **autoimmune antibodies.** These

---

*The terms immunization and sensitization are generally used interchangeably. However, the term sensitization has a bad connotation, whereas the term immunization has a good one. Since isoantibody formation serves no physiologically useful purpose as far as is known, the term isosensitization may be more appropriate, especially in cases of maternofetal incompatibility (erythroblastosis fetalis).

have been found in some hemolytic anemias, in thyroid disorders, in systemic lupus erythematosus, in rheumatoid arthritis, perhaps in pernicious anemia, and in other autoimmune diseases.

Sensitization against the Rh antigen is one of the best examples of intraspecies antibodies. If an individual lacks the Rh factor and receives a transfusion of blood having the Rh agglutinogen that he lacks, he can form anti-Rh antibodies. These persist for years and probably for life. A second stimulus, no matter how much later in life, by the same Rh agglutinogen that sensitized the individual in the first place, will result in a sharp rise in titer against that antigen; if Rh-positive blood is then transfused, a severe hemolytic reaction will ensue.

Ehrlich and Morgenroth were the first to demonstrate isoimmunization, or **intraspecies immunization,** or isosensitization, in their experiments with goats. They injected goats, which have no natural isoantibodies, with blood cells from other goats and produced immune isoantibodies in the injected goats. The isoantibodies thus formed hemolyzed the red cells from the goats that had supplied the original inocula and also the cells of some, but not all, the other goats with which they experimented. The serum of the injected goats did not contain an autolysin; that is, it did not affect or combine with the cells of the animal in which the antibodies were formed. These experiments, conducted in 1900 to 1901, showed that a considerable number of different antigens might exist in similar cells of different individuals in a single species, as well as that an animal will not ordinarily produce antibodies against antigens present in its own blood. It is true that some animals can form antibodies against some of their own proteins or other tissue components such as the substance of the crystalline lens, casein, and an alcoholic extract of brain, but these materials are considered blood-foreign and thus satisfy one of the primary prerequisites for antigenicity. By the use of **Freund's**

adjuvant (Difco), antibodies can readily be prepared against thyroid, brain, and other tissue.

Immune isoantibodies have since been produced in many other animals besides goats.

In man, intramuscular injections of small volumes of A-B-O incompatible blood have not resulted in significant rises in antibody titer. However, after transfusions of 500 ml or more of incompatible blood, which is sufficient to produce a severe hemolytic reaction, there is first a negative phase due to in vivo absorption of isoagglutinins. This is generally followed by a marked rise in titer. There are also examples of isoimmunization of a subgroup A_2 individual by transfusions of group A_1 blood cells. Also, anti-**H** isoagglutinins have been observed in group A_1B individuals after transfusions.

To produce anti-**Rh** sera in donors, Wiener[5] found that at least two exposures to the antigen are required, with an interval of several months between them. The first injection generally produces no demonstrable antibodies but acts as a "primer," whereas the second injection 4 months later elicits the production of antibodies in almost half the donors. Continuous stimulation with huge quantities of the antigen over a short period of time is less effective in bringing about the formation of isoantibodies.

Group-specific substance[6,7]

Anti-**A** and anti-**B** titers can be increased in group O individuals by injection of group-specific substances A and B, also termed **Witebsky substances**. A-like specific substances have been isolated from group A specific carbohydrate-like compounds from horse saliva and in commercial preparations of pepsin and peptone. B-like specific substance has been obtained from the stomach juice of group B subjects. Group A–like specific substances, if added to blood serum of group B (anti-**A**), markedly inhibits agglutination of human blood cells of group A by that serum. Both A and B blood group specific substances are available commercially. A-like and B-like specific substances will reduce a high isoagglutinin titer of bivalent antibodies to low levels in group O blood, but they will have less effect on the titer of IgG (7S) anti-**A** and anti-**B**. Both substances can stimulate antibody formation in a human being even when they are in combination with the natural anti-**A** and anti-**B** agglutinins of group O people.

Both substances have been used by serum manufacturers to produce high-titered anti-**A** and anti-**B** serum, that is, commercial antisera for use by laboratories engaged in testing blood prior to transfusions.

REFERENCES

1. Wiener, A. S., Gordon, E. B., and Unger, L. J.: Bull. Jewish Hosp. 3:46, 1961.
2. Mourant, A. E., Kopeć, A. C., and Domaniewska-Sobczak, K.: The distribution of the human blood groups and other polymorphisms, ed. 2, London, 1976, Oxford University Press.
3. Wiener, A. S.: Personal communication, 1971.
4. Wiener, A. S.: Proc. Soc. Exp. Biol. Med. **56:** 173, 1944.
5. Wiener, A. S., and Sonn-Gordon, E. B.: Am. J. Clin. Pathol. **17:**67, 1947.
6. Tisdall, L. H., Garland, D. M., Szanto, P. B., Hand, A. M., and Bennett, J. C.: Am. J. Clin. Pathol. **16:**193, 1946.
7. Tisdall, L. H., Garland, D. M., and Wiener, A. S.: J. Lab. Clin. Med. **31:**437, 1946.

4 □ Genetic principles in blood grouping

Much of the progress in the field of blood grouping serology, as well as the classification of blood groups into systems, has been possible because of earlier and continuing studies into the hereditary nature of transmission. It was Epstein and Ottenberg who in 1908 first suggested that the A-B-O blood groups are hereditarily transmitted. In 1910 von Dungern and Hirszfeld postulated that the blood groups are inherited in accordance with Mendel's laws by two pairs of independent genes, *A-a* and *B-b*. In 1924 Bernstein, using methods of population genetics, demonstrated that the inheritance of the A-B-O blood groups is actually by triple allelic genes, *A*, *B*, and *O*. Wiener, in the third edition (1943) of his classic text *Blood Groups and Transfusion*, reported investigations in over 10,000 family studies of the hereditary transmission of the A-B-O blood groups. Andresen in 1947 wrote of the results of 20,000 tests he had conducted on the A-B-O blood groups of mothers and their children.

After the work of Wiener on the heredity of the Rh-Hr types, beginning in 1941, it became evident that blood groups of all systems are inherited by means of multiple allelic genes. All blood group systems so far discovered have conformed to the men-

delian laws of heredity, and only one, the Xg system, has proved to be sex-linked. During the past 53 years, despite many publications purporting to dispute the allelic gene theory of transmission of blood group characteristics, no adequate evidence has ever been found to disprove it. There are, to be sure, modifying genes that have posed problems in these studies; in addition, there are reports so marred by technical laboratory errors that their results are unreliable.

GREGOR JOHANN MENDEL
(Fig. 4-1)

Modern work in the field of genetics began with Mendel's contributions and discoveries. Johann Mendel was born in 1822 of German parents in Heinzendorf in Silesia. He entered the Augustinian Monastery at Brünn, Austria, at the age of 21 and remained there for the balance of his life. When he entered the monastery, he became Gregor and is presently known as Gregor Johann Mendel. Mendel cultivated a small strip of garden behind the monastery building to experiment on hybridization in plants and used his own rooms to hybridize mice. Along the edge of the garden he experimented with bees, and in the garden itself he crossed many kinds of plants—garden peas, columbine, snapdragons, slipperworts, pumpkins, four o'clocks, beans, etc. His work with garden peas is the most widely known.

Mendel chose peas having seven pairs of contrasting characteristics, including

---

□ For the study and understanding of the heredity of the blood groups, knowledge of the genetic code and the structure of DNA and RNA is not required. Interested readers are referred to standard texts on genetics.

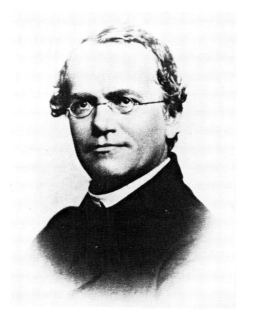

Fig. 4-1. Gregor Johann Mendel.

smooth seeds and wrinkled seeds, yellow cotyledons and green cotyledons, inflated pods and constricted pods, yellow pods when unripe and green pods when unripe, flowers in the axils of the leaves and flowers at the ends of the stems, white seed coats and brown seed coats, and tall plants and dwarf plants. So meticulous was he in his studies that he has often been called the perfect scientist. Although some knowledge has been added to the basic facts he discovered, no one has ever been able to disprove anything that he reported. He kept copious notes and made his reports only after he had satisfied himself that the conclusions he reached were correct. Although his work was performed during the nineteenth century and published in 1866, it was not until 1900 that this work was rediscovered and not until 30 years after publication that he was finally given credit for his contributions.

He crossed tall plants with dwarf plants and produced a first filial generation, called by him F_1, in which all the plants were tall. These tall plants were "selfed"; that is, they were crossed with each other, and they produced both tall and dwarf plants

—three times as many tall as dwarf plants. In the second generation, two thirds of the tall plants, when selfed, produced tall and dwarf plants in a 3:1 ratio, just like the F_1 plants. All the F_1 plants were tall, according to Mendel, because the factor that determines tallness in plants is **dominant** over the factor for dwarfness; when the two characteristics occur together, the plants develop along the tall line. When the hybrid tall plants were selfed, tallness developed in a proportion of three tall for each one dwarf plant. The factor that did not produce its effect in the presence of the contrasting factor was called by Mendel a **recessive** characteristic. Tallness, in other words, was dominant, and dwarfness was recessive. If two recessive characteristics were inherited, one from each parent, the offspring developed as a recessive. Likewise, if the offspring inherited two dominant characteristics, it developed as a dominant, and if one characteristic from one parent were dominant and the like characteristic from the second parent were recessive, the offspring also developed as a dominant but could transmit to its offspring both dominant and recessive characteristics.

The terms dominant and recessive do not imply either good or bad or strong or weak. They simply indicate which characteristic will develop when the two determinants come together in an offspring.

BASIC FACTS AND TERMINOLOGY IN HEREDITY

When cells divide, the pairs of chromosomes separate, one half going to one of the new (daughter) cells, the second half to the other. Each species of animals and plants is marked by a certain characteristic number of chromosomes. Man has 23 pairs, or 46 chromosomes altogether. These pairs have been classified and grouped according to similarity and size: chromosome pairs 1, 2, and 3 belong to group A; 4 and 5 to group B; 6 to 12 to group C; 13 to 15 to group D; 16 to 18 to group E; 19 and

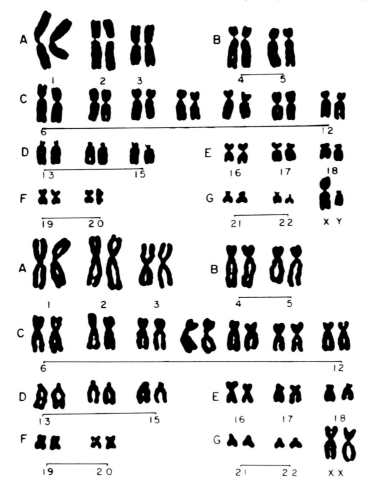

Fig. 4-2. Human chromosomes. Top: *A* to *G*, from a male; bottom, *A* to *G*, from a female. (Photograph of enlargement and classification of chromosomes courtesy Dr. John D. Bauer, DePaul Hospital Division, St. Louis, Mo.)

20 to group F; and 21, 22, and the sex pair XY to group G (Fig. 4-2).

In every living organism the **somatic cells** that comprise it produce the body tissues, and the **segregated germ cells** produce the **gametes**—the spermatozoa and ova. When the **ovum,** or female germ cell, is fertilized by the **spermatozoon,** or male germ cell, a **zygote** is formed, consisting of hereditary factors derived in equal numbers from the male and the female parent —half from each. The inherited characteristics are transmitted through the **genes,** which lie in the chromosome, each occupying a specific position, or **locus.** Each characteristic of an individual is determined by two genes, or **alleles,** located at corresponding loci on each of the paired chromosomes. The gametes, or germ cells, contain only one member of each pair of chromosomes. During fertilization of the ovum by the sperm, the two gametes combine their respective 23 single chromosomes, resulting in restoration of the 23 pairs of chromosomes for the new cell. The zygote, or fertilized cell, therefore has the full complement of 23 pairs of chromosomes, and the new individual, or **offspring,** begins with the zygote. The pair of genes together constitutes the **genotype.** Agglutinogens, like other traits, are determined by the genes.

The **observable characteristics,** or **phenotypes,** of an individual must not be confused with his genotype. This means that a group A person could have inherited one gene *A* and one gene *O* (genotype *AO*), or he may have inherited two *A* genes (genotype *AA*); in either case his blood reacts in the laboratory as group A (phenotype A). There is no laboratory test at present that will distinguish reliably between bloods from individuals of genotypes *AA* and *AO*. However, a genotype *AO* person can be recognized from the fact that he can transmit the *O* gene to his offspring and therefore can have a group O child, which a genotype *AA* person cannot.

Each parent therefore contributes half of each chromosome pair to the offspring, and every chromosome carries hundreds of genes that determine the individual characteristics. When an individual has two identical genes for a characteristic, he is said to be **homozygous** for that characteristic; if the two genes are different, then he is **heterozygous** for that characteristic.

As stated, **allelic genes,** also called **allelomorphic genes** or simply **alleles,** are situated alternately at corresponding loci in a pair of chromosomes, each gene for a certain characteristic being at its own specific locus. (The loci of some genes have been mapped.) All the alternate genes that can be located at a given locus are called alleles. The locus for the allelic genes of the A-B-O groups, for example, is on a different pair of chromosomes from that for the allelic genes of the M-N-S system, and the allelic genes of the Rh-Hr system are on still another pair of chromosomes, and so on. These three blood group systems therefore are inherited independently of one another.

Since the genes that determine each of the different blood group systems are located on different pairs of chromosomes, in the **independent assortment** that takes place, the combinations of the several genes that make up the blood group systems are **random** in each individual. For example, the same parents can have children with several different combinations of agglutinogens but only those agglutinogens determined by genes present in the parents.

The **law of independent assortment** does not apply to the genes that are located on the same chromosome, since each chromosome tends to be inherited as a whole. An exception is the occurrence of **crossing over,** which has never been observed for the genes that determine blood groups of the same system. When nonallelic genes for two distinctly different characteristics are located on the same pair of chromosomes and are so close that they almost always pass from parent to child together, although determining different characteristics that are inherited together, it is called complete or close **linkage.** Evidence has been offered that the A-B-O secretor genes are linked to the Lutheran blood group gene. Agglutinogens of the different blood group systems are inherited independently of one another by multiple alleles, each set at its specific blood group locus in its own pair of chromosomes. Separation, or cross-over, among serologic specificities of a single agglutinogen does not occur.

Some genes can be detected only by their effect on the expression of other genes. These are called **modifying genes,** or **suppressor genes.** For example, there is a rare gene *x*, which, if present in **double dose,** or homozygous form *xx*, will prevent the expression of the A-B-O blood group antigens both in the saliva and on the red cells. This is what takes place with the so-called Bombay blood type, which is described later. Bombay-type persons have their inherited A-B-O genes, but they are also homozygous for the inhibitor gene *x*, genotype *xx*. This prevents the A-B-O genes from placing their respective antigens onto the red cells and into the saliva.

Except for factor **Xg,** which is the subject of discussion later in the book, blood group genes are not sex-linked.

So-called **chimeras** have been observed by Owen[1] in bovine nonidentical twin embryos due to vascular anastomoses in utero, in which the primordial blood cells of each twin become implanted in the bone marrow of the other, where they survive, multiply, and develop. This occurrence has also been observed in humans, although much more rarely. These individuals then have a mixture of cells of two sets of blood groups. For more detailed information, see Dunsford et al.[2] See also mixed agglutination, p. 229ff.

Gene frequency refers to the number of times a gene occurs in the population as a whole or in any given population group. This is discussed in Chapter 23.

The genes reside in the chromosome as previously stated, and in the case of the blood groups they are **allelic;** that is, the two genes that determine any given blood group or type occupy the corresponding **locus,** or place, in a pair of chromosomes. **Alleles** are genes that are members of such a corresponding gene pair, each kind of allele affecting the particular character somewhat differently from the other. All the different possible alleles that can be present in a gene pair, or genotype, make up a series of **multiple alleles.**

Since genes O, A, and B are alleles and therefore have the same locus on a chromosome, if an individual has two B genes (genotype BB), for example, he cannot have an O or an A gene because the locus for either of these is already occupied by a B gene. A group B person can also have in addition to the one B gene a second gene O (genotype BO), since the O is not expressed in laboratory tests and is considered an **amorph.** Similarly, the genes for the various Rh-Hr, M-N-S, P-p, K-k, etc. agglutinogens have their own specific locus on their chromosome and are not in close proximity to the genes for the other types.

It has generally been the custom for geneticists to use a single base letter for a series of allelic genes, for example, the A-B-O blood group genes have been designated as I^A, I^B, and I^O, respectively, the letter I being derived from "isoagglutinogen." Since the gene O is an amorph, the alternative suggestion has been made to designate the genes as I^A, I^B, and i, respectively.

However, for the sake of simplicity, the I is generally omitted, although some purists continue to use it.

HEREDITARY TRANSMISSION OF THE A-B-O GROUPS

If the genotypes of the parents are known, the genotypes and also phenotypes of their possible offspring can be forecast. At present no tests but extensive family studies will identify genotypes, except for blood groups such as O, AB, M, N, MN, rh, and rh'rh, each of which has only a single corresponding genotype.

The following diagram is an example of the transmission of the genes from parents to offspring if both parents are group O. In this case the genotype of each parent will necessarily be OO.

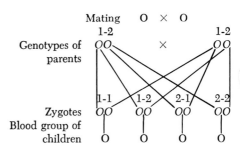

The numbers 1 and 2 represent the two genes of each parent, gene 1 of the first parent combining with gene 1 of the second; gene 1 of the first parent with gene 2 of the second; gene 2 of the first parent with gene 1 of the second; and gene 2 of the first parent with gene 2 of the second.

Children not possible to this mating are A, B, and AB. Obviously, in any single family no more than four different genotypes are possible among the children for any blood group system. When one of the parents is homozygous, only two genotypes can occur in the children; when both are homozygous, only one genotype can occur.

The genotypes in the various blood group systems are now fairly well known. For example, group A_1 can be of genotype A^1A^1, A^1A^2, or A^1O (Table 4-2), but in any single individual only one of these genotypes is possible. However, in determining the possibilities of the blood groups of the offspring, since the exact genotype of the parent cannot be identified by laboratory testing available to date, the serologist must allow for all possibilities. Thus in a mating between a group A_1 and a group O individual, there will necessarily be three diagrams. Possible combinations of genotypes of parents A_1 and O are (1) $A^1A^1 \times OO$, (2) $A^1A^2 \times OO$, and (3) $A^1O \times OO$.

Three diagrams are needed to illustrate these combinations:

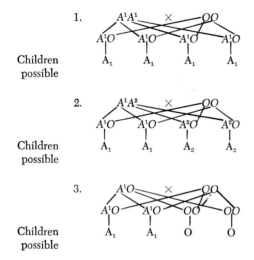

In the mating of parents $A_1 \times O$, if all three possibilities are combined, the children possible to this mating are A_1, A_2, and O but not B, A_1B, or A_2B. It must be noted, however, that both groups A_2 and O cannot occur in this case in one and the same family.

The genotypes in the A-B-O system have been determined as in Tables 4-1 and 4-2. For an exception, see blood group "cis AB," p. 76.

Some authors refer to the gene for O as an **amorph,** stating that it does not exert or produce any recognizable effect. In support of this idea, group A_2 blood from genotype A^2O individuals reacts much more strongly with anti-A sera than does group A_2B blood, genotype A^2B, even though in both cases the individual has only a single dose of gene A^2. In the A_2B individual the genes

Table 4-1. Genes in the four A-B-O blood groups

Blood group	Possible genotypes
O	*OO*
A	*AA* or *AO*
B	*BB* or *BO*
AB	*AB*

Table 4-2. Genes in the A-B-O system, including subgroups[*]

Blood group	Possible genotypes
O	*OO*
A_1	A^1A^1 or A^1A^2 or A^1O
A_2	A^2A^2 or A^2O
B	*BB* or *BO*
A_1B	A^1B
A_2B	A^2B

[*]The subgroup symbols for the phenotypes and agglutinogens use subscripts, and the gene symbols use only superscripts in conformity with the practice of geneticists.

A^2 and B apparently compete with one another for the common precursor substance to produce their respective gene products, whereas in the case of genotype A^2O, since gene O is an amorph, the A^2 gene can achieve its fullest expression. A practical consequence of this is the frequent misgrouping of group A_2B blood as group B.[3]

The genotypes in each system are presented in the various chapters in which each blood group system is discussed and will not be repeated here.

BASIC LAWS OF HEREDITY OF THE BLOOD GROUPS

The inheritance of the blood groups is subject to certain laws; the following is a brief outline:

1. No child can have a gene absent from both parents. For example, a child with both parents of group O cannot belong to group A, since a group A child would necessarily have gene A, which is lacking in both parents.

2. An individual belonging to blood group AB cannot be the parent of a group O child* because such a parent will transmit either *A* or *B*, neither of which is present in the genotype of group O. In general, every individual must transmit to every child one of the two genes that make up his genotype.

3. An individual of group O cannot be the parent of a group AB child, since such a child must have inherited one *A* gene from one parent and one *B* gene from the other.*

4. If a child is type M, the M characteristic must have been present in both parents, since a type M person is genotype *MM*, one *M* gene being derived from each parent. The parents could be type M or MN.

5. A type MN person must have received the *M* gene from one parent (type M or MN), and the *N* gene from the other (type N or MN).

6. The **M** specificity cannot appear in a child unless it is present in at least one parent, and likewise the **N** specificity cannot appear in a child unless present in at least one parent.

7. If either or both parents are type M, there can be no type N child; if either or both parents are type N, there can be no type M child.

8. Oversimplifying the Rh-Hr system by regarding individuals as either Rh positive or Rh negative, if both parents are Rh negative, all the children will be Rh negative. There can be an Rh-negative child in a union between two Rh-positive persons, provided that both parents are heterozygous for the Rh factor *(Rhrh)*.

9. None of the Rh factors can appear in a child unless present in the blood of at least one parent. Each Rh agglutinogen has many serologic specificities (blood factors) inherited as a set, or block, so that if the Rh-Hr type is to be determined, the genotype possibilities in any given case

should be known. For details of this complex system see Chapter 8.

In the Rh-Hr system at least ten distinct varieties of genes have been completely identified, and each determines a corresponding agglutinogen. Thus gene *r* determines rh; R^1 determines agglutinogen Rh_1, which has a number of different blood group factors or serologic specificities such as Rh_o, Rh^A, Rh^B, Rh^C, Rh^D, **rh′**, and **hr″**. It is essential to learn the difference between serologic specificities (blood factors) and agglutinogens. Theoretically a single agglutinogen can have innumerable serologic specificities (Wiener). In naming the genes in the Rh-Hr system, the "h" has been dropped from Rh and the genes designated by the use of *italics;* the symbols make use of superscripts. Symbols for agglutinogens and blood groups are printed in regular type, using subscripts. Symbols for red cell specificities, or factors, and for antibodies are expressed in **black** or **boldface type**, and these also use subscripts.

Interest in the heredity of blood groups has led investigators into a number of different methods of discovery such as injecting animals with human erythrocytes, absorbing out certain of the antibodies that are formed, and studying those remaining in the serum after absorption. New blood group factors and systems have thus been found, first the M-N types of Landsteiner and Levine, then the P-p system, also of Landsteiner and Levine (1927). From a clinical standpoint, the most important of all investigations since Landsteiner's discovery in 1901 of the A-B-O blood groups was the discovery of the Rh factor in humans by Landsteiner and Wiener in 1937, with publication of the results in 1940.

This discovery was followed in rapid succession by the work of Levine, Katzin, Vogel, and Burnham on the relationship between sensitization of the mother to a blood group factor inherited by her fetus and the resulting erythroblastosis fetalis; rapidly thereafter the K-k (Kell-Cellano), Lewis, Lutheran, Duffy, Kidd, Diego, Vel, and other systems, were found and identi-

---

*For a rare exception see blood group "cis AB," p. 76.

fied. All these blood groups systems demonstrated beyond any doubt that the inheritance of the various blood groups is through allelic genes and follows the mendelian laws of heredity.

The discoveries of the various blood group systems and the conclusions drawn from the research into families have led to laboratory tests in cases of disputed paternity and maternity, cases of supposedly mixed babies in hospitals and nurseries, kidnapping cases, and suits of kinship in immigration and citizenship claims, as well as an opening of new fields in anthropology and personal identification. Criminology has benefited from these studies, especially as new technics and methods had to be devised for identification of the various blood group factors and attributes, which aided in the investigation of crimes, particularly in the identification of blood groups of stains, saliva, semen, sweat, nasal secretions, and even urine.

None of this progress would have been possible had not the original workers in this field been so meticulously dedicated to the scientific aspects of their investigations and had they not been willing to study thousands of families before drawing any conclusions about their findings or publishing their surmises. Thus blood grouping, with all its various facets, remains a bulwark of scientific investigation even today, and most workers in this field are imbued with the knowledge that strict adherence to technic and to details are mandatory if the results of their tests are to be of any value.

Blood group antibodies in the A-B-O system are developed by the age of 6 months. In 1928 Furuhata[4] proposed his theory that the antibodies, like the agglutinogens, are inherited. He modified Bernstein's theory of triple alleles *A*, *B*, and *O*

and postulated instead three pairs of completely linked genes *(Ab)*, *(aB)*, and *(ab)*, respectively, in which the dominant genes *A* and *B* determine agglutinogens A and B, respectively, and the alternate genes *a* and *b* the corresponding isoagglutinins. Furuhata's theory has the same practical consequences as Bernstein's theory and at the same time could accout for reciprocal relationship between agglutinogens and isoagglutinins (**Landsteiner's law**). However, antibodies are serum globulins formed or modified in response to an antigenic stimulus so that the theory of control by genes in antibody formation appears to be incorrect. The isoagglutinins are probably the result of exogenous stimuli and represent cross-reacting antibodies. This view has now been accepted. Wiener[5] has called attention to the heterogenetic origin of anti-**A** and anti-**B** isoagglutinins. See Chapter 13 for a discussion of heredity of the various blood group systems.

REFERENCES

1. Owen, R. D.: Science **102**:140, 1945.
2. Dunsford, I., Bowley, C. C., Hutchinson, A. M., Thompson, J. S., Sanger, R., and Race, R. R.: Br. Med. J. **2**:81, 1953.
3. Wiener, A. S.: Advances in blood grouping, vol. 3, New York, 1970, Grune & Stratton, Inc.
4. Furuhata, T.: Jpn. Med. World **7**:197, 1927.
5. Wiener, A. S.: J. Immunol. **66**:679, 1951.

RECOMMENDED READINGS

Colin, E. L.: Elements of genetics, New York, 1956, McGraw-Hill Book Co.
Levine, L.: Biology of the gene, ed. 3, St. Louis, 1977, The C. V. Mosby Co.
Levitan, M., and Montagu, A.: Textbook of human genetics, New York, ed. 2, 1977, Oxford University Press.
Moody, P.: Genetics of man, New York, 1967, W. W. Norton Co.
Stern, C.: Principles of human genetics, ed. 2, San Francisco, 1960, W. H. Freeman & Co.
Strickberger, M. W.: Genetics, New York, 1968, The Macmillan Co.

5 □ The A-B-O blood group system

HISTORY

Until 1900 the existence of blood groups was neither established nor suspected. In that year, Karl Landsteiner observed that there were differences among the bloods of humans and through his research not only identified the A-B-O blood groups but also initiated methods of examination that are still in use. Three of the four blood groups were discovered by Landsteiner—group zero (later called O), group A, and group B. The rarest group, AB, was discovered by von Decastello working with Sturli, who was a pupil of Landsteiner. Landsteiner's method of investigation was to mix the serum of one normal individual with the red blood cells of other normal individuals. Certain bloods mixed without any visible effect, but in other cases the cells were strongly agglutinated. The blood group that he termed zero was so named because the cells were not agglutinable by any of the other blood sera and therefore did not have any agglutinable substance. The serum of this blood, however, could clump the cells of all other blood groups except those bloods belonging to that same group.

The blood that he designated A had cells that were clumped by sera of groups O and B, and its serum caused agglutination of cells of groups B and AB. Likewise the cells of group B were agglutinated by the sera of groups O and A, and the serum caused clumping of the cells of groups A and AB. Group AB cells were agglutinated by the sera of the other three groups, but its serum did not cause agglutination of any cells. Table 5-1 gives this in a simple form.

Jansky in 1907 and Moss in 1910 designated the four groups by the Roman numerals I, II, III, and IV and IV, II, III, and I, respectively, but this numbering of the groups gave no clue to their composition and only added confusion to the subject. The numbers were eventually dropped from the literature.

GENERAL CHARACTERISTICS

Each member of a blood group system has some characteristics in common with the other members of that system, although the members differ from one another. When a gene is present for a given agglutinogen, there cannot be a gene for any other agglutinogen of the same system at that locus on that chromosome. For example, if gene B is present, no gene A could occupy that locus on the same chromosome, or if gene A is present, there could be no gene B at that locus on that chromosome. However, the allelic gene for either of the two given here as an example could be present at the corresponding locus

Table 5-1. Nature of the four A-B-O blood groups

Blood group	Cells agglutinated by serum of groups	Serum causes agglutination of cells of groups
O	None	A, B, and AB
A	O and B	B and AB
B	O and A	A and AB
AB	O, A, and B	None

for that allelic gene on the other chromosome of the pair. The genotypes corresponding to the four principal blood groups (phenotypes) of the A-B-O system are presented in Table 4-1.

This same principle holds true in the other blood group systems, which enables investigators to postulate the allelic genes and to determine the genotypes corresponding to the observed phenotypes. Tabulation of genotypes and phenotypes, as in Table 4-1, helps investigators to understand the genetics of the blood group systems.

The terms **blood groups** and **blood types** are used interchangeably by many authors, although some make the distinction of referring to the A-B-O phenotypes as the blood groups and to the phenotypes in other blood group systems as the blood types. An example would be group AB, type MN, type Rh₁rh.

As explained, the blood groups are all identified by means of **antigen-antibody reactions,** usually agglutination reactions, that is, the clumping of the red cells as a result of the action of serum agglutinins on red cell agglutinogens. When the antibodies in the serum are known to be anti-**A,** the cells have the specificity **A** if they agglutinate in this serum, and the agglutinogen is thus identified as A. On the other hand, if a serum agglutinates group A but not group B cells, the specificity of the antibody in the serum is anti-**A** and so on for the other antigens and antibodies.

Identification of the groups

In determining the A-B-O blood groups, only two antisera are needed—anti-**A,** which detects specificity **A** and agglutinogen A, and anti-**B,** which identifies specificity **B** and agglutinogen B. Other antisera are used as a check over the laboratory reactions, notably group O serum, as detailed in the section on methods; still other antisera are used to determine the subgroups of A and AB in this system. (Subgroups are described later in this chapter.) Table 5-2 shows how the identity of the four blood groups is established when the cells are tested with anti-**A** and anti-**B** sera; it also shows their distribution in the United States and the binary code symbols.* It is understood and accepted that each antiserum reacts only with the antigen for which it is named; anti-**A** reacts only with A but not with B, and anti-**B** reacts with B only and not with A.

In addition to determining the agglutinogens of the cells to identify the blood groups, it is also possible to identify the groups by determining what antibodies or

---

*These binary symbols are to code the reactions and blood groups for computer use, in which 1 represents a positive reaction and 0 a negative reaction.

Table 5-2. Identifying the A-B-O blood groups by testing the cells

Known anti-A serum + unknown cells	Known anti-B serum + unknown cells	Blood group	Population in United States (%)	Binary code symbols
−	−	O	45	00
+	−	A	42	10
−	+	B	10	01
+	+	AB	3	11

+ = agglutination; − = absence of agglutination.

Explanation: Anti-**A** detects agglutinogen A, found on the cells of groups A and AB. Anti-**B** detects agglutinogen B, found on the cells of groups B and AB. Note that group O cells, which have neither A nor B agglutinogen, do not react with either anti-A or anti-B serum. Group A cells, which have A but not B agglutinogen, react only with anti-**A.** Group B cells, which have B but not A agglutinogen, react only with anti-**B.** Group AB cells, which have both A and B agglutinogens, react with both anti-**A** and anti-**B.**

agglutinins are present in the serum. To do this, the sera are tested with cells having the specific antigens; in the A-B-O system these are cells of groups A and B. All four A-B-O blood groups can be identified by testing the unknown serum with known A and B cells, respectively, as shown in Table 5-3.

In practice, direct grouping of red cells and reverse grouping of serum are both done routinely to ensure accuracy of the results. Table 5-4 summarizes the complete results of such tests.

Anti-C and specificity C

In addition to the agglutinins anti-**A** and anti-**B**, other natural agglutinins occur in the serum of group O, notably anti-**C**, often called the **cross-reacting antibody.** In the usual description of group O serum, the isoagglutinins are designated as anti-**A** and anti-**B**, implying that group O serum is comparable to a simple mixture of anti-**A** and anti-**B** sera, but this is not correct. Absorption experiments have proved that in group O serum there is a third antibody that **cross reacts** with both group A and

group B cells; for example, absorption of group O serum with group A cells removes the reactivity for A and also usually reduces the titer for group B cells. Some workers have assumed that this is due to fusion of anti-**A** and anti-**B** molecules or that there are antibody molecules which have two different combining sites—one for A and the other for B. This does not explain, however, why injection of group A blood or blood group substance A into group O individuals causes not only the anti-**A** but also the anti-**B** titer to rise. Wiener demonstrated the nonexistence of **heteroligating antibodies,** that is, antibodies with two different combining groups, but believed instead that group O serum has also a third isoantibody which he termed anti-**C**. This anti-**C** determines a serologic specificity C, shared by red blood cells of groups A, B, and AB but absent from the cells of group O. This does not mean that group A has two agglutinogens, A and C, or that group B has two agglutinogens, B and C. It means simply that agglutinogens A and B share a serologic specificity, or blood factor (extrinsic attribute) C, that is

Table 5-3. Identification of the A-B-O blood groups by testing the serum

Known group A cells + unknown serum	Known group B cells + unknown serum	Agglutinins identified in unknown serum	Blood group
−	−	Neither anti-**A** nor anti-**B**	AB
+	−	Anti-**A**	B
−	+	Anti-**B**	A
+	+	Both anti-**A** and anti-**B**	O

+ = agglutination; − = absence of agglutination.

Table 5-4. Agglutinogen and agglutinin content of the A-B-O blood groups

Blood group	Agglutinogens of cells	Agglutinins in serum
O	Neither A nor B	Both anti-**A** and anti-**B**
A	A	Anti-**B**
B	B	Anti-**A**
AB	Both A and B	Neither anti-**A** nor anti-**B**

responsible for their reactions with anti-C of blood group O serum. Anti-C combines with both agglutinogens A and B because of this factor. Wiener's explanation should not be confused with Moss' two early hypotheses postulating three agglutinogens and three corresponding antibodies, both of which have been proved to be incorrect. Wiener, like Landsteiner, later postulated only two agglutinogens, but he also postulated three corresponding antibodies and specificities.[1]

To understand specificity **C**, as well as the antiserum that detects it, the **difference between an agglutinogen and a specificity, or blood factor,** must be appreciated. An **agglutinogen** is the reacting substance (**intrinsic attribute**) on a red blood cell, which is determined by a corresponding allelic gene. Each agglutinogen, however, may have a multiplicity of different **serologic specificities** (**extrinsic attributes**) that make the cells agglutinable by more than one kind of antibody. Thus agglutinogen A has two principal specificities, **A** and **C**, with the **C** specificity also being shared by agglutiogen B. Groups A, B, and AB have either A or B agglutinogen or both. Since factor **C** is a serologic specificity of both A and B agglutinogens, groups A, B, and AB cannot have anti-C in their sera. However, group O, which lacks A and B agglutinogens and therefore has no **C** specificity, can and usually does have agglutinin anti-**C** (in addition to anti-**A** and anti-**B**); the anti-C can detect the **C** factor of groups A, B, and AB. Table 5-5 shows the composition of the A-B-O groups.

If blood group O serum is titrated for its anti-A and anti-B content and is then absorbed with group A cells, the anti-A titer is lowered or eliminated as expected but often so is the titer for group B cells. Similarly, if group O serum is titrated and then absorbed with group B cells, the titer is lowered not only for group B but also for group A cells. Group A cells must therefore remove some antibody for a factor found also in group B cells, and group B cells must remove some antibody for a factor found also in group A cells. Since A and B cells share the factor **C**, it can be assumed that they both remove anti-C from group O serum, which would lower the titer against both A and B cells.[2]

Further evidence of the specific antibody anti-C peculiar to group O serum is provided by the existence of certain rare bloods variously designated as A_x, A_4, A_o, C_A,[3] etc. but preferably as group C, which are not agglutinated by anti-**A** or anti-**B** sera but are agglutinated by group O serum.

Variant group C, also called A_o or A_x

Group C, also designated A_x, A_4, or A_o, as well as A_z and A_5, was first clearly described by Dunsford and Aspinal[4] in 1952. The cells fail to clump when mixed with ordinary anti-**A** or anti-**B** sera, but they are agglutinated by blood group O serum, showing that such serum must contain a third antibody (agglutinin) specific for these red cells. The antibody in question is obviously anti-**C**.

Table 5-5. Composition of the four A-B-O blood groups*

Blood group	Agglutinogens on cells	Specificities, or blood factors	Agglutinins in serum
O	Neither A nor B	None	Anti-**A**, Anti-**B**, and Anti-**C**
A	A	**A** and **C**	Anti-**B**
B	B	**B** and **C**	Anti-**A**
AB	A and B	**A**, **B**, and **C**	None

*Modified from Wiener, A. S., and Ward, F. A.: Am. J. Clin. Pathol. **46:**27, 1966.

When blood cells are not agglutinated by anti-**A** and anti-**B** sera, they are routinely identified as blood group O. Many laboratories test all bloods not only by mixing the cells with known anti-**A** and anti-**B** sera but also with group O serum that contains, in addition to anti-**A** and anti-**B**, a third antibody, anti-**C**. (Some authors erroneously refer to group O serum as "anti-**A,B**.") Cells of the variant group C, unlike group O cells, will clump in group O serum but not in anti-**A** or anti-**B**, showing that they are not group O. The cells are not agglutinated by anti-**A** or anti-**B** sera because these antisera lack anti-**C**. If group O serum is not used in testing, variant group C blood is erroneously typed as group O.

The serum of group C agglutinates cells of groups A_1, A_2, B, and AB but not O.

The **incidence** of C is only one in 60,000 Caucasoids, but it is not uncommon among the Bantu. **Secretors** of C have H but no A substance in their saliva. The **inheritance** of the blood group C is by an allele in some families or by a modifying gene in other families. The peculiar properties of group C seem to be due to a predominance of the specificity **C** on the red blood cells.

IMPORTANCE OF THE A-B-O GROUPS IN TRANSFUSION

Of all the blood group systems, the A-B-O is the most important in transfusions because the isoantibodies exist preformed, and strong reactions take place when incompatible bloods are mixed with each other not only in vitro but especially in vivo. Even an initial transfusion of group A blood into a group B subject would be disastrous because the natural anti-**A** in the blood of the group B patient reacts promptly with the incoming group A cells, causing agglutination or hemolysis of the cells, or both; this results in a so-called **hemolytic transfusion reaction**. In addition, the incoming anti-**B** of the plasma of the group A donor, if present in high titer, could react with the recipient's own group B cells and cause them to hemolyze.

In **hemolytic reactions,** red cells are destroyed with release of free hemoglobin. The plasma or serum becomes colored, and a color change may be observed in the urine. Since the reaction of the urine is ordinarily acid, the red of the hemoglobin changes to dark brown or even black in a severe hemolytic crisis. The free hemoglobin in the blood plasma is converted to bilirubin, increasing the bilirubin levels of the serum, and jaundice may be evident. There may also be lower nephron nephrosis, characterized by oliguria, hematuria, anuria, and increase in blood urea. In extreme cases death ensues.

Noticeable reactions occur at times even when a small amount of **incompatible blood** has been administered but usually only after introduction of 50 ml or more of the blood. The **symptoms** are a tingling sensation, a feeling of great discomfort and anxiety, fullness in the head, precordial oppression, a constricting feeling in the chest, and difficulty in breathing, along with severe pain in the back of the neck, chest, and especially in the lumbar region. Signs of collapse follow, with rapid feeble pulse, cold clammy skin, marked flushing of the face, dyspnea, cyanosis, drop in blood pressure, dilatation of the pupils, and nausea and vomiting. There may also be less severe cases with little complaint from the patient.

When a hemolytic reaction is suspected, red counts or hematocrit tests should be made, as well as tests for free hemoglobin in the blood serum or plasma, for serum bilirubin, and for urine volume. Bilirubin values rise during the first 24 hours after transfusion if there has been a hemolytic reaction.

When a transfusion reaction due to incompatibility is suspected, the cause should be investigated. The pretransfusion specimens of both the patient and all the donors must be tested (assuming that all laboratories save the specimens until at least after the patient has shown no signs of reaction), and the tests must always include retyping of the blood. Cross-matching tests must also be repeated. (See Part three.)

The reaction of anti-**A** against cells with agglutinogen A and anti-**B** against cells with agglutinogen B is rapid and strong. In incompatible transfusions, this reaction occurs within the blood vessels, destroying the cells and eventually blocking the renal tubules. Prevention of such a reaction is the reason for making so many tests on the blood of the donors and of the recipient before a transfusion.

Unlike other blood group systems, when an individual lacks one or more of the A-B-O agglutinogens, he almost invariably has antibodies against the agglutinogen(s) that is lacking. In the other blood group systems, agglutinins against an agglutinogen lacking in an individual develop in an artificial manner, that is, by transfusions of incorrect blood or by pregnancy with a fetus of an incompatible blood type. For example, in transfusion of an Rh-negative person with Rh-positive blood, the recipient develops anti-Rh agglutinins. Unlike the A-B-O system, there are no naturally occurring antibodies for the Rh-Hr agglutinogens. This is true also of the other blood group systems such as Fy, K-k, and Lu. Only in the A-B-O system are there regularly occurring natural isoagglutinins in the absence of immunization by transfusion or pregnancy. Irregularly occurring natural isoagglutinins of specificities anti-**P**, anti-**Le**, and, rarely, anti-**M** and anti-**N** may also be encountered, however.

The importance of the **A-B-O groups in erythroblastosis fetalis** is discussed in detail in Chapter 9 and will not be repeated here.

Universal donors and recipients

The subject of donors and recipients is discussed in detail in Chapter 21 and will not be repeated here, except to state that group O was formerly designated universal donor and group AB universal recipient. This idea is not in use generally at present, especially since untoward reactions have been reported after transfusions of group O blood given to patients of differ-

ent blood groups from the donors. A fatal hemolytic reaction due to the use of group O donor blood with high-titer anti-**A** and anti-**B** for a group A recipient was reported by Wiener and Moloney.[5]

It is best, when selecting a donor for transfusion, to give blood of the same A-B-O blood group as that of the recipient.

SUBGROUPS OF A AND AB

In 1911 von Dungern and Hirszfeld[6] called attention to the fact that when group B serum, which has anti-**A** agglutinin, is treated with certain group A blood cells until it loses its power to clump the absorbing cells, the absorbed serum will still cause agglutination of most other group A and AB bloods. These experiments suggested subdivision of the A and AB groups. This was confirmed in 1923 by Coca and Klein,[7] and at present these subgroups are known as A_1, A_2, A_1B, and A_2B. Other subgroups and variants of the A agglutinogen have also been found.

In the sera of blood groups B and O there are agglutinins that react against agglutinogen A, present on the cells of blood groups A and AB. These agglutinins are not the single entity anti-A but are composed of many qualitatively different fractions. The two **principal varieties of anti-A** are (1) anti-A proper, which reacts with both agglutinogens A_1 and A_2 with about equal intensity, and (2) agglutinin anti-A_1, which reacts preferentially with agglutinogen A_1 but hardly at all with agglutinogen A_2. These two fractions occur in different proportions in groups B and O sera, so that two anti-A (group B) sera that react at the same titer against A_1 cells may have quite different titers for A_2 cells and especially A_2B cells. Some rare group B sera (anti-A) have been reported that react strongly against A_1 cells but hardly at all against A_2. It would be quite dangerous to use such antisera for testing purposes to identify the blood groups, since if a person is subgroup A_2 or especially A_2B, his blood would be only weakly agglutinated by such an anti-A serum. Any anti-A serum used for testing purposes must therefore be

Table 5-6. Distribution (%) of the A-B-O groups and subgroups*

Groups	O	A₁	A₁,₂	A₂	A₃, A₄, etc.	B	A₁B	A₁,₂B	A₂B
Caucasoid	41.7 to 45.8	26.8 to 29.0	0 to 0.4	7.4 to 8.9	0 to 0.03	12.4 to 13.0	4.0 to 5.8	0 to 0.4	1.0 to 1.4
Negroid	45.2 to 48.4	15.2 to 20.0	0.8 to 5.8	4.3 to 7.2	0 to 0.2	21.5 to 22.8	1.6 to 3.2	0 to 0.4	1.1 to 3.2
Chinese	31.2 to 43.0	27.0 to 32.6	0	0	0	25.2 to 27.5	4.75 to 8.7	0	0

*Modified from Wiener, A. S.: Am. J. Clin. Pathol. **51**:9, 1969.

Table 5-7. Theory of multiple alleles for subgroups of A

Genes	Corresponding agglutinogens	Specificities
O	None	None
A¹	A₁	**A₁** and **A**
A²	A₂	**A**
B	B	**B**

titrated and tested not only against A₁ but also against A₂ and especially A₂B cells.

Distribution of the subgroups

Subgroup A₂ comprises approximately one fifth to one fourth of all group A individuals among Caucasoids. This subgroup is also common in Negroids, but all group A and group AB blood from Mongoloids tested are subgroup A₁. The distributions of A-B-O groups and subgroups in representative populations are shown in Table 5-6.

Heredity of the A-B-O subgroups

As with the four principal A-B-O groups, the subgroups A₁ and A₂ are determined by hereditary factors. The phenotypes and genotypes in the A-B-O blood groups system are presented in Table 4-2.

Importance of the subgroups of A and AB

Although there are records of some group A₂ individuals becoming sensitized to the A₁ agglutinogen and forming anti-A₁ agglutinins, these are extremely rare, and the subgroups of A are ordinarily disregarded when selecting donors for blood transfusions. The subgroups are important, however, in cases of disputed parentage.

Identification of the subgroups

The subgroups of A and AB are identified by mixing the cells with an anti-A₁ serum (absorbed B) or anti-A₁ lectin obtained from the seeds of *Dolichos biflorus* (Chapter 18) and observing the results. The A₁ and A₁B cells react with these reagents and clump, but A₂ and A₂B cells do not. (See lectins in Chapter 17.)

Agglutinogen A₁ has at least two specificities, **A₁** and **A**, whereas agglutinogen A₂ has only the specificity **A**. This has often been misinterpreted when, for example, subgroup A₁ cells are said to have the two antigens or two agglutinogens A and A₁, which is not true. That A₁ and A do not represent separate agglutinogens in subgroup A₁ blood has been proved by genetic studies. For example, in the mating AB × O, each child inherits either **A** or **B** but not both; on the other hand, in the mating A₁ × O, each child either inherits *both* **A₁** and **A** from the A₁ parent or he inherits *neither;* the two specificities *do not separate* but are inherited *as a set.* (See Table 5-7.)

Subgroup A₁,₂ (A₍ᵢₙₜ₎)

Subgroup A₁,₂ gives reactions of intermediate intensity. Anti-A serum derived from group B human subjects causes strong clumping of cells having A_1 as well as A_2 agglutinogens. This characteristic is present in all commercial anti-**A** sera certified by the National Institutes of Health (NIH). In subgroup $A_{1,2}$ the cells react strongly with anti-**A** serum, only weakly with anti-A_1, and strongly with anti-**H** lectin (although there are exceptions). Anti-**H** lectin often causes no reaction or only weak agglutination of A_1 cells but regularly produces strong agglutination of cells of groups O and A_2.

Because the reactions in this subgroup are **intermediate** between subgroup A_1 and subgroup A_2, the blood group they define has been named subgroup $A_{1,2}$, or intermediate A (A_{int}). This subgroup is seen most frequently in Negroids, and it is not uncommon among them. Since $A_{1,2}$ appears to be closely related serologically to A_2, in **statistical analyses** of the various blood groups and subgroups the subgroup $A_{1,2}$ should be classified together with A_2. It is possible that A_2 and $A_{1,2}$ may be merely different products or expressions of the same gene (A^2).*

Pitfalls in subgrouping

Subgroup A_1 blood from **newborn infants** may give weak or even negative reactions with anti-A_1 reagents, like $A_{1,2}$ adult blood, but differs because it reacts weakly or not at all with anti-**H**. Therefore subgrouping of infant's blood should be

*Wiener, A. S.: Unpublished data.

deferred until the infant is at least 3 months old and the agglutinogens are fully developed. Just as anti-**A** serum reacts more weakly with A_2B cells than with A_2 (p. 60), so anti-A_1 reagents react more weakly with A_1B cells than with A_1. An explanation for this phenomenon is offered on p. 69, and it is significant in this connection that A_2B cells are more strongly agglutinated than A_1B cells by anti-**B** reagents.

It may be pointed out that the anti-**B** agglutinins from subgroup A_2 individuals generally have higher titers and a broader span of reactivity than do anti-**B** from subgroup A_1 individuals.*

Serum of subgroups A_2 and A_2B may have the **cold anti-A_1 agglutinin.**

CODING OF BLOOD GROUP REACTIONS IN THE A-B-O SYSTEM

Wiener suggested a simple method of coding reactions in various blood group systems, making use of the digits of the binary code. Applying this to the A-B-O system, the binary numbers for coding are used not only for the reactions of the phenotypes, but also for genes, agglutinogens, and genotypes. (See Table 5-8.)

AGGLUTINOGENS A_3 AND A_4

It was noted by Fisher and Hahn[8] in 1935 that certain rare group A individuals gave atypical reactions even when the

*Wiener, A. S.: Personal communication, 1971.

Table 5-8. Coding reactions in the A-B-O system*

Blood group	Reactions of cells with			Specificities (blood factors) detected	Agglutinogens present	Binary code reactions
	Anti-A	Anti-B	Anti-A_1			
O	−	−	−	None	None	000
A_1	+	−	+	**A** and A_1	A_1	101
A_2	+	−	−	**A**	A_2	100
B	−	+	−	**B**	B	010
A_1B	+	+	+	**A**, A_1, and **B**	A_1 and B	111
A_2B	+	+	−	**A** and **B**	A_2 and B	110

*Modified from Wiener, A. S.: Haematologia 2:205, 1968.

most potent anti-**A** sera were used in testing their cells. A characteristic reaction of the blood cells of such persons consists of large clumps of cells on a background of unagglutinated cells. Friedenreich[9] in 1936 described the agglutination reaction when such cells are mixed with anti-**A** serum and with group O serum, which contains both anti-**A** and anti-**B** agglutinins, as consisting of clumps of red cells on a background of unagglutinated cells. He designated the agglutinogen as A_3, giving rise to two additional subgroups of A, A_3, and A_3B, which are hereditarily transmitted by another allelic gene A^3. It is the consensus that the identification of blood as belonging to subgroup A_3B should not be made without family evidence of such subgroups.

The presence of A_3 presents a problem for the laboratory, since it must be differentiated from chimeras and other mixtures of blood, as well as from changes brought about by leukemia. The serum of subgroup A_3 contains anti-**B** agglutinins just as ordinary blood group A serum does. Cold agglutinins anti-A_1 may be present in these sera and in the sera of subgroup A_3B.

In 1941 Wiener and Silverman[10] described a subgroup A_3 patient. Even though the patient was group A, her red cells were incompletely agglutinated by anti-**A** sera from group B persons as well as from rabbits previously immunized against human group A blood, although these sera promptly and completely agglutinated subgroups A_1 and A_2 cells. Microscopically, the A_3 patient's cells showed small clumps on a background of many free cells. Her serum gave strong and prompt agglutination of group B cells but did not clump the cells of group O or A_2 individuals. There was a weak reaction against A_1 cells, demonstrating the presence of an irregular agglutinin, anti-A_1.

The subgroups A_3 and A_3B have been extensively studied by Gammelgaard and Marcussen,[11] to whose excellent monograph the reader is referred.

Wiener and Cioffi[12] in 1972 observed the counterpart of A_3 in a group B mother and her son, both of whom were nonsecretors of the A-B-H substance. Their red cells were not agglutinated by anti-**A** serum, and in tests with anti-**B** or with group O serum only about one tenth of the cells formed agglutinates in a background of free red cells. Their sera agglutinated the red cells of groups A_1 and A_2 but not of groups O or B, but their red cells were strongly agglutinated by anti-**H** lectin. The blood groups of this mother and her son could therefore be designated as subgroup B_3.

BLOOD GROUP SPECIFICITIES AND BLOOD GROUP–SPECIFIC SUBSTANCES
Specificity H

Group O cells are characterized not merely by the absence of agglutinogens A and B but also by the regular presence of a special specificity **H**, at one time mistaken for the expected specificity **O**. Only rarely do antibodies of specificity anti-**H** occur in human sera, and then they are found only in the plasma of subgroups A_1B and A_1. Anti-**H** antibody was first found by Schiff in animal sera, especially in sera from cattle and eels; it has also been produced artificially by heterogenetic immunization of goats with Shiga bacilli.

Anti-**H** cannot be used to determine the genotypes of groups A and B persons as was thought when the reagent was still designated as anti-**O**. Actually, only family studies can identify genotypes in the A and B groups. In subgroups A_1B and A_2B, however, genotypes are always A^1B and A^2B, respectively, and in group O they are *OO*. For an exception, see cis AB, p. 76.

The A-B-O agglutinogens all share specificity **H** (H substance), and all body fluids and secretions in humans also share this specificity, provided that the subject is a secretor. However, the **H** specificity occurs in unequal amounts on the red cells of the various A-B-O blood groups; the cells of groups O and A_2 react regularly and have the highest degree of **H** reactivity. **H** is variable and usually less well developed in agglutinogen B, and in agglutinogen A₁ it is also variable and tends to be least developed.

The relationship of the **H** specificity to the A-B-O factors on red cells has been studied in detail by Wiener et al.[13] Some of the results are shown in Table 5-9. More recently (1972), Wiener et al.[14] showed that the relationship of **H** to A-B-O on red cells varies according to race, based on studies on Negroids, Caucasians, and Chinese in New York City.

Specificity **H** is due to a substance H, which is distinct from the A and B substances but similar in chemical structure. According to Wiener, H and A-B develop in parallel, but the genes that determine the H substance and those that determine the A and B agglutinogens apparently compete with one another for the same substrate from which the substances are formed. The alternate view of Watkins et al.[23] regarding the relationship between H and A-B, is detailed in Chapter 6. The serologic reactions of Table 5-9 are ascribed by Wiener and Karowe[15] to the relative positions of the H and A-B determinant groups on the final blood group macro-molecule, with resulting steric interference.

Antibodies of specificity anti-**H** were originally designated anti-**O** because they were believed to be specific for agglutinogen O, but when it was found that all the A-B-O blood groups share this specificity, even though in unequal degree, the antiserum was renamed anti-**H**. Reagents having anti-**H** specificity are most easily derived from extracts of seeds, especially the seeds of *Ulex europeus*, and instead of being called antiserum, these anti-**H** reacting extracts are termed **lectins**. They are valuable in determining the A-B-H secretor types. They give sharp reactions despite their low titers and are useful in testing saliva of individuals of any of the A-B-O groups.

Springer[16] distinguishes between **blood group substances** and **blood group–active substances**. If animals raised under germ-free conditions had antibodies to the A-B-H substances, these antibodies could be gene products. If, however, antibodies are caused by environmental factors, they should be absent in germfree animals. Normal chickens of certain varieties form antibodies reactive for human group B cells by the time they reach the age of

Table 5-9. Reactions of anti-**H** *(Ulex europeus)* lectin on a random series of blood specimens from 400 adults*

A-B-O group	Strength of reaction†						Totals‡	
	I	II	III	IV	V	VI	Number	Percent
O	168	1	0	0	0	0	169	42.25
A₁	1	21	21	18	24	24	109	27.25
A₂	25	1	0	0	0	0	26	6.50
A₁,₂	5	0	0	0	0	0	5	1.25
B	6	35	15	3	3	8	70	17.50
A₁B	0	0	0	1	2	14	17	4.25
A₂B	1	2	0	0	0	1	4	1.00
Totals	206	60	36	22	29	47	400	100.00

*Modified from Wiener, A. S., Moor-Jankowski, J., and Gordon, E. B.: Vox Sang. 29:82, 1966.
†Class I—Complete clumping, no free cells.
Class II—Marked clumping, minority of cells unagglutinated.
Class III—Moderate clumping, about half the cells unagglutinated.
Class IV—Distinct agglutination, majority of cells unagglutinated.
Class V—Weak or doubtful reactions.
Class IV—No agglutination.
‡If subgroup A₁,₂ is counted as subgroup A₂, the calculated gene frequencies by the square root formulas are $O = 0.650$; $A^1 = 0.172$; $A^2 = 0.057$; $B = 0.125$.

about 20 days. Springer et al.[17] kept some white Leghorn chickens in a germfree environment and at the same time permitted others to live under ordinary conditions. The germfree chickens produced no anti-**B** blood group–specific antibodies even 45 days after hatching, but those raised under ordinary conditions showed the same anti-**B** titer as other normal chickens. Springer and his associates also observed that when blood group B–active meconium extracts were fed to the germfree chickens or when the chickens were sprayed with the extracts, they developed a moderate anti-**B** titer in their sera. A single feeding of live, blood group B–active *Escherichia coli* O_{86} caused them to produce an extremely high anti-**B** titer, but bacteria with no blood group activity had no effect. Feeding this same strain *E. coli,* killed by desiccation, to infants with severe diarrhea caused the infants to produce a highly significant thirty-two–fold increase in anti-**B** antibody titer, which began to decrease slightly only after several months. Even ingestion of dead *E. coli* O_{86} stimulated de novo iso-agglutinin formation in infants or increased the titer of preexisting antibodies in adults suffering from severe intestinal disorders. So-called normal hemagglutinins can develop as a result of immunogenic stimuli, as shown by these experiments of Springer. He concluded that the *apparatus* for producing antibodies is inherited, but the specific antibodies themselves are not.

Not only do *E. coli* O_{86} bacteria specifically stimulate formation of anti-**B** antibodies, but they also absorb anti–blood group B antibodies. Hyperimmune anti-**B** sera retard the growth of *E. coli* O_{86} in the absence of complement and kill the bacteria if complement is present. This work of Springer was the first demonstration of a pathophysiologic role of blood group antibodies outside the field of the blood groups proper. Springer's experiments point to an oligosaccharide structure in *E. coli* O_{86} that is responsible for its blood group B specificity, although rigorous chemical proof of such a structure is lacking.

Øyen et al.[18] showed that the somatic antigens A and B of *E. coli* O_{86}:B7 could be used to remove unwanted anti-**B** from serum. This is particularly important in the preparation of such reagent sera as anti-**Lu**^{b}, anti-**k**, and anti-**Vel**, which can be rendered free of anti-**B** without loss of antibody titer or avidity. Absorption of anti-**A** is less efficient, especially from group O sera. Absorption of antisera with these *E. coli* organisms caused slight loss in activity of an anti-**P**$_1$ serum but in no other human antisera tested by the authors.

As shown by Springer, **blood group–specific substances** of **H** specificity occur in higher plants and viruses, as well as in bacteria, and these must not be confused with **plant agglutinins.** The blood group agglutinating substances from plants (**lectins**) are believed to be globulins or glycoproteins, whereas the H group–specific substances of plants are polysaccharides that neutralize human, rabbit, or plant anti-**H** agglutinins only weakly or not at all, although they are antigenic. However, blood group H substances of man, as well as from yew and sassafras, are immunologically equivalent when measured with **eel serum** (which has a natural anti-**H**), even though these three substances differ in their chemical properties. The blood group H molecules from plants contain neither nitrogen nor fucose, which the human substances do. The close immunologic relationship between the blood group H–specific macromolecules of man and of higher plants may seem surprising, since the substances in man and in these plants are chemically different. According to Springer,[16] these findings point to the limitations of immunologic methods, particularly when heterologous reagents such as most blood group antibodies are used, although the unreliability of immunochemical reactions may be more apparent than real when one bears in mind the nature of serologic specificity.

Some cardiac glycosides and antibiotics share certain serologic specificities when compared with certain reagents like the human blood group substance H, even though they differ chemically. Myxoviruses also have some blood group–active substances, as Springer[74] has shown. Influenza viruses specifically destroy the principal antigens of the M-N system, and *Vibrio cholerae* and *Clostridium perfringens* have **receptor-destroying enzymes (RDE)**.

In quantitating bacterial blood group activity, the choice of culture media is an important factor.[19] The blood group activity is often a property of the bacterium per se, but it is also affected by the cultural environment of the organism. With high concentrations of peptones (made with hog pepsin), the media could transfer their own blood group A activity to the bacteria in proportion to the concentration of the peptones. Low concentrations of peptones seem to have no effect on the blood group activity levels.

The blood group substances A, B, and H are not limited to the red blood cells of man. They are found in water-soluble form in human body fluids of **secretors** and are also ubiquitous, being present in microorganisms, animals, higher plants, and other sources. Blood group–specific substance is also found among the gram-negative intestinal bacteria that constitute the normal flora in man. **Immunologic mimicking** of human blood group A-B-H substances by toxic bacterial lipopolysaccharides is so great that when these substances are adsorbed onto human erythrocytes, the cells acquire their blood group specificity; this can be the cause of problems in the laboratory in grouping blood when selecting donors for transfusion. A notable example of this is the occasional acquisition by group A_1 cells of a weak B reactivity, mostly in elderly patients with gastrointestinal pathology. The red cells usually react most clearly with anti-**B** derived from individuals of subgroup A_2, and a clue to the fact that these individuals are not group AB is provided by the presence in their serum of anti-**B**. Obviously, such patients should be transfused only with group A blood.

The ability of the red cells, which have enormous surface area, to bind toxic substances of the type mentioned previously suggests a transport and detoxifying function for the blood group antigens on the red cells that has still to be investigated.[20,21]

A-B-H substances

The A-B-H substances are not restricted to red cells but are present in the cells of most tissues and organs, except for nerve tissue, epidermis, skin appendages, bone, and cartilage. The A-B-H blood group substances in red cells and tissues can be extracted with alcohol and other lipid solvents but only in quite small amounts. These substances, as already explained, also occur in water-soluble form and are secreted by certain individuals and not by others. The A-B-H substances of red cells appear to be lipopolysaccharides (glycolipids), but those of secretions are mucopolysaccharides (glycoproteins); however, the determinant chemical groups on the antigen molecule responsible for their blood group specificities appear to be identical for both kinds of blood group substances—*N*-acetyl-D-galactosamine for the specificity **A**, D-galactose for specificity **B**, and L-fucose for specificity **H**. Since the blood group substances can be extracted in pure form more easily and in larger amounts from secretions than from red cells, almost all the biochemical studies are based on analyses of preparations of water-soluble group substances, obtained especially from saliva and the contents of ovarian cysts and stomachs of animals.

Although the A-B-O and H-h systems are inherited independently of one another, many workers believe that the H substance must be present for the formation of A and B substances.

Tests for water-soluble blood group substances are made by mixing the water-soluble substances in body fluids with appropriate antisera. The substances are able to combine specifically with the blood group antibody and neutralize it; when the corresponding red cells are subsequently added as indicators, they fail to agglutinate. Because of such methods of identification, these substances are often referred to as **inhibitory substances** in the laboratory, and the tests are known as **inhibition tests.** (See Table 5-10.) Substances of like nature are also found in some plants and bacteria, which serve as sources for laboratory studies (pp. 65 and 66).

Chemistry of the A-B-H group substances

The A-B-H blood group substances are glycoproteins with an average molecular weight of about 300,000 to 1,000,000. The substances are composed of about 85% carbohydrate and 15% amino acids. The carbohydrate moiety of the A, B, H, or Lewis substances is composed of five sugars: (1) L-fucose (Fuc), (2) D-galactose (Gal), (3) N-acetyl-D-glucosamine (GNAc), (4) N-acetyl-D-galactosamine (Gal NAc), and (5) a 9-carbon sugar, N-acetylneuraminic acid (NANA) (sialic acid), which apparently does not participate in the specificity of the blood group antigens. The sugars are arranged in a large number of fairly short chains attached by covalent linkage to a peptide "backbone" composed of fifteen amino acids, four of which—threonine, serine, proline, and alanine—comprise two thirds of the amino acids present. Sulfur-containing amino acids are virtually absent. Aromatic amino acids are present in only small amounts. The peptide component apparently maintains correct spacing and orientation of the carbohydrate chains. The complete macromolecule must retain its integrity for maximal serologic reactivity. The blood group antigenic specificity depends on the terminal nonreducing ends of the chains, as seen in Fig. 5-1.

According to Wiener and Socha[22]:

"Fig. [5-1] is based on the information and diagrams in the paper of Watkins.[23] All blood group substances are presumed to have a basic tetrasaccharide that acts as a precursor, to which are added the appropriate determinant sugars in nonreducing form at the location and in the proper linkage, as shown in Fig. [5-1]. Actually, the precursor is believed to be of two kinds: one with a $\beta1,3$, and the other with a $\beta1,4$ linkage between the two terminal sugars, galactose and N-acetyl-D-glucosamine (1).* These considerations apply only to blood group substances derived from secretions rather than from red cells, for reason of limited availability of the materials. Serologically, the precursor substance of A-B-H and Lewis is said to have a type XIV specificity because of its cross-reactivity with rabbit antisera against type XIV pneumococci. The fucose determinant

---

*The number in parentheses (1) refers to the various structures in the right-hand column in the figure.

Table 5-10. Results of inhibition tests on saliva

	Is mixed with a drop of:		
	Anti-A serum	**Anti-B serum**	**Anti-H lectin**
	To the mixture are then added:		
Drop of saliva from	**A red cells**	**B red cells**	**O red cells**
Secretor of			
Group O	+	+	−
Group A	−	+	−
Group B	+	−	−
Group AB	−	−	−
Nonsecretor of			
any group	+	+	+

+ = agglutination, i.e., no inhibition; − = no agglutination, i.e., inhibition.

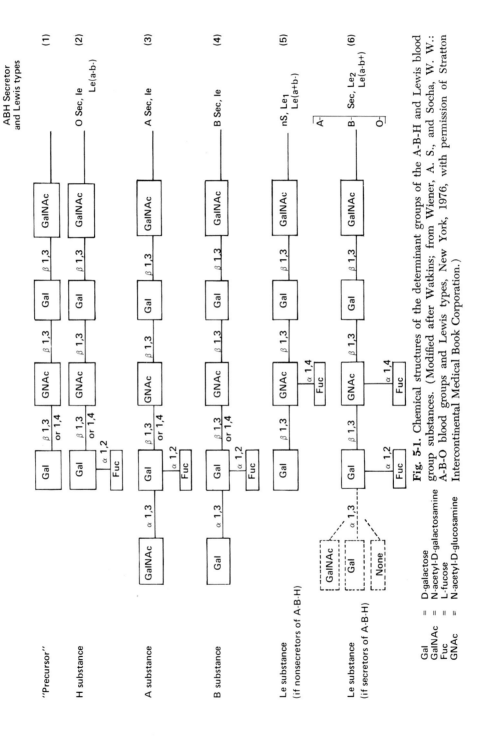

Fig. 5-1. Chemical structures of the determinant groups of the A-B-H and Lewis blood group substances. (Modified after Watkins; from Wiener, A. S., and Socha, W. W.: A-B-O blood groups and Lewis types, New York, 1976, with permission of Stratton Intercontinental Medical Book Corporation.)

groups responsible for the H specificity are attached to the terminal galactose in $\alpha1,2$ linkage. Presumably, this occurs in group substances from all secretors, since, aside from individuals of the so-called Bombay type, all humans have the H antigen. Carriers of the *A* gene are presumed to produce a specific transferase that adds *N*-acetyl-D-galactosamine in $\beta1,3$ linkage to the terminal galactose, to which fucose is also necessarily attached in secretors. The B substance differs from the A substance only in that terminal galactose is present instead of *N*-acetyl-D-galactosamine.

"The Lewis substance resembles H substance except that the fucose is attached in $\alpha1,4$ linkage to the subterminal *N*-acetyl-D-galactosamine, and the precursor chain is exclusively the one with the $\beta1,3$ linkage.

"In Lewis-positive individuals who are A-B-H secretors, the additional fucose determinant that is responsible for the H specificity is also present in the oligosaccharide chain. The simultaneous presence of the two fucose determinant groups give rise to the additional serologic specificity Le^b (Le$_2$) in the same way that the simultaneous presence in the same molecule of the hr' and hr" determinants of the Rh-Hr system gives rise to the specificity hr."

Readers interested in the historical background of the biochemical nature of the blood group substances may consult a 1970 article by Wiener.[24]

Watkins and Morgan have made no attempt to provide a biochemical explanation for the subgroups of A; according to Wiener's hypothesis[15] the determinant group is the same in both subgroups, *N*-acetyl-D-galactosamine, and the difference in reactions is due to the length of the subjacent oligosaccharide chain. Wiener's hypothesis explains why it is not possible to distinguish serologically between the A$_1$ and A$_2$ blood group substances in secretions such as saliva (Moreno et al.[25]) (Fig. 5-2).

Wiener visualized the blood group hapten as having a basic structure, probably

polysaccharide in nature. In group O (genotype *OO*), only this rudimentary structure with its rather weak polar groups is assumed to be present. Agglutinogen A, however, would have the basic structure, plus a certain relatively complex, strongly polar group. If the group A is genotype *AO*, only one such group would be present in the molecule. In genotype *AA* the polar group would be duplicated at each end of the hapten. Agglutinogen B is similarly represented but with a different polar group of related structure. In group AB it is assumed that there is only a single type of molecule with two different polar groups, A and B, respectively, rather than a mixture of two kinds of molecules. Wiener and Karowe[15] assumed also that in the red cells these haptens are combined with lipids or lipoproteins, whereas in the secretions they occur free in molecular form or in relatively small molecular aggregates.

A good source of material for chemical analysis of the blood group–specific substance is the meconium.

VARIANTS OF AGGLUTINOGEN A
Variant A$_m$

Landsteiner's rule of agglutinins in the A-B-O system is that those agglutinins are regularly present in the plasma for which the corresponding agglutinogen(s) is absent from the red cells, except during the neonatal period, in which there usually are no antibodies, and in agammaglobulinemia, in which antibody production does not occur.

The A$_m$ phenotype is very rare. In this group, first described by Wiener and Gordon,[26] the red cells react like those of group O in that they fail to clump in anti-A and anti-B sera, whereas the serum of A$_m$ clumps group B cells and not group A, including cells of subgroup A$_1$. Group O serum has both anti-A and anti-B agglutinins; thus these individuals manifestly do not belong to group O. Wiener and Gordon described a patient whose cells were not agglutinated by anti-A or anti-B sera

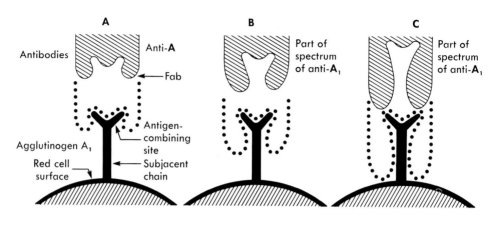

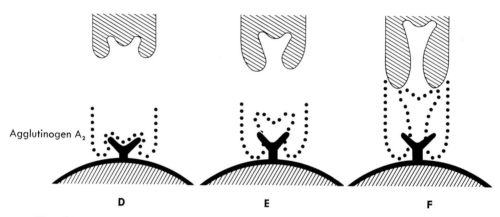

Fig. 5-2. Diagrammatic representation of reactions of spectrum of anti-**A** antibodies with various A agglutinogens. **A** to **C**, Good fit of entire spectrum of anti-**A** antibodies with combining site of agglutinogen A₁, which is possible because of greater length of chain subjacent to combining site. **D** to **F**, In contrast, only part of the spectrum of anti-**A** antibodies can fit the combining site of agglutinogen A₂, because shortness of subjacent chain prevents proper combination of antigen and antibody in **E** and **F**. (From Wiener, A. S., and Socha, W. W.: Int. Arch. Allergy Appl. Immunol. **47:**946, 1974; with permission of S. Karger AG, Basel.)

but whose serum strongly clumped group B cells. The gamma globulin concentration was normal or even slightly above normal, and tests on saliva showed strong inhibition of anti-**A**. Anti-**B** was not affected. The saliva therefore contained the A substance. The blood cells also failed to react with extremely high-titered anti-**A** serum from both human and animal sources.

These findings resembled those observed in the lower monkeys and gorillas, whose red cells are not agglutinated by anti-**A**, anti-**B**, or anti-**H** reagents. (The A-B-O blood groups of monkeys are determined by test-ing their saliva for A, B, and H human substance, and their sera for the reciprocal agglutinins. See Part Two, pp. 207 and 208, and Part Three, p. 361.) Wiener and Gordon therefore designated the agglutinogen A_m to show that the reactions resembled those of lower monkeys. According to one theory, the A_m type is due to homozygosity for a special suppressor gene independent of the A-B-O genes.

Specificity A_{hel}; specificity A_{HP}

Prokop et al.[27] in 1965 extracted a potent reagent of anti-**A** specificity from the albumin glands of snails of the genus *Helix*, species *H. hortensis*. The agglutinin is of high potency and titer and makes an excellent anti-**A** reagent. It reacts with almost equal intensity against A_1 and A_2 erythrocytes, although A_2B cells react more weakly. It detects a specificity Prokop called A_{hel}, the hel being derived from *Helix*. Similar anti-**A** agglutinins have been found in *H. pomatia* (Weinbergschnecke). These are designated anti-A_{HP}. Snail anti-**A** has been used for studies of the blood groups in nonhuman primates. Wiener[24] found that anti-A_{HP} is inhibited by *N*-acetyl-D-galactosamine and by *N*-acetyl-D-glucosamine but not by other simple sugars tried.

Specificity Ac (a different specificity detected by snail agglutinins)

Extracts of another snail species, *Achatina granulata*, also have hemagglutinating properties.[28] These antibodies detect a blood factor designated **Ac**, short for *Achatina*, shared by the red cells of all humans and mice tested to date but absent from the red cells of nonhuman primates, rats, and rabbits.[29] The saliva of all nonhuman primate species tested has been able to neutralize this hemagglutinin to some degree when the hemagglutination-inhibition technic was used. The inhibition titers in the saliva of man are relatively low or give little or no inhibition. Nonhuman primates show considerably higher titers than the highest inhibition titers observed with human saliva. There appears to be no relationship between Ac and the A-B-H substances, except that Wiener found that the agglutinin of the snail *A. granulata* is inhibited by all three sugars: *N*-acetyl-D-galactosamine, *N*-acetyl-D-glucosamine, and *N*-acetyl-mannosamine.

Variant A_{end}

W. Weiner et al. in 1959[75] described a weak variant, apparently due to an allele of A-B-O, but which did not fit into the category C or A_m. It was later designated A_{end}.[76] It was present in two generations of a family and appeared at first to be similar to an abnormally weak A_3, except that the saliva of all three carriers had H but not A substance. Other examples have been reported.

Variant A_{el}

Even weaker than the A_{end} antigen is that designated A_{el}. This antigen can be demonstrated only by absorption and elution. The saliva of secretors of A_{el} contains H but no A substance. Examples of this extremely rare characteristic have been found in an Italian Canadian donor and his sister, in three generations of one American family, in Sweden and West Germany, and in other American families.

Variant A_{bantu}

A variation of agglutinogen A has been found in 4% of Bantu group A blood. The original studies were those of Brain.[30] The agglutination pattern is the same as that of A_3, except that the saliva of secretors contains H but no A. Anti-**A** is regularly present in the serum.

A_P component

A component of human A antigen complex, called A^P, was described because group A pig cells absorb the hemolytic fraction of "immune" anti-**A** but do not absorb the agglutinin of "natural" anti-**A**. The two anti-**A** fractions appear to have different specificities. According to Konugres and Coombs,[31] the anti-A^P fraction of immune anti-**A** is that fraction which fails to be inhibited by the A substance in the Witebsky partial neutralization test for immune anti-**A**.

Other variants of A

No doubt there are other variations in the agglutinogen A that only await discovery. It should be noted that tests must be made of the cells not only with anti-**A** and anti-**B** sera but also with group O serum, and the saliva must be tested with anti-**H** reagents if these unusual and rare blood subgroups are to be recognized.

Agglutinogen A in nonhuman primates

Chapter 15 dealing with the blood groups of animals, discusses agglutinogen A in nonhuman primates so that no further presentation will be given here.

THE BOMBAY BLOOD TYPE O$_h$

The Bombay blood type, called O$_h$, is of great theoretical and practical interest in blood group serology and genetics because it provides the best example of the so-called **modifying genes** among various blood groups. One rare gene, *x*, if present in double dose, or homozygous form, *xx*, can prevent the expression of the A-B-O blood group antigens not only in the saliva but also on the red blood cells. Whereas Bombay type people have normal A-B-O genes, they are also homozygous for the inhibitor gene, or genotype *xx*, that prevents the A-B-O genes from placing their respective antigens onto the red cells and into the saliva. Bhende et al.[32] in 1952 reported three individuals in whom the red cells were not agglutinated by anti-**A**, anti-**B**, or anti-**H** sera. If these had been group O individuals, their blood cells would have reacted with anti-**H** serum or with anti-**H** lectin, and their sera could not then have contained anti-**H**. This type of blood was found first in Bombay; hence its name. Several families in Bombay were of this group.

Ceppellini et al.,[33] in 1952, postulated that these were examples of an inhibitory mechanism involving both red cells and saliva. The characteristics of this blood presumably result from the action of a pair of modifying genes *X-x*. The Bombay type was found by Levine et al.[34] in three members of an American family of Italian extraction. As Levine explained, when he postulated the **suppressor,** or **epistatic gene,** human individuals in general are homozygous for a gene *X*, located on a different pair of chromosomes from those that contain A-B-O genes. It is hypothesized that gene *X* acts on the blood group precursor substance and converts it to a form susceptible to the action of the *A*, *B*, and *H* genes.

A clear explanation of the nature of the Bombay type has been given by Wiener[35] in Table 5-11. This shows the manner by which the Bombay type is identified, together with the probable genotype of the father, mother, and child, respectively.

Recapitulating, the red blood cells and secretions in Bombay individuals lack H as well as the A-B substances, irrespective of the A-B-O genotype, so that the cells fail

Table 5-11. The Bombay blood group*

A. Results of tests carried out in routine fashion

Blood of	Reactions of red cells with antiserum		Reaction of serum with red cells of		Indicated blood group
	Anti-A	Anti-B	Group A	Group B	
Father	−	−	+	+	O
Mother	−	−	+	+	O
Child	−	+	+	−	B

B. Results of more thorough examination of same family

Blood of	Reaction of red cells with antiserum (or lectin)			Reaction of serum with red cells of group				Indicated blood group	Probable genotype	
	Anti-A	Anti-B	Anti-H	O	A$_1$	A$_2$	B			
Father	−	−	+	−	+	+	+	O	XX	OO
Mother	−	−	−	+	+	+	+	O$_h$	xx	BO
Child	−	+	±	−	+	+	−	B	Xx	BO

*Modified from Wiener, A. S.: Advances in blood grouping, vol. 3, New York, 1970, Grune & Stratton, Inc.

to agglutinate in anti-**H** as well as in anti-**A** and anti-**B** reagents, and the serum of such people contains anti-**H** as well as anti-**A** and anti-**B** agglutinins.

The Bombay group is now designated group O_h to show the absence of the H substance, which distinguishes these people from ordinary group O individuals. If only routine blood group tests are made, such subjects will be classified as belonging to blood group O. (It should be noted that the X and x genes are often regarded as the same as H and h, and the genotypes are given as HH, Hh, and hh.)

Some authors give the Bombay types as O_h^A, $O_h^B m$, O_h^{AB}, A_h, B_h, O_{Hm} or O_m^h, O_{Hm}^A or O_m^h, O_{Hm}^A or A_m^h, O_{Hm}^P or B_m^h, if family studies show which antigen has been suppressed.

Fig. 5-3 illustrates the hereditary transmission of the Bombay blood group.

Elution studies by Lanser et al.[36] indicate that the suppressed A and B antigens of O_h red cells are present in some form, even though they do not participate in agglutination.

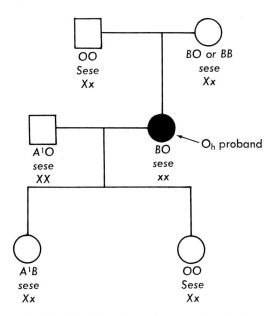

Fig. 5-3. Hereditary transmission of the Bombay blood group. (From Wiener, A. S., and Socha, W. W.: A-B-O blood groups and Lewis types, New York, 1976; with permission of Stratton Intercontinental Medical Book Corporation.)

The gene **frequency** for the Bombay type in India seems to be around 0.0066. Even though more than a million donors or patients have been tested for the Bombay type in England, not a single example has been found to date.

MULTIPLICITY OF SPECIFICITIES* OF AGGLUTINOGENS A AND B

The agglutinogens A and B are not simple substances. Rather, they and all other agglutinogens are characterized by multiple serologic specificities. As has already been emphasized repeatedly, each agglutinogen (an intrinsic attribute of the red cell membrane) is characterized by multiple **serologic specificities** (extrinsic attributes of the agglutinogen molecule demonstrable by serologic tests), and this applies also to the agglutinogens A and B. For example, as has been previously shown, the gene A^1 determines an agglutinogen having at least three serologic specificities: (1) specificity A_1, which is peculiar to the agglutinogen A_1; (2) specificity **A,** which it shares with agglutinogen A_2; and (3) a specificity **C,** which it shares with agglutinogen B.

Tests for A-like and B-like agglutinogens on the red cells of lower mammals have disclosed the existence of still other specificities; for example, injection of group A human blood into rabbits stimulates the production not only of anti-**A** agglutinins but also of **hemolysins** for sheep red blood cells, which are adsorbable by the red cells used for immunization. Conversely, immunization of the rabbit with sheep red blood cells may give rise to production of anti-**A** agglutinins or hemolysins. This shows that agglutinogen A has other specificities that it shares with sheep red cells; these have been designated F_A, after Forssman, who described the first heterogenetic sera for sheep red cells produced by immunization

---

*Blood factors (serologic specificities of red cells), which are **extrinsic** attributes, must not be confused with determinant groups, which are **intrinsic** attributes of the agglutinogen molecule.

with guinea pig kidney containing the so-called **Forssman antigen.** Similarly, human anti-**B** sera cross-react with red cells from rabbits and other species of rodents. By absorption with red cells of these various mammalian species the anti-**B** agglutinin of human groups A and O sera could be fractionated, and each antibody fraction defines a different B specificity, designated as B_i, B_{ii}, and B_{iii}, etc. For example, taking into account only rabbits, at least two beta (anti-**B**) antibodies must be considered—anti-B_i, reactive only with human group B red cells, and anti-B_{ii}, reactive for rabbit red cells as well as for human red cells. Since rabbits have B-like agglutinogens, they do not respond readily to immunization with group B blood; when they do, the antibody they produce is of specificity anti-B_i. In contrast, the anti-**B** produced by chickens, whose red cells share the specificity B_i with human B cells, is anti-B_{ii}. Since normal human group B cells have all the specificities B_i, B_{ii}, B_{iii}, etc., anti-B_i of rabbits and anti-B_{ii} of chickens give parallel reactions with anti-**B** sera in tests on human blood. These various specificities of human group B blood—B_i, B_{ii}, and B_{iii}—must not be confused with the subgroups of group B and the variants of agglutinogen B now to be described.

Factor C. As explained on pp. 57 to 59, agglutinogen B is also characterized by specificity **C.**

SUBGROUPS OF AGGLUTINOGEN B
Weak B of Mäkelä and Mäkelä

In 1955 O. Mäkelä and P. Mäkelä[37] in Finland described a blood group antigen, a weak B, present on the red blood cells of a patient with an antibody of B-like activity in the serum. The patient's B cells were not agglutinated by the anti-**B** in his own serum. This patient had five group O siblings. Boorman and Zeitlin[38,39] found two generations of an English family in which the cells reacted with anti-**B** serum, although weakly. In the serum of one member of this family was also an anti-**B** agglutinin that reacted with all B cells tested

except her own, her father's, and those of the Mäkeläs' propositus. This weak B-like antigen has also been found in three members of a Polish family, in one French donor with no living relatives, and in four members of another Finnish family.

B_w of Levine et al.[40]

Levine et al. found a weak B antigen, which they designated B_w, in the blood of several members of a Negroid family. It reacted with anti-**B** serum to produce the "extremely weak agglutination seen in artificial mixtures of 99 parts of group O blood and 1 part of normal group B blood." Both the B and H substances were present in the saliva of those individuals who were carriers of B_w and who were also secretors. Weak B reactions are more easily detected when group O serum, erroneously called anti-**A,B**, is used along with the anti-**A** and anti-**B** routinely employed in testing for blood groups.

B_3, the weak B of Moullec et al.[41]

In 1955 Moullec et al. described a patient whose red blood cells reacted weakly with anti-**B** serum and absorbed anti-**B** poorly, but eluates from these cells demonstrated more anti-**B** activity than did eluates prepared from normal B cells. The authors traced the gene for this agglutinogen through three generations. The saliva showed the presence of H substance but no demonstrable B substance.

More recently (1972), an individual of group B was described[12] whose red cells gave weak reactions with anti-**B** reagents comparable to those of agglutinogen A_3 with anti-**A** sera. In tests with potent anti-**B** reagents, only about one tenth of the red cells of this individual were agglutinated, and the same phenomenon was observed in the tests on his mother's blood. See p. 63.

B^3 gene of Sussman et al.[42]

Sussman et al. described an example of an unusual B^3 gene, discovered during routine preoperative blood grouping and cross matching. The serum and cells gave different blood group results by laboratory tests. The cells reacted as group O, but the serum contained only anti-**A** and no anti-**B** agglutinins. The blood also seemed to be compatible with group O blood donors, not only in the tests employing saline-suspended cells but with the antiglobulin and high-protein methods as well. The cells were agglutinated by potent anti-**B** sera and in some group O sera after incubation at 25° C for several hours, but the agglutinates were barely visible clumps with only about five to ten cells surrounded by many unagglutinated cells.

Neutralization tests showed that the serum had no demonstrable B substance. Even though the saliva contained H substance, no B substance was present.

Reports of this nature restress the importance not only of testing the cells against known anti-**A** and anti-**B** sera, but also of testing the serum against at least known group A and group B cells and, preferably, also group O cells.

OTHER SEROLOGIC SPECIFICITIES OF THE A-B-O SYSTEM
Specificity Z

Much research has recently (1971) been directed toward finding reagents, other than human sources usually employed, that react with human A, B, and H substances. Such substances as antisera prepared in rabbits, agglutinins from snails, and seed extracts (lectins)—especially those having the specificities anti-**A₁** and anti-**A** (*Dolichos biflorus, Phaseolus limensis,* etc.), anti-**H** (*Ulex europeus, Lotus tetragonolobus,* etc.), and anti-**B** (also anti-**C**) (*Crotolaria striata,* etc.)—have been tried. Wiener et al.[43] were successful in producing immune hemagglutinins against human blood cells by injecting human secretor saliva into certain catfish (*Ictalurus nebulosus*). In direct tests these antisera proved to differ in specificity from anti-**H,** since they agglutinated in very high titer human red cells of all the A-B-O groups to approxi-

mately the same titer, whereas anti-**H** clumped cells of groups O and A₂ to higher titers than cells of the other groups. Nevertheless, the antisera detected a specificity related to the A-B-O system, which is shared by all four groups but not those of the Bombay type. This specificity has been designated as **Z,** and the antiserum that defines it is termed anti-**Z.** Saliva from secretors but not from nonsecretors strongly inhibits the anti-**Z** agglutinin.

In 1949 Grubb[44] and in 1964 Bhatia[45] described antibodies that reacted similarly to anti-**Z.** Bhatia immunized chickens with human group O cells and produced an antiserum that reacted in high titer with human red cells of all A-B-O groups but in much lower titer with human blood cells of the Bombay type. When the antisera were absorbed with Bombay type red cells, the reagents no longer reacted with Bombay type cells but were still highly reactive with human red cells belonging to all A-B-O groups. Since they did not cause agglutination of Bombay red cells, Bhatia thought that they were of specificity anti-**H.** However, they seem to be similar to the anti-**Z** antibody of catfish immunized with secretor saliva.

The **Z** antibody thus defines an antigen or blood factor common to the red blood cells of all humans except those of the Bombay type. It is present in all anthropoid apes except gorillas and is absent in monkeys; it is well developed in the red cells of newborn humans. It has been postulated by Wiener, Chuba, Gordon, and Kuhns that the blood group **Z** substance is possibly a basic blood group substance on which the genes *A, B,* and *H* impose their respective specificities, presumably with the aid of specific transferases. It is postulated that the blood group substance Z may be hereditarily determined by a pair of allelic genes *Z* and *z,* independent of genes A-B-O and *H-h.* In those rare individuals who are homozygous for gene *z,* the Bombay type of blood results, designated "type z," which is devoid of the blood specificities **A, B,** and **H.**

Blood group "cis AB" (AB*)

According to the Bernstein theory, a group AB person cannot be the parent of a group O child, nor can a group O person be the parent of a group AB child. In 1930 Haselhorst and Lauer[46] reported the case of a woman who was subgroup A_2B and who had given birth to a group O child. This exception to the Bernstein theory was well documented and was ascribed by different authors either to mutation or to nondisjunction. Wiener et al.[47] offered two alternative explanations of this phenomenon: "Such exceptions could be explained by postulating the existence of four *completely linked* pairs of genes: *(AB), (Ab), (aB), (ab),* or what amounts to the same thing, by assuming the existence of four allelomorphic genes, of which three are the genes *A, B,* and *O* of the Bernstein theory, while the fourth allelomorphic gene acts like the genes *A* and *B* together, insofar as it determines the presence of both agglutinogens, A and B, in the erythrocytes." It seemed therefore conceivable that very rare families could exist with parents O × AB in which, instead of half the children being group A and half group B, half could be group O and half group AB if the group AB parent were heterozygous for the postulated extremely rare fourth allelic gene. This would be comparable to the mating rh × rh'rh", which in some families results in half the children being type rh' and half rh" and in other families half the children being type rh and half rh'rh" like the parents.

When no similar examples such as those of Haselhorst and Lauer were found at first, the authenticity of the case was doubted, and the Bernstein law was applied without reservation in cases of disputed parentage. In 1966, however, Reviron et al.[48] and in 1968 Reviron and Salmon[49] reported transmission of blood group AB in a family as if by a single chromosome or allele, instead of by two separate chromosomes or genes. They called the newly discovered very rare blood group "cis AB." Similar cases were later reported

from Japan. It was subsequently shown that cis AB can occur in two forms—cis A_1B and cis A_2B.

The reactions of cis AB blood with anti-**A** reagents appear to be typical. With anti-**B** reagents, however, they tend to be weak. With anti-**B** derived from group A_2 individuals the reactions are stronger than with anti-**B** from group A_1 persons, similar to the reaction of red cells of group A_1 having "acquired B."

The B agglutinogen of cis AB red cells does not have all the specificities of ordinary group B red cells, and the serum usually has an anti-**B** isoagglutinin that reacts with ordinary group B and AB red cells but not with red cells of the cis AB individual himself. This resembles Rh-Hr types in that type rh'rh" blood of genotype *r'r"* is agglutinated by anti-**rh'** and anti-**rh**ᵢ reagents, but blood of genotype *rʸr* is agglutinated only by anti-**rh'** reagents (pp. 112, 121, and 122).

To indicate the unusual nature of the B agglutinogen in cis AB blood, the blood group has been designated (1971) as AB* by Salmon,[50] or A_1B* or A_2B*, depending on the subgroup. Cis AB (AB*) individuals who are secretors have group-specific substances A and H in normal amounts in their saliva, but B cannot be demonstrated.

Blood specificity Cl

A "new" blood factor, **Cl**, was demonstrated by Wiener and Moon,[51] using extracts of seeds of the Korean *Clerodendron trichotomum* (Thunberg). One advantage of using seed extracts, or lectins, as diagnostic reagents for blood grouping and for biochemical studies is their presumed chemical simplicity; that is, it has been tacitly assumed that seed extracts consist of a homogeneous population of lectin molecules in contrast to blood serum antibodies, which have an entire spectrum of molecules of related structure. Wiener et al.[52] showed that seed extracts can be fractionated into lectins of more than one specificity by absorption with properly selected red cells. In this way, Moon and Wiener[53] fractionated a potent anti-**N** lectin from the leaves of the Korean *Vicia unijuga,* which proved useful as a diagnostic reagent for laboratory tests and for blood group research.

Absorbed seed extract, designated as anti-**Cl** lectin, identified a blood specificity **Cl** that proved to be different not only from **A, B,** and **H** but also from the blood specificities **M, N, S, s, P, Lu**[a]**, K, k, Jk**[a]**, Fy**[a]**, Fy**[b]**, Le**[a]**, Le**[b]**, Xg**[a]**, Rh**[o]**, rh′, rh″, hr′, hr″,** and **hr.** No striking differences were observed in the distribution of the blood factor **Cl** among Caucasoids, Negroids, and Chinese.

Most of the strong reactions occurred with blood specimens of group O and most of the negative reactions with blood of group A, superficially resembling the behavior of anti-**H** reagents. Further tests showed that anti-**Cl** is not identical to anti-**H,** since it failed to agglutinate many group O cells, although a probable association exists between **Cl** and **H,** detected by *Ulex europeus* seed extracts. In further tests it was found that anti-**Cl** clearly detects another specificity of the A-B-H molecule, but due to a combining group distinct from A and H, or else due to a structure closely connected with the A-B-H macromolecule.

Saliva was tested by the standard inhibition method with anti-**H** and anti-**Cl** reagents, using group O as indicator red cells. Bombay cells, which were also used, were strongly agglutinated by crude extracts of *Clerodendron* seeds but not by the absorbed or purified anti-**Cl** reagent. This showed two lectins in the extracts of *Clerodendron* seeds—one a panagglutinin, the other the anti-**Cl** lectin that detects a "new" blood group specificity.

Ficin treatment of red cells increases their activity with anti-**H** lectin but destroys their reactivity with anti-**Cl** lectin.

The specificity **Cl** appears to be due to a structure on or closely connected to the A-B-H-Le macromolecule, but distinct from the combining groups for **H, A, B,** and **Le.** Sialic acid may play an important role in this newly found (1975) specificity,

just as it does for the specificities **M** and **N.**

Acquired B (pseudo-B)

In 1959 Cameron et al.[54] reported the presence of a weak B antigen in seven group A_1 blood specimens that they had tested over the years. All seven were group A_1, and four of these had group O children; their genotype therefore was A^1O, and there was no room at the A-B-O locus for a weak *B* allele. Moreover, their sera contained anti-**B.** Those who were secretors of the A-B-H substance had A and H but not B in their saliva. Marsh et al.[55] were able to induce a similar change in vitro by treating A_1 cells with a bacterial filtrate (Garratty et al.[56]).

As explained on p. 65, a close serologic relationship exists between *Escherichia coli* O_{86} and blood group B. It is known that purified lipopolysaccharides and protein-lipopolysaccharides from *E. coli* O_{86} and other organisms can be adsorbed onto A and O red cells, so that they have a B-like antigen. This has been proved by exposing the cells to anti-**B** serum and later eluting the antibody. The cells are polyagglutinable after adsorption of the polysaccharides so that elution is necessary. It has also been found that a bacterial filtrate that is a powerful **T** activator can induce the B change in group O, as well as in A, cells. The T changing factor can be separated from the B changing factor. The B-like antigen is probably acquired through action of a bacterial enzyme.

In all, thirty-three examples of acquired B were found, thirty-two that were group A_1, and one group A_2. Most of the individuals had carcinoma of the colon or rectum, a few had carcinoma of the cervix, prostate, or peritoneum, and the others had infection of the intestine or gangrene of the legs.

The occurrence of acquired B is important, especially when typing patients for transfusion. If the patient has any of the previously mentioned conditions and the blood appears to have a weak B antigen, testing of the serum will reveal an anti-**B** agglutinin if this is a case of acquired B. For transfusion, of course, such patients should be given group A and not group AB blood.

Blood group antigen modification

A number of instances of modification of the A antigen to a weak A have been reported in patients with myeloblastic leukemia, acute monoblastic leukemia, hypoplastic anemia, Hodgkin's disease, and erythroleukemia. Modification not only of A but also of B, H, I, i, and Rh_o has been reported. The same effect has likewise been noted in some otherwise healthy old (79 years) patients.

In these cases, for example, a patient who has previously been grouped as A_1 without difficulty is found to have lost the strong A_1 antigen and in its place to have an extremely weak A_1 or no A_1 at all. The cells have lost their ability to be agglutinated by their specific anti-A_1 antiserum but they retain their power to absorb the anti-A_1 from the reagent. During remission, however, the number of agglutinable cells increases.

Salmon et al.[57] suggested that chromosome inactivation may be responsible for these results, but the reason for the change has not, in fact, been elucidated.

When the laboratory is aware that one of the above-mentioned diseases is present and there is some question as to the validity of the blood grouping test results, absorption tests must be carried out for proper blood grouping, using the patient's cells. It has been noted that the unagglutinable cells react more strongly with anti-H *Ulex* lectin than did the cells that were agglutinated by anti-A serum.

CROSS REACTIVITY OF ANTISERA[58-60]

Anti-A and anti-B sera differ in their reactions with red cells of lower mammals, and the antibodies can be fractionated by absorption with mammalian red cells. Studies on cross-reactions of antisera in other systems, for example, anti-M, anti-N, and anti-Rh_o reagents, with red cells of nonhuman primates also show that such antisera do not really detect unit specificities but actually contain a **spectrum of antibodies** having a multiplicity of related serologic specificities. This is also true of anti-H reagents and other antisera (pp. 177 and 178).

PRECAUTIONS CONCERNING TESTING FOR BLOOD GROUP OF A RECIPIENT IMMEDIATELY AFTER TRANSFUSION

Transfusion of blood cells may result in a mixture of groups in a patient, as when group O cells have been transfused into individuals of the other A-B-O blood groups, but this admixture is only temporary. Provided that the transfused cells are compatible and fresh, their **life span** is the same as that of naturally produced cells. Ashby[61] traced the **survival** of group O cells in group A and group B individuals and in this way showed the life of the red cells to be about 120 days. Mollison[62] has taken small amounts of blood from volunteers, tagged the red cells with ^{51}Cr, and then reinjected the blood. In this way the half life of normal red cells has also been determined.

By **differential agglutination** tests the survival of donor's cells even of the same A-B-O group can be followed, for example, if they are of different M-N or Rh-Hr blood types, as pointed out by Wiener. Wiener[63] has also used the differential agglutination test in cases of suspected hemolytic transfusion reaction to determine whether the donor's red cells have actually been hemolyzed.

Wiener[64] has also pointed out that some cases of severe anemia in the newborn are due to massive occult transplacental blood loss in utero into the maternal circulation. In such cases, as shown by Chown,[65] the fetal red cells are demonstrable in the maternal blood by differential agglutination tests. In the more common instances of **transplacental fetal bleeding**, the amount of fetal blood is too small to be demonstrable by such tests, but it can be shown by the Kleihauer[66] method (pp. 294 and 295).

CHIMERAS

In Greek mythology the chimaera was a fire-breathing monster—part lion, part goat, and part serpent—killed by Bellerophon. Biologically, a chimera is an unusual organism with tissue characteristic of two or more types. In blood grouping a chimera exhibits a mixture of cells of different generic constitution, derived from two or more distinct zygote lineages. Chimeras have often been noted in bovines but seldom in man, until fairly recently. Vascular anastomoses are usually present between dissimilar bovine twin embryos; the primitive red cells of one twin take root in the bone marrow of the other twin and continue throughout the life of the second twin to produce red blood cells having genetically foreign antigens. The cow or bull with such a mixture of blood can transmit to its offspring only those genes that were derived through heredity but not the genes for the antigens that are present due to the anastomoses.

Chimeras among humans can be detected by the differential agglutination test to identify the two populations of red cells.

Two types of chimeras have been noted —**twin** and **dispermic.** In twin chimeras, anastomoses are usually present between dissimilar twin embryos. The young red cells in the hematopoietic organs from one twin grow in the bone marrow of the other twin. These primitive cells persist throughout life. Thus there are red cells of different genetic antigens in one and the same person.

In 1953 Dunsford et al.[67] reported a mixture of two kinds of blood in a healthy donor who was later found to be a twin. Her twin brother had died in infancy 25 years prior to this examination. Twenty sets of such twins are described by Race and Sanger.[68]

When a chimera is known to be a twin, classification as a twin chimera is not difficult. But there are recorded cases in which a twin has been aborted or assimilated, and in such cases the classification is difficult to make.

Chimeras may result artificially, as from a bone marrow graft or an intrauterine transfusion. In the latter, donor lymphocytes have been known to persist for as long as a year or more.

In dispermic chimeras there is evidence of two sets of paternal genes with or without mosaicism, such as different color of skin patches or different-colored eyes. Battey et al.[69] in 1974 reported a female chimera who had two red cell populations, 93% O and 7% A_1, with an overwhelming preponderance of lymphocytes with the normal male karyotype 46XY. This patient is referred to in the literature as the **Birmingham chimera.** She was said not to be a twin and there was no evidence of dispermy. She transmitted to her offspring genes that determined her minor red blood cell population. In a later report on the Birmingham chimera, Bird et al.[70] stated that although this patient had said she was not a twin, she could have been a twin and the other twin could have been aborted or assimilated. There was no evidence that dispermy was responsible for the two cell populations. If she is a twin, her true blood group is that represented by her minority red blood cell population (A_1), and her true sex is that represented by her minority lymphocyte population (46XX). If she is in reality a dispermic chimera, she would have two true red cell populations.

Erythrocytic mosaicism in disease

Erythrocytic mosaicism, two different red cell populations in one individual, occurs in certain malignant diseases of lymphoreticular tissue (polycythemia vera, erythroleukemia), somatic mutation, and in monosomy with no apparent disease. In this type of mosaicism, a modification of the erythrocytic membrane occurs. In 1972 Kahn et al.[71] reported a patient having erythroleukemia with a normal A and weak A mosaicism. Callender et al.[72] reported examples of Rh mosaicism in 1971. In 1976

Bird[73] described a male patient having acute erythroleukemia with mixed-field agglutination. At first this appeared to be 60% O and 40% B cells, but it was shown later to be a mixture of normal B and very weak B cells. For more information, see the section on polyagglutinability, p. 229ff.

REFERENCES

1. Socha, W. W., and Wiener, A. S.: N.Y. State J. Med. **73**:2144, 1973.
2. Wiener, A. S., Socha, W. W., and Gordon, E. B.: Br. J. Haematol. **24**:195, 1973.
3. Wiener, A. S., and Ward, F. A.: Am. J. Clin. Pathol. **46**:27, 1966.
4. Dunsford, I., and Aspinall, P.: Ann. Eugen. (Lond.) **17**:32, 1952.
5. Wiener, A. S., and Moloney, W. C.: Am. J. Clin. Pathol. **13**:74, 1943.
6. von Dungern, E., and Hirszfeld, L.: Immunitätsforsch. **8**:526, 1911.
7. Coca, A. F., and Klein, H.: J. Immunol. **8**:477, 1923.
8. Fischer, W., and Hahn, F.: Z. Immunitätsforsch. **84**:177, 1935.
9. Friedenreich, V.: Z. Immunitätsforsch. **89**:409, 1936. (Translation available from Blood Transfusion Research Division, U.S. Army Medical Research Laboratory, Fort Knox, Ky.)
10. Wiener, A. S., and Silverman, L. J.: Am. J. Clin. Pathol. **11**:45, 1941.
11. Gammelgaard, A., and Marcussen, P. V.: Z. Immunitätsforsch. **98**:411, 1940.
12. Wiener, A. S., and Cioffi, A. F.: Am. J. Clin. Pathol. **58**:693, 1972.
13. Wiener, A. S., Moor-Jankowski, J., and Gordon, E. B.: Int. Arch. Allergy **29**:82, 1966.
14. Wiener, A. S., Socha, W. W., and Gordon, E. B.: Vox Sang. **22**:97, 1972.
15. Wiener, A. S., and Karowe, H.: J. Immunol. **49**:51, 1944.
16. Springer, G. F.: Angew. Chem. (Engl.)**5**:909, 1966.
17. Springer, G. F., Horton, R. E., and Forbes, M.: J. Exp. Med. **110**:221, 1959.
17a. Springer, G. F., Nagai, Y., and Tegtmeyer, H.: Biochemistry **5**:3254, 1966.
18. Øyen, R., Colledge, K. I., Marsh, W. L., and Wainfan, E.: Transfusion **12**:98, March-April, 1972.
19. Moody, M. R., Young, V. M., and Faber, J. E.: J. Appl. Microbiol. **181**:262, 1969.
20. Springer, G. F., and Horton, R. E.: J. Gen. Physiol. **47**:1229, 1964.
21. Springer, G. F., Wang, E. T., Nichols, J. H., and Shear, J. M.: Ann. N.Y. Acad. Sci. **316**:17, 1966.
22. Wiener, A. S., and Socha, W. W.: A-B-O blood groups and Lewis types, New York, 1976, Stratton Intercontinental Medical Book Corporation.
23. Watkins, W. M. In Wiener, A. S., editor: Advances in blood grouping, vol. 3, New York, 1970, Grune & Stratton, Inc.
24. Wiener, A. S.: Haematologia (Budap.) **4**:157, 1970.
25. Moreno, C., Lunblad, S., and Kabat, E. A.: J. Exp. Med. **134**:439, 1971.
26. Wiener, A. S., and Gordon, E. B.: Br. J. Haematol. **2**:305, 1956.
27. Prokop, O., Rackwitz, A., and Schlesinger, D.: J. Forensic Med. **12**:108, 1965.
28. Brain, P., and Grace, M. J.: Vox Sang. **15**:297, 1968.
29. Wiener, A. S., Brain, P., and Gordon, E. B.: Haematologia (Budap.) **3**:9, 1969.
30. Brain, P.: Vox Sang. **2**:686, 1966.
31. Konugres, A., and Coombs, R. R. R.: Br. J. Haematol. **4**:261, 1958.
32. Bhende, Y. M., Deshpande, C. K., Bhatia, H. M., Sanger, R., Race, R. R., Morgan, W. T., and Watkins, W. M.: Lancet **1**:903, 1952.
33. Cepellini, R., Nasso, S., and Tecilazich, F.: La malattie emolitica del neonato, Milan, 1952, Istituto Sieroterapice Milanese Serafino Belfanti.
34. Levine, P., Robinson, E., Celano, M., Briggs, O., and Falkenberg, L.: Blood **10**:1100, 1955.
35. Wiener, A. S.: Advances in blood grouping, vol. 3, New York, 1970, Grune & Stratton, Inc.
36. Lanser, S., Ropartz, C., Rousseau, P. Y., Guerbet, Y., and Salmon, C.: Transfusion (Paris) **9**:255, 1966.
37. Mäkelä, O., and Mäkelä, P.: Ann. Med. Exp. Biol. Fenn. **33**:33, 1955.
38. Boorman, K. E., and Zeitlin, R. A.: Proceedings of the 7th Congress of the International Society of Blood Transfusion, 1959.
39. Boorman, K. E., and Zeitlin, R. A.: Vox Sang. **9**:278, 1964.
40. Levine, P., Celano, M., and Griset, T.: Proceedings of the 6th Congress of the International Society of Blood Transfusion, 1958.
41. Moullec, J., Sutton, E., and Burgade, M.: Rev. Hématol. **10**:574, 1955.
42. Sussman, L. N., Pretshold, H., and Lacher, M.: Blood **15**:1788, 1960.
43. Wiener, A. S., Chuba, J. V., Gordon, E. B., and Kuhns, W. J.: Transfusion **8**:226, 1968.
44. Grubb, R.: Acta Pathol. Microbiol. Scand. **84**(supp.):10, 1949.
45. Bhatia, H. M.: Indian J. Med. Res. **52**:5, 1964.
46. Haselhorst, A., and Lauer, A.: Z. Konstit. **15**:205, 1930, and **16**:277, 1931. Cited in

Wiener, A. S.: Blood groups and transfusion, ed. 3, 1943; reprinted, New York, 1962, Hafner Publication Co.

47. Wiener, A. S., Lederer, M., and Polayes, S. H.: J. Immunol. **18**:201, 1930.

48. Reviron, J., Salmon, C., Salmon, D., Delarue, F., and Schenmetzler, C.: 6th Congress of the National Transfusion Sanguinis, 1966. Tours.

49. Reviron, J., and Salmon, C.: Nouv. Rev. Fr. Hématol. **8**:323, 1968.

50. Salmon, C.: Nouv. Rev. Fr. Hématol. **11**:858, 1971.

51. Wiener, A. S., and Moon, G. J.: Haematologia (Budap.) **9**(3-4):235, 1975.

52. Wiener, A. S., Moor-Jankowski, J., and Gordon, E. B.: Int. Arch. Allergy **36**:582, 1969.

53. Moon, G. J., and Wiener, A. S.: Vox Sang. **26**:167, 1974.

54. Cameron, C., Graham, F., Dunsford, I., Sickles, G., MacPherson, C. R., Cahan, R., Sanger, R., and Race, R. R.: Br. Med. J. **2**:29, 1959.

55. Marsh, W. L., Jenkins, W. J., and Walther, W. W.: Br. Med. J. **2**:63, 1959.

56. Garratty, G., Willbanks, E., and Petz, L. D.: Vox Sang. **21**:45, 1971.

57. Salmon, C., Jacquet, A., Kling, C., and Salmon, D.: Nouv. Rev. Fr. Hématol. **7**:755, 1967.

58. Wiener, A. S.: Blood groups and transfusion, ed. 3, 1943; reprinted, New York, 1962, Hafner Publication Co.

59. Wiener, A. S., Moor-Jankowski, J., Cadigan, F. C., Jr., and Gordon, E. B.: Transfusion **8**:235, 1968.

60. Wiener, A. S., Moor-Jankowski, J., Gordon, E. B., and Kratochvil, C. H.: Proc. Natl. Acad. Sci. U.S.A. **56**:458, 1966.

61. Ashby, W.: Arch. Intern. Med. **29**:527, 1922.

62. Mollison, P. L.: Blood transfusion in clinical medicine, ed. 3, Philadelphia, 1961, F. A. Davis Co.

63. Wiener, A. S.: J.A.M.A. **102**:1779, 1934.

64. Wiener, A. S.: Am. J. Obstet. Gynecol. **56**:717, 1948.

65. Chown, B.: Lancet **1**:1213, 1954.

66. Kleihauer, C., Broun, H., and Betke, K.: Klin. Wochenschr. **35**:637, 1957.

67. Dunsford, I., Bowley, C. C., Hutchison, A. M., Thompson, J. S., Sanger, R., and Race, R. R.: Br. Med. J. **2**:81, 1953.

68. Race, R. R., and Sanger, R.: Blood groups in man, ed. 6, Oxford, England, 1975, Blackwell Scientific Publications.

69. Battey, D. A., Bird, G. W. G., McDermott, A., Mortimer, C. W., Mutchinick, O. M., and Wingham, J.: J. Med. Genet. **11**:283, 1974.

70. Bird, G. W. G., Battey, D. A., Greenwell, P., Mortimer, C. W., Watkins, W. W., and Wingham, J.: J. Med. Genet. **13**:70, 1976.

71. Kahn, A., Boivin, P., Wroklans, M., and Hakins, J.: Rev. Fr. Hématol. **12**:609, 1972.

72. Callender, S. T., Kay, H. E. M., Lawler, S. D., Millard, R. E., Sanger, R., and Tippett, P.: Br. Med. J. **1**:131, 1971.

73. Bird, G. W. G.: Rev. fr. Transfus. Immunohématol. **19**:247, 1976.

74. Springer, G. F., Nagai, Y., and Tegtmeyer, H.: Biochemistry **5**:3254, 1966.

75. Weiner, W., Sanger, R., and Race, R. R.: Proceedings of the 7th Congress of the International Society of Blood Transfusion; cited in Race, R. R., and Sanger, R., ed. 6.

76. Sturgeon, P., Moor, B. P. L., and Weiner, W.: Vox Sang. **9**:214, 1964.

6 □ Secretors of blood group substances; the Lewis system

At the time of Landsteiner's discovery of the A-B-O groups, divisions into the various blood groups were made simply by agglutination reactions between antiserum and cells, the serum containing the specific antibody and the cells the specific antigen with which the antibody reacted. Later it was discovered that the A-B-O antigens, or blood group substances, are not limited to the red cells but that they can be found in soluble form in the body fluids of individuals who are secretors of these substances.

SECRETOR GENES AND THE H SUBSTANCE

Five blood group specificities are detectable in human secretions—**A, B, H, Le**[a], and **Le**[b]. The gene systems *ABO, Hh, Lele,* for these specificities, are closely interrelated, but the specificities have certain chemical structures that differentiate them (p. 67ff). The A, B, and H substances are found in secretions in man only when the corresponding antigen is present on the surface of the red cells, but in Old World monkeys and gorillas they are present in saliva and absent from the red cells. About 20% of Caucasoids with A-B-H antigens on their red cells fail to secrete the corresponding substances in their body fluids. The ability to secrete the A-B-H antigens in the saliva was first reported by Schiff and Sasaki,[1] who showed that the genes responsible for such ability are inherited as mendelian dominants. The allelic genes that control this ability are *Se* and *se;* these

are inherited independently of the *ABO* genes.

It is now accepted that whenever the gene *Se* appears in either single or double dose, the individual will be a secretor of the A-B-H substances; that is, the A-B-H substance will be present in the saliva and other body fluids. When the *se* gene is present in double dose, the individual will not be a secretor (nonsecretor). Secretors are designated Sec, and nonsecretors are nS.

There are two distinct forms of the A-B-O antigen: (1) a water-soluble form not present in red cells or serum but present in most of the body fluids and organs of secretors and (2) an alcohol-soluble form present in all tissues except the brain and on the red cells but absent from the secretions. The water-soluble form is determined by the secretor gene *Se;* the alcohol-soluble form is not influenced by this gene. Absence of *Se* gene is designated *se.*

Secretors of A must have at least one *A* gene, at least one *Se* gene, and at least one *H* gene.

Three combinations of A-B-H secretor genes are possible: homozygous *SeSe,* heterozygous *Sese,* and homozygous *sese.* *SeSe* and *Sese* people are secretors; *sese* people are not. Nonsecretors among American Indians comprise about 1%, whereas 40% of Negroids are nonsecretors of the A-B-H substance. According to Race and Sanger,[2] the gene frequencies are 52.33% for *Se* and 47.67% for *se.* The genotype frequencies obtained in Liverpool were as follows: of the secretor types, 35.4% were *SeSe* and 64.6% were *Sese;* 22.72% of the population proved to be nonsecretors *(sese).*

If both parents are homozygous *SeSe,* all the children will be *SeSe.* If one parent is *SeSe* and the other is *Sese,* all children will be secretors, but half will be homozygous *SeSe,* the other half *Sese.* If both parents are heterozygous *Sese,* one fourth of the children will be homozygous *SeSe,* one half will be *Sese,* and one fourth will be *sese*— nonsecretors (three fourths will be secretors).

The *Se-se* genes are transmitted independently of the A-B-O genes, as illustrated in Table 6-1, which presents the results of a mating of a group AB Sec male with a group AB nS female. The symbols Sec and nS designate phenotypes, secretor and nonsecretor, respectively.

Watkins and Morgan,[3] Ceppellini,[4] and others pointed out that the formation of H substance is apparently controlled by a pair of allelic genes, *H* and *h.* When the *H* gene appears in single or double dose, the H character is present; when the very rare allele *h* is present in double dose, the H character is absent, as in individuals of the Bombay types. According to Watkins and Morgan, the H-active material, under the influence of the *A* and *B* genes, is

mostly converted into the **A- and B-active substances.** The existence of large quantities of H substance in group O persons seems to be due to the absence of the *A* and *B* genes in that group. A, B, and H antigens are well developed in the saliva of the newborn.

Individuals who secrete the substances are termed **secretors;** the others are **nonsecretors.** The blood group substances can be extracted with aqueous solutions from tissues and organs of secretors, especially from their salivary glands and gastric mucosa; these substances are also present in high concentration in the saliva, gastric juice, and semen. A-B-H group substances have also been found on spermatozoa of secretors, most probably adsorbed from the seminal fluid.[5] Water-soluble group substances are not demonstrable in the body fluids or secretions of nonsecretors. The terms secretor and nonsecretor apply only to the A, B, and H antigens, although Le[a] and Le[b] antigens are present in the saliva of the respective Le type, as is antigen Sd[a].

THE LEWIS SYSTEM

In their review on the Lewis blood group in 1964, Wiener et al.[6] pointed out that Landsteiner and Levine[7] had described in 1929 an irregular isoagglutinin, which in retrospect can be recognized as having the **Lewis** specificity. Cases of severe and fatal hemolytic transfusion reactions that, also in retrospect, can be recognized as having been due to Lewis sensitization were described by Parr and Krischner[8] in 1932, by Neter[9] in 1936, and by Levine and Polayes[10] in 1941. It was not until 1946, however, when Mourant[11] described the same antibody in the serum of a patient, Lewis, that the antibody received its name, anti-**Le.** When Andresen[12] in 1948 described an antibody of related specificity, Mourant's antibody was designated anti-**Le**[a] and Andresen's anti-**Le**[b].

It was Grubb[13] who in 1948 first pointed out that practically all persons who have the **Lewis** factor on their red blood cells

Table 6-1. Independent transmission of genes for the A-B-O blood groups and the ABH secretor types[*]

Germ cells	Sperm cells			
	A Se	*A se*	*B Se*	*B se*
A se	*AA Sese*	*AA sese*	*AB Sese*	*AB sese*
Ova				
B se	*AB Sese*	*AB sese*	*BB Sese*	*BB sese*

As shown, in the mating of group AB secretor father with a group AB nonsecretor mother, among the children there should be ⅛ A Sec, ⅛ A nS, ¼ AB Sec, ¼ AB nS, ⅛ B Sec, and ⅛ B nS.

[*]Modified from Wiener, A. S., and Socha, W. W.: A-B-O blood groups and Lewis types, New York, 1976, with permission of Stratton Intercontinental Medical Book Corporation.

are nonsecretors of the A-B-H substances and that those who lack the **Lewis** factor on their red cells are almost always secretors. Wiener et al.[6,14] have contributed to the knowledge of the Lewis blood group system with their studies on nonhuman primates, and they have proposed a new system of nomenclature. Watkins,[15] in her studies on the biochemistry of the A, B, H, and Le substances, further clarified the subject of secretors and nonsecretors of blood group substances.

Although the Lewis blood group system was not discovered until 1946, and the M-N, P, and Rh-Hr systems had been reported earlier than that year, the Le system and the knowledge of the H substances are so closely linked with the A-B-O blood groups that they are discussed here and not in a later chapter.

Lewis antigen and A-B-H secretor genes

The Lewis antigen and A-B-H secretor genes must not be confused. The genes for the Lewis antigen and for secretors are present on different chromosomes. It was originally believed that the Lewis substances, Le^a and Le^b, were determined by corresponding allelic genes, *Le^a* and *Le^b*, respectively. In fact, that is why the symbols Le^a and Le^b were introduced. However, if Le^a and Le^b were due to allelic genes, there should be three types analogous to the three M-N types: Le(a+b−), Le(a−b+), and Le(a+b+). Actually, type Le(a+b+) is nonexistent or is rare in adults, but there is a type Le(a−b−), contrary to expectations. It is now realized that Le^b is not due to a gene *Le^b* allelic to *Le^a* but instead is a specificity of the product of the combined action of the *Lewis* and *H* genes. Le^b is therefore better designated, as noted by Wiener, as Le^H or even as H^{Le}. However, most workers continue to use the original nomenclature, and this remains a source of misunderstanding and errors. According to the present concept, the Lewis types are determined by a pair of allelic genes *Le* and *le*, so that Lewis-positive in-

dividuals can be homozygous *(LeLe)* or heterozygous *(Lele)*, and Lewis-negative individuals are genotype *lele*.

The **genes for the Lewis types** are inherited independently of the *ABO* and the *Sese* genes, but there is a close relationship between the A-B-O and Lewis systems insofar as the secreted substances are concerned. The reason for this appears to be that the determinant groups responsible for the **Le** specificities are on the same macromolecules as the determinant groups responsible for the specificities **H, A,** and **B.** In single or double dose the *Le* gene gives rise to the **Le** (or Le^a) specificity. The *le* gene in double dose results in its absence. The expression of the *Le* gene is *not* controlled by the *Se-se* genes. The **Le** and **H** specificities are due to separate L-fucose determinant groups on the same molecule. The juxtaposition of the two fucose groups evidently gives rise to the specificity **Le^H** (**Le^b**). The null type Le(a−b−) is homozygous recessive and is due to the *le* gene.

Nature of the Lewis types

The Lewis types differ from the usual blood groups in that in this system there is no agglutinogen as such, but instead there is a **water-soluble Lewis substance,** present in body fluids and secretions such as saliva, semen, and vaginal fluid, and the Lewis group substances are only secondarily adsorbed onto the red blood cells. This adsorption renders the red cells reactive when they are mixed with anti-**Lewis** serum.

The Lewis and A-B-H substances are chemically similar, and for that reason they are believed to be derived from the same substrate. When the *Le*, or *Lewis*, genes and the *Se*, or *secretor*, genes occur together in the same person, they compete for this same substrate, a mucopolysaccharide. Lewis secretors who are A-B-H nonsecretors will therefore generally have more Lewis substance in their body fluids than will those who are A-B-H secretors. (See Fig. 5-1.)

Since the Lewis antigen is not an agglutinogen intrinsic to the red cells but rather a substance adsorbed onto them, individuals who are **Lewis** secretors but not secretors of the A-B-H substance will have more highly reactive cells with anti-**Lewis** serum than will individuals who have both the Lewis and the A-B-H substances. The red cells of those who are nonsecretors of the Lewis substance, whether or not they are secretors of the A-B-H substance, *do not react* with anti-**Lewis** serum.

Importance of the Lewis factors

In addition to contributing to the knowledge of secretors and nonsecretors and to the study of the biochemistry of the blood group substances, the Lewis groups are important because of their role in certain transfusion reactions and in genetic studies, as well as in investigation of the blood groups in nonhuman primates and other animals.

Clinically, the Lewis system is important primarily in transfusions because individuals who lack the substance in their saliva are Lewis negative, and they can become sensitized to the **Lewis** factor if transfused with Lewis-positive cells. If a subsequent transfusion is performed using Lewis-positive cells, the antibodies produced as a result of the first transfusion are capable of reacting with the incoming Lewis-positive cells, which could result in a serious or even fatal hemolytic transfusion reaction. According to Wiener and Socha,[16] production of Lewis antibodies and hemolytic transfusion reactions caused by Lewis sensitization are much more common in Negroids than in whites, which is not surprising since the Lewis type le occurs in nearly 23% of Negroids against only 3% of whites (in New York City). No cases of erythroblastosis fetalis due to Lewis sensitization have been reported for the reason that the **Lewis antibodies** are of the 19S variety and thus do not pass through the placenta. Another reason is that in **newborn infants** the Lewis substance is not yet on the red cells, and all

newborn infants react as Lewis negative in tests on their red cells.

When an Le(a−) recipient is transfused with Le(a+) blood, differential agglutination tests with anti-**Le**[a] serum after a relatively short period of time show that all the red cells in the recipient's circulation react as Le(a−), even though the donor's red cells survive normally, as shown by blood grouping sera of anti-**M** and other specificities. Likewise, when an Le(a+) recipient is transfused with Le(a−) blood, the Le(a−) red cells are not demonstrable in the recipient's circulation by differential agglutination with anti-**Le** serum.

Red cells of fetuses and newborn infants react as Le(a−), even when the Lewis substance can be demonstrated in their saliva and serum by inhibition tests. By the time the infants reach the age of 3 months, 80% will react with anti-**Le**[a] serum.[17] By the age of 2 years, the adult frequency of 20% is attained. The agglutinability · of maternal cells decreases during pregnancy.

When Le(a−) red cells are transfused to an Le(a+) recipient, the incoming Le(a−) cells adsorb the Lewis substance from the recipient's plasma and then react as Le(a+). When Le(a+) cells are introduced into an Le(a−) subject, the Lewis substance of the incoming Le(a+) cells is eluted by the recipient's plasma and the cells become Le(a−). For these reasons, anti-**Le** serum is not used to trace survival of transfused red cells, and for the same reasons, in chimeras, tests with anti-**Le** sera fail to show the mixture of Lewis blood types.[16]

Once the Lewis substance is adsorbed onto the red cells, the cells become agglutinable by anti-**Le** sera. The reaction is not as sharp as the reactions with anti-A and anti-B sera.

Red cells with adsorbed Lewis substance can be hemolyzed by anti-Le sera, which is a source of dangerous hemolytic transfusion reactions.[7-9] Sensitized le recipients should first be given transfusion of Le-positive plasma or purified Lewis substance when type le donors are not available, until the patient's antibodies have been neutralized, after which the incompatible Lewis-positive blood can be transfused safely. By the time the antibodies reappear in the recipient's circulation, the transfused Le-positive red cells have lost their coat of Lewis substance and will survive normally.

Sources of Le substance. Le[a] substance is present in the saliva of more than 90% of Europeans. Milk is a richer source of Le[a] substance than is saliva in recently delivered women who have an *Le* gene.[18] Le[a] substance is present in gastric juice in the same amount as in saliva. Urine is a rich source of Le[a] substance. Le[a] is also present in seminal fluid.

Although the nomenclature is now accepted as Lewis types, the Japanese workers by 1939 identified an antigen in nonsecretor saliva using a precipitin reaction with certain normal chicken sera.[19] The antigen was termed T and the antibody anti-T. These terms are not to be confused with Friedenreich's 1930 antigen T and its antibody anti-**T** (refer to index). The Japanese T and anti-**T** apparently are the same as the Lewis and anti-**Lewis.** They found the T substance present in saliva, serum, milk, urine, seminal fluid, amniotic fluid, meconium, gum arabic, etc.

Nomenclature in the Lewis system

The nomenclature in the Lewis system is confusing mainly because when the Le factors were first discovered, the nature of the Lewis substance and its relationship to the secretor types were not fully understood. The factors, for example, were originally designated **Le**[a] and **Le**[b], and some texts still use this nomenclature, although it is now known that the **Le** factors are not due to allelic genes. The symbol Le(a+) is used to designate cells that are agglutinated by anti-**Le**[a] serum, and Le(a−) is used for cells that are not so agglutinated. **Le**[b] was at first considered to be the antithesis of **Le**[a] because it usually occurs on the red cells when **Le**[a] is absent. As previously shown, however, the so-called

anti-**Le**[a] and anti-**Le**[b] sera identified only three types, Le(a+b−), Le(a−b+), and Le(a−b−), but no type Le(a+b+). If *Le*[a] and *Le*[b] were actually alleles, as the nomenclature seems to imply, then the nonexistence or rarity of type Le(a+b+) would be a paradox.

It is now generally accepted that the **genes for the Lewis system** are *Le* and *le*, and there is no special gene *Le*[b]. Genotypes with at least one *Le* present result in either red cell phenotype Le(a+b−) or Le(a−b+). Genotype *lele* results in the red cell phenotype Le(a−b−). Since the *se* gene cannot act on Le[a] substance, individuals with an *Le* and two *se* genes have red cell type Le(a+b−). Those with two *le* genes do not form Le[a] so that whether or not the *Se* gene is present, *lele* persons will be red cell phenotype Le(a−b−).

Some authors maintain that the *A* and *B* genes not only convert H substance to A and B but also convert some Le[b] into A or B substance: group A or B persons have fewer Lewis antigens than group O persons of the same Lewis type.

This complex system has been clarified by the work of Grubb and Ceppellini[20] and by Wiener et al.,[6] who introduced a **new and simpler nomenclature** that eliminates the Le[b] paradox.

SALIVA TYPES

Adopting the notations of previous workers, Wiener et al.[6] presented the following classification of the Lewis types:

1. Presence of the Lewis substance in the saliva—Les
2. Absence of the Lewis substance from the saliva—nL
3. Secretors of the H substance—Sec
4. Nonsecretors of the H substance—nS

Since, as Ceppillini has shown, the Lewis and the H substances are genetically independent of one another, in combination they determine **four saliva types:** (1) Les Sec, (2) Les nS, (3) nL Sec, and (4) nL nS.

Not only must the **blood type** in the Lewis system be designated but also must the **saliva type.** The preceding classification refers only to the saliva type.

BLOOD TYPES

Le₁. Since the Lewis and H substances are both derived from the same substrate, Le secretors who are A-B-H nonsecretors (saliva type Les nS) will generally have more Le substance in their body fluids than will A-B-H secretors (saliva type Les Sec); therefore their blood cells will be highly reactive with anti-**Lewis** serum. These individuals are blood type Le₁.

Le₂. In individuals of saliva type Les Sec, the blood cells are less reactive with anti-**Lewis** serum and therefore are designated blood type Le₂. These persons are secretors of both the Le and the H substance.

le. The red cells of individuals of either saliva type nL Sec or saliva type nL nS are nonreactive with anti-**Lewis** serum, since the cells have not adsorbed any Lewis substance, which is not present in the saliva or other body fluids. These individuals are designated as blood type le.

Nomenclature of the Lewis antisera

Some **Lewis** antisera react with cells of both blood types Le₁ and Le₂, and these antisera are designated simply as anti-**Le.** They were formerly called anti-**Le**^{x}.

Anti-**Le₁** designation has been assigned to the antisera formerly called anti-**Le**^{a}. These are reactive only with cells of type Le₁.

The red cells of type Le₂ are agglutinated specifically by certain other rare sera originally designated anti-**Le**^{b}. Persons whose blood cells react with these antisera carry both dominant genes *Le* and *Se,* and they are **saliva type** Les Sec. They have both the Lewis and the H substances in their saliva, as well as a third specificity that results from the presence of both Le and H on the same macromolecule. Since this specificity identifies a hybrid of Lewis and H, it should be designated **Le**^{H} (or **H**^{Le}). The antigen is present in the body fluids and is only secondarily adsorbed onto the red cells of type Le₂ individuals. Anti-**Le**^{H} serum as a rule reacts most intensely with red blood cells of group O and subgroup A₂ individuals. These sera, formerly called anti-**Le**^{b}, should now be designated anti-**Le**^{H}. By adopting this designation, the incorrect implication of allelism between *Le*^{a} and *Le*^{b} is eliminated.

Production of Lewis antibodies

Only those who lack the Lewis substance can form anti-**Lewis** antibodies. Such individuals would be of saliva type nL and blood type le. Although to date all sensitized Lewis-negative patients have been A-B-H secretors, there is no reason to believe that A-B-H nonsecretors could not also form anti-**Le** antibodies, that is, if they are nonsecretors of the Lewis substance.

Anti-**Le**^{H} antibodies are formed by subjects who are saliva type nL and are also A-B-H nonsecretors. Except among Negroids, this type is relatively rare, so that sensitization to **Le**^{H} occurs infrequently.

General considerations in Lewis typing

Lewis typing can be done without the use of anti-**Le**^{H} antiserum. Typing of saliva and of the red cells is carried out using ordinary anti-**Le** serum, plus a suitable anti-**H** reagent like anti-**H** lectin made from extracts of seeds of *Ulex europeus.*

The reactions of red cells may vary even in the same individual when Lewis tests are made on cells. The reactions are dependent to a great degree on the age of the subject and the methods used in the tests. This is especially true of tests made during the neonatal period and during pregnancy. Tests on saliva, on the other hand, usually yield consistent and reproducible results.

Lewis donors

When seeking compatible donors for patients who have become sensitized to the **Lewis** factor, tests of the red cells should be made on all prospective donors, along with inhibition tests of the saliva, to establish both the saliva and blood types. The methods are described in Chapter 18.

Frequency of the Lewis types

Based on the figures of McConnell[21] relating to Caucasoids in England and on the figures of Ceppellini and Siniscalco[22] from their work with Negroids in Charleston, West Virginia, the frequency of the Le saliva types is as presented in Table 6-2.

As has already been mentioned, according to the theory of Ceppellini, the Lewis and secretor genes are independent of one another; that is, they are located on different pairs of chromosomes. This theory implies the following relationship among the frequencies of the four saliva types: $\overline{\text{Les Sec}} \times \overline{\text{nL nS}} = \overline{\text{Les nS}} \times \overline{\text{nL Sec}}$. (The fact that the analogous formula for the four

A-B-O groups, $\overline{AB} \times \overline{O} = \overline{A} \times \overline{B}$, does not hold was used by Bernstein as proof that the A and B agglutinogens are not inherited independently of one another, as postulated by von Dungern and Hirszfeld.)

In the case of the saliva types, the following results are obtained for Caucasoids: $\overline{\text{Les Sec}} \times \overline{\text{nL nS}} = 73.5 \times 0.6 = 42.1$, while $\overline{\text{Les nS}} \times \overline{\text{nL Sec}} = 23.1 \times 2.8 = 65.7$. Thus the fit with the theoretical expectation is reasonably close. For Negroids $\overline{\text{Les Sec}} \times \overline{\text{nL nS}} = 58.5 \times 5.9 = 345$, and $\overline{\text{Les nS}} \times \overline{\text{nL Sec}} = 18.6 \times 17.0 = 316$, so that in this case the fit is even closer.

The **Wiener classification of the Lewis blood types** in man, including their reactions and possible genotypes, is given in Table 6-3.

Designation Le^c

In 1972 Gunson and Latham[23] found in the serum of a patient a cold agglutinin that reacted only with cells of Le(a–b–) nonsecretor persons. This patient had been transfused once and had had four pregnancies. This antibody had been predicted by Potapov[24] and named by him anti-**Le^c**.

Table 6-2. Frequency of the Le-Se saliva types

Designation	Caucasoids (%)	Negroids (%)
Les nS	23.1	18.6
Les Sec	73.5	58.5
nL Sec	2.8	17.0
nL nS	0.6	5.9

Table 6-3. Lewis blood types in man (after Wiener) *

Present symbol	Previous symbols	Reactions of red cells with anti-Le serum	Le substance in saliva	A-B-H substance in saliva	Possible genotypes†
Le₁	Lewis positive Le(a+) Le(a+b−)	+	Present (type Les)	Absent (type nS)	*LeLe sese* *Lele sese*
Le₂	Lewis negative Le(a−) Le(a−b+)	±‡	Present (type Les)	Present (type Sec)	*LeLe SeSe* *Lele SeSe* *LeLe Sese* *Lele Sese*
le	Lewis negative Le(a−) Le(a−b−)	−	Absent (type nL)	Present (type Sec) Absent (type nS)	*lele SeSe* *lele Sese* *lele sese*

*From Erskine, A. G. In Frankel, S., Reitman, S., and Sonnenwirth, A. C., editors: Gradwohl's clinical laboratory methods and diagnosis, vol. 1, ed. 7, St. Louis, 1970, The C. V. Mosby Co.
†Theory of Ceppellini. In International Society of Blood Transfusion: Proceedings of the 5th Congress, Paris, **1955**, pp. 207-211.
‡Red cells may react either positively or negatively, depending on the potency and freshness of the reagent.

The Le^c:anti-Le^c reaction was strongly inhibited by saliva of Le(a–b–) nonsecretors, less strongly by Le(a–b–) secretors as well as Le(a+b–) nonsecretors, and hardly at all by Le(a–b+) secretors. Anti-Le^c serum agglutinates the cells of Le(a–b–) nonsecretors but not those of Le(a–b–) secretors.

Designation Le^d

Potapov[25] immunized a goat with group O saliva from a group O Le(a–b+) individual and obtained an antiserum that had a strong anti-Le^b antibody, as well as other antibodies, after absorption with Le(a+b–) trypsinated cells. The other antibodies consisted of IgG(7S), cold-reactive antibodies, titers 8 to 16, which did not agglutinate Le(a+b–) cells or Le(a–b–) cells from nonsecretors but did agglutinate Le(a–b–) cells from secretors. This new Lewis antigen, characteristic of Le(a–b–) A-B-H secretors, was designated Le^d. Two designations have been suggested for the Lewis system to include this new antiserum—one by Potapov and one by Wiener.

According to Potapov, type Les nS gives rise to specificity Le^a (Le_1), and type Les Sec gives rise to Le^b (Le_2), and there is evidence that type nL nS has a specificity Le^c, and type nL Sec has a specificity Le^d.

A **simplified nomenclature** was proposed by Wiener. Table 6-4 shows this nomenclature (new designations of genotypes) and frequencies as presented by Potapov.[24] In this simplified table the four **saliva types** are Les Sec, Les nS, nL Sec, and nL nS, and the corresponding **red cell types** are LH, Lh, lH, and lh, respectively.

Designation Le^x

Wiener and Socha[16] reviewed the work of Arcilla and Sturgeon[25] who, in 1974, reported their findings with respect to anti-Le^x. Wiener and Socha postulated that Le^x occupies a position in the Lewis system similar to that of **C** in the A-B-O system. Anti-Le^x agglutinates red cells that have Le^a or Le^b but does not react with red cells that lack both specificities. The three Lewis blood types, if tested with anti-Le^a, anti-Le^b, and anti-Le^x sera, would show the following results:

1. $Le_1 = Le(a+b-x+)$
2. $Le_2 = Le(a-b+x+)$
3. $le = Le(a-b-x-)$

The principal value of anti-Le^x serum is its use in testing cord red cells. Arcilla and Sturgeon showed that red cells of newborn infants that characteristically fail to agglutinate with anti-Le^a or anti-Le^b sera do react with anti-Le^x sera. It seems, there-

Table 6-4. Simplified designation of the Lewis saliva and red cell types (Wiener nomenclature)*

Genotypes	Saliva types designation	Percent	Anti-Le (Le^x)	Anti-Le^h (Le_1 or Le^a)	Anti-Le^H (Le^b)	Anti-le^H (anti-Le^d)	Symbol of blood type
LL SS Ll SS LL Ss Ll Ss	Les Sec	74.2	+	–	+	–	LH (Le_2)
LL ss Ll ss	Les nS	13.9	+	+	–	–	Lh (Le_1)
ll SS ll Ss	nL Sec	9.8	–	–	–	+	lH ⎫
ll ss	nL nS	2.1	–	–	–	–	lh ⎭ (le)

*Modified from Wiener and Potapov.[16,24]

Anti-le^H or anti-Le^d is the new antibody of Potapov. The hypothetical le^h (Le^c) is omitted from the table.

fore, that it is now possible to distinguish the Lewis positive from the Lewis negative newborn infants by the use of anti-**Le**^{x} sera, as follows: Le$_1$ or Le$_2$ are Le(a–b–x+), whereas le is Le(a–b–x–).

It is strongly suggested that **Le**^{x} may be a precursor of Le$_1$ and Le$_2$.

Nature of the Lewis reactions

Approximately 20% of individuals give positive reactions with anti-**Lewis** sera against their red cells independently of their A-B-O blood groups. This agglutination is equally intense at 20° and 37° C with many antisera. The clumps vary in size over a background of unagglutinated cells. If **fresh serum** from a Lewis-sensitized person is used, the Lewis-positive red cells dissolve, or hemolyze, when tested at 37° C in vitro, and this generally incomplete hemolysis masks agglutination. If the test is performed at room temperature, which is about 20° C in the temperate zones, agglutination occurs and hemolysis is usually not observed. If the serum has been inactivated before use, that is, if the complement is rendered inactive by heat, agglutination takes place at both 20° and 37° C. Antiglobulin tests and tests using ficinated red cells give readable reactions, although the strongest reactions occur when the ficinated cell antiglobulin technic is employed.

When the stronger Lewis antisera are used fresh, **hemolysis** occurs with saline-suspended Lewis-positive red cells, especially if the red cells have been ficinated. If the antisera are allowed to stand in a refrigerator or at room temperature for several days, they lose their hemolytic properties but retain their agglutinating ability using the antiglobulin and ficinated cell technics. A few lose all reactivity except by the **ficinated cell antiglobulin method.** Eventually, the antisera will react only with ficinated type Le$_1$ cells, which includes approximately 20% of the population, that is, those who have the Lewis substance in their saliva and are nonsecretors of A-B-H substance.

Nature of the Lewis antibodies

Anti-**Lewis** antibodies may be either naturally occurring or isoimmune. Those that occur naturally react best at low temperature. Isoimmune **Lewis** antibodies react best at 37° C. The natural anti-**Le** antibodies react almost exclusively with type Le$_1$ cells, originally called Le(a+b–). Isoimmune **Le** antibodies react with both the Le$_1$ and Le$_2$ cells.

The Lewis factor in infants

In newborn infants the red cells usually are not agglutinated by anti-**Le** serum, except the rare anti-**Le**^{x} (p. 89). During the first year after birth, positive reactions rise in frequency to nearly 90%, then decrease again to the adult frequency of 20%.

REFERENCES

1. Schiff, F., and Sasaki, H.: Klin. Wochenschr. **2**:1426, 1932.
2. Race, R. R., and Sanger, R.: Blood groups in man, ed. 6, Oxford, England, 1975, Blackwell Scientific Publications.
3. Watkins, W. M., and Morgan, W. T. J.: Vox Sang. **4**:97, 1959.
4. Ceppellini, R.: In Wolstenholme, G. E. W., and O'Connor, C. M., editors: Symposium on the Biochemistry of Human Genetics, London, 1959, J. & A. Churchill, Ltd.
5. Edwards, R. G., Ferguson, L. C., and Coombs, R. R. A.: J. Reprod. Fertil. **7**:153, 1964.
6. Wiener, A. S., Gordon, E. B., and Moor-Jankowski, J.: J. Forensic Med. **11**:67, 1964.
7. Landsteiner, K., and Levine, P.: J. Immunol. **17**:1, 1929.
8. Parr, L. W., and Krischner, R. H.: J.A.M.A. **98**:47, 1932.
9. Neter, E.: J. Immunol. **30**:225, 1936.
10. Levine, P., and Polayes, S. H.: Ann. Intern. Med. **14**:1903, 1941.
11. Mourant, A. E.: Nature (Lond.) **158**:237, 1946.
12. Andresen, P. H.: Acta Pathol. Microbiol. Scand. **25**:728, 1948.
13. Grubb, R.: Nature (Lond.) **162**:933, 1948.
14. Wiener, A. S.: Am. J. Clin. Pathol. **43**:388, 1965.
15. Watkins, W. M.: Science **152**:172, 1966.
16. Wiener, A. S., and Socha, W. A.: A-B-O blood groups and Lewis types, New York, 1976, Stratton Intercontinental Medical Book Corporation.
17. Andresen, P. H.: Acta Pathol. Microbiol. Scand. **24**:616, 1948.

18. Lawler, S. D.: Proceedings of the 7th Congress European Society of Haematology, London, Part II, 1219, 1959.

19. Ueyama, R.: Hanzaigaku-Zasshi, 13:51, 1939 (in Japanese), and Jpn. J. Med. Sci. Sect. VII, Social Med. Hyg. 3:23, 1940.

20. Ceppellini, R.: Proceedings of the 5th International Congress of Blood Transfusion, Paris, 1955.

21. McConnell, R. B.: Conference on Human Genetics, Rome, 1961 (abstract available from Excerpta Medica Foundation, Amsterdam).

22. Ceppellini, R., and Siniscalco, M.: Rev. Istituto Sieroterap. Ital. 30:431, 1955.

23. Gunson, H. H., and Latham, V.: Vox Sang. 22:344, 1972.

24. Potapov, M. I.: Probl. Hematol. (Moscow) 15(11):45, 1970.

25. Arcilla, N. B., and Sturgeon, P.: Vox Sang. 26:425, 1974.

7 □ The M-N-S blood group system

The M-N blood group system was discovered in 1927 by Landsteiner and Levine[1,2] when they immunized rabbits with human red blood cells. This was the second blood group system to be discovered, and it differed from the manner in which the A-B-O blood groups had been found in that the antibodies were artificially produced by injection of blood cells into an animal and were not naturally occurring like anti-**A** and anti-**B** agglutinins.

DISCOVERY OF THE M-N TYPES

Landsteiner and Levine injected rabbits with human blood cells and produced certain antibodies in these animals. When these rabbits' blood sera were absorbed with the cells of certain individuals other than the ones whose blood had been used for the injections, the resulting absorbed antiserum agglutinated the blood cells of other humans, as well as those of the person(s) whose blood was used to produce the antiserum. Two different antisera were produced—one designated anti-**M**, the other anti-**N**—and these identified two corresponding human blood group antigens M and N. The symbols M and N were taken from the word "iMmuNe" to indicate the manner in which the antisera had been produced. These two antisera determined three distinct blood types in humans—type M, in which the blood cells were agglutinated by anti-**M** and not by anti-**N**; type N, in which the cells were agglutinated by anti-**N** and not by anti-**M**; and MN, in which the cells were agglutinated by both anti-**M** and anti-**N**. No bloods have been found lacking both the M and N agglutinogens. Table 7-1 shows the reactions of the three principal M-N types, together with their suggested binary code numbers.

The approximate **frequencies** among Caucasoids have been found to be 30% for M, 20% for N, and 50% for MN. The **distribution** in some other representative racial groups is shown in Table 7-2.

The three types are named for their agglutinogen content, according to convention. Natural anti-**M** and anti-**N** antibodies have been found in human sera but are rare, especially anti-**N**, and the M and N antigens are relatively weakly antigenic for humans. For this reason, the M and N blood types are seldom considered when selecting donors for blood transfusions.

The method of preparing anti-**M** and anti-**N** sera for testing purposes is essentially the same at present as that described by Landsteiner and Levine in their original report, except that now the blood used for injecting rabbits is not selected "blind" but contains *known* M or N agglutinogen. Blood group O, which lacks the A and B

Table 7-1. The three M-N types

Anti-M serum + cells	Anti-N serum + cells	Type	Binary code number
+	−	M	10
−	+	N	01
+	+	MN	11

+ = agglutination; − = no agglutination.

agglutinogens, is used for the injections to prevent formation of immune antibodies against the A or B agglutinogens.

After sufficient injections over a period of time, the rabbit serum is first tested for anti-**M** or anti-**N** agglutinins. If they are present in sufficiently high titer, all the blood is removed from the rabbit, and the serum is separated, diluted, and then absorbed with pooled group O, A, and B cells to remove species-specific antibodies, as well as any anti-**A** and anti-**B** agglutinins that may be present. The serum is then titrated for its anti-**M** or anti-**N** content against known M, N, and MN cells. If the antisera are not absorbed with A and B cells, they might cause agglutination of human cells because of their anti-**A** and anti-**B** content and not because of anti-**M** or anti-**N**.

IMPORTANCE OF THE M-N TYPES

Because the M-N types are only weakly antigenic for man, they are usually of little importance in blood transfusions. They are of considerable importance in forensic medicine, however, especially in tests in cases of disputed parentage (pp. 94 to 96).

DIFFERENTIAL AGGLUTINATION

The M and N types are considered **natural tags** for incoming donor cells in the patient's circulation. Often the donors and recipient in a transfusion belong to different M and N types, and, when this is so, these types can be useful in tracing survival of the donor cells within the patient's circulation (pp. 78 and 324). These **survival tests,** also designated **differential agglutination,** aid in the study of transfusion reactions and in comparing the relative merits of different methods for storing blood in blood banks.

THE M-N BLOOD GROUP SYSTEM

The three M-N types have proved to be related and thus form the basis for the M-N blood group system. By family studies, Landsteiner and Levine proved that the M and N characteristics are inherited by means of **allelic genes** *M* and *N*. Individuals of genotype *MM* are type M, those of genotype *NN* are type N, and those of genotype *MN* are type MN.

According to Allen[3] and Metaxas and Metaxas-Buehler,[4] there is a null gene at

Table 7-2. Racial distribution and gene frequencies in the M-N types*

Race or nationality	Number tested	Types (%)			Gene frequencies	
		M	**N**	**MN**	*M*	*N*
Ainu	504	17.86	31.94	50.20	43.0	57.0
Australian aborigines	730	3.0	67.4	29.6	17.8	82.2
Chinese	1,029	33.24	18.17	48.59	57.5	42.5
English	1,522	30.48	21.36	48.16	54.6	45.4
Eskimos†	569	83.48	0.88	15.64	91.3	8.7
Eskimos‡	1,063	66.2	2.9	31.0	81.6	18.4
Germans	40,255	30.22	19.73	50.04	55.2	44.8
Hindus	300	42.7	10.7	46.7	76.0	24.0
American Indians	140	59.29	7.85	32.86	75.7	24.3
Japanese	7,551	28.99	21.09	49.93	54.0	46.0
Negroes (NYC)	278	28.42	21.94	49.64	53.2	46.8

*From Wiener, A. S.: Blood groups and transfusion, ed. 3, 1943; reprinted New York, 1962, Hafner Publication Co.
†East Greenland.
‡Southwest Greenland.

the M-N locus, but the null type has never been found. This gene produces no M, N, S, s, or U, and is clearly a recessive gene. It has been postulated that homozygosity for such a gene may be a lethal condition.

CLINICAL SIGNIFICANCE

Although the M and N types are regarded as of little clinical significance, there are cases of hemolytic transfusion reactions due to anti-**M** and anti-**N** agglutinins.[5,6] Yoell[7] reported a hemolytic transfusion reaction due to anti-**N** in the serum of a group O type Rh₀ type M patient as a result of multiple transfusions of packed type MN cells. Masters and Vos[8] described anti-**N** formation in a 10-week-old infant. If a patient is to receive blood transfusions over a period of months, it is best to use blood of the same M-N type as that of the recipient.

M sensitization due to incompatible M-N transfusions in individuals of type N has also been reported by a number of authors.[9,10] A patient with multiple stillbirths ascribed to anti-**M** erythroblastosis fetalis was reported by MacPherson and Zartman.[11] This woman had one living normal M-negative child. The patient had formed anti-**M** antibodies during her numerous pregnancies, and these seemed to be predominantly 7S gamma globulin. The antibody titer was essentially the same in the mother and the child. Most antibodies that cause agglutination of cells suspended in saline are of the 19S variety. This antibody did cause agglutination of saline-suspended cells, and so at first it appeared to be of the 19S variety. It was suggested that perhaps it was of a smaller molecular size than the usual 19S antibodies. As previously stated, 19S antibodies do not pass readily through the placenta, but 7S antibodies do. As a rule therefore, even though the mother might form anti-**M** antibodies, they are of the 19S variety and so do not affect the child.

In testing for M-N blood types, the cells must *not* be treated by proteolytic enzymes.

BLOOD FACTORS S AND s OF THE M-N-S SYSTEM

In 1947 Walsh and Montgomery[12] discovered an antibody that could not at the time be identified with any known blood group antibody or system. Sanger and Race[13] and later Sanger et al.[14] found that this antibody was associated with the M and N agglutinogens. The antibody was designated anti-**S**, and the blood specificity (factor) it identified was called **S**. This antibody was present in the serum of a mother of an erythroblastotic baby. The mother had previously been isosensitized to the **Rh₀** factor so that her serum contained anti-**Rh₀** antibodies along with the anti-**S**.

Although it was noted that S could not be an allele of *M* and *N*, it was related to the **M** and **N** factors in the same manner that **A₁** and **A** are related in agglutinogen A₁ of the A-B-O system.

When **S** was first discovered, the small letter "s" was used to note its absence from the blood. However, in 1951 Levine[15] found in the serum of a mother of an erythroblastotic infant an antibody that gave reactions reciprocally related to those of anti-**S** and thus corresponded to the antibody expected for specificity s. Other workers later found additional samples of like antisera. Sera of specificity anti-s are not easily available, although there have been many satisfactory anti-**S** sera.

The discovery of the **S** specificity complicated the previously, seemingly simple M-N system. It has been shown that S and *s* act like alleles. According to some authors, the linkage between *M-N* and *S-s* is so close that these genes are inseparable; others maintain that there are four allelic genes at the M-N locus—*M*ˢ, *M*ˢ, *N*ˢ, and *N*ˢ.

Frequency of specificity S

Specificity **S** had a frequency of 56.1%, whereas S negative had a frequency of 43.9% among 393 donors tested in New York City.

If persons of types M, N, and MN are subdivided according to their reactions with anti-**S** serum alone, six types can be distinguished—M.S, M.s, N.S., N.s, MN.S, and MN.s. When anti-**s** as well as anti-**S** is used, nine phenotypes can be recognized—M.SS, M.Ss, M.ss, N.SS, N.Ss, N.ss, MN.SS, MN.Ss, and MN.ss. The **incidence** of the **S** specificity is not the same in all three M-N types; two thirds of type M but only one third of type N Caucasoids are S positive.

Clinical significance of the S-s specificities

Anti-**S** was originally found, as stated above, in the blood serum of a mother of an erythroblastotic infant. Anti-**s** hemolytic disease was reported in 1966 by Lucher et al.[16] in the baby of a mother who had been sensitized by a previous pregnancy. The antibody proved to be 7S IgG. The baby displayed a compensated hemolytic anemia with minimal icterus. The **S** and **s** specificities have thus been shown to be antigenic to those who lack them.

Significance of S-s in medicolegal investigations

In exclusion tests in disputed paternity suits, if tests are conducted for the **S** blood specificity as well as for the M-N factors, the efficiency of the M-N system is considerably enhanced. According to Wiener,[17] if only anti-**M** and anti-**N** sera are used, the calculated probability that a falsely accused man in parentage suits will be excluded is 18.75%. If all four antisera—anti-**M**, anti-**N**, anti-**S**, and anti-**s**—are used, the probability of exclusion would be increased to 31.58%.[18] Unfortunately, anti-**s** sera are difficult to obtain, and their reactions are generally not clear-cut. If only anti-**M**, anti-**N**, and anti-**S** are used, the probable exclusion rate is 23.9%.

The blood factor **S** cannot be present in the blood of a child unless it is present in the blood of at least one of the parents. When factor **S** is associated with blood specificity **M** in a parent, it is associated in like manner in the blood of the children of this parent and in other members of his family. This is also true of specificity **S** when it is associated with factor **N**, and it is likewise true of factor **s** in association with **M** or **N** in a parent.

It must always be kept in mind that specificities (factors) **S** and **s**, as well as **M** and **N**, are not attributes of separable substances but are specificities of single agglutinogens. This favors the multiple allele theory of the blood group factors **M-N-S-s**. Sussman has stressed the fact that the multiple allele theory enables the inheritance of the *M-N-S* gene complex to be accurately followed through the generations, and any deviation from their anticipated transmission indicates nonparentage. (See Tables 7-3 and 7-4.)

In 1954 Greenwalt et al.[19] described S–s– erythrocytes. Most such bloods are also U–.

Table 7-3. Children possible to matings in the M-N-S system, testing for **S** but not for **s**[*]

Mating	Children possible
MS × MS	MS, M
MS × M	MS, M
M × M	M
MS × MNS	MS, MNS, M, MN
MS × MN	MS, MNS, M, MN
M × MNS	MS, MNS, M, MN
M × MN	M, MN
MS × NS	MNS, MN
MS × N	MNS, MN
M × NS	MNS, MN
M × N	MN
MNS × MNS	MS, M, NS, N, MNS, MN
MNS × MN	MS, M, NS, N, MNS, MN
MN × MN	M, N, MN
MNS × NS	MNS, MN, NS, N
MNS × N	MNS, MN, NS, N
MN × NS	MNS, MN, NS, N
MN × N	MN, N
NS × NS	NS, N
NS × N	NS, N
N × N	N

[*]Modified from Sussman, L. N.: Blood grouping tests, medicolegal uses, Springfield, Ill., 1968, Charles C Thomas, Publisher.

Table 7-4. Genotypes of M-N-S-s*

Phenotype	Anti-M	Anti-N	Anti-S	Genotype
MS	+	−	+	*MSMS, MSMs*
Ms	+	−	−	*MsMs*
NS	−	+	+	*NSNS, NSNs*
Ns	−	+	−	*NsNs*
MNS	+	+	+	*MSNS, MSNs, MsNS*
MNs	+	+	−	*MsNs*

*Modified from Sussman. L. N.: Blood grouping, medicolegal uses, Springfield, Ill., 1968, Charles C Thomas, Publisher.

BLOOD SPECIFICITY (FACTOR) U

In 1953 Wiener et al.[20] found an abnormal antibody in the serum of a Negroid woman. The antibody strongly agglutinated the cells of the two donors whose blood had been used in transfusing her. The patient had received a transfusion after a diagnosis of bleeding peptic ulcer, but the transfusion was terminated after 100 ml of blood had been administered because the patient developed chills and fever. One week later another transfusion was attempted. The woman died shortly thereafter, apparently as a result of another hemolytic reaction.

The antibody found in her serum was of high titer and avidity—400 units at 37° C but only 40 units at refrigerator temperature. It was active by ordinary agglutination tests in saline medium, and so it was assumed to be 19S (IgM) type antibody.

An original series of 690 Caucasoids and 425 Negroids was tested. There were no negative reactions among the whites and only four negative reactions among the Negroids. In another series the red cells of all 1,100 Caucasoids tested were agglutinated by the antibody, but in twelve out of the 989 Negroids tested in New York there was no agglutination of the cells. Because of its **almost universal occurrence,** the antigen was designated as U by the authors, and the antibody that detects it was called anti-U. Wiener et al.[20] reported that all U-negative individuals tested by them were either type N or type MN, and all tested were S negative, indicating a relationship between U and the M-N system. A second example of anti-U was found in 1954 by Greenwalt et al.,[19] who showed that the two available examples of blood not agglutinated by anti-U were also not agglutinated by anti-S or anti-s. As already shown, the factors S and s are also closely associated with specificities M and N. The association of U with S and s thereby confirmed the theory of Wiener that factor U belongs in the M-N-S system.

Wiener and Unger performed a series of tests on another U-sensitized patient and demonstrated that the anti-U antibodies failed to clump cells that had been ficinated and then suspended in saline, again showing a relationship of U with the M-N-S system. Anti-M, anti-N, and anti-S generally fail to agglutinate saline-suspended ficinated cells having the blood factors for which they are specific.

The second sensitized patient studied by Wiener and Unger had 7S (IgG) anti-U antibodies, whereas the first patient's antibodies were of the 19S (IgM) type.

Individuals who lack specificity U, which is a rare occurrence, have been designated as type uu. Family studies on such individuals[21] seemed to indicate that the antigen is inherited by a pair of allelic genes *U* and *u*—the *U* determining the presence of the antigen and the *u* its absence.

Among nearly 10,000 Milwaukee Caucasoids,[22] no U-negative individuals were found. U-negative individuals are found more frequently among African Negroes than among American blacks. Of 126 Congo Pigmies tested, 35% proved to be U negative, according to Fraser et al.[23]

Clinical significance of blood specificity U

The U specificity is important only when it is absent from the blood, since only those who lack the factor can become sensitized to it. Hemolytic transfusion reactions have been observed in such subjects, and in other cases isosensitization of the pregnant woman has been reported. Another interesting observation, made by Wiener and Unger, was that there is a similar antiglobulin titer for red cells maximally coated with U antibodies and with Rh_0 antibodies, which indicates that the number of antigenic sites per red cell is approximately equal for the two blood group agglutinogens.

THE HUNTER SPECIFICITY (Hu)

The **Hu,** or **Hunter,** specificity was described in 1934 by Landsteiner et al,[24] who obtained an antiserum after injecting the blood of a Negroid subject, named Hunter, into a rabbit. This agglutinin caused clumping of the blood cells of 7.3% of all Negroids tested and of only 0.5% of the Caucasoids. The antigen has also been found in 22% of West Africans tested. It is rare in Europeans, although it does occur in some. When Wiener[25] found that all the blood samples which gave distinct positive reactions with the antiserum were either type N or MN, the association with the M-N system was established. To date, no isoimmune **Hu** antibodies have been reported in man.

THE HENSHAW SPECIFICITY (He)

In 1951 Ikin and Mourant[26] found another antibody present in rabbit anti-**M** serum. Later Chalmers et al.[27] produced a similar antibody by injecting the blood of a Nigerian male subject named Henshaw into a rabbit. The antibody was designated anti-**He** (for **Henshaw**), and the antigen it identified as He. The He antigen was found in 38, or 2.7%, of 1,390 West Africans tested, but it was not found in the blood of 1,500 Europeans.

Most of the bloods that were positive for He specificity were also found to have the specificities N and S as well, placing He in the M-N-S system. Tests made with anti-**Hu** and anti-**He** on the same specimens of blood showed the two factors to be distinct.

No natural or isoimmune antibodies of the He specificity have been found to date in humans, but the antigen is important in genetic studies. When **Hu** or **He** is associated with the **M** or **N** specificity in the parents, there is a similar association in the children. **Hu** and **He** are therefore additional specificities of unit agglutinogens of the M-N-S system.

Specificity M^e

A blood specificity has been found that appears to be shared by the M and He antigens, which can lead to mistakes in cases of disputed parentage. Discrepancies were observed by Wiener and Rosenfield[28] in reactions obtained when using two different anti-**M** reagents for tests on blood cells of a Negroid subject in a case of disputed parentage. Both reagents had been prepared in the usual manner of injecting rabbits with group O, type M cells, then absorbing the diluted serum with type N cells until the serum no longer agglutinated the absorbing cells. On further examination, it was found that the blood cells that gave the conflicting reactions had been those of a type N.He (Henshaw)-positive Negroid individual. The immunized rabbits had surely not received He-positive cells in error. These findings were like those of Mourant and his associates that led to the discovery of the He antigen.

The anti-**M** reagent had been believed to be ordinary, standard anti-**M** serum before this individual of type N.He was encountered. This antiserum also agglutinated five more unrelated type N.He bloods. All other type N bloods that were also Henshaw negative, even if they were Hu (Hunter) positive, were not agglutinated. When this anti-**M** reagent was absorbed with type M cells, it lost all its agglutinating activity, including that for type N.He cells. When the antiserum was absorbed with an equal amount of type N.He cells, the activity for the absorbing cells was removed, but some weak residual activity for the M antigen remained. This could be removed by additional absorption with N.He cells. This anti-**M** reagent presumably contained a single antibody for a specificity shared by cells having the M antigen and cells of type N.He. The designation of this specificity then was proposed as **M**^{e} and the corresponding antibody that identifies it as anti-**M**^{e}.

Thus specificity **M**^{e}, by definition, is shared by the M and He antigens. It could be a definite source of error in laboratory tests for the M-N types. In cases of **disputed paternity,** if both the father and the child are type N, He-positive and the mother is type N, He-negative, a false exclusion of paternity could result if the subjects involved are tested at different times and with different reagents. If, for example, the putative father is tested with ordinary anti-**M** and the child with anti-**M**^{e}, the putative father and the mother would both be reported as type N and the child as type MN, which would lead to a false exclusion of paternity.

OTHER VARIANTS OF AGGLUTINOGEN M
Variant M^c

At times, blood cells react in a manner contrary to what might be expected. In such a case, Dunsford et al.[29] described a blood that reacted with twenty-five out of twenty-seven anti-**M** sera and with five out of twenty-eight anti-**N** sera. The antigen of this blood was designated M^c. The antigen had been found in only one family. Since the publication of the original paper by Dunsford et al., anti-**M** and anti-**N** reagents have been classified as reactors or nonreactors with variant M^c by Metaxas and his colleagues. Two more examples of variant M^c have been found in Zurich—one aligned with **S** and the other, like the original family in England, with **s**. The patients of Metaxas had blood that reacted

with the anti-**M**$_1$ (p. 101), but the original M^c blood did not.

Variant M^g

Allen et al.[30] encountered a patient whose red cells were not agglutinated by anti-**M** or anti-**N** sera. When the patient needed a transfusion, it was found that her red cells were agglutinated by the prospective donor's serum due to an antibody designated anti-**M**^{g} by Allen. Antigen M^g occurred only once in 40,000 individuals tested, but the antibody was found much more frequently—in one out of 100 individuals. Recognizing this variant is important because if the facts regarding it are not completely appreciated, an erroneous exclusion of parentage could result when the alleged parent and child are of opposite M-N types. An example could be a father who is M negative and N positive, or type N, with a child who is typed as M positive and N negative, or type M. Normally, no person who is type N would be the parent of a type M child so that the putative parent would be excluded. If, however, the type N parent is of genotype M^gN and the type M child is M^gM, there would be no exclusion because the M^g gene would have come from the putative parent, and the M from the other parent (in this case the mother). Instead, since M^g is an extremely rare gene, its simultaneous appearance in a child and also in a man suspected of being the father would be strong circumstantial evidence of paternity. Whenever there is doubt regarding an M-N exclusion test therefore, one should test the various bloods with anti-**M**^{g} serum if it is available.

Anti-**M**^{g} reacts with cells suspended in saline. The reaction is much easier to read if the test is incubated 5 minutes at 37° C and then centrifuged and read again.

The gene for **M**^{g} appears to be allelic to genes M and N. If blood of a genotype M^gM person is tested only with anti-**M** and anti-**N** standard antisera, the reaction would be interpreted as type M. Similarly, blood representing genotype M^gN would react as type N with standard anti-**M** and anti-**N** sera.

OTHER SPECIFICITIES OF THE M-N SYSTEM
Factors Mi^a and Vw

Levine et al.[31] found a "new" antibody in the blood serum of a patient with hemolytic disease. Because the patient's name was Miltenberger, the antigen defined by the antiserum was called Mi^a and the antibody anti-Mi^a. The specificity Mi^a was found in the blood of the husband and in two of the children of the propositus but not in 425 random group O and group A Caucasoids tested.

Anti-Mi^a has been found as a cause of hemolytic disease. It has also been found in sera of patients with acquired hemolytic anemia but not in the sera of random healthy people. Mi^a is a low-frequency antigen.

There seems to be a multiplicity of antigens having specificities related to **Mi^a**, all of which are complex in their relationships to each other and about which not all the facts are known. Some authors group the specificities **Mi^a** (Miltenberger), **Vw** (Verweyst), **Gr** (Graydon), **Mur** (Murrell, also called **Mu**), and **Hil** (Hill) together. Anti-**Mi^a** and anti-**Gr** are relatively new terms, and both antibodies may be present in the same serum and can be at least partially fractionated by absorp-

tion. Some sera have been found with both anti-**Mi^a** and anti-**Mur**. Other sera have related antibodies that have not been named. Consult Table 7-5. The new names were proposed by Cleghorn.[32]

The anti-**Vw** antibody was described in 1954 by van der Hart et al.[33] This antibody coated the cells of a baby, and the direct antiglobulin test on those cells was positive. The specificity was called **Vw**. It was found to be associated with the M-N-S system. At first it was believed that **Vw** and **Mi^a** were identical, but later half of the **Mi^a**-positive persons proved to be **Vw** positive, and half were **Vw** negative. (See Table 7-5.) No Mi^a-negative, Vw-positive person has been found to date. It appears that the *Vw* gene produces an agglutinogen having specificities **Mi(a+)Vw(+)**, whereas the *Mi^a* gene produces an agglutinogen with the specificities **Mi(a+)Vw(−)**.

Specificities M$_i$, M$_{ii}$, M$_{iii}$, M$_{iv}$ . . . etc.

Most anti-**M** sera react with the red cells of anthropoid apes and many species of monkeys. Occasional anti-**M** sera react with human type M blood exclusively and detect an **M** specificity, **M$_i$**, not shared by nonhuman primates.

Furthermore, most anti-**M** sera react with red cells of all chimpanzees, as well as with human type M but not human type N blood. These contain the antibody fraction designated anti-**M$_{ii}$**, which detects a

Table 7-5. Some reactions of cells and sera within the Mi^a complex of antigens*

New cell type	Old phenotype	Reaction of cells with			
		Anti-Gr	Anti-Mi^a	Anti-Mur	Anti-Hil
Designation	**Notation**	**Anti-Vw**	**Anti-Mi^a**	**Anti-Mu**	**Anti-Hill**
Cell Class I	Mi(a+)Vw+	+	+	−	−
Cell Class II	Mi(a+)Vw−	−	+	−	−
Cell Class III	Mi(a+)Vw−Mur+	−	+	+	+
Cell Class IV		−	+	+	−

*From Issitt, P. D.: Applied blood group serology, Oxnard, Calif., 1970, Spectra Biologicals, Division of Becton, Dickinson & Co.

specificity shared by chimpanzees and human red cells, either alone or together with the antibody fraction anti-M_i. This is comparable to the presence in group A sera of the antibody fractions anti-B_i, specific exclusively for human B blood, and the antibody fraction anti-B_{ii} for a specificity shared by rabbit blood and human B blood. By extending the tests with anti-M reagents to other species of apes and monkeys, using multiple anti-M sera and resorting to absorption experiments when necessary, evidence has been obtained for a virtually unlimited series of M specificities, designated as M_i, M_{ii}, M_{iii}, M_{iv}, etc. (p. 212ff). By definition, all these specificities are possessed by the human agglutinogen M as proved by the fact that absorption of the various anti-M reagents with human type M cells removes their reactivity also for nonhuman primate red cells.[34,35]

At the same time, by comparative tests with anti-N sera on red cells of man and chimpanzees, it is possible to demonstrate that the agglutinogen N also has multiple specificities, as described in greater detail on p. 101 and in Chapter 15.

The multiplicity of specificities of the agglutinogens M and N demonstrated by these comparative tests on nonhuman primate blood serves as an aid in the understanding of the difference between an agglutinogen and its blood factors or specificities. See Table 7-6.

Pursuing this line of investigation, Landsteiner and Wiener,[35] and later Wheeler et al.[51] injected rhesus monkey red cells into rabbits and showed that after absorption with human type N cells, the antisera had anti-M specificity. Even though the anti-rhesus anti-M reagents were, of course, not identical in specificity to the antihuman anti-M reagents, they gave parallel reactions in tests on human red cells.

Landsteiner and Wiener then reasoned that, since injection of sheep blood into rabbits produced reagents of anti-A specificity (see F_A, p. 73), and since injection of rhesus monkey cells into rabbits produced reagents having anti-M specificities,

Table 7-6. Homologues of the human agglutinogen M in nonhuman primate blood*

Source of specimen	Anti-M testing fluid					
	M5	M1	M21	M35	M2	M82
Human M	+++	+++	++±	++±	++±	++±
Human N	−	−	−	−	−	−
Chimpanzee	+++	+++	+++	++	+++	±
Old World monkeys (Cercopithecidae)						
Sphinx baboon	+++	++	++±	−		−
Drill baboon	+++	+++	++±	(±)	(+)	(+±)
Chacna baboon	+++	+++	++±	−	tr.	−
Rhesus macaque	+++	+++	++±	−	tr.	−
Java macaque	+++	+++	++±	(+±)	±	−
Sooty mangabey	+++	+++	++±	−	−	−
Green monkey	+++	+++	++±	tr.	±	±
New World monkeys (Platyrrhini)			−	−	−	−
White spider monkey	++±	−	−	−	−	−
Black spider monkey	±	−	−	tr.	−	−
Wooly monkey	−	−	(±)	−	−	−
Brown ringtail (Capuchin) monkey	−	−	−		−	−
Moss monkey	−	−	f. tr.	±	−	−
Lemur	−	−	−	−	−	−
Average titer of testing fluids	64	64	52	24	16	16

*From Wiener, A. S.: Blood groups and transfusion, ed. 3, 1943; reprinted New York, 1962, Hafner Publication Co.

perhaps if the anti-**rhesus** sera were absorbed, antibody fractions detecting new specificities might be separated. This is, in fact, how the Rh factor was discovered by Landsteiner and Wiener in 1937 and why the antigen was given the symbol Rh, obviously because it was first detected with anti-**rhesus** monkey serum. (See p. 13ff.)

SUBGROUPS OF M
Subgroup M_1

Some human anti-**M** sera contain an antibody designated anti-M_1 because it is comparable to the antibody fraction anti-A_1 of group B human anti-**A** serum. This antibody was found in six out of twenty human anti-**M** sera by Jack et al.,[36] although it was not present in anti-**M** sera from eight rabbits or from one horse. All examples of anti-M_1 have been found in the sera of type N people. Anti-M_1 behaves in a manner analogous to that of anti-A_1 of the A-B-O blood group system. Type M_1 is found more frequently in Negroids than in whites. As many as one fourth of the M genes of American Negroids have proved to be M^1. Among whites, about one out of twenty individuals has the gene M^1.

The N antigen of type M_1N blood is weaker than that of type MN blood lacking specificity M_1. Some authors regard antigen M_1 as a "**super**" M, because a weak, cold-reacting, agglutinating anti-**M** may cause clumping of all M-positive cells at 4° C, but of only M_1-positive cells at 22° C.

Subtype M_2

Subtype M_2, a weak form of the **M** factor, was described by Friedenreich and Lauridsen,[37] who found that red cells which carried the antigen were agglutinated by five out of nine rabbit anti-**M** sera.

SPECIFICITIES AND SUBTYPES OF AGGLUTINOGEN N
Specificities N_i, N_{ii}, etc.

Agglutinogen N has a **mosaic structure** just as M has. Only two specificities have been clearly demonstrated,[38] N_i, which is peculiar to human type N cells only, and N_{ii}, which is shared by human N cells and

chimpanzee red cells having **N**-like agglutinogens. The M and N agglutinogens of humans have all the serologic specificities that can and do characterize each agglutinogen.

Subtype N_2

Crome[39] described the subtype of N designated N_2. Type N_2 blood is characterized by its weak reactivity with anti-**N** sera. Many anti-**N** reagents fail to clump N_2 cells, or in other cases the reaction may be extremely weak and so overlooked. This has led to serious errors in medicolegal cases. All N-negative bloods must therefore be checked with more than one anti-**N** serum, otherwise serious errors might arise due to failure to detect this subtype. Blood type MN_2 appears to be most common among Chinese and has been a source of error in blood grouping tests in immigration cases based on claims of **derivative citizenship**.

Allele M^k

In 1964 an allele that produces no M, N, S, or s antigen was found in a Swiss family by Metaxas and Metaxas-Buehler,[40] and named M^k. No M, N, or M^g antigen was produced by members of this family. The cells of the propositus were apparently N, but gave only a single dose reaction with anti-**N** reagents. One of her children was later found to be type M. It was not determined at that time whether or not this allele produced S or s antigen. However, in a Danish family reported by Henningsen[41] in which the same allele was found, it was shown that this new allele produced no S or s. This family shows the effect that this allele can have on a pedigree. In no less than three successive generations the established M-N-S-s groups would appear to exclude the maternity of all five of these children. An MS–s+ grandmother has an NS–s+ daughter married to an MS+s+ man and they have an MS+s– and two MS–s+ daughters, one of whom has an NS–s+ child. Seven more M^k families have been reported.

The frequency of M^k is estimated at

0.00064, based on tests of 3,895 Swiss families.

The M^k allele results in no M, N, S, or s antigens, and no M^k antigen is produced. Metaxas et al.[42] suggest that "M^k may be an amorph whose presence at the MNSs locus leaves unconverted a basic substance from which the MNSs antigens normally arise." They liken it to Rh_{null} and K_o. (See Table 11-1.)

OTHER ANTIGENS IN THE M-N-S SYSTEM

In addition to the specificities (factors) and subtypes already listed in the M-N-S system, other possible alleles at the M-N locus or other possible specificities of the M and N agglutinogens have been described. All are dominant characters.

1. M^V is an agglutinogen that reacts with all anti-N sera and a few anti-M sera.

2. M^A specificity is part of the "normal" M mosaic. The rare M^a cells react with all anti-M sera, except that formed (anti-M^A) by an M^a subject (one who lacks specificity M^A). Almost all M-positive cells also have the M^A specificity; therefore M^A is a cognate of the specificity M, just as Rh^A, Rh^B, Rh^C, and Rh^D are cognates of Rh_o of the Rh-Hr system.

3. Vr, also called Vr^a, has been found in three out of 1,200 Dutch donors.

4. Ny^a has been found in 1 out of 600 Norwegian donors.

5. Mt^a is rare.

6. Ri^a is found in fewer than 1 out of 1,000 English donors.

7. Cl^a is found in fewer than 1 out of 1,000 Scottish donors.

8. Sul is rare, having been found as a dominant in only one large family.

9. Tm was found to be present in 25% of Caucasoids and in 30% of Negroids tested. The antibody is weak, and the tests are poorly reproducible.

10. Sj is present in 2% of Caucasoids and 3% of Negroids. All Sj-positive bloods so far have been Tm positive, and most anti-Tm sera also contain anti-Sj.

11. St^a may have an effect on an M anti-gen with which it travels. Two M types, M^z and M^r, have both been found to be St(a+). St^a was found in 14 of unrelated 220 Japanese, and in 6 of 420 Chinese.

12. M^z reacts with most anti-M and a few anti-N sera. It does not react with anti-M_1 but does react with anti-M'. It is St(a+). The only known family with this antigen was typed as M^zs.

13. M^r is a very rare variant of M. It is St(a+).

14. Far is recognized by specific antibodies.

15. M^c has no specific antibody.

For details, see especially papers by Nordling et al.[43] and Metaxas et al.[40,44]

SEROLOGY OF THE M-N TYPES

The M and N agglutinogens are highly antigenic for rabbits. Anti-M and anti-N testing sera are therefore readily prepared in rabbits by injection with pooled group O human blood cells containing either the M or the N agglutinogen. In testing a number of anti-M sera not only with human blood cells but also with the cells of non-human primates, it was found that at least four or five distinct specificities exist, based on cross-reactions with nonhuman primate red cells. At least two different specificities were also found to exist, as detected by anti-N.[35,38] (See factors M_i, etc. and N_i, etc. preceding.)

Nevertheless, different anti-M (and anti-N) reagents generally give parallel results when tested against human red cells. If, however, the blood of lower primates is tested, the reagents often give differing results, showing that these reagents actually have different serologic specificities. As stated, there are at least four or five different M and at least two different N specificities that were found by Wiener in this way. When testing human blood, this can be disregarded because all human bloods with M agglutinogen have all the M specificities, and all human bloods with N agglutinogen have all the N specificities, so all anti-M and anti-N reagents give essentially the same results with appropriate human bloods. One exception is anti-M^c reagent because it gives strong reactions with the blood of type N.He persons, mostly Negroids. If anti-M^e is used unwittingly, errors could result in the interpretation of the laboratory tests—type N.He people would be reported as type MN.

Extracts of seeds of *Vicia graminea* were shown by Ottensooser and Silberschmidt[45] to give reactions paralleling anti-N in specificity, and these extracts make excellent anti-N reagents also for testing red cells of nonhuman primates. Specific anti-N reagents prepared from rabbits' antisera seldom exceed a titer of 10 units, but it is possible to prepare anti-M reagents with titers as high as 256 units from rabbit antisera. Type M blood, in addition to the multiple M specificities, also has a weakly reacting N-like specificity so that when anti-N immune rabbit serum is absorbed by type M blood to remove species-specific agglutinins, the anti-N reagent is weakened at the same time by the N-like factor in the M cells. On the other hand, if the antiserum is underabsorbed during the preparation process, the reagent will be nonspecific. This same result occurs on absorption with type M red cells of anti-N reagent made from extracts of *Vicia graminea* seeds. The weak N-like specificity of agglutinogen M was observed by Landsteiner and Levine at the time of their original discovery, when they prepared anti-N reagent by absorbing the raw rabbit antisera with human M cells. Some workers have suggested[46] therefore that N may be the precursor of M. Wiener pointed out that the relationship of N to M is analogous to that of H to A-B and has made this the basis for a **newer genetic theory of the M-N types.**

According to the original genetic theory of Landsteiner and Levine, type M blood is homozygous for *M*, genotype *MM;* type N is homozygous for *N*, genotype *NN;* and type MN blood is heterozygous for both *M* and *N*, genotype *MN*. The difference in reactivity of type M and type MN blood with anti-M reagents is only slight, but type N blood reacts strikingly stronger than type MN blood with anti-N reagents

so that with weak anti-N reagents, type MN blood may fail to agglutinate at all. The great difference in reactivity of N and MN with anti-N reagents has generally been ascribed to a **gene dose effect** and attributed to differences in zygosity for gene N.

According to Wiener's newer genetic theory, on the other hand, the agglutinogen N is determined by a pair of genes independent of the agglutinogen M, just as genes *H-h* are independent of *A-B-O*. All humans are assumed to be homozygous for *N*, genotype *NN*, just as they are assumed to be homozygous for *H*, genotype *HH*.

Gene *M*, instead of being allelic to *N*, is transmitted independently, but it has an amorphic gene, *m*, as its allele. The three M-N types would thus correspond to three possible genotypes as follows: type M, genotype *MMNN;* type N, genotype *mmNN;* and type MN, genotype *MmNN*. N, therefore, appears to be related to M in the same manner as H is related to A and B, rather than as A is related to B.

Whereas, according to this theory, all humans are assumed to be homozygous for gene *N*, the expressivity of the agglutinogen N is postulated to be affected by the *M-m* genotype. The interaction between the independently transmitted genes *M* and *N* is postulated to occur at the phenotypic level and is ascribed to the proximity of the structures responsible for the M and N specificities, which are either on the same molecule or on adjacent molecules. In individuals of genotype *mmNN*, there would be no determinant group for M, so that the N specificity would have its maximum expressivity in determining type N individuals. In persons of genotype *MMNN*, in contrast, the M determinant group would be maximally expressed, rendering the N determinant group (presumably located deeper in the agglutinogen molecule) virtually inaccessible for anti-N reagents, thus determining type M individuals. In genotype *MmNN* there are presumably fewer M determinant groups so that the N determinant groups are more readily accessible, giving rise to an intermediate reactivity with anti-**N** reagents, thus determining MN types.

Not only would this genetic theory account for the results of absorption experiments cited above, but it would also explain the much higher reactivity of type N red cells with anti-**N** reagents by comparison with the reactivity of type MN red cells with the same reagent, and the much smaller difference in reactivity between red cells of types M and MN in tests with anti-**M** reagents. The newer genetic theory receives its strongest support from the observations on homologues of the human M-N type in apes,[52] which cannot be explained in terms of the classic genetic theory. (See Part Two, Chapter 15.) Wiener stated that he had this theory in mind as long ago as 1945 when he published his article with Karowe on the diagrammatic representation of the A-B-O groups.[*]

Anti-**N** is extremely rare in human serum, probably because type M cells have, in addition to the M agglutinogen, this weak N-like antigen, which prevents formation of anti-**N** antibodies by those whose blood cells contain this weak antigen. On the other hand, proportionally many more type N individuals have natural anti-**M** agglutinins. Wiener showed that anti-**M** can be produced fairly readily in type N persons by isoimmunization.

The M-N system, far from being a simple one, is extremely complex because of the multiple serologic specificities such as **S, s, U, He, Hu,** and **M^e. One outstanding characteristic of this system is the fact that the agglutinins generally fail to cause clumping of cells having the corresponding serologic specificity if the cells have been treated with proteolytic enzymes.**

BIOCHEMISTRY OF THE M-N SUBSTANCES

The present status of knowledge of the biochemistry of M-N is mainly due to the work of Springer and his team,[47] as well as that of Prokop and Uhlenbruck.[48] According to these investigators, the M-N

[*]Wiener, A. S.: Personal communication, Aug., 1971.

substances are glycoproteins having a polypeptide backbone and protruding oligosaccharide chains that determine the serologic specificities. However, unlike the A-B-H substances, the M-N substances do not occur in water-soluble form in body fluids or secretions. In fact, so far they have been found only on the surface of erythrocytes, which is the usual source of materials used for chemical analysis of the blood group substances. It will be recalled that red cells treated with proteases lose their ability to react with M-N reagents. Uhlenbruck has shown that this is due to splitting off of the specific substances that go into solution in the supernatant fluid, where their presence can be demonstrated by the inhibition test.

Springer's technic of extracting the N substance from red cell stromata entails the use of phenol at an acid pH. He has also prepared from meconium a highly purified material, which he calls the **Me-Vg substance** because of its reactivity with anti-**N^V** lectin. (The V refers to *Vicia* seed extracts.)

Of the sixteen amino acids present in the preparation, threonine is the predominant one, followed by serine. Among the sugars isolated were N-acetylneuraminic acid (sialic acid), N-acetylgalactosamine, N-acetylglucosamine, galactose, and fucose. Although N-acetylneuraminic acid (NANA) appears to be essential for the serologic activity, it apparently is not involved in its specificity.

Receptor-destroying enzymes (RDE), that is, neuraminidase from cholera bacilli, inactivate the M-N blood group antigens, as well as the receptors on the red cell surface for influenza virus.[49] Thus the M-N agglutinogens and influenza virus receptors are closely related, although they may not be the same.

Summarizing their findings, Springer et al.[50] state that sialic acid and galactose are involved in the **N** specificities, as determined by tests with human and rabbit sera, whereas the specificity determined by anti-**N^V** lectin apparently depends on a β-galactopyranosyl group. The myxovirus receptor activity on red cells is also dependent on the presence of sialic acid, according to Springer. Based on his biochemical findings, Springer has proposed a genetic theory for the M-N types similar to the theory of Wiener just described.

REFERENCES

1. Landsteiner, K., and Levine, P.: Proc. Soc. Exp. Biol. Med. **24**:600, 941, 1927.
2. Landsteiner, K.: J. Exp. Med. **47**:757, 1928.
3. Allen, F. H., Jr.: Bibl. Haematol. Part I (No. 38), p. 186, 1971.
4. Metaxas, M. N., and Metaxas-Buehler, M.: Nature (Lond.) **202**:1123, 1974.
5. Wiener, A. S., Gordon, E. B., and Mazzarino, C. A.: Proc. Soc. Exp. Biol. Med. **69**:8, 1948.
6. Wiener, A. B., and Gordon, E. B.: Rev. Hématol. **5**:3, 1950.
7. Yoell, J. H.: Transfusion **6**:592, 1966.
8. Masters, P. L., and Vos, G. H.: Lancet **2**: 641, 1942.
9. Wiener, A. S., and Forer, S.: Proc. Soc. Exp. Biol. Med. **47**:215, 1941.
10. Broman, B.: Acta Paediatr. (supp. 2) **31**:1, 1944.
11. MacPherson, C. R., and Zartman, E. R.: Am. J. Clin. Pathol. **43**:544, 1965.
12. Walsh, R. M., and Montgomery, C.: Nature (Lond.) **160**:504, 1947.
13. Sanger, R., and Race, R. R.: Nature (Lond.) **160**:505, 1947.
14. Sanger, R., Race, R. R., Walsh, R. J., and Montgomery, C.: Heredity **2**:131, 1948.
15. Levine, P., Kuhmichel, A. B., Wogod, M., and Koch, E.: Proc. Soc. Exp. Biol. Med. **78**: 218, 1951.
16. Lucher, L. M., Zuelzer, W. W., and Parson, P. J.: Transfusion **6**:590, 1966.
17. Wiener, A. S.: J. Immunol. **19**:259, 1930.
18. Wiener, A. S.: Am. J. Hum. Genet. **4**:37, 1952.
19. Greenwalt, T. J., Sasaki, T., Sanger, R., Sneath, J., and Race, R. R.: Proc. Natl. Acad. Sci. U.S.A. **40**:1126, 1954.
20. Wiener, A. S., Unger, L. J., and Gordon, E. B.: J.A.M.A. **153**:1444, 1953.
21. Wiener, A. S., and Unger, L. J.: Exp. Med. Surg. **162**:213, 1958.
22. Greenwalt, T. J. In Tocantins, L. M., editor: Progress in hematology, vol. 3, New York, 1962, Grune & Stratton, Inc.
23. Fraser, G. R., Giblett, E. R., and Motulsky, A.: Am. J. Hum. Genet. **18**:546, 1966.
24. Landsteiner, K., Strutton, W. R., and Chase, M. W.: J. Immunol. **27**:469, 1934.
25. Wiener, A. S.: Blood groups and transfusion, ed. 3, 1943; reprinted New York, 1962, Hafner Publication Co.
26. Ikin, E. W., and Mourant, A. E.: Br. Med. J. **1**:456, 1951.
27. Chalmers, J. N. M., Ikin, E. W., and Mourant, A. E.: Br. Med. J. **2**:175, 1953.
28. Wiener, A. S., and Rosenfield, R. E.: J. Immunol. **87**:376, 1961.
29. Dunsford, J., Ikin, E. W., and Mourant, A. E.: Nature (Lond.) **172**:688, 1953.
30. Allen, F. J., Corcoran, P. A., Kenton, H. B., and Breare, N.: Vox Sang. **3**:81, 1958.
31. Levine, P., Stock, A. H., Kuhmichel, A. B., and Bronikovsky, N.: Proc. Soc. Exp. Biol. Med. **77**:402, 1951.
32. Cleghorn, T. W.: Vox Sang. **11**:219, 1966.
33. van der Hart, M., Bosman, H., and van Longhem, J. J.: Vox Sang. **4**:108, 1954.
34. Wiener, A. S.: J. Immunol. **34**:87, 1938.
35. Landsteiner, K., and Wiener, A. S.: J. Immunol. **33**:19, 1937.
36. Jack, J. A., Tippett, P., Noades, J., Sanger, R., and Race, R. R.: Nature (Lond.) **186**: 642, 1960.
37. Friedenreich, V., and Lauridsen, A.: Acta Pathol. Microbiol. Scand. (supp. 38) **15**:155, 1938.
38. Wiener, A. S.: J. Immunol. **34**:11, 1938.
39. Crome, W.: Deutsch. Z. Ges. Gerichtl. Med. **24**:147, 1935.
40. Metaxas, M. N., and Metaxas-Buehler, M.: Nature (Lond.) **202**:1123, 1964.
41. Hunningsen, K.: Acta Genet. **16**:239, 1966.
42. Metaxas, M. N., Metaxas-Buehler, M., and Romanski, Y.: Vox Sang. **20**:509, 1971.
43. Nordling, S., Sanger, R., Gavin, J., Furuhjelm, U., Myerlyä, G., and Metaxas, M. N.: Vox Sang. **17**:300, 1969.
44. Metaxas, M. N., Metaxas-Buehler, M., and Ikin, E. W.: Vox Sang. **15**:102, 1968.
45. Ottensooser, F., and Silberschmidt, J.: Nature **172**:914, 1953.
46. Wiener, A. S., Moor-Jankowski, J., and Gordon, E. B.: Kriminalistik und foreniche Wissenschafter (Berlin, DDR) **6**:63, 1971.
47. Springer, G. F., Nagai, Y., and Tegtmeyer, H.: Biochemistry **5**:3254, 1966.
48. Prokop, O., and Uhlenbruck, G.: Human blood and serum groups, New York, 1969, John Wiley & Sons, Inc.
49. Springer, G. F.: Naturwissenschafter **57**: 1621, 1970. (Complete articles of Springer available in Wiener, A. S., editor: Advances in blood grouping, vol. 3, New York, 1970, Grune & Stratton, Inc.)
50. Springer, G. F., Huprikar, S. V., and Tegtmeyer, H.: Z. Immunitaetsforsch. **142**:99, 1971.
51. Wheeler, K. M., Sawin, P. B., and Stuart, C. A.: J. Immunol. **37**:159, 1939.
52. Wiener, A. S., Gordon, E. B., Moor-Janowski, J., and Socha, W. W.: Haematologia (Budap.) **6**:419, 1972.

8 □ The Rh-Hr blood group system

DISCOVERY OF THE Rh FACTOR

The discovery of the Rh factor by Landsteiner and Wiener constituted the most important advance in blood grouping since the discovery of the four principal A-B-O blood groups. The manner in which it was found differed from previous immunologic research in that there was a conscious intention to find a "new" blood factor in human blood, utilizing an unusual method of investigation. Landsteiner and Wiener were trying to obtain more information about the agglutinogens M and N, employing nonhuman primates as test animals. As shown in Chapter 7, the M agglutinogen of human blood has a large number of serologic specificities, some of which are shared by the red cells of various nonhuman primates, but all of which are present in the human M agglutinogen. All the anti-M reagents at Wiener's disposal gave parallel reactions in tests with human red cells, but they were not identical in that some strongly agglutinated the red cells of rhesus monkeys and others did not. When these antisera were absorbed with human type M cells, the antibodies for the monkey blood were completely removed, proving that the reactions with rhesus red cells were actually due to the anti-M in the reagent and not to some other antibody. (See pp. 13 and 14.)

Landsteiner and Wiener then immunized rabbits with rhesus monkey red cells. The antisera produced were then absorbed with human type N cells and yielded good anti-M reagents as expected; these reagents could be used in place of the anti–human

M reagents, with which they gave parallel reactions in tests on human blood. The anti-M agglutinin was then removed from the anti-rhesus rabbit sera by absorption, which resulted in a reagent that agglutinated the cells of 85% of the Caucasoids tested but failed to agglutinate the cells of the remaining 15%. Because the blood factor defined by this new reagent differed from any previously found, it was given the name rhesus, or Rh factor, using the first two letters of the word rhesus. The discovery of this factor in 1937 was not reported until 1940 so that methods of producing the antiserum could be improved. This delay unfortunately contributed to a controversy over who was to be credited with the discovery of the Rh factor. It has now been resolved, and Landsteiner and Wiener[1] are rightfully credited with the discovery.

Rh-Hr NOMENCLATURE

Three methods of designation of types in the Rh-Hr system have been in use for some time and are still in use. These are the designations of Wiener, the C-D-E notations of British workers, and the numbering by Rosenfield. The Committee on Medicolegal Problems of the American Medical Association[2] studied the available information in an attempt to resolve the nomenclature problem, and "therefore recommend(ed) that the C-D-E notations for the Rh-Hr types be discarded, and that the original Rh-Hr nomenclature of Wiener be retained as the sole nomenclature for this blood group system." Despite this recom-

Table 8-1. Comparisons of the designations for phenotype Rh_1rh in three currently used nomenclatures*

Wiener's Rh-Hr nomenclature	Fisher and Race's C-D-E notations†	Rosenfield's numbered notations‡
Rh_1rh	1. $+++$ or $++-++$, etc.	Rh: 1, 2, -3, 4, 5, 6, 7, -8, -9,
	2. $C+D+E-c+d?e+$	-10, -11, 12, 13, 14, 15, 16,
	3. $\begin{cases} + + - + + \\ C \ D \ E \ c \ e \end{cases}$	17, 18, 19, -20, 21
	4. CDe/cde or CDe, cde, etc.	
	5. $\dfrac{CDe}{cde}$ ("most likely" genotype)	
	6. $\begin{cases} CDe/cde \\ CDe/cDe \\ Cde/cDe \end{cases}$	
	7. CcDee	
	8. CDce	
	9. CcD or DCc	
	10. DCe/dce or DCe, dce, etc.	
	11. DCcee	
	12. D-Ccee, CcD-ee, etc.	
	13. CDe/ce, DCe/ce, etc.	
	14. CDe/c-e	
	15. CDeF/cdef, DCeF/dcef, etc.	
	16. CcDeef, etc.	
	17. CcDeefG, etc.	

*From Wiener, A. S.: Am. J. Hum. Genet. **17**:457, 1965.
†Partial listing only.
‡As of 1962; present approved listing is not known. This system depends on the use of a list of the Rh-Hr blood factors, arranged in a particular order. Since the exact arrangement of the blood factors is largely a matter of taste and has no scientific basis, 6 different blood factors could give rise to as many as 240 different systems of notations, while with more than 30 factors, as are known at present, the number of possibilities becomes astronomical.

mendation, the other nomenclatures still appear in the literature, and commercial antisera for testing purposes continue to bear at least two different symbols on their labels.

The choice of nomenclature in the Rh-Hr system is in part a choice between the Wiener theory of allelic genes and the Fisher-Race theory of completely linked genes. The Fisher-Race theory conceives of a simple 1:1 correspondence, or relationship, among genes, agglutinogens, antibodies, and serologic specificities (blood factors). According to Fisher and Race, each new serologic specificity must be the product of another gene. So many new serologic specificities are being discovered that this would suggest a highly improbable genetic system, with chromosomes carrying **cistrons** having more than thirty **subloci** at the count in 1971.

Fisher and Race, in their **linked gene**

hypothesis, originally proposed that there are three loci for allelic genes, which they designated as *Dd, Cc,* and *Ee,* with *D* determining the Rh_o or "D" agglutinogen, *C* determining rh' or "C" agglutinogen, and *E* determining the rh'' or "E" agglutinogen. In their nomenclature, d would correspond to nonexistent Hr_o, c to hr', and e to hr'', as follows:

$$D = Rh_o \qquad d = Hr_o \text{ (nonexistent)}$$
$$C = rh' \qquad c = hr'$$
$$E = rh'' \qquad e = hr''$$

The agglutinogens (not the phenotypes) in the Wiener and the Fisher-Race nomenclatures would be rh = cde, rh' = Cde, rh'' = cdE, rh_y = CdE, Rh_o = cDe, Rh_1 = CDe, Rh_2 = cDE, and Rh_z = CDE. So many different phenotypes have been used by different authors that only those for Rh_1rh will be given here. See Table 8-1.

This nomenclature supposedly simplified the Rh-Hr system. However, even though at first it seemed to solve the problem of difficult nomenclature, as the various specificities were found, as family studies revealed that the linked gene theory is incorrect with respect to the blood groups, and especially as different antisera became available, this nomenclature, instead of simplifying the subject, actually complicated and confused it. In implying a 1:1 correspondence between gene, agglutinogen, and serologic specificities, this nomenclature disregards the fact that certain basic antisera required by the C-D-E theory have never been found, such as anti-d and anti-F. With the Wiener nomenclature, "f" is specificity **hr,** and there is definitely an anti-**hr** serum, but anti-F serum is not included in the Wiener nomenclature because no such specificity as "F" has ever been found. In addition, the "intermediate" factors, like C^W, C^V, and C^u of Race and associates, cannot be placed in the linked gene scheme unless it is assumed that C and C^W are multiple alleles.

Miale[3] believes that the scientific evidence overwhelmingly supports the Wiener theory of multiple allelic genes, and he has suggested that the Wiener nomenclature be adopted exclusively, especially because of the genetic and serologic principles on which it is based.

The Wiener nomenclature can be learned within a short time, as can the composition of each agglutinogen in the Rh-Hr system, primarily because each symbol has within itself an abbreviated description, or **terse mnemonic,** of the specificities of each agglutinogen and the reactions with the antisera of blood having such specificities. An example is phenotype Rh_1rh. It can readily be perceived that phenotype Rh_1 has at least the specificities **Rh_o** and **rh′** (combination Rh_1) and that the rh half shows the specificities **hr′** and **hr″** to be present, both of which are found when gene r or R^o is present. The symbol on the left-hand side of the phenotype indicates the reactions with anti-Rh sera, and that on the right in-

dicates reactions with anti-Hr sera. Such blood will therefore react positively with anti-**Rh_o,** anti-**rh′,** anti-**hr′,** and anti-**hr″** sera but negatively with anti-**rh″.**

The essential difference between the two systems of nomenclature is a serologic and not a genetic one. Considering blood factors as serologic attributes of agglutinogens is different from considering them as products of specific genes that produce specific agglutinogens, each having a single corresponding antibody. In the blood groups the theory of complete linkage with multiple subloci does not take into consideration that a difference exists between an agglutinogen and its serologic attributes.[4]

A system of nomenclature should be uniform throughout the world, regardless of language differences, like the symbol H for hydrogen, pH for hydrogen ion concentration, Na for sodium, and Hg for mercury. Except for the Rh-Hr system for which three different nomenclatures have been suggested, the blood groups O, A, B, AB, Lewis, Lutheran, M-N-S, etc. have uniform terse symbols that are universally employed. This should also be true of the Rh-Hr system. Ranganathan[5] states, "It is high time that the prolonged and acrimonious controversy about the Rh nomenclature was ended and a single, unified scientific nomenclature was adopted for the Rh-Hr blood types. In this connection, international scientific organizations have a major responsibility to call for a fact-finding meeting of experts in the field to solve the problem on a basis of free discussion, not by vote. . . . The delay (in adopting a single, simple nomenclature) has not been in vain. It has helped confirm the scientific superiority of the original Rh-Hr nomenclature and its ability to accommodate the 25 or more new Rh blood factors discovered during the interval. At the same time, it has demonstrated the inadequacy of the C-D-E notations to embrace the newly discovered blood factors without causing further confusion."

In the Wiener nomenclature, *italics* are used for genes and genotypes; **boldface**

type for serologic specificities (blood factors) and their corresponding agglutinins; and lightface, or regular, type for agglutinogens and phenotypes. The more antigenic factors in the Rh-Hr nomenclature are written with a capital "R" and the less antigenic with the small "r." The Rh-Hr symbols lend themselves to a logical arrangement when tables of phenotypes and genotypes are constructed, comparable to the arrangement in the A-B-O blood group system, in the order O-A-B-AB. Thus elaborate tables need not be memorized but can be produced by reasoning. The Wiener Rh-Hr nomenclature will be followed throughout this text.

Rosenfield numerical code for the Rh-Hr blood types

Rosenfield[6] suggested a third method of designating the Rh-Hr blood types using numbers after the symbol Rh to represent the blood factors present (or absent) in each blood. The numbers refer merely to the order of the discovery of the different factors and give no hint as to the composition of the agglutinogens. For example, Rh2 and Rh4, which are **rh'** and **hr'**, give no indication of the reciprocal relationship of the two factors. Table 8-4 lists the most important Rh-Hr specificities (factors), but not in the numerical order used by Rosenfield. The Rosenfield scheme does not differentiate among agglutinogens, phenotypes, and genes and genotypes. For example, phenotype Rh₁rh would be written Rh: 1, 2, –3, 4, 5, 6, 7, –8, –9, –10, –11, 12, 13, 14, 15, 16, etc, with the minus sign indicating absence of a factor. (The numerical subscripts to indicate graded differences between some of the subgroups such as A_1 and A_2 should not be confused with the Rosenfield numbers used to identify types.)

Decimal numbers do not constitute a nomenclature, but they may be used for coding, although using the numbers of the binary system for such a purpose seems better, as explained in Chapter 21.

INTRAGROUP TRANSFUSION REACTIONS

In 1939 Wiener and Peters,[7] investigating three cases of severe hemolytic transfusion reaction in which the patients had been transfused with blood from donors of their own A-B-O blood group (**intragroup transfusion reaction**), found irregular agglutinins in the patients' sera. These agglutinins clumped the red cells of the donors whose blood had caused the hemolytic reactions, as well as those of approximately 85% of all Caucasoids examined, irrespective of their A-B-O blood groups or of the **M, N,** or **P** factors, This suggested that the factor responsible for the production of the antibody could be the **rhesus** factor, and parallel tests with anti–**rhesus monkey** rabbit antisera showed this surmise to be correct. All three patients proved to be rhesus negative, and all donors were rhesus positive. This was the first report on intragroup hemolytic transfusion reactions in which an antibody of a new specificity was clearly demonstrated in the blood serum of a recipient. Intragroup hemolytic transfusion reactions had been reported previously, but they were ascribed merely to "irregular" isoagglutinins of undefined specificity.

Within a year ten more cases of intragroup transfusion reactions due to the rhesus factor were found.[8] Such reports then became rather numerous, showing sensitization to the rhesus factor to be the cause of most of such reactions. As a result, Rh blood typing of recipients and prospective donors was then adopted as a routine laboratory procedure in pretransfusion examinations, and Rh-negative patients were given only Rh-negative blood, thus preventing Rh isosensitization.

DISCOVERY OF THE ROLE OF ISOSENSITIZATION IN ERYTHROBLASTOSIS FETALIS

In 1939 Levine and Stetson[9] reported the case of a mother of a stillborn fetus who suffered a severe hemolytic reaction when transfused with her husband's blood. Her serum agglutinated her husband's red cells and those of eighty out of 104 donors who were compatible with her A-B-O group. The antigen that her antiserum identified proved to be different from and independent of the A-B-O, M-N, and P groups, but when her blood was injected into rabbits, the rabbits did not produce antibodies. Levine and Stetson concluded that the mother lacked an antigen of undefined specificity, which was present in her husband's blood and in that of her fetus, and that this antigen, inherited from the fetus' father, had caused the mother to form antibodies against it. Thus, when she was transfused with her husband's blood containing the antigen, the antibody already in her serum reacted against the incoming cells, and these were agglutinated or hemolyzed, with a resulting hemolytic reaction. As in other previously reported cases of intragroup hemolytic transfusion reactions,[10-14] Levine and Stetson did not identify the antibody, but they laid the foundation for the present knowledge of **erythroblastosis fetalis** and **isoimmunization of pregnant women** by their fetuses. The antibody was never positively identified because, as noted in the report, the patients' serum had lost its reactivity after a few months, as in the previously reported cases.

In 1941 Levine, Burnham et al.[15-18] showed that erythroblastosis fetalis (EBF) is usually the result of Rh incompatibility between mother and fetus. This finding has been elaborated, and at present it is known that there are many other antigenic factors besides Rh which, when lacking in the mother and present in the child, can also result in EBF.

The finding of the Rh factor and the association of this factor with hemolytic transfusion reactions, as well as its role in EBF, opened a new field in blood grouping, leading to new methods and new discoveries in genetics and in other branches of immunohematology, including prevention of EBF and more recently attempts at treatment of hemolytic transfusion reactions once they become manifest. (See pp. 13 to 16.)

In 1941 Landsteiner and Wiener[19] published their findings that the Rh antigen was present in approximately 85% of all Caucasoids tested and that tests on members of sixty families showed the Rh factor to be a dominant characteristic, independent of the A-B-O and M-N systems.

DISCOVERY OF IgG (7S) (BLOCKING, OR INCOMPLETE) ANTIBODIES

The original anti-Rh sera used for testing purposes were obtained either from Rh-isoimmunized women after delivery of an erythroblastotic infant or were prepared by injecting rabbits or guinea pigs with rhesus monkey red cells. Some means of manufacturing anti-Rh testing serum that would give strong reactions was necessary before tests for the Rh factor could become routine in the laboratory. Some seeming anomalies needed explanation, particularly why no anti-Rh antibodies could be demonstrated in the sera of some women who had manifestly become isosensitized and who were Rh negative mated to an Rh-positive man. In 1944 Wiener[20] published his test for a so-called **blocking antibody,** and Race[21] independently reported on an **incomplete antibody** found in human serum. The blocking and incomplete antibodies are now known to be 7S immunoglobulins that coat the red cells but do not cause them to agglutinate (IgG).

DISCOVERY OF rh′

Division of all humans into two groups—Rh positive or Rh negative—at first seemed simple, but in 1941 Wiener discovered an Rh-like agglutinin in the serum of a patient who had had a hemolytic transfusion reaction. Although apparently related to the Rh system, this antibody caused agglutination of cells of only approximately 70% of Caucasoids examined instead of the expected 85%. The question then arose of the serologic and genetic relationships between the original Rh factor and the newly discovered factor. Wiener postulated that there were two, not one, serologic specificities—

one designated Rh_o, the original Rh factor, and the other **rh'**, detected by the new 70% antiserum—and these could be detected by agglutinins subsequently designated anti-Rh_o and anti-**rh'**, respectively. The small letter in rh' was used to show its relatively low antigenicity by comparison with Rh_o.

To understand the many ramifications of the Rh-Hr system, one must always keep in mind the **difference between an agglutinogen and a blood factor, or serologic specificity.** The agglutinogen is the substance on the red cell that reacts with the agglutinin. It may have many serologic factors that are identified by the reactions of the red cells with the respective specific agglutinins. Red cells can therefore have both specificities Rh_o and **rh'** due to a single agglutinogen designated Rh_1, just as agglutinogen A has blood factors **A** and **C**, and agglutinogen M of humans has the multiple specificities M_i, M_{ii}, M_{iii}, M_{iv}, and others. Each gene determines an agglutinogen having more than one serologic specificity. The Wiener theory of multiple alleles is based on this concept, and this is the difference between the Wiener theory and the linked allele theory later proposed by the British workers. The theory of Wiener has been confirmed by family studies.[22]

HEREDITARY TRANSMISSION OF Rh FACTORS

Anti-Rh_o and anti-**rh'** detected four types: rh, Rh_o, Rh_o' (or Rh_1), and rh'. The problem then arose as to the mechanism of hereditary transmission of these four types. Because of the historic importance of the manner in which Wiener solved the problem, that is, by using methods of population genetics, his own words will be quoted directly. To understand the quotation, one must keep in mind that the antibody Wiener,[23] in 1943, tentatively called "anti-Rh_1" is presently known as anti-Rh_o, and "anti-Rh_2" is now anti-**rh'**. "The reactions could be explained most simply by assuming the existence of two qualitatively different agglutinogens, Rh_1 and Rh_2, in the blood cells, corresponding to the aggluti-

nins anti-Rh_1 and anti-Rh_2. The four sorts of blood would then have the composition Rh_1Rh_2, Rh_1, Rh_2, Rh-negative, respectively. This assumption would imply the existence, however, of two corresponding genes Rh_1 and Rh_2, which would have to be either independent, linked, or allelic. The first two possibilities are excluded since the product of the frequencies $Rh_1Rh_2 \times$ Rh-negative is much greater than $Rh_1 \times Rh_2$. Moreover, the existence of allelic genes Rh_1 and Rh_2 in individuals whose bloods react with both anti-Rh_1 and anti-Rh_2 would necessitate that this class not exceed 50 per cent, while the actual frequency is 70 per cent. Accordingly, the observations are best explained by assuming the existence of 3 qualitatively different Rh agglutinogens instead of only 2, one type reacting with anti-Rh_1 serum but not anti-Rh_2, a second reacting with anti-Rh_2 but not anti-Rh_1 and a third reacting with both sorts of anti-Rh sera." Wiener had considered the possibility of linkage but disproved it. Two years later Fisher reintroduced the linkage theory and made it the basis of a different notation system for the Rh-Hr types.

After discovery of the **rh'** factor, Wiener postulated the existence of four allelic genes: (1) *r*, which gives rise to agglutinogen rh that lacks both factors Rh_o and **rh'**; (2) *r'*, which gives rise to agglutinogen rh', with only specificity **rh'**; (3) R^o, which gives rise to agglutinogen Rh_o having only specificity Rh_o; and (4) R^1, which gives rise to agglutinogen Rh_1 that has both Rh_o and **rh'** specificities. This hypothesis was also confirmed by family studies.[22]

OTHER DISCOVERIES IN THE Rh-Hr SYSTEM

In 1943 Wiener described a third Rh antiserum that agglutinated the red cells of 30% of Caucasoids tested, which he later designated as anti-**rh''**.

Tests using three instead of two antisera divided the population into eight instead of four phenotypes. To account for their heredity, Wiener[27] postulated six allelic genes, presently designated *r*, *r'*, *r''*, R^o, R^1, and

R^2, and later added the rare genes r^y and R^z. From the following observations, it will become clear that as many as eight alleles must be invoked. There are two types of families in which one parent is type rh, that is, lacks all three Rh factors, **Rh₀**, **rh'**, and **rh"**, and the other is type rh_y, that is, has factors **rh'** and **rh"** but not **Rh₀**. In one type, half the children are type rh' and half are type rh", which is comparable to the situation in the mating O × AB. In these families the type rh_y parent is evidently genotype $r'r''$, and since the type rh parent must be genotype rr, half the children must be genotype $r'r$ and half $r''r$. In the second type of family, rh × rh_y, half the children are type rh and half are rh_y like the parents. It is therefore necessary to invoke a special allelic gene r^y which determines agglutinogen rh_y and has both specificities **rh'** and **rh"**. In the second type of family therefore the rh_y parent is genotype r^yr and the type rh parent is of course genotype rr, so that half the children must be genotype r^yr and half genotype rr.[28,29]

The eight phenotypes consist of two sets —four lacking factor **Rh₀** and four having the principal factor **Rh₀** (Table 8-2). The eight types and their corresponding thirty-six genotypes under the Wiener multiple allele theory are included in Table 8-3. The accuracy of this theory was established by a long series of family studies by Wiener et al.[30] and also by Race and associates.

DISCOVERY OF Hr FACTOR

It was also in 1941 that Levine and Javert reported that they had detected in the serum of an Rh-positive mother of an erythroblastotic infant an antibody with the property of agglutinating all Rh-negative bloods. This antibody, with reactions seemingly reciprocal to those of the Rh antibody, was named **anti-Hr**,[18] and the antigen it detected was called "Hr." The anti-**Hr** serum of Levine[24] gave approximately 30% positive reactions.* Levine also stated that all Rh-positive bloods which were not agglutinated by anti-**rh'** reacted with the anti-**Hr** serum. He postulated that Rh and Hr were allelic and that **Hr** incompatibility must be considered as a possibility whenever an Rh-positive mother gave birth to an Rh-negative child. Because of the reciprocal relationship of Hr to rh', the original symbol was later changed by Wiener from Hr to hr'.

At about the same time that Levine de-

*Whereas the general principle stated by Levine in his original report was correct, there seem to be some inaccuracies in his observations. Sera of the specificity he described, now called anti-hr', give 80% positive reactions instead of only 30%. Levine's original serum was evidently weak and probably failed to agglutinate red cells from heterozygotes for hr'. Similarly, in cases of erythroblastosis fetalis due to hr' sensitization, the mother is usually type Rh₁Rh₁ and the baby type Rh₁rh, but somehow the baby in Levine's case was typed as Rh negative. In his first case the mother may perhaps have been genotype R^1r and the baby $r'r$.

Table 8-2. The eight standard Rh blood types (phenotypes)

Phenotypes	Reaction of red cells with			Binary code number
	Anti-Rh₀	Anti-rh'	Anti-rh"	
rh	−	−	−	000
rh'	−	+	−	010
rh"	−	−	+	001
rh_y	−	+	+	011
Rh₀	+	−	−	100
Rh₁	+	+	−	110
Rh₂	+	−	+	101
Rh_z	+	+	+	111

Table 8-3. Wiener nomenclature of the Rh-Hr phenotypes and genotypes

2 Rh phenotypes — Designations	Approximate frequencies in N.Y.C. whites (%)	Reaction with anti-Rh$_o$ (or anti-rhesus)	12 Rh phenotypes — Designation†	Expected frequencies in N.Y.C. whites (%)§	Anti-rh'	Anti-rh''	Anti-rh^w	28 phenotypes — Designation	Expected frequencies in N.Y.C. whites (%)§	Anti hr'	Anti hr''	Anti hr	55 Genotypes*
Rh negative	15	−	rh	14.4	−	−	−	rh	14.4	+	+	+	rr
			rh'	0.46‡	+	−	−	rh'rh	0.46	+	+	+	$r'r$
								rh'rh'	0.0036	−	+	−	$r'r'$
			rh'^{w}	0.004	+	−	+	rh'^{w}rh	0.004	+	+	+	$r'^w r$
								rh'^{w}rh'	0.00006	−	+	−	$r'^w r'$ or $r'^w r'^w$
			rh''	0.38	−	+	−	rh''rh	0.38	+	+	+	$r''r$
								rh''rh''	0.0025	+	−	−	$r''r''$
			rh$_y$	0.01	+	+	−	rh'rh''	0.006	+	+	−	$r'r''$
								rh$_y$rh	0.008	+	+	+	$r^y r$
								rh$_y$rh'	0.0001	−	+	−	$r^y r'$
								rh$_y$rh''	0.0001	+	−	−	$r^y r''$
								rh$_y$rh$_y$	0.000001	−	−	−	$r^y r^y$
			rh$_y^w$	0.00005	+	+	+	rh'^{w}rh''	0.00005	+	+	−	$r'^w r''$
								rh$_y^w$rh'	0.000001	−	+	−	$r'^w r^y$
Rh positive	85	+	Rh$_o$	2.8	−	−	−	Rh$_o$	2.8	+	+	+	$R^o R^o$ or $R^o r$
			Rh$_1$	50.7	+	−	−	Rh$_1$rh	33.4	+	+	+	$R^1 r$, $R^1 R^o$ or $R^o r'$
								Rh$_1$Rh$_1$	17.3	−	+	−	$R^1 R^1$ or $R^1 r'$
			Rh$_1^w$	3.3	+	−	+	Rh$_1^w$rh	1.6	+	+	+	$R^{1w} r$, $R^{1w} R^o$ or $R^o r'^w$
								Rh$_1^w$Rh$_1$	1.7	−	+	−	$R^{1w} R^1$, $R^1 r'^w$, or $R^{1w} r'$ / $R^{1w} R^{1w}$, or $R^{1w} r'^w$
			Rh$_2$	14.6	−	+	−	Rh$_2$rh	12.2	+	+	+	$R^2 r$, $R^2 R^o$ or $R^o r''$
								Rh$_2$Rh$_2$	2.4	+	−	−	$R^2 R^2$ or $R^2 r''$
			Rh$_z$	13.2	+	+	−	Rh$_1$Rh$_2$	13.5	+	+	+	$R^1 R^2$, $R^1 r''$ or $R^2 r'$
								Rh$_z$rh	0.2	+	+	+	$R^z r$, $R^z R^o$ or $R^o r^y$
								Rh$_z$Rh$_1$	0.03	−	+	−	$R^z R^1$, $R^z r'$ or $R^1 r^y$
								Rh$_z$Rh$_2$	0.07	+	−	−	$R^z R^2$, $R^z r''$ or $R^2 r^y$
								Rh$_z$Rh$_z$	0.0008	−	−	−	$R^z R^z$ or $R^z r^y$
			Rh$_z^w$	0.6	+	+	+	Rh$_1^w$Rh$_z$	0.008	−	+	−	$R^{1w} R^z$, $R^{1w} r''$ or $R^z r'^w$
								Rh$_1^w$Rh$_2$	0.6	+	+	+	$R^{1w} R^2$, $R^{1w} r^y$ or $R^2 r'^w$

*This table does not include hypothetical genes R^{zw} and r'^w, which, if they exist at all, are very rare.

†In this table Rh$_1$ is used as a short designation for Rh$_o$', Rh$_2$ is short for Rh$_o$'', rh$_y$ is short for rh', and rh$_z$ is short for rh$_o$'.

‡The reduction in the frequency of type rh' as compared with that given in earlier charts can be attributed to recognition of bloods of type Rh$_1$ (containing Rh$_o$ variant), which are now included in type Rh$_1$ instead of rh'. The agglutinogens $\Re$h$_o$, $\Re$h$_1$, and $\Re$h$_2$ and their corresponding genes $\Re^o$, $\Re^1$, and $\Re^2$ are not given here because this would serve unnecessarily to complicate the chart by increasing the number of possible genotypes to 91. Also, no attempt is made to include certain rare, exceptional bloods such as those lacking both factors rh' and hr' or lacking both hr'' and hr'', etc.

§Based on the estimated gene frequencies, $r = 0.38$, $r' = 0.006$, $r'' = 0.005$, $r^y = 0.0001$, $r'^w = 0.00005$, $R^o = 0.005$, $R^1 = 0.41$, $R^2 = 0.15$, $R^z = 0.002$, and $R^{1w} = 0.02$.

Table 8-4. Serologic specificities of the Rh-Hr system

Antiserum	Specificity defined	Comments
1. Anti-**rhesus**	**rhesus** factor	Original antiserum of Landsteiner and Wiener; 85% positive in Caucasoids
2. Anti-**Rh$_o$**	**Rh$_o$**	Demonstrated by Wiener and Peters in posttransfusion sera, closely parallels anti-**rhesus**; 85% positive in Caucasoids; most important Rh factor; also called D
3. Anti-**rh′**	**rh′**	Described by Wiener in 1941; 70% positive in Caucasoids; also called C; so called because first factor found related to **Rh$_o$** but less antigenic
4. Anti-**rh″**	**rh″**	Described by Wiener and Sonn in 1943; 30% positive in Caucasoids; also called E; so called because second factor found related to **Rh$_o$**
5. Anti-**hr′**	**hr′**	Independently discovered by Levine working with Javert and Race working with Taylor; 80% positive in Caucasoids; also called c; so called because antithetical to **rh′**
6. Anti-**hr″**	**hr″**	First identified by Mourant; 98% positive; so called because antithetical to **rh″**; also called e
7. Anti-**Rh^A**	**Rh^A**	Cognates of **Rh$_o$**; first cognate found but not named by Shapiro; **Rh^A** first
8. Anti-**Rh^B**	**Rh^B**	of a series of cognates found by Wiener and Unger et al.(this family of
9. Anti-**Rh^C**	**Rh^C**	specificities closely associated with **Rh$_o$** was thoroughly studied and ex-
10. Anti-**Rh^D**	**Rh^D**	plained by Wiener and Unger); so designated to indicate their relationship to **Rh$_o$**
11. Anti-**hr**	**hr**	First identified by Rosenfield; specificity shared by products of genes r and R^o only; simulates somewhat specificity of factor **Hr$_o$** (d) predicted by Fisher; also called f and ce
12. Anti-**rh$_i$**	**rh$_i$**	First identified by Rosenfield and Haber; reacts only with agglutinogens determined by genes $r′$ and R^1, therefore simulates **rh′**; also called Ce
13. Anti-**rh$_{ii}$**	**rh$_{ii}$**	Described by Keith, Corcoran, Caspersen, and Allen; reacts with agglutinogens determined only by genes $r″$ and R^2; also called cE
14. Anti-**rh**	**rh**	Described by Dunsford; reacts with products only of genes r^y and R^z; also called CE
15. Anti-**rh^{w1}**	**rh^{w1}**	Found by Callender and Race; infrequent specificity associated with factor **rh′** in some type Rh$_1$ individuals, Rh$_1^w$, etc; also called C^w
16. Anti-**rh^x**	**rh^x**	Described by Stratton and Renton; another rare factor found associated with **rh′** in type Rh$_1$ blood
17. Anti-**rh^{w2}**	**rh^{w2}**	Described by Greenwalt and Sanger; rare specificity found associated with **rh″**, as in type Rh$_2^w$ blood; also called E^w
18. Anti-**hr^V**	**hr^V**	Described by DeNatale, Cahan, Jack, Race, and Sanger; specificity found associated with products of genes r and R^o, especially in type Rh$_o$ in Negroids; also called V and ce^s
19. Anti-**hr^H**	**hr^H**	Found by Shapiro; another specificity often associated with type Rh$_o$ in Bantu
20. Anti-**rh^G**	**rh^G**	Found by Allen and Tippett; specificity shared by red cells having factor **Rh$_o$**, **rh′**, or both and also individuals of rare type rh^G
21. Anti-**hr^S**	**hr^S**	Defined by Shapiro; cognate specificity of **hr″** factor; blood that is **hr″** positive but lacks **hr^s** is found mostly in Negroids
22. Anti-**hr^B**	**hr^B**	Another cognate specificity of **hr″** with similar properties to **hr^s** (Shapiro)
23. Anti-**Rh^{Wi}**	**Rh^{Wi}**	Described by Chown, Lewis, and Kaita; rare specificity associated with factor **Rh$_o$**; named after patient, Wiel; also called D^w
24. Anti-**rh^T**	**rh^T**	Found by Vos and Kirk; specificity associated with **rh″**; also called E^T
25. Anti-**Hr**	**Hr**	Antibody of very broad specificity, produced by isosensitization of persons of very rare types $\overline{R}$h$_o$ and $\overline{R}$h^w; has been designated incorrectly as anti-C+c+E+e
26. Anti-**RH**	**RH**	Specificity shared by all bloods except the Rh$_{null}$ type
27-32.		These additional specificities have not been thoroughly studied and so are not listed here.
Anti-**LW**	**LW**	Described by Levine; high-frequency factor incorrectly assigned to the Rh-Hr system, simply because the antiserum was originally produced by immunizing guinea pigs with rhesus monkey red cells; exact nature of the **LW** blood factor still not clearly understood because of lack of potent, specific reagents and the rarity of LW-negative blood (pp. 177 to 179)

scribed his Hr factor, Race and Taylor[25] described a blood factor they called **St,** which occurred in approximately 80% of all individuals. Wiener et al.[26] showed that **St** and **Hr** were the same and that the differences in percentage of positive reactions were due to differences in potencies of the reagents used.

By 1944, therefore, four blood specificities belonging to the Rh-Hr blood group system had already been identified—the original **Rh**$_0$ (and closely related rhesus factor of Landsteiner and Wiener), **rh′**, **rh″**, and **hr′**. Shortly thereafter additional Rh and Hr factors were discovered in rapid succession. At present more than thirty serologic specificities belonging to the Rh-Hr system have been identified. A list of the more important of these and their corresponding antibodies, with some comments, is given in Table 8-4. Of well over thirty Rh-Hr specificities known to date and listed in Table 8-4, some are extremely rare and have only theoretical interest because of unavailability of appropriate typing sera. Table 8-3, on the other hand, lists Rh phenotypes defined by reagents commonly used in blood grouping laboratories.

BLOOD SPECIFICITY Rh$_0$

The discovery of the Rh factors in human blood marked the beginning of a new era in blood grouping, transfusion, blood group genetics, serology, immunohematology and immunogenetics, as well as in the finding of more and more blood group specificities. This number now exceeds a hundred and seems to be limitless.

The **Rh**$_0$ factor is present in approximately 85% of all humans, occurring either alone or in combination with other factors in the system. The two other Rh factors, **rh′** and **rh″**, occur in 70% and 30% of the population, respectively.

Cognates of Rh$_0$—Rh^A, Rh^B, Rh^C, Rh^D [31,32]

Wiener, Unger, and associates showed that Rh$_0$ is not an agglutinogen with only a single blood factor (specificity). It is a complex agglutinogen having a multiplicity of factors. Some of these have been identified by antibodies in the sera of persons who seem to have typical Rh agglutinogens or variants of the **Rh**$_0$ factor, as in types Rh$_0$, Rh$_1$, Rh$_2$, and Rh$_Z$. However, these persons have had a hemolytic transfusion reaction or have given birth to an erythroblastotic infant, even though they were classified as **Rh**$_0$ positive. The antibody found in such sera at first appears to be identical to anti-**Rh**$_0$, but it does not react with the patient's own **Rh**$_0$-positive cells or with cells of certain other **Rh**$_0$-positive individuals.

To date at least four such antibodies have been discovered and identified—anti-**Rh**^{A}, anti-**Rh**^{B}, anti-**Rh**^{C}, and anti-**Rh**^{D}, respectively. The so-called "standard" anti-**Rh**$_0$ serum reacts with all bloods that have any or all of these specificities.

"Normal" Rh-positive blood has all the associated specificities **Rh**^{A}, **Rh**^{B}, **Rh**^{C}, and **Rh**^{D}. The existence of these specificities, called **cognates** of Rh$_0$ because of their close association with **Rh**$_0$ in Rh-positive blood, was discovered only because there are rare Rh-positive individuals who lack one or more of the cognate factors and become sensitized after transfusion of ordinary Rh-positive blood or during pregnancy with an Rh-positive fetus. The resulting antibody—anti-**Rh**^{A}, anti-**Rh**^{B}, etc. or combinations—closely parallels anti-**Rh**$_0$ in specificity, and hence arose the paradox of an Rh-positive person with anti-**Rh** in the serum, at times cited as "D with anti-D." Actually, this is not D with anti-D, otherwise the patient's serum would agglutinate his own cells, which does not occur.

Theoretically, any combination of the factors **Rh**^{A}, **Rh**^{B}, **Rh**^{C}, and **Rh**^{D} should be possible, which would give rise to as many as sixteen kinds of Rh-positive blood. Actually, not all have been found, and some varieties appear to be more common than others. As for terminology, since normal Rh positive has all the cognate factors, their presence is implied even when the simple symbol of the type is employed in the usual way. **Special symbols** are therefore required only for the rare bloods that lack one or more of the cognate factors; this was accomplished by using the small letter to indicate the missing specificity. As an example, type Rh_o^d, not uncommon in the South African Bantu, is blood of type Rh_o that lacks the specificity Rh^D. Similarly, blood of type $\mathfrak{R}h_1^{acd}$, which is the most common variant type in Caucasoids, has an Rh_o variant that lacks the cognate factors Rh^A, Rh^C, and Rh^D. The blood in question has the factor rh' as well.

Limited family studies have shown that the variant types such as Rh_o^d, not uncommon among Bantu, are transmitted by corresponding allelic genes, the gene in this case being R^{od}.

For fuller details, the reader should consult the original papers of Wiener, Unger et al.[32-36]

Another unusual antibody in the Rh-Hr system, involving the antigen Rh_o, was described in 1964 by Sussman and Wiener[37] in a group O Rh-positive Caucasian female. At admission her serum was screened by routine methods, and no antibodies were found. She then received two units of compatible group O Rh-positive blood, after surgery. Six months later she was readmitted to the hospital, and her serum was again tested for antibodies. At that time the serum revealed the presence of an irregular antibody resembling anti-Rh_o, and subsequently she was given group O Rh-negative blood in a transfusion. Her tests showed her to be group O, type Rh_1rh, Kell negative. Her serum sensitized all available Rh_o-positive cells except her own. An eluate from her agglutinated cells sensitized all available Rh_o-positive cells, including her own. Her cells thus divided all anti-Rh_o sera into two fractions—one that could agglutinate all Rh_o-positive cells *including* her cells, and one that was capable of agglutinating all Rh_o-positive cells *except* her own. Tests with anti-Rh^A, anti-Rh^B, anti-Rh^C, and anti-Rh^D were all negative, even though her red cells were strongly agglutinated by all anti-Rh_o sera

used, by the saline method, and by anti-rh' and anti-hr' sera, as well as by the standard anti-Rh_o. Her red cells were therefore classified as $Rh_1^{abcd}rh$ because they lacked the four cognates of Rh_o but did have Rh_o, rh', and hr'.

Using the atypical Rh-positive bloods that lack one or more of the cognate Rh factors, it has been possible to prove that anti-Rh_o sera are not monospecific as they seem to be but contain an entire spectrum of antibodies of Rh_o-like specificity. Many, but not all, when absorbed by Rh_1^{ab}blood, for example, until they no longer react with the absorbing red cells, have a fraction of antibodies remaining that gives parallel reactions with unabsorbed anti-Rh_o serum. This fraction appears to be of specificity anti-Rh^A, anti-Rh^B, or a mixture of the two. An analogous kind of fractionation of anti-Rh_o sera has been produced by Wiener et al.[38] by absorption with red cells of chimpanzees and gorillas.[39] Anti-Rh sera in general therefore contain a spectrum of antibodies with closely related specificities just like other sera such as human anti-A, which can be fractionated by absorption with human A_2 cells or sheep red cells, etc.

The simple factor Rh_o has a capital "R" because it is the most antigenic of the Rh-Hr factors and the most important clinically. To emphasize the central position of Rh_o in the Rh-Hr system, the capital "R" is used in contrast to the small "r" in symbols like rh', rh'', etc. Because specificities Rh^A, Rh^B, Rh^C, and Rh^D are cognates of Rh_o, the capital "R" is used for their symbols as well.

Other unusual Rh_o blood types

Variant $\mathfrak{R}h_o$. Variant $\mathfrak{R}h_o$ was discovered by Wiener[39] in 1944 and later was called factor D^u by British workers. To show its relationship to the standard Rh_o factor, the Germanic capital R is utilized in the terminology of Wiener. Certain blood specimens give weak but distinct reactions with most Rh_o antisera and therefore appear to occupy a position intermediate between negatively reacting bloods and those that give sharp positive reactions. This particular variant was originally designated an **intermediate Rh factor,** but that term is seldom used now. Family studies have shown that these variants are transmitted in most cases by corresponding allelic genes. The genes that determine them have been called **Rh₀** variant genes. The **Rh₀** variants, however, are not always due to allelic genes but may also result from suppressor genes. A common example is provided from blood of individuals of the genotype R^1r', in which case the r' gene seems to have a suppressor effect so that the blood reacts in the laboratory as Rh_1Rh_1, but its reactions with anti-**Rh₀** sera are weaker than usual.

According to Cepellini et al.,[40] there are two types of the Rh_0 variant ($\mathfrak{R}h_0$): the hereditary type, transmitted by a corresponding allelic gene as a weak Rh_0, and a second type resulting from gene interaction, as in genotype R^1r', which leads to suppression of Rh_0 by gene r' on the opposite chromosome.

The agglutinogen $\mathfrak{R}h_0$ belongs to a group of antigens with intermediate intensity of reaction with anti-**Rh₀** sera. Bloods that react typically with most anti-**Rh₀** sera but give slightly weaker reactions with a number of other anti-**Rh₀** sera are known as **high-grade variants.** Those that react consistently weakly with all anti-**Rh₀** sera are called **low-grade variants.**

Characteristic of the reactions of this variant are the following: When the tests are performed with the cells suspended in a saline medium, they fail to react with anti-**Rh₀** sera no matter how potent the antisera are. Almost every time, but not necessarily at all times, they do react with IgG(7S) anti-**Rh₀** serum if the conglutination method of testing is used; they also react by the antiglobulin technic, although the avidity and titer of the reactions are generally lower than those for typical Rh₀-positive bloods. Before identifying these cells as an **Rh₀** variant, however, a direct antiglobulin test should first be made to be certain that the cells were not coated

to begin with, as in cases of autohemolytic anemia.

The bloods of chimpanzees give reactions resembling those of high-grade **Rh₀** variants.[41]

The $\mathfrak{R}h_0$ factor is antigenic and can sensitize Rh-negative subjects; the specificity of the resulting antibodies resembles ordinary anti-**Rh₀**. There is no such thing therefore as an anti-$\mathfrak{R}h_0$ serum.

Bloods having an **Rh₀** variant are most common among Negroids and are more apt to lack one or more of the cognate factors **Rh^A**, **Rh^B**, **Rh^C**, or **Rh^D** than ordinary Rh-positive blood. $\mathfrak{R}h_0$ is relatively rare among Caucasoids.

When $\mathfrak{R}h_0$ is present in an agglutinogen along with the factors **rh'** and **rh″**, four other Rh types may be determined: (1) $\mathfrak{R}h_0$ has only factor $\mathfrak{R}h_0$, (2) $\mathfrak{R}h_1$ has factors $\mathfrak{R}h_0$ and **rh'**, (3) $\mathfrak{R}h_2$ has factors $\mathfrak{R}h_0$, and **rh″**, and (4) $\mathfrak{R}h_z$ has factors $\mathfrak{R}h_0$, **rh'**, and **rh″**. The corresponding allelic genes determining these agglutinogens are designated as $\mathfrak{R}^0$, $\mathfrak{R}^1$, $\mathfrak{R}^2$, and $\mathfrak{R}^Z$, respectively.

If the **Rh₀** variant is not detected by laboratory tests, an $\mathfrak{R}h_0$ individual will be mistyped as Rh negative, $\mathfrak{R}h_1$ will be mistyped as **rh'**, $\mathfrak{R}h_2$ as **rh″**, and $\mathfrak{R}h_z$ as **rh_y**. If blood of any of these individuals is used to transfuse an Rh-negative patient, that patient could develop anti-**Rh₀** antibodies, and after a second transfusion of the same type of blood could no doubt undergo a severe transfusion reaction or even die. In addition, if this Rh-negative patient who erroneously received $\mathfrak{R}h_0$ blood is a female in the childbearing age, she could become sensitized to the Rh factor to such extent that her chances of bearing a normal Rh-positive child become greatly lessened. Unfortunately, as already explained, the anti-**Rh₀** agglutinins formed as a response to this variant react not only with $\mathfrak{R}h_0$ but also with any blood having the **Rh₀** specificity. There are also reports of **low-grade** $\mathfrak{R}h_0$ persons who have formed anti-**Rh₀** agglutinins when erroneously transfused with Rh-positive blood.[42] Many of those who work in or operate blood banks consider any $\mathfrak{Rh}_o$ person as Rh positive if a donor and as Rh negative if a recipient.

Type $\bar{\bar{Rh}}_o$. Type $\bar{\bar{Rh}}_o$ was discovered by Race et al.[43] in 1951 when they found in the serum of a mother of an erythroblastotic infant an antibody that clumped 1,400 consecutive blood specimens but failed to clump the mother's own cells. Her red cells reacted with anti-Rh_o serum but appeared to lack the contrasting factors of the two pairs **rh′-hr′**, and **rh″-hr″**. Wiener suggested the use of a double bar over the R to indicate the absence of these two pairs of factors. The British workers called this **type —D—**. Race et al.[44] postulated that a **deletion** had occurred in the Rh "chromosomes" and asserted that the genotype of the mother was –D– / –D–. Wiener, on the other hand, postulated the existence of a **special rare allele,** $\bar{\bar{R}}^o$ so that the rare person of type $\bar{\bar{Rh}}_o$ would be homozygous, that is, $\bar{\bar{R}}^o\bar{\bar{R}}^o$. It is noteworthy, in the case of the study of Race and his associates, that not only was this propositus the product of a consanguineous marriage but also that among twenty other individuals of this type, thirteeen proved to be the results of consanguineous marriages, the parents of four more were related, and there was no information about the remaining three. This is a high rate of consanguinity by comparison with incidence for factors in other blood groups.

The red cells of this patient were agglutinated in saline media by anti-Rh_o(IgG) serum, which will not clump ordinary Rh_o-positive cells but instead coats them. It was assumed that this patient had an agglutinogen similar to agglutinogen Rh_o, except that it had a much higher reactivity with anti-Rh_o serum. This is one of the fundamental characteristics of this agglutinogen. It is understandable when one considers that there are no combining groups on the molecule for **rh′, hr′, rh″, hr″,** or **hr** so that the absence of steric interference from such groups permits readier access of anti-Rh_o to the Rh_o combining site. This is comparable to the case of group O blood that lacks combining sites

for **A** and **B** and therefore reacts most intensely with anti-**H**.

Evidence that the combining site for Rh_o is distinct from that for **rh′** and **rh″** was provided when Wiener showed, for example, that when type Rh_1Rh_2 blood is coated, or blocked, with Rh_oIgG antibodies, it still can be agglutinated by anti-**rh′** or anti-**rh″** saline agglutinating (IgM) reagents.[45]

In 1962 Unger[46] described a type $\bar{\bar{Rh}}_o$ blood that he found after deliberately searching for such a type for approximately 10 years and after testing many thousands of bloods. His patient was a Puerto Rican woman 82 years of age. All donor bloods tested with her serum were incompatible. Her blood group was O, MN $\bar{\bar{Rh}}_o$. Her serum contained a high-titered antibody that clumped the cells of all prospective donors but not her own cells. On further investigation,[47] the antibody was classified as anti-**Hr**, which is produced by isosensitized persons homozygous for the so-called double bar genes $\bar{\bar{R}}^o$, $\bar{\bar{R}}$, etc. Members of her family whose blood types were studied demonstrated clearly that not only was the rare gene $\bar{\bar{R}}^o$ transmitted by heredity but so also was another rare gene, $\hat{R}^{od}$. (See $\hat{R}^o$ gene under Hr factors, p. 124.)

Since the antibody in the serum of sensitized type $\bar{\bar{Rh}}_o$ reacts with all red cells except those of types $\bar{\bar{Rh}}_o$, $\bar{\bar{Rh}}^w$, and Rh_{null}, Wiener designated such antibodies "anti-**Hr**" (Table 8-4). In the Fisher-Race notations it was called anti-C+c+E+e, even though no antibody fractions such as anti-C, anti-c, etc. can be separated from it by absorption.

Individuals of genotype $\bar{\bar{R}}^o\bar{\bar{R}}^o$ are readily recognized by direct tests because they react as type $\bar{\bar{Rh}}_o$, but individuals who are heterozygous for the gene $\bar{\bar{R}}^o$ present a serious pitfall in medicolegal cases of disputed parentage. For example, a person of genotype $R^1\bar{\bar{R}}^o$ will react as phenotype Rh_1Rh_1, whereas if the genotype is $R^2\bar{\bar{R}}^o$, the person reacts as type Rh_2Rh_2. When therefore the putative father is type Rh_1Rh_1 and the child is type Rh_2Rh_2, paternity is not necessarily excluded; instead, if the putative father can be shown to be genotype $R^1\bar{\bar{R}}^0$ and the child genotype $R^2\bar{\bar{R}}^0$, there would be strong circumstantial evidence that this man actually is the father. This can sometimes be done by titration tests for gene dose effects; for example, a person of genotype R^2R^2 has a double dose of the gene for **hr'**, whereas a person of genotype $R^2\bar{\bar{R}}^0$ has only a single dose.

Type $\bar{R}h_0$. The single bar Rh_0 type was first described by Wiener et al.[47] It refers to individuals whose Rh_0 agglutinogen is characterized by absence of only the single pair of contrasting blood factors **rh″** and **hr″**. The British workers[48] call this cD–. This type was found in an inbred Caucasoid family in which three members were homozygous for the corresponding gene, genotype $\bar{R}^0\bar{R}^0$.

Type $\bar{\bar{R}}h^w$.[49] See specificity **rh^w**, following.

In type $\bar{\bar{R}}h^w$ the red cells react strongly with anti-**Rh_0** and anti-**rh^w** sera, but they also lack both contrasting pairs of blood factors, **rh'-hr'** and **rh″-hr″**. A corresponding gene, $\bar{\bar{R}}^w$, has been postulated. Type $\bar{\bar{R}}h^w$ persons presumably are homozygous, or genotype $\bar{\bar{R}}^w\bar{\bar{R}}^w$, and like type $\bar{R}h_0$ are generally the result of consanguineous marriage.

Type Rh_{null}. Rh_{null}, the first example of a blood with **no demonstrable Rh antigens**, was found by Vos et al.[50] in 1961. Later other examples were found—eleven in one year. In this rare type the red cells fail to clump in tests with any of the Rh-Hr antisera—anti-**Rh_0**, anti-**rh'**, anti-**rh″**, anti-**hr**, anti-**hr'**, anti-**hr″**, etc.; they also are not clumped by anti-**rhesus** serum produced in guinea pigs by injection of monkey blood.

Wiener[1] called attention to the fact that **two kinds of Rh_{null} bloods** have been described.[51,52] (1) type $\bar{r}h$, determined by a special corresponding allelic gene so that these individuals are homozygous genotype $\bar{r}\bar{r}$, and (2) type $\dot{r}h$, which includes individuals of any Rh-Hr genotype who are homozygous for an independently inherited **suppressor gene** comparable to the

suppressor genes for the Bombay blood group O_h of the A-B-O system. The suppressor gene affects not only Rh-Hr agglutinogens but also agglutinogens of other blood group systems, and it may so damage the envelope of the red cells as to cause a hemolytic anemia, with stomatocytosis, spherocytosis, and high reticulocyte count. Allen[54] suspects that the Rh_{null} genes are close to being lethal, and in fact some of them are lethal. Schmidt et al.,[53] in discovering this **frailty of the red cell envelope**, suggested that the red cells may have a shortened life span in vivo. In addition, these workers found that the Rh_{null} blood of one person was s positive and U negative, which is the only case on record with this combination of blood factors.

This observation may be related to the known fact that Rh_{null} individuals often show marked weakening of such antigens as C of the A-B-O system, some of the M-N antigens such as s and U, and also one of the Fy antigens.

SPECIFICITIES RELATED TO BLOOD FACTOR rh'
Specificity rh^w

Variants of each of the three so-called standard Rh factors have been found, and each of the factors also has related or **associated factors**. The **rh^w** specificity is an example of a factor associated with **rh'**. This factor is also designated **rh^{w1}** to avoid confusion with an analogous factor associated with **rh″** and assigned the same qualifying superscript, factor **rh^{w2}**. The **rh^w** antigen was identified by an antibody found by Callender and Race[55] in the serum of a woman with disseminated lupus erythematosus, which had evidently been formed as a result of numerous transfusions. The patient was phenotype Rh_1Rh_1 (Table 8-4). As a consequence of the multiple transfusions, she had developed antibodies against specificity **hr'**, which is reciprocally related to **rh'**, to specificity **N**, and to three previously undescribed blood specificities, one of which was **rh^w**. The superscript w was assigned to designate the name of the patient in whom the antibody was found (Willis). All persons with the specificity **rh**[w] also have specificity **rh'**. Blood having specificity **rh**[w] reacts more weakly with anti-**rh'** serum than does blood without the factor, and this can be a source of error in Rh-Hr typing.

The **incidence** of specificity **rh**[w] is only about 3% to 7% among Caucasoids so that it is easy to find donors who lack **rh**[w] when this type of blood is needed for transfusion.

Since **rh**[w] is found only in association with **rh'**, the only types in which the "w" factor is found are Rh_1 (specificities **Rh**$_0$ and **rh'**), Rh_Z (specificities **Rh**$_0$, **rh'**, and **rh''**), **rh'**, and rh_y (specificities **rh'** and **rh''**). These types, if they also have factor "w", would be designated as Rh_1^w, Rh_Z^w, rh'^w, rh_y^w, respectively. Actually, although rh_y^w and Rh_Z^w do exist, they are extremely rare. In place of Rh_Z^w, the symbol $Rh_1^wRh_2$ is preferred to indicate that in this type the **rh**[w] specificity is almost always associated with an Rh_1 agglutinogen. These various types are identified by using anti-**rh**[w] serum along with the three standard Rh antisera —anti-**Rh**$_0$, anti-**rh'**, and anti-**rh''**.

When bloods of type Rh_1 have been tested for the **hr'** factor and classified either as Rh_1Rh_1 (**hr'** negative) or Rh_1rh (**hr'** positive) (Table 8-3), they may be further divided by testing with anti-**rh**[w] serum according to Table 8-5.

The incidence of positive reactions is considerably higher among individuals belonging to phenotype Rh_1Rh_1 than among those who are Rh_1rh, which is to be expected.

The **rh**[w] factor is important in family studies, in transfusion reactions, and in

Table 8-5. Subdivision of types Rh_1Rh_1 and Rh_1rh

Rh type	Reaction with anti-rh^w serum	Rh subtype
Rh_1Rh_1	+	$Rh_1^wRh_1$
	−	Rh_1Rh_1 (proper)
Rh_1rh	+	Rh_1^wrh
	−	Rh_1rh (proper)

cases of erythroblastosis fetalis or isosensitization in pregnancy. It is therefore possible for a type Rh_1 individual to have a hemolytic transfusion reaction even if given type Rh_1 blood, provided the patient lacks **rh**[w] and the donor cells have this specificity. A type Rh_1 pregnant woman may become sensitized to **rh**[w] if it is present in her fetus' blood but not in her own. In this case the Rh-positive fetus could be either Rh_1^w or $Rh_1^wRh_2$ and the mother Rh_1 but lacking **rh**[w]. Some laboratories now test for the **rh**[w] factor routinely because of its potential danger to individuals lacking it.

Specificity rh^x

Another rare blood type specificity that occurs only in association with **rh'** is designated as **rh**[x], and the antibody that defines it is anti-**rh**[x]. The antigen was reported by Stratton and Renton[56] in 1954 and has been found in only 4 out of 3,391 unrelated people. The original antibody was found in the serum of a mother. The antibody has also been found in patients with acquired hemolytic anemia.

Together with anti-**rh**[w], anti-**rh**[x] further subdivides Rh_1 agglutinogens into three sharply defined types—Rh_1^x, Rh_1^w, and Rh_1 proper. The most common of these types, of course, is Rh_1 proper.

Specificity rh^G

In 1949 a serum was obtained from an immunized donor that reacted with almost equal titer on type Rh_0 and type rh' bloods and could be completely absorbed with either. There seems therefore to be a specificity, assigned the symbol **rh**[G], shared by agglutinogens having the specificity **Rh**$_0$, **rh'**, or both in much the same manner that specificity **C** of the A-B-O blood groups is shared by agglutinogens A and B (pp. 57 and 58), as **M**[e] is shared by M and He (pp. 97 and 98), and U by S and s (pp. 96 and 97).

It has been shown that some **Rh**$_0$-negative individuals (types rh or rh''), when sensitized with type Rh_0 blood, which lacks the **rh'** specificity, can produce antibodies (anti-**rh**^{G}) that react with type rh' blood, which lacks the **Rh**$_o$ specificity. This has occurred after transfusions. One such serum was that reported by Waller and Waller[57] in 1949.

Allen and Tippett[58] in 1958 had described the reaction of blood of an apparently type rh donor whose red cells nevertheless reacted with most anti-**Rh**$_o$ sera and therefore called this rare type rh^G. Using the serum they had described and obtained in which the cells of the same type rh^G blood were found to react with most anti-**Rh**$_o$ sera, Allen and Tippett prepared eluates of anti-**rh**^{G} specificity with which they showed that all the Rh agglutinogens have the specificity "G," except those determined by the genes r and r".

The factor just described has been designated **rh**^{G} by Wiener and antigen G by the British workers. The antibody that defines it is termed anti-**rh**^{G}. The genotypes corresponding to the rare type rh^G are obviously $r^G r$ and $r^G r^G$.

The **rh**^{G} factor is important in further

elucidating the complex nature of the serologic specificities in the Rh-Hr system and also because it is antigenic and can cause antibody production by transfusion or pregnancy in individuals whose blood cells lack the specificity.

Specificity rh$_i$

Another specificity in the Rh-Hr system was described in 1958 by Rosenfield and Haber.[59] This blood factor gives positive results using specific antisera, that is, sera that react with agglutinogens produced by genes r' and R^1 but not with any of the other six "standard" Rh-Hr agglutinogens, as seen in Table 8-6.

Since genes r^y and R^z and their corresponding agglutinogens are rare, it can easily be seen that anti-**rh**$_i$ closely parallels anti-**rh'** in its specificity. The two reagents —anti-**rh'** and anti-**rh**$_i$—can therefore easily be confused, and there are reasons to believe that a number of commercially prepared sera labeled anti-**rh'** are in reality anti-**rh**$_i$. This has given rise to serious errors in a number of medicolegal cases of disputed paternity described by Wiener —one case in 1964[60] and others in 1968.[61]

In the first case the putative father was reported to be type Rh$_z$Rh$_1$ and the child Rh$_2$rh. Paternity was excluded on the basis that an **hr'**-negative individual cannot be the parent of an **rh'**-negative child. Table 8-7 gives the results of the first report, together with the corrections. Actually, the child proved to be **rh'** positive and type Rh$_z$rh, as shown when both anti-**rh'** and anti-**rh**$_i$ sera were used to determine the phenotypes. Apparently, anti-**rh**$_i$ had in-

Table 8-6. Reactions of agglutinogens with anti-**rh'** and anti-**rh**$_i$ sera

Gene	Corresponding agglutinogen	Reaction with	
		Anti-rh'	Anti-rh$_i$
r	rh	−	−
r'	rh'	+	+
r"	rh"	−	−
r^y	rh$_y$	+	−
R^o	Rh$_o$	−	−
R^1	Rh$_1$	+	+
R^2	Rh$_2$	−	−
R^z	Rh$_z$	+	−

Table 8-7. False exclusion of paternity*

Blood of	Original report	Correct report		Reactions with		
		Phenotype	Genotype	Anti-rh'	Anti-rh$_i$	Anti-hr
Putative father	Rh$_z$Rh$_1$	Rh$_z$Rh$_1$	$R^z R^1$, $R^z r'$, or $R^1 r^y$	+	+	−
Mother	Rh$_1$rh	Rh$_1$rh	$R^1 r$, $R^1 R^o$, or $R^o r'$	+	+	+
Child	Rh$_2$rh	Rh$_z$rh	$R^z r$, $R^z R^o$, or $R^o r^y$	+	−	+

*From Wiener, A. S.: Acta Genet. Med. Gemellol. (Roma) **13:**340, 1964.

advertently been used instead of anti-**rh'** in the original tests, and since the child's cells did not react with this anti-**rh**$_i$ serum, the mistake was made of reporting the **rh'** factor missing, as seen in Table 8-8. The mother and father both had positive reactions with anti-**rh**$_i$ as well as with anti-**rh'** so that only the child's phenotype was in doubt.

From the results of the corrected examinations, it can be seen that the tests, instead of excluding paternity, gave strong circumstantial evidence in favor of paternity (see possible genotypes in Table 8-7), since both the father and the child carry the rare gene R^z (or r^y) that is lacking in the mother.

In another case involving the use of anti-**rh**$_i$ instead of anti-**rh'** serum, the husband left his wife on the strength of the original erroneous report before the error was discovered.

The principal usefulness of testing for reactions with anti-**rh**$_i$ therefore is to differentiate phenotypes **rh'rh''** from **rh**$_y$**rh** and **Rh**$_1$**Rh**$_2$ from **Rh**$_z$**rh**. In the case of **Rh**$_z$**rh** the individual could erroneously be typed as **Rh**$_2$**rh**. Anti-**rh**$_i$ differs from anti-**rh'** only in its inability to react with cells having the rare agglutinogens **rh**$_y$ and **Rh**$_z$. Most so-called anti-**rh'** sera have a mixture of varying proportions of anti-**rh'** and anti-**rh**$_i$. If the antiserum is predominantly anti-**rh**$_i$, errors will result. This can be avoided by testing the reagent against blood of the rare type **Rh**$_z$**rh**, which is **rh'** positive but **rh**$_i$ negative. Unfortunately this test is seldom done by serum manufacturers who distribute Rh-Hr antisera.

SPECIFICITIES RELATED TO BLOOD FACTOR rh''

Blood factor **rh''** is identified by its reaction with anti-**rh''** serum. Type **rh''** cells do not agglutinate in anti-**Rh**$_o$ or anti-**rh'** sera. Specificity **rh''** is also shared by types **Rh**$_2$ and **Rh**$_Z$, in addition to types **rh''** and **rh**$_y$.

Specificity rh^{w2}

In 1955 Greenwalt and Sanger[62] described a rare antigen that they called E^w, which is preferably designated **rh**^{w2}. The antibody had been the cause of hemolytic disease of the newborn, or erythroblastosis fetalis. Cells having this specificity are agglutinated by sera containing anti-**rh**^{w2} antibodies and by most but not all anti-**rh''** sera. In 1964 and again in 1966 there were reports of two more families[63] in which the blood cells reacted only with certain anti-**rh''** sera as well as with the original anti-**rh**^{w2} (anti-E^w) serum.

Specificity rh$_{ii}$

Blood specificity **rh**$_{ii}$ is a serologic specificity shared by agglutinogens **rh''** and **Rh**$_2$ but absent from the other six "standard" Rh-Hr agglutinogens. In specificity anti-**rh**$_{ii}$ therefore closely parallels anti-**rh''** serum, with which it may be confused. This would give rise to errors similar to those described for factor **rh**$_i$. If anti-**rh**$_{ii}$ is erroneously used in place of anti-**rh''**,

Table 8-8. Results of tests on child's blood in original and corrected examinations

Blood of child	Antisera used in original examination						
	Anti-Rh$_o$	**Anti-rh**$_i$*	**Anti-rh''**	**Anti-hr'**	**Anti-hr''**		
Results	+	−	+	+	+		
	Antisera used in corrected examination						
	Anti-Rh$_o$	**Anti-rh'**	**Anti-rh''**	**Anti-hr'**	**Anti-hr''**	**Anti-hr**	**Anti-rh**$_i$
Results	+	+	+	+	+	+	−

*Mistaken for anti-**rh'**.

blood belonging to type Rh_Zrh would be classified as type Rh_1rh. Anti-rh_{ii} serum appears to be extremely rare, and so this type of error is less likely to occur than that due to using anti-rh_i in place of anti-**rh′**.

THE Hr BLOOD FACTORS
Hr factors hr′ and hr″

The original Hr factor was discovered in 1941 by Levine and Javert[15-18,64,81] (p. 112ff). They had detected an antibody in the serum of an Rh-positive mother of an erythroblastotic infant that agglutinated all Rh-negative bloods. Because this antibody seemed to give reactions reciprocal to those of anti-Rh sera, it was designated anti-Hr, Hr being the reverse of Rh. Levine also noted that all Rh-positive bloods that were not agglutinated by anti-**rh′** sera did react with anti-Hr. He then postulated that Rh and Hr are allelic and asserted that Hr incompatibility must be considered as a possibility whenever an Rh-positive woman gave birth to an Rh-negative child and was sensitized. He also believed that people of phenotype Rh_1Rh_2 are invariably Hr negative, but this has been disproved. Levine's original serum gave positive reactions with 30% of all bloods tested by him, but in 1943 Race and Taylor found a serum of an Rh-positive mother of an erythroblastotic infant that had an agglutinin which reacted with all Rh-negative bloods but gave 80% instead of 30% positive reactions. The antiserum used by Levine was weaker than that used by Race and Taylor,[65] which Wiener and Davidsohn believe accounts for the errors in Levine's report.

Further study showed that the **Hr** factor is related to **rh′** in the same manner that **M** and **N** are related to one another; that is, individual bloods are either **rh′** positive or **Hr** positive, or both, just as bloods are either **M** positive or **N** positive, or both, but no bloods lack both these specificities.

Table 8-9. Identification of the Rh-Hr phenotypes by use of five standard antisera*

Rh phenotypes	Reactions with Rh antisera			Rh-Hr phenotypes	Reactions with Hr antisera		Binary code number (after Wiener)
	Anti-Rh_o	Anti-rh′	Anti-rh″		Anti-hr′	Anti-hr″	
Blood lacking Rh_o rh	−	−	−	rh	+	+	00011
rh′	−	+	−	rh′rh′	−	+	01001
				rh′rh	+	+	01011
rh″	−	−	+	rh″rh″	+	−	00110
				rh″rh	+	+	00111
rh_y	−	+	+	rh_yrh	+	+	01111
				rh_yrh′	−	+	01101
				rh_yrh″	+	−	01110
				$rh_y rh_y$	−	−	01100
Blood having Rh_o Rh_o	+	−	−	Rh_o	+	+	10011
Rh_1	+	+	−	Rh_1Rh_1	−	+	11001
				Rh_1rh	+	+	11011
Rh_2	+	−	+	Rh_2Rh_2	+	−	10110
				Rh_2rh	+	+	10111
Rh_z	+	+	+	Rh_zRh_o	+	+	11111
				Rh_zRh_1	−	+	11101
				Rh_zRh_2	+	−	11110
				Rh_zRh_z	−	−	11100

*Modified from Erskine, A. G. In Frankel, S., Reitman, S., and Sonnenwirth, A. C., editors: Gradwohl's clinical laboratory methods and diagnosis, ed. 7, St. Louis, 1970, The C. V. Mosby Co.

Because of its reciprocal relationship to **rh'**, Levine's Hr factor was designated **hr'** by Wiener. When the specificity **rh'** is determined by a gene at a locus, **hr'** is absent from the gene product. If **rh'** is absent, **hr'** is present. This is true except in extremely rare instances, for example, blood of type $\bar{\bar{R}}h_0$ or $\bar{\bar{R}}h^w$.

In 1945 Mourant[66] found a serum that gave reactions reciprocal to anti-**rh''**. The antibody was later designated anti-**hr''** and the specificity it detects, **hr''**.

Ever since the discovery of the reciprocal Hr factors, researchers have been searching for a possible antibody reciprocally related to Rh₀, which would then be called anti-Hr₀, but no such antibody has been found in the ensuing 35 years, and it must be assumed that Hr₀ is nonexistent.

The Hr factors are specificities reciprocally related to the Rh factors, and they are present in agglutinogens only when the corresponding, or reciprocal, Rh factor is absent from the same agglutinogen. The use of anti-**hr'** and anti-**hr''** sera establishes the right half of the phenotype symbol in the Rh-Hr system, as explained later.

The **hr'** factor is present in 80% of the population and **hr''** in 98%. In other words, only 20% of the population lack **hr'** and only 2% lack **hr''**. Both these factors·are antigenic so that when **hr'** is absent from a patient's red cells, that patient can be isosensitized to the **hr'** factor either through transfusions or by pregnancy, and if **hr''** is absent, that patient can be sensitized to the **hr''** factor. The relative infrequency of transfusion reactions and cases of erythroblastosis fetalis due to **hr'** or **hr''** sensitization is no doubt due to their weak antigenicity, but they are important and must not be ignored.

Phenotypes beyond the standard eight Rh blood types can be determined by testing the red cells also with anti-**hr'** and anti-**hr''** sera as shown in Table 8-9.

Individuals who are **rh'** negative are almost invariably **hr'** positive, and those who are **rh''** negative are almost invariably **hr''** positive, as already shown. There are ex-

tremely rare exceptions in types $\bar{\bar{R}}h_0$, $\bar{\bar{R}}h^w$, and $\bar{\bar{R}}h_0$. On the other hand, if the **rh'** or **rh''** factor is present, the corresponding Hr factor, **hr'** or **hr''**, may or may not be present. This is the basis for the results in Table 8-9.

Other specificities of the Hr complex have been discovered, which has made it possible to trace the **etiology of erythroblastosis fetalis** in some unusual cases and to explain certain transfusion reactions.

Other Hr specificities

Specificity hr^S (and bloods having agglutinogen $\hat{R}h_0$, $\hat{\mathfrak{R}}h_0$, or $\hat{r}h$). One of the most important discoveries in the Hr category was made by Shapiro[67] in 1960 when he announced his finding of a "new" blood factor he designated **hr^S**. This specificity was discovered during an investigation of an unusual case of hemolytic disease of the newborn. The superscript "S" was given because the patient's name was Shabalala.

The blood factor **hr^S** is related to factor **hr''** in much the same way as blood factors **Rh^A**, **Rh^B**, **Rh^C**, and **Rh^D** are related to the blood specificity **Rh₀**, that is, **hr^S** is a cognate of **hr''**.

Anti-**hr^S** reacts like anti-**hr''** except that occasional **hr''**-positive bloods give negative reactions with anti-**hr^S**. Shapiro reported that among the Bantu there were occasional individuals of type Rh₀ who had blood specificity **hr''** without the associated factor **hr^S**, and he designated these bloods $\hat{R}h_0$. The caret above the R designates absence of the expected **hr^S** factor. Shapiro showed that individuals of type $\hat{R}h_0$ are homozygous for a corresponding Rh-Hr allelic gene; that is, they are genotype $\hat{R}^0\hat{R}^0$. Type Rh₀ persons who are heterozygous for gene $\hat{R}^0$ would have to be genotype $R^0\hat{R}^0$ or $\hat{R}^0r$, and their blood necessarily gives reactions resembling those of ordinary phenotype Rh₀. Heterozygous genotype $R^2\hat{R}^0$ persons, on the other hand, give distinctive reactions because they have specificity **hr''** but lack factor **hr^S**. This phenotype has been assigned a distinctive symbol, $\mathfrak{R}h_2\hat{R}h_0$.

Most commercially available antisera labeled anti-**hr″**, as well as those made in individual laboratories, have both anti-**hr″** and anti-**hr**^{S} antibodies, but many are actually predominantly or almost completely anti-**hr**^{S}. If anti-**hr**^{S} serum is used in place of anti-**hr″**, blood of type Rh$_2$R̂h$_o$ would be incorrectly classified as type Rh$_2$Rh$_2$. Such an error can easily be made. This individual, if involved in a suit of disputed parentage, could be falsely excluded if the child is type Rh$_o$, genotype $R^o\hat{R}^o$. Anti-**hr**^{S} has been found in all sera tested that hitherto were regarded as **monospecific** for **hr″**.

Bloods lacking **hr**^{S} in the presence of **hr″** are fairly common in the Bantu. Discovery of the **hr**^{S} factor suggests that at least some persons previously designated R̄h$_o$ were actually type R̂h$_o$.

Sensitization of an **hr″**-positive individual with resultant anti-**hr″**–like antibodies is thus analogous to the anti-**Rh$_o$**–like antibody produced by some Rh$_o$-positive individuals (see cognates of Rh$_o$, pp. 115 and 116).

Population and family studies show absence of **hr**^{S} only in certain rare rh and Rh$_o$ agglutinogens. Four types distinguished by this anti-**hr**^{S} antiserum, along with their genotypes, are shown in Table 8-10. It is likewise possible that other agglutinogens like Rh$_1$ and Rh$_1^w$ might lack **hr**^{S}, but these have not as yet been reported.

In 1952 Wiener cautioned against using anti-**hr″** sera in tests for exclusion of parentage, citing a case in which the mother was type Rh$_o$ but her child appeared to be type Rh$_2$Rh$_2$. Taken at face value, it would have been assumed that this child was not hers. With the knowledge that **hr**^{S} antibody is present in most anti-**hr″** sera, it is possible that the serum Wiener used was actually anti-**hr**^{S} and not anti-**hr″**. It is especially important when testing the blood of Negroids to make sure that the anti-**hr″** serum is not anti-**hr**^{S} because some such persons occasionally lack **hr**^{S}, although they have **hr″**. Lack of **hr**^{S} is an inherited characteristic.

Specificity hr. In 1953 Rosenfield[68] announced the finding of an antiserum that at first was believed to be the predicted anti-**Hr$_o$**. Further studies showed, however, that the antibody in the serum reacted with blood cells from all individuals carrying the genes R^o and r, but it did not react with blood from persons lacking these genes. Originally this antibody was called anti-**f**,[69] but the Rh-Hr symbol assigned to it by Wiener is anti-**hr**. Because **hr** is a serologic specificity exclusively of the agglutinogens determined by genes r and R^o, reactions of anti-**hr** serum can subdivide phenotypes rh$_y$rh and Rh$_Z$Rh$_o$ into two subtypes each, as in Table 8-11.

Since the Fisher-Race triple-linked gene hypothesis did not allow for the specificity f, a new closely linked locus F-f was postulated, producing the enlarged "cistron" DCEF. However, the thus predicted **anti-**

Table 8-10. Four types distinguished by anti-**hr**^{S} serum

Type	Genotypes
Rh$_2$r̂h	$R^2\hat{R}^o$, R^2R̂h^o, and $\hat{R}^o r''$
R̂h$_o$	$\hat{R}^o\hat{R}^o$, $\hat{R}^o$R̂h^o, and $\hat{R}^o\hat{r}$
R̂h$_o$	R̂h^{o}R̂h^o, and R̂h$^o\hat{r}$
r̂h	$\hat{r}\hat{r}$

Table 8-11. Subdivisions of types rh$_y$rh and Rh$_Z$Rh$_o$ using anti-**hr** serum

Type	Reaction with anti-hr	Genotypes	Subtype
rh$_y$rh	+	$r^y r$	rh$_y$rh
	−	$r'r''$	rh′rh″
Rh$_Z$Rh$_o$	+	$R^Z r$, $R^Z R^o$, or $R^o r^y$	Rh$_Z$rh
	−	$R^1 R^2$, $R^1 r''$, or $R^2 r'$	Rh$_1$Rh$_2$

thetical antigen F has never been found. It was then noticed that the so-called f antigen occurred in blood of individuals carrying the chromosome complex *dce* (corresponding to the *r* gene of Wiener) or *Dce* (corresponding to Wiener's gene R^o) but not in the blood of individuals carrying any of the other six chromosome complexes. Factor f was therefore renamed ce on the postulation that there is an interaction product of the genes *c* and *e* in the cis position on the same chromosome. Unfortunately, the position taken regarding terminology was not firm so that the symbol f continues to be used alongside of ce. The same hypothesis was used by the British investigators to explain the properties of other Rh-Hr specificities. For example, factor **rh**$_i$ corresponds to the Fisher-Race Ce complex, **rh**$_{ii}$ corresponds to their complex cE, whereas specificity **rh** corresponds to CE. (See Table 8-4.) The multiple allele theory readily accounts for these specificities, provided one bears in mind the difference between agglutinogens and blood factors (specificities), and this eliminates the need to invoke additional hypotheses.

Anti-**hr** serum is in short supply and so cannot be used routinely to subtype all type Rh$_Z$Rh$_o$ blood. It must therefore be reserved for cases in which it appears likely from the various Rh-Hr types of the putative parents and child that the results of the **hr** test would yield useful information.

The bulk of persons of phenotype Rh$_Z$Rh$_o$ are **hr** negative and thus belong to subtype Rh$_1$Rh$_2$. Gene R^Z is rare in comparison with genotype R^1R^2. Type rh$_y$rh is about evenly subdivided between genotypes r^yr and $r'r''$, since even though gene r^y is very rare, so is the combination of the two uncommon genes r' and r''.

The value of anti-**hr** serum is primarily its use in medicolegal cases.

Anti-**hr** and anti-**rh**$_i$ sera are useful in **resolving parentage disputes** involving type Rh$_Z$Rh$_o$ putative parents or children, that is, bloods that give positive reactions with all five of the standard anti-Rh sera: anti-**Rh$_o$**, anti-**rh'**, anti-**rh''**, anti-**hr'**, and anti-**hr''**. As an example, a type Rh$_Z$Rh$_o$ person

with a type rh or type Rh$_o$ child, or vice versa, would be excluded if he belonged to one of the more common genotypes, R^1R^2, or R^1r'', or R^2r', but not if he belonged to one of the rare genotypes, R^Zr, or R^ZR^o, or R^or^y. If the blood of a type Rh$_Z$Rh$_o$ individual is hr negative and rh$_i$ positive, he is excluded. If the blood is negative with anti-**rh**$_i$ serum and positive with anti-**hr**, he is not excluded.

Specificity V, or hr^V. A blood factor, apparently related to the Rh-Hr blood group system, was discovered in 1954 by DeNatale et al.[70] and was designated **V**. It was common in Negroids but rare in Caucasoids. The antigen is inherited as a mendelian dominant. It is associated exclusively with genes *r*, $\mathfrak{R}^o$, and R^o. In 1960 Geiger[71] reported finding antibodies in the serum of a Caucasoid male who had had twenty-five transfusions without any reported reactions. The serum reacted with red cells having the specificity **V** by both the antiglobulin and the ficinated cell method. The antibodies were found in a routine examination of the patient's serum using a panel of cells with various antigens, as is now customary in many blood banks and hospitals. Apparently the patient was V negative and had received blood from a donor whose blood had the **V** specificity. The blood factor **V** is designated as **hr^V** in the Wiener terminology.

Anti-**hr^V** serum separates hr-positive red cells of Negroids into two subgroups—hr^V negative and hr^V positive, for example, Rh$_o$ proper and Rh$_o^V$.

Specificity hr^H. In 1960 Sanger et al.[72] reported finding an antibody, anti-VS, in the blood of a woman they had examined. The serum reacted with all bloods that had the V antigen and with most **type rh' bloods of the type seen most commonly in Negroids,** rh'^{n}, which differs from type rh' of whites by its failure to react with anti-**rh**$_i$ sera.

Later, in 1964, Shapiro[73] presented serologic and genetic evidence that anti-VS sera of Sanger et al. actually contained two antibodies—one anti-**hr^V** (anti-**V**) and a second antibody that he designated anti-hr^H after the donor, a woman named Hernandez, in whose serum the antibody had been found. In examining 511 blood specimens of South African Bantu, it was found that 3.3% had only **hr**^{V}, 14.5% had only **hr**^{H}, and 29.9% had both factors. Shapiro showed that **hr**^{V} and **hr**^{H} occur in various combinations in the products of genes r'^n, R^o, and r in Negroids but seldom if ever in the products of R^1 and R^2 genes. Each Rh gene determines agglutinogens having one, both, or neither of the specificities.

OTHER UNUSUAL VARIANTS

Other Rh agglutinogens have been found. These are of interest scientifically, but they are not of much practical clinical importance. They have been assigned special designations such as rh^M, rh^L, and rh$'^N$.[74]

NEW SOURCE OF ANTI-Rh ANTIBODIES

It may be recalled that the first anti-Rh reagent was obtained from the sera of rabbits immunized with red cells of rhesus monkeys. Later it was found that the sera obtained from guinea pigs immunized with rhesus blood cells gave sharper reactions and were therefore more satisfactory as reagents for typing human blood. In fact, at one time guinea pig antisera were the only readily available diagnostic anti-Rh sera and were described as the preferred reagent in clinical laboratory texts as late as 1948.[75] However, when the existence of "blocking" antibodies in human anti-Rh sera was demonstrated and methods were devised for circumventing their interference with the tests as ordinarily performed at that time in saline media,[76] human anti-Rh sera became the preferred reagent and guinea pig anti-rhesus sera are now hardly ever used for clinical work.

Nevertheless, guinea pig anti-rhesus sera still remain of considerable theoretical interest and have been used in sporadic investigative work. Recently (1977), the idea of using primate red cells for production of anti-Rh sera was revived by the discovery that potent and highly specific anti-**Rh**$_o$ antibodies could be produced by iso-

immunizing a chimpanzee with the red cells of another appropriately selected chimpanzee.[77] The reagent proved to give results exactly paralleling those obtained with anti-**Rh**$_o$ from a human source, not only in tests with typical Rh-positive and Rh-negative bloods but also in tests with the rare Rh phenotypes.[78] It is of interest that the chimpanzee anti-**Rh**$_o$ serum detects on chimpanzee red cells a simian-type specificity called **L**^{c} (for details see Chapter 16).

THE LW FACTOR

The **LW** factor is a blood group factor, discovered by Levine, which is found in more than 99% of all persons tested. It was mistakenly confused with the **Rh**$_o$ factor discovered by Landsteiner and Wiener. Since convincing evidence that it bears any relationship at all to the Rh-Hr system of blood groups is lacking, it will not be discussed further in this chapter but instead is in Chapter 11, on high- and low-frequency blood factors.

BIOCHEMISTRY OF THE Rh-Hr AGGLUTINOGEN

The Rh blood group substances occur solely on the surface of red cells, despite some early claims of their presence in amniotic fluid and other secretions, which could not be confirmed. In his earlier experiments, Wiener used autoclaved saliva to neutralize the A and B isoagglutinogens when preparing anti-Rh reagents from the sera of isosensitized humans. Attempts to extract the Rh substance in pure form from the red cell stromata have been unsuccessful or inconclusive, and so it is not surprising that little or nothing is known about the biochemistry of those substances. There is evidence that expression of the Rh antigens depends on a complex interaction of lipid and protein.[79,80]

IMPORTANCE OF THE Rh-Hr BLOOD GROUP FACTORS
Transfusion

Next to A-B-O, Rh-Hr is the most important blood group system. Individuals who lack one or more of the Rh-Hr factors can be isosensitized to that specificity through transfusion, and a pregnant woman can be isosensitized to a factor lacking in her blood cells but present in those of her fetus. Isosensitization therefore can result from two events. The first is transfusion or injection of Rh-positive red cells or red cell stromata into an Rh-negative individual. (A serious hemolytic reaction may follow transfusion of Rh-positive blood into an Rh-sensitized person or transfusion of blood having the factor(s) lacking in the recipient's blood.) The second is sensitization from pregnancy with a fetus having a factor(s) lacking in the red cells of the mother.

In transfusing an Rh-negative patient, no Rh-positive subject should be selected as a donor. This is most important in transfusing women, for a person once Rh-sensitized remains so for life. A woman who is already sensitized to the Rh factor as a result of a transfusion may have difficulty in bearing a normal child if the father is Rh positive. If blood having a particular Rh factor lacking in the red cells of the patient is transfused to that patient, antibodies against that factor are formed, and, as stated, these persist for life. If that same person, now sensitized, receives a transfusion of blood having that factor, the antibodies already present react with the incoming donor cells, and a severe hemolytic transfusion reaction most likely will ensue, or death might follow. In selecting donors, therefore, follow the rule that *all Rh-negative persons should receive only Rh-negative blood in a transfusion.*

If a patient is Rh positive but lacks Rh_o —that is, if he belongs to type rh', rh'', or rh$_y$ and if blood having Rh_o is used to transfuse him—he most likely will form anti-Rh_o antibodies. If he later receives any blood having this factor such as type Rh_o, Rh_1, Rh_2, Rh_Z, or even $\mathfrak{Rh}_o$ $\mathfrak{Rh}_1$, $\mathfrak{Rh}_2$, or $\mathfrak{Rh}_Z$, the antibodies formed after the initial transfusion will react with the incoming donor cells, and a serious reaction will occur. Similarly, if an individual of type rh, that is, a person lacking Rh_o, rh', and rh'', is transfused with blood having any of these specificities, he can form antibodies and thus become isosensitized so that a subsequent transfusion of blood having the same specificity could cause a serious reaction.

Discovery of the various Rh-Hr specificities has come as a result of transfusion of blood having such factors into a recipient who lacked them, with formation of antibodies of the same specificity as the factors that stimulated their production. These are **intragroup transfusion reactions,** so named because they occur between individuals of the same A-B-O groups, for example, group O blood transfused to a group O recipient but of different Rh-Hr types. This is in contrast to those **intergroup reactions** in which the wrong A-B-O donor blood was erroneously used.

In modern laboratories it is becoming increasingly more difficult to select the wrong donor blood, since not only are the red cells of donor and recipient screened with a battery of different antisera containing many different types of antibodies, but also the sera of both donor and recipient are likewise tested for antibodies against a battery of selected blood cells, each having certain definite antigens. This is detailed in Chapter 19.

Although the most antigenic of all the Rh factors is Rh_o, found in 85% of the population, the other Rh-Hr factors are also antigenic, and this must be kept in mind. Many laboratories, in dealing with blood types rh', rh'', and rh$_y$, consider any person of these three types as Rh negative if that person is the **recipient** of a transfusion, and they will use only type rh blood for transfusion; but if that individual is a **donor,** he is considered Rh positive, and his blood is given only to Rh-positive patients.

Routinely, patients are now tested for the Rh_o factor, and if it is not present, an Rh-negative donor is chosen. If it is present, Rh-positive blood may be used.

The Hr factors are also antigenic, but to a lesser degree than Rh_o. Of the Hr factors, **hr′** is believed to be the most antigenic. Type rh blood has both **hr′** and **hr″**, and this is one of the reasons why it is not desirable to transfuse Rh-positive patients with Rh-negative blood.

Pregnancy

Transfusion of the mother. In the chapter on erythroblastosis fetalis (p. 133ff), the mechanism by which the fetal cells may enter the maternal circulation is presented in detail and will not be given here. Suffice it to say that in cases in which the mother is Rh negative and the fetus is Rh positive, the cells of the fetus may enter the maternal circulation and cause her to form anti-Rh antibodies, in other words, to become isosensitized to the Rh factor. If this mother is in need of a blood transfusion and if she is transfused with Rh-positive blood, the antibodies that she has already formed by reason of the presence of an Rh-positive fetus will react against the incoming Rh-positive donor red cells, and a serious transfusion reaction undoubtedly will occur. If Rh-negative blood is used, her antibodies will be harmless against the cells because they do not have the Rh antigen, and no reaction due to Rh incompatibility will ensue. Therefore, even in the primary transfusion of an Rh-negative pregnant or postpartum woman, always select only Rh-negative donors of the same A-B-O blood group as the patient.

Erythroblastosis fetalis. Erythroblastosis fetalis (EBF) is the subject of Chapter 9.

Anthropology

As with the A-B-O groups, the Rh-Hr types show significant differences in their distributions among various races and populations throughout the world. As an example, Table 8-12 shows the differences in frequencies of the Rh-Hr types observed among whites, Negroids, and Chinese in New York City. Study of such differences constitutes an invaluable tool for anthropologists for tracing origins and affinities of human races and populations. See also seroanthropology, p. 211.

Table 8-12. Distribution of the Rh-Hr blood types in the New York City metropolitan area[*]

Population	rh	rh′rh	rh″rh	rh_yrh	$\Re h_o$	Rh_o	Rh_1Rh_1	Rh_1rh	$Rh_1^wRh_1$	Rh_1^wrh	Rh_2Rh_2	Rh_2rh	Rh_2Rh_o	Rh_2Rh_1	Rh_zRh_2	Total tested
Caucasoid																
Number	60	4	4	1	0	11	111	162	5	5	9	47	90	1	0	500
Percent	12.0	0.8	0.8	0.2	0	2.2	22.2	32.4	1.0	1.0	1.8	9.4	16.0	0.2	0	
Negroid																
Number	34	5	0	0	3	229	10	104	0	1	1	93	20	0	0	500
Percent	6.8	1.0	0	0	0.6	45.8	2.0	20.8	0	0.2	0.2	18.6	4.0	0	0	
Chinese																
Number	0	0	0	0	0	1	213	30	0	0	19	6	126	4	1	400
Percent	0	0	0	0	0	0.25	53.25	7.5	0	0	4.75	1.5	31.5	1.0	0.25	

[*]Modified from Wiener, A. S.: Advances in blood grouping, vol. 3, New York, 1970, Grune & Stratton, Inc.

REFERENCES

1. Wiener, A. S.: Advances in blood grouping, vol. 3, New York, 1970, Grune & Stratton, Inc.
2. Medicolegal Applications of Blood Grouping Tests, Supplementary Report; a report of the Committee on Medicolegal Problems, American Medical Association, prepared by A. S. Wiener, R. D. Owen, C. Stormont, and I. B. Wexler: J.A.M.A. 164:2036, 1957.
3. Miale, J. B.: Trans. N.Y. Acad. Sci. (ser. II) 29:887-891, 1967.
4. Wiener, A. S., and Socha, W. W.: Haematologia (Budap.) 5:461, 1971.
5. Ranganathan, K. S.: Antiseptic 50(28):1-6, 1968.
6. Rosenfield, R. E., Allen, F. H., Swisher, S. N., and Kochwa, S.: Transfusion 2:287, 1962.
7. Wiener, A. S., and Peters, H. R.: Ann. Intern. Med. 13:2306, 1940.
8. Wiener, A. S.: Arch. Pathol. 32:227, 1941.
9. Levine, P., and Stetson, R. E.: J.A.M.A. 113:126, 1939.
10. Unger, L. J.: J.A.M.A. 84:591, 1925.
11. Neter, E.: J. Immunol. 30:255, 1936.
12. Culbertson, C. J., and Ratcliffe, A. W.: Am. J. Med. Sci. 192:471, 1936.
13. Zacho, A.: Z. Rassenphysiol. 8:1, 1938.
14. Pondman, A.: Nader. Tidjschr. Geneesk. 82:611, 1938.
15. Levine, P., Katzin, E. M., and Burnham, L.: J.A.M.A. 116:825, 1941.
16. Levine, P., Vogel, P., Katzin, E. M., and Burnham, L.: Science 94:371, 1941.
17. Burnham, L.: Am. J. Obstet. Gynecol. 42:389, 1941.
18. Levine, P., Burnham, L., Katzin, E. M., and Vogel, P.: Am. J. Obstet. Gynecol. 42:925, 1941.
19. Landsteiner, K., and Wiener, A. S.: J. Exp. Med. 74:309, 1941.
20. Wiener, A. S.: Proc. Soc. Exp. Biol. Med. 56:173, 1944.
21. Race, R. R.: Nature (Lond.) 153:771, 1944.
22. Wiener, A. S., and Landsteiner, K.: Proc. Soc. Exp. Biol. Med. 53:167, 1943.
23. Wiener, A. S.: Blood groups and transfusion, ed. 3, Springfield, Ill., 1943, Charles C Thomas, Publisher; reprinted New York, 1962, Hafner Publishing Co.
24. Levine, P.: J. Pediatr. 23:656, 1943.
25. Race, R. R., and Taylor, G. L.: Nature (Lond.) 152:300, 1943.
26. Wiener, A. S., Davidsohn, I., and Potter, E. L.: J. Exp. Med. 81:63, 1945.
27. Wiener, A. S.: Proc. Soc. Exp. Biol. Med. 54:316, 1943.
28. Wiener, A. S.: Nature (Lond.) 2:735, 1948.
29. Wiener, A. S., and Hyman, M. A.: Am. J. Clin. Pathol. 18:921, 1948.
30. Wiener, A. S.: Rh-Hr blood types, New York, 1954, Grune & Stratton, Inc.
31. Wiener, A. S., Geiger, J., and Gordon, E. B.: Exp. Med. Surg. 15:75, 1957.
32. Unger, L. J., and Wiener, A. S.: Blood 14:522, 1959.
33. Unger, L. J., Wiener, A. S., and Weiner, L.: J.A.M.A. 170:1380, 1959.
34. Unger, L. J., and Wiener, A. S.: J. Lab. Clin. Med. 54:835, 1959.
35. Sacks, M. S., Wiener, A. S., Jahn, E. F., Spurling, C. L., and Unger, L. J.: Ann. Intern. Med. 51:740, 1959.
36. Wiener, A. S., and Gordon, E. B.: J. Forensic Med. 14:131, 1967.
37. Sussman, L. N., and Wiener, A. S.: Transfusion 4:50, 1964.
38. Wiener, A. S., Moor-Jankowski, J., and Gordon, E. B.: Am. J. Hum. Genet. 16:246, 1964.
39. Wiener, A. S.: Science 100:595, 1944.
40. Cepellini, R., Dunn, L. C., and Turri, M.: Proc. Natl. Acad. Sci. U.S.A. 44:283, 1955.
41. Wiener, A. S., and Wexler, I. B.: Heredity of the blood groups, New York, 1958, Grune & Stratton, Inc.
42. Argall, C. I., Ball, J. M., and Trentelman, E.: J. Lab. Clin. Med. 41:895, 1953.
43. Race, R. R., Sanger, R., and Selwyn, J. G.: Br. J. Exp. Pathol. 32:124, 1951.
44. Race, R. R., and Sanger, R.: Blood groups in man, ed. 5, Philadelphia, 1968, F. A. Davis Co.; ed. 6, Oxford, England, 1975, Blackwell Scientific Publications.
45. Wiener, A. S., and Wexler, I. B.: An Rh-Hr syllabus, ed. 2, New York, 1963, Grune & Stratton, Inc.
46. Unger, L. J.: Transfusion 4:173, 1964.
47. Wiener, A. S., Gordon, E. B., and Cohen, L.: Am. J. Hum. Genet. 4:363, 1952.
48. Tate, H., Cunningham, C., McDade, M. G., Tippett, P. A., and Sanger, R.: Vox Sang. 5:398, 1960.
49. Gunson, H. H., and Donohue, W. L.: Vox Sang. 2:320, 1957.
50. Vos, G. H., Vos, D., Kirk, R. L., and Sanger, R.: Lancet 1:14, 1961.
51. Ishimori, T., and Hasekura, H.: Proc. Jpn. Acad. 42:658, 1966.
52. Ishimori, T., and Hasekura, H.: Transfusion 7:84, 1967.
53. Schmidt, P. J., Lostumbo, M. M., English, C. T., and Hunter, O. B., Jr.: Transfusion 7:33, 1967.
54. Allen, F. H., Jr.: Am. J. Clin. Pathol. 66:467, 1976.
55. Callender, S. T., and Race, R. R.: Ann. Eugen. (Lond.) 13:102, 1946.

56. Stratton, F., and Renton, P. H.: Br. Med. J. 1:962, 1954.
57. Waller, R. K., and Waller, M. J.: J. Lab. Clin. Med. 34:270, 1949.
58. Allen, F. H., and Tippett, P. A.: Vox Sang. 3:321, 1958.
59. Rosenfield, R. E., and Haber, G. V.: Am. J. Hum. Genet. 10:474, 1958.
60. Wiener, A. S.: Acta Genet. Med. (Rome) 13:304, 1964.
61. Wiener, A. S.: J. Forensic Med. 15:106, 1968.
62. Greenwalt, T. J., and Sanger, R.: Br. J. Haematol. 1:52, 1955.
63. Winter, N., Milkovich, L., and Konugres, A. A.: Transfusion 6:271, 1966.
64. Levine, P.: J. Pediatr. 23:656, 1943.
65. Race, R. R., and Taylor, G. L.: Nature (Lond.) 152:300, 1943.
66. Mourant, A. E.: Nature (Lond.) 155:544, 1945.
67. Shapiro, M.: J. Forensic Med. 7:96, 1960.
68. Rosenfield, R. E., Vogel, P., Gibbel, N., Sanger, R., and Race, R. R.: Br. Med. J. 1:975, 1953.
69. Sanger, R., Race, R. R., Rosenfield, R. E., Vogel, P., and Gibbel, N.: Proc. Natl. Acad. Sci. U.S.A. 39:824, 1953.
70. DeNatale, A., Cahan, A., Jack, J. A., Race, R. R., and Sanger, R.: J.A.M.A. 159:247, 1955.
71. Geiger, J.: J.A.M.A.: 173:1590, 1960.
72. Sanger, R., Noades, J., Tippett, P., Race, R. R., Jack, J. A., and Cunningham, C. A.: Nature (Lond.) 186:171, 1960.
73. Shapiro, M.: J. Forensic Med. 2:52, 1964.
74. Sussman, L. N.: Blood grouping tests, Springfield, Ill., 1968, Charles C Thomas, Publisher.
75. Todd, J. C., Sanford, S. H.: Clinical diagnosis by laboratory methods, ed. 11, Philadelphia, 1948, W. B. Saunders Co.
76. Wiener, A. S.: Rh-Hr blood types; application in clinical and legal medicine and anthropology, New York, 1954, Grune & Stratton, Inc.
77. Socha, W. W., and Moor-Jankowski, J.: Int. Arch. Allergy Appl. Immunol. (In press 1977.)
78. Marsh, W. L.: Personal communication, 1977.
79. Green, F. A.: Biol. Chem. 243:5519, 1968.
80. Green, F. A.: Nature (Lond.) 219:86, 1968.
81. Levine, P., and Javert, C.: N.Y. State J. Med. 42:1928, 1942.

9 □ Erythroblastosis fetalis

EBF, HEMOLYTIC DISEASE OF THE NEWBORN, ICTERUS GRAVIS NEONATORUM

CHARACTERISTICS OF THE DISEASE

The term **erythroblastosis** refers literally to the presence of considerable numbers of nucleated red cells (erythroblasts) in the circulating blood. **Fetalis,** literally translated, means "of the fetus." One would expect, therefore, that this disease is a condition in which there are a larger number than normal of nucleated red cells in the blood of a fetus. Actually, erythroblastosis fetalis (EBF) is the name given to a disease of the newborn, a severe hemolytic anemia due to the presence in the baby of antibodies derived from the mother by transplacental transfer. The two principal varieties of the condition are Rh-Hr and A-B-O hemolytic disease. The **blood film** of the newborn erythroblastotic infant shows many changes, and the more severe the condition, the more severe the blood picture is likely to be. There will be macrocytosis, reticulocytosis over 6%, and ordinarily all types of nucleated red cells. The white cells are also affected, with greater than normal numbers of young leukocytes. The principal finding, however, is the tremendous increase in the blood **bilirubin level,** almost all of which is the indirect variety, since the immaturity of the hepatic enzyme system prevents the liver from converting it to the direct type. The amniotic fluid also contains bilirubin pigment, which is the basis for a prenatal test to determine the probability that erythroblastosis fetalis will develop in the child.

The disease is characterized by abnormal destruction and regeneration of erythrocytes. The findings vary, depending on the severity of the disease. It is believed that intravascular hemolysis, clumping, or both, initiates all the other pathologic changes. The degree of pathologic changes depends on the attempt by the body to compensate for the excessive destruction of erythrocytes. The most commonly observed **signs** are anemia, increased bilirubin in the blood and various fixed tissues of the body, abnormal islands of erythropoiesis in many organs including the spleen and liver, and an increase in immature forms of erythrocytes in the circulating blood. The condition, when severe, is also accompanied by extreme edema (hydrops), which has not as yet been satisfactorily explained, except that it might be due to renal failure and injury of the general capillary bed, along with the decrease in plasma proteins that occurs in conjunction with cellular hemolysis. Other signs are jaundice, hepatosplenomegaly, and varying degrees of purpura. The infant may have all, some, or none of these signs. Those infants most severely affected are stillborn or die shortly after birth. Untreated infants who survive the immediate postnatal period almost invariably show a steady rise in serum bilirubin. This is believed to be due to the fact that the liver of the newborn infant is unable to convert indirect into direct bilirubin, as already stated.

Wiener and Wexler[1] stated that the **clinical course** can be predicted in only a general way. Those infants with severe anemia, petechiasis, high cord blood icterus index, edema, and hepatosplenomegaly generally die within a few hours or days of pulmonary hemorrhage after becoming extremely jaundiced. Postmortem examination almost always shows bilirubin staining of the basal nuclei of the brain, or **kernicterus.** Less severely affected infants that have a more moderate anemia, 10 to 14 gm/100 ml of hemoglobin and elevated cord blood icterus index of more than 16 units, frequently die within 3 to 5 days with nuclear jaundice. Some of these babies may survive, but the brain is damaged; such babies often later exhibit retarded physical and mental development.

Some infants are only mildly affected, and those with normal cord blood hemoglobin concentration and a cord blood icterus index of less than 16 units are not in jeopardy as a rule, although nuclear staining may still occur and some degree of cerebral damage may become manifest within a few days after birth. It is recommended therefore that all such mildly affected infants in jeopardy be treated with exchange transfusion—the only therapy to date that has proved effective in saving the lives of these infants and preventing neurologic sequelae.

Those infants whose general condition remains good and whose jaundice never becomes intense enough to cause concern may be treated expectantly. However, in case of doubt it is much better to perform an exchange transfusion than to leave the child untreated, for he could then sustain irreversible brain damage. The success of treatment by exchange transfusion depends to a large degree on the promptness with which it is initiated and the thoroughness with which it is carried out.

The cause of EBF was not understood until publication of an article by Darrow[2]

in 1938. She believed that both the hemolysis of the baby's red cells and the liver dysfunction were due to an antigen-antibody reaction in the fetus and newborn infant, and she discarded the theory that nutritional, toxemic, or infectious disease of the mother or primary liver or blood disease of the fetus were the cause of this disease.

ISOIMMUNIZATION

Isoimmunization was first noted by Ehrlich and Morgenroth in 1900; they immunized goats with the blood of other goats and produced an antibody that would react with the blood of some goats, including the blood of the goats whose blood was used for the immunizing injections. The antibodies were isohemolysins, which in vitro as well as in vivo dissolved the red cells of the goats that had furnished the immunizing blood cells. Beginning with the observations of these two authors, scientists were shown the possibility that a vast number of different antigens might exist in similar cells of different individuals in a species. They also found that an animal will not ordinarily produce antibodies against antigens that are present in its own blood (Ehrlich's principle of *horror autotoxicus*).

Performing isoimmunization experimentally in man has always been difficult, although it has been done. As a matter of fact, that is how commercial anti-Rh sera are produced. Despite the difficulty of intentionally producing isoimmunization, there is nevertheless the constant danger of inadvertent isosensitization from transfusions involving intragroup incompatibilities as well as from pregnancy.

In the following discussion, individuals will be considered as either Rh positive or Rh negative, but the mechanism is the same whether the isoimmunization is due to Rh_o or to any of the other Rh-Hr factors.

In 1946 Pieri and Schwartz[3] (Figs. 9-1 and 9-2) explained the mechanism by which gases, water, and nourishment are interchanged between the mother and her fetus. This interchange takes place through

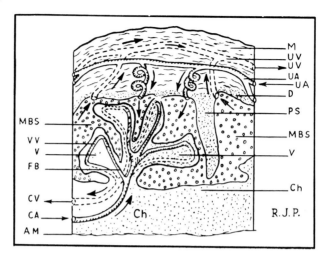

Fig. 9-1. Diagrammatic section through a human placenta. *M,* Uterine muscle; *UV,* branch of uterine veins; *UA,* branch of uterine artery; *D,* decidua; *PS,* decidual septum; *MBS,* maternal blood sinus; *V,* villus; *Ch,* chorion frondosum; *AM,* amnion; *CA,* branch of umbilical artery; *CV,* branch of umbilical vein; *FB,* villus branch of umbilical artery; *VV,* vein withdrawing blood from villus. (From Pieri, R. J., and Schwartz, R. C.: N.Y. State J. Med. **46:**387, 1946.)

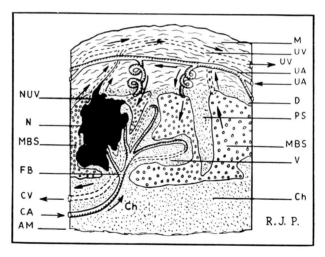

Fig. 9-2. Diagrammatic illustration of rupture of placental villus. *N,* Fetal blood from villus vessels pouring into maternal blood sinus, *MBS.* Fetal blood enters maternal uterine vein at *NUV,* to gain access to general circulation of the mother. (See Fig. 9-1 and text.) (From Pieri, R. J., and Schwartz, R. C.: N.Y. State J. Med. **46:**387, 1946.)

the fragile membrane of the placental villus, a trophoblastic projection of the chorion frondosum itself. Each villus is supplied through an arteriole with fetal blood by a branch from an umbilical artery, and a corresponding venule eventually returns the blood to the fetal circulation. The delicate placental villi are bathed in pools of maternal blood in the intervillous spaces, and this blood is carried to these spaces by minute branches of the uterine artery, usually found in relation to the decidual septa. Corresponding veins return it eventually to branches of the uterine vein. Constant circulation is assisted by uterine contractions occurring at intervals throughout the pregnancy.

Normally, the blood of the fetus circulates inside the villus and the maternal blood circulates outside, but the relationship is so close that dialysis readily takes place through the villous wall. There are great numbers of villi. The placenta is extremely susceptible to the effects of tumors, trauma, and disease. Careful scrutiny of the placenta will reveal in nearly every instance the unmistakable evidences of single or multiple areas of old or recent pathologic alteration. These scars vary in size from pinhead to several cubic millimeters. Each scar represents the evidence of a previous placental injury, and since the most delicate portion of the placenta is the villus, it is the most susceptible to injury. Whatever the cause, any break in the continuity of the vessels of one or more villi could result in hemorrhage of fetal blood cells into the maternal circulation. The fetal blood elements, after hemorrhage into the maternal circulation, are carried into the uterine veins and from there into the mother's general circulation.

If the fetal cells have an Rh factor that the mother's cells lack, a variable degree of isoimmunization of the mother results. To be specific, if the mother is Rh negative and the fetal blood cells are Rh positive, the influx of Rh-positive cells into the mother's circulation causes her to form anti-Rh antibodies. She is then isosensitized to the Rh factor. This is not harmful to her unless she is in need of a blood transfusion and is erroneously transfused with Rh-positive blood. In such a case the antibodies she formed as a result of isosensitization to her Rh-positive fetus will react against the incoming Rh-positive blood cells and agglutinate or hemolyze them, or both. In any event, she will undergo a serious transfusion reaction, often of the hemolytic variety, which could result in damage to her renal tubules, uremia, or even death. It is imperative therefore in transfusions, especially of an Rh-negative pregnant woman, that the patient be given only Rh-negative blood, which lacks the antigen for which her newly formed antibodies are reactive. This blood, then, will be safe to use in transfusing her.

In 1965 Freese,[4] in studies with monkeys on the mechanism by which interchange of food, oxygen, and wastes between the blood of the mother and fetus takes place in the placenta, found that although the fetus receives its nourishment from the mother's bloodstream, the mother's intact blood cells do not normally enter the fetal circulation. Using x-ray motion pictures and other means, Freese showed the exact route by which such interchange takes place.

The placenta is a disk-shaped vascular organ about 10 inches in diameter, which develops against the uterine wall during pregnancy. Blood vessels from the fetus enter the placenta through the umbilical cord. The surface of the placenta that is attached to the uterine wall is divided into lobes, or cotyledons. The blood vessels from the fetus pass through the umbilical cord and then branch out into a treelike formation within the placenta. The branches and innumerable twigs are called villi. The villi are densely packed around the circumference of each cotyledon, but at the center of the cotyledon there are no villi.

The arteries that enter the placenta from the mother also divide into small branches, but the walls of these blood vessels are eroded by the villi of the fetal circulatory system, so that the villi are bathed in a lake of the mother's blood. The villi are so closely packed together, however, that fluid cannot move freely between them. The spaces, according to Freese's studies, have been shown to be no wider than ordinary capillaries.

Using radiopaque dye for injection into the blood vessels of a pregnant monkey and then taking x-ray motion pictures, the points of entry of the dye into the placenta were shown. As the maternal blood enters the cotyledons, the center of each fills first, and then the dye disperses laterally in a kind of "smoke ring." There are a considerable number of portals of entry of maternal blood.

After the baby monkeys had been born, Freese examined the placentas and found that the number of cotyledons in each corresponded to the number of "smoke rings" found in the radiographic studies. The maternal blood first enters the center of each cotyledon and then passes through the spaces between the villi, proving that each cotyledon is supplied with blood from a separate maternal arteriole.

The maternal blood is under considerable pressure when it encounters the villi nearest the center of the cotyledon, which is probably where the nutrient exchange occurs. Freese's work implies that the maternal pressure drops as the blood seeps through the capillary-sized spaces between villi, and this explanation answers the question of how transfer of nutrients can take place. The blood pressure in the fetus is equivalent to about 30 mm Hg, but in the spaces between the villi it is believed to be only 5 to 10 mm Hg.

Levine and Stetson[5] are often credited with being the first to link EBF with blood group incompatibilities; however, their article did not mention EBF but dealt instead with a hemolytic transfusion reaction, which they ascribed to sensitization of the mother to some antigen in the body of the fetus. Darrow[2] thought that sensitization of the mother to fetal hemoglobin was the cause of EBF. It was not until the publication of the work of Landsteiner and Wiener on their discovery of the Rh factor that the etiology of this disease was fully appreciated. Not only was the cause of EBF then determined but so also was the reason for intragroup hemolytic transfusion reactions. Later, the discovery by Wiener of two kinds of antibody—the large molecule type (IgM, or 19S) that does not traverse the placenta and the small molecule variety (IgG, or 7S) (also described independently by Race) that can pass through an intact placenta—led to new tests for detection of the antibodies. Wiener called the small

molecule variety **univalent** and the large type **bivalent**. Race called the small type **incomplete**. These are now more precisely termed IgG(7S) and IgM(19S) **immunoglobulins,** respectively.

MECHANISM OF ISOSENSITIZATION OF THE MOTHER AND OF EBF (Fig. 9-3)

The **mechanism of isosensitization of the mother** is as follows: If a pregnant woman who lacks a particular blood group factor, for example, Rh (she is Rh negative), is mated to a man who has the factor (he is Rh positive) and if he is homozygous for the Rh factor, all the offspring of this mating will have the same Rh factor as that of the father (all the offspring would be Rh positive). If the father is heterozygous for the Rh factor, only half the possible children will be Rh positive. The Rh-positive blood of the fetus may enter the circulation of the Rh-negative mother and cause her to form anti-Rh antibodies, in other words, to become isosensitized to the Rh factor present in her fetus.

If this mother has not previously received an Rh-positive blood transfusion and if this is her first pregnancy with an Rh-positive fetus, she may develop anti-Rh antibodies, but usually under these circumstances they are not potent enough to harm the fetus. Such antibodies will, however, make it dangerous for her to receive an Rh-positive blood transfusion. Once formed, the Rh antibodies generally persist for life so that if she becomes pregnant again with an Rh-positive fetus, her antibodies will most likely increase in titer. If they are of the 7S, small molecule variety, IgG, as they usually are, they will pass through the placenta, enter the fetal circulation, coat the fetal red cells, and give rise to disease. If the extent of the damage to or hemolysis of the fetal red cells is considerable, the infant may be stillborn, or, if born alive, may survive for only a short time. If born alive and not treated, the infant may develop EBF, resulting perhaps in brain damage or even death. Often the infant has a severe

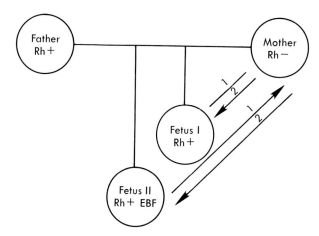

Fig. 9-3. Isoimmunization of the mother in incompatible pregnancies and development of EBF in offspring. *1.* Transplacental passage of the fetal Rh-positive red cells into maternal circulation, with the resultant production by the mother of anti-**Rh** antibodies. *2.* Transplacental passage of maternal anti-**Rh** IgG antibodies into fetal circulation with development of EBF in the second and in subsequent Rh-positive offspring.

anemia in addition to very high bilirubin, and both conditions must be treated.

MANAGEMENT OF EBF

Three abnormalities in the infant must be corrected: (1) the anemia, if present, which can be overcome by transfusion; (2) removal of the coated red cells and free antibodies in the infants plasma, which is accomplished by exchange transfusion; and (3) quick removal of the bilirubin that forms in hemolytic reactions. Otherwise, irreversible brain damage, or **kernicterus,** can result.

As soon as the infant is born, tests must be made to determine if the red cells are coated with 7S anti-Rh antibodies. This is the **direct antiglobulin,** or **Coombs, test;** it is made by thoroughly washing the cells to remove free globulin, then applying antiglobulin serum to test whether the cells will agglutinate. This will determine if the cells of the newborn infant have been coated with IgG (7S) antibodies. (The specificity of the antibodies is not established by this test.) For details of the technic, see p. 252.

When the direct antiglobulin test is positive, the infant is transfused by the exchange method, using Rh-negative blood in cases of Rh-Hr incompatibilities. When compatible cells are not available or in emergencies, the mother's cells can be washed several times, suspended in A-B-O compatible plasma, and used; even the mother's whole blood can be used because her antibodies are considered harmless if they persist after the exchange. The father's blood must not be used because his Rh-positive cells will react with the free anti-Rh antibodies in the infant's circulation. If an Rh-negative donor is available, his blood should be of the same A-B-O blood group as that of the mother. The ideal choice of donor is an Rh-negative person with no antibodies against the infant's blood factors.

In the **management of erythroblastosis fetalis,** it is necessary to know the possible genotypes of the prospective mother and father, so that the probable genotypes and hence phenotypes of the unborn infant can be anticipated. If both parents are Rh negative, the infant will be Rh negative. If the mother is Rh positive and the father Rh negative, the fetus, even though Rh positive, cannot sensitize the Rh-positive mother. If the mother is Rh negative and the father is Rh positive and heterozygous for the Rh factor, the infant may be either Rh positive or Rh negative. If the father is Rh positive and homozygous for the Rh factor, all the children born of this union will be Rh positive, and senstization of the mother can occur.

The mother's serum should be tested periodically throughout the pregnancy to determine if she is forming antibodies or, if she already has antibodies, whether the titer is rising. If it is (excluding laboratory error), she must be carrying an Rh-positive fetus. If the titer is not rising, the fetus could be either Rh negative or Rh positive.

Antibody concentration

At what concentration of antibodies does it become necessary to prepare for delivery and treatment of an erythroblastotic infant? This has never been answered satisfactorily, since in some instances the titer is lower than could be expected to cause such results, and in others it is high. Generally, however, the higher the titer the more severe the manifestations.

Laboratory tests

The principal tests to determine the likelihood of development of this disease are (1) prenatal examination of the mother's serum for antibodies, titration when present, and repeating the titrations at intervals; (2) examination of the infant's cells or cord blood immediately after birth to determine if the cells have been coated with antibody; (3) study of bilirubin content of amniotic fluid obtained by amniocentesis; and (4) the Kleihauer test for fetal cells in the maternal circulation. The appearance of antibodies in the first full-term pregnancy in the absence of prior history of abortion or blood transfusion is quite rare. In cases with the first pregnancy after abortion, 4.3% of the women form antibodies during the first half of the first full-term pregnancy, but 6% of Rh-positive abortions result in antibody formation.[6] For details of the technic, see Chapter 17.

A **direct antiglobulin test** on the cord or infant's cells as soon after birth as possible

is recommended, and if the test is positive and the cord bilirubin is significantly elevated, an exchange transfusion should be performed promptly. Some physicians prefer to wait 8 to 12 hours or longer after the baby is born for any signs or symptoms that may indicate EBF; if there are no clinical signs, that is, no severe jaundice and no significant anemia, they withhold the exchange transfusion.

The principle of the antiglobulin test on cord or infant's blood (**direct Coombs test**) is based on the fact that in EBF the infant's red cells are coated with 7S antibody derived from the isosensitized mother. If all the excess protein is washed from the baby's cells and these same cells are then mixed with antiglobulin serum, the cells will agglutinate if they have been coated with antibody. If they have not been so coated, the red cells remain evenly suspended and the test is negative.

In prenatal tests of the mother's serum, if she has formed antibodies, it is necessary to determine the type and specificity by testing her serum against an entire panel of cells having as many as possible of the known red cell antigens. When antibodies are detected, the serum must be titrated to determine the titer, or concentration. Titrations are then made at intervals throughout the pregnancy, and when the titer is rising, the physician should be prepared for delivery of an erythroblastotic infant. The titer of the mother's antibodies determines the degree of coating of the fetal cells, as shown in Tables 9-1 and 9-2.

For EBF to develop, not only must the infant's cells be coated with antibody but also there must be sufficient **conglutinin** in the blood to cause clumping. Complement and complement-like substances such as conglutinin are not fully developed before birth. If the mother's antibody titer is very high over a long period of time, however, the child may be stillborn, or if born alive he may manifest severe EBF. At times the baby appears normal at birth but early in the neonatal period develops signs of the disease.

Although the infant's red cells are coated

Table 9-1. Rh antibody titration of expectant mother showing no significant change in titer antenatally but rise in titer postpartum[*][†]

Date of test	Agglutinin method	Albumin-plasma method	Antiglobulin method	Ficinated cell method
6/1/66	0	3	13	32
11/4/66	0	2	7	14
11/23/66	0	4	9	46
1/6/67	0	7	11	36
3/1/67	0	4	7	24
Average of 5 antenatal titers	0	4	9	30
5/6/67 (postpartum)	0	28	40	56

[*]From Erskine, A. G. In Frankel, S., Reitman, S., and Sonnenwirth, A. C., editors: Gradwohl's clinical laboratory methods and diagnosis, ed. 7, St. Louis, 1970, The C. V. Mosby Co. (Patient I. B. of Dr. A. S. Wiener, baby Rh positive, treated by exchange transfusion.)
[†]Error of titration method in *skilled* hands is one doubling serum dilution.

Table 9-2. Rh antibody titration of expectant mother showing two rises in titer antenatally and comparative titration of baby's cord serum[*][†]

Date of test	Agglutina-tion method	Albumin-plasma method	Anti-globulin method	Ficinated cell method	Comments
Antenatal tests on mother					
1/8/69	0	½	4	9	EDC‡ 3/20/69
1/30/69	0	0	2	6	
Average of above 2 titers	0	¼	3	7½	
2/11/69	0	4	12	18	Titer apparently rising
2/18/69	0	12	48	56	
2/21/69	0	4	36	80	
Average of above 2 titers	0	8	42	68	Marked rise in titer
2/25/69	0	24	72	160	Amniocentesis and induction of labor tried unsuccessfully
3/3/69 at delivery	0	48	128	384	
Average of above 2 titers	0	36	100	272	Further rise in titer
3/25/69	0	60	320	160	No further significant change in titer postpartum
Cord blood of baby at delivery	0	6	26	48	Baby successfully treated by exchange transfusion

[*]From Erskine, A. G. In Frankel, S., Reitman, S., and Sonnenwirth, A. C., editors: Gradwohl's clinical laboratory methods and diagnosis, ed. 7, St. Louis, 1970, The C. V. Mosby Co. (Patient F. G. of Dr. A. S. Wiener, baby Rh positive, treated by exchange transfusion.)
[†]Each titration was carried out against at least two different Rh-positive red cell suspensions so that each reported titer represents the average of two or more titration results.
‡Expected date of confinement.

at birth, they can survive and function like uncoated cells, but, according to Wiener, when conglutinin (or complement) is produced by the baby's own body after birth, the coated cells clump or lyse, with resultant pathology. Once the coated cells, free antibody, and excess bilirubin in the baby's blood have been removed and the coated red cells are replaced by uncoated ones, EBF becomes a self-limited disease. According to W. Weiner and Wingham,[7] Rh antibodies that are detectable by enzyme-treated cells only, not by albumin or antiglobulin methods, do not usually result in EBF.

The **jaundice** in hemolytic disease of the newborn is both hemolytic and hepatogenous in origin. The **brain damage,** although it occurs more often in severely jaundiced babies, is not always seen with severe jaundice. There are occasional severely jaundiced infants who may recover completely, just as there are others with only lighter jaundice who may die or exhibit brain damage. According to Wiener,[8] the tissue damage is due primarily to vascular injury resulting from intravascular conglutination of the baby's coated cells. Damage to the liver results in jaundice. Sludging of red cells in the circulation of the brain produces blood vessel damage, permitting the bilirubin to cross the bloodbrain barrier more readily and kill the nerve cells in basal ganglia of the brain, which then take up the bilirubin stain (**kernicterus**). If, however, the coated cells are removed before intravascular clumping occurs and if they are replaced by cells that cannot be coated with free antibody, tissue damage can be prevented. The rapidly developing jaundice and organic injury seen in infants with EBF may possibly be due to increase in the concentration of conglutinin in the infant's circulation during the early neonatal period, resulting in intravascular clumping and red cell destruction in the spleen.

Exchange transfusion

Exchange transfusion was introduced in 1944 by Wiener et al.[9-11] It is a method of simultaneously withdrawing and injecting blood, that is, withdrawing the baby's blood and at the same time injecting the donor blood.

The principal purpose of the exchange transfusion is to remove the baby's coated cells and to replace them with other red cells that cannot react with the passively acquired antibodies. It is not sufficient, however, to simply remove the baby's coated red cells, which cause the disease, because the disease process has a certain momentum and it may require a few days for the damage to be reversed. Meanwhile, bilirubin may accumulate in the baby's body because of poor liver function. If the bilirubin concentration reaches a high enough level, irreversible brain damage can result. A second exchange transfusion is therefore necessary at times to counteract the hyperbilirubinemia until the infant's liver can cope with the excess bilirubin.

If the baby's cord blood already has a bilirubin concentration of 5 mg/100 ml, the infant will most likely develop kernicterus if left untreated, even in the absence of anemia. Exchange transfusion should therefore be carried out immediately. If the baby is less severely affected, the bilirubin test should be repeated twice daily for the first two days and then at least once daily. If the rate of rise in bilirubin indicates that it probably will exceed 20 mg/100 ml, the exchange transfusion should be initiated without delay. Brain damage rarely results before the icterus index exceeds 120 to 150 units, corresponding to a bilirubin level of about 20 to 25 mg/100 ml (icterus index divided by 6 = approximate bilirubin concentration). A figure of 120 icterus index units, or about 20 mg/100 ml of bilirubin, would therefore be an indication for repeating an exchange transfusion.

If therapy is withheld, bilirubin tests should be made twice daily or more often for at least 5 days or until the peak has been passed and the bilirubin content is declining.

Severely affected babies should be treated as quickly after birth as possible.

The indications for exchange transfusion are not always clearcut.

Some physicians have used as many as seven exchange transfusions on successive days for treating severely affected infants, using only 1 unit of blood for each transfusion. Wiener and Wexler prefer to use 2 units (1000 ml) of blood, in which case it is seldom necessary to perform more than two such exchange transfusions.

Additional facts about exchange transfusion

The antibody in the baby's circulation, derived from the isosensitized mother, has a half-life of about 30 to 35 days.[12] In erythroblastotic babies this half-life may appear to be shorter because newly formed Rh-positive cells (in cases of Rh sensitization) absorb the free Rh antibodies, and these babies are Rh positive. (The babies do not produce any antibodies.) Since the infants increase in size as they grow, the antibodies in their larger blood volume are further diluted.

Prevention of fetal death in utero

When EBF appears likely to develop, some obstetricians perform a preterm delivery. There has always been a need for tests to forecast the optimum time for such procedure. Some use amniocentesis to predict hemolytic disease of the newborn, and still others have advocated administering blood to the fetus while still in utero. The only justification for early or premature induction of labor in Rh-isosensitized pregnancy is prevention of fetal death in utero. Freda et al.[13] pointed out that this assessment must be based on past obstetric history, probable zygosity of the father, estimated fetal weight and expected date of confinement, and spectrophotometric scanning of amniotic fluid in selected cases.

Despite all the tests to determine the Rh genotypes of the parents, it is not always possible to predict whether the baby will be Rh positive. Only the probable genotype can be determined in the absence of family investigations. For this reason and others, screening tests for abnormal antibodies in the mother's serum should be made at the first antepartum visit to the physician. The test should be repeated at monthly intervals in the second trimester and at 2-week intervals in the third trimester. If possible, all titrations should be made in parallel with a previously drawn specimen stored in the frozen state. The **critical titer level** of the indirect antiglobulin test is said to be 16 units ±1 doubling dilution. If this level is not exceeded, according to Freda, there is no indication to perform amniocentesis or to induce labor prematurely.

If the antibody level or titer is higher, spectrophotometric scanning of the amniotic fluid could aid in predicting the severity of the hemolytic process.

About one third of Rh-negative mothers carrying an Rh-positive fetus will produce a rise in antibody titer during gestation according to Wiener et al.[14] Moreover, if the Rh antibody appears for the first time during a particular pregnancy or if there is a significant rise in titer, such as 2 tube dilutions or more, it is reasonably certain that there will be an affected Rh-positive baby.

Photetherapy

Bilirubin is present in the erythroblastotic infant not only in the blood plasma but also in the extravascular tissue spaces, from which it diffuses into the circulation during the transfusion. The concentration is not static, for even in normal babies it tends to rise during the first 2 to 4 days of life (**physiologic icterus**). When bilirubin is exposed to light, it is altered chemically and, apparently, then becomes harmless. This is the underlying principle in the treatment of neonatal hyperbilirubinemia through phototherapy. The child's eyes must be protected while his entire body is exposed to the light. (Phototherapy equipment is available commercially.) This type of treatment has been successful in a number of instances but must not be used as a substitute for exchange transfusion when indicated.

Amniocentesis

Fetal or neonatal death is frequently associated, in Rh-Hr incompatibilities, with a steadily rising anti-Rh_0 antibody titer in an Rh_0-negative pregnant woman. Increased bilirubin pigment in amniotic fluid of erythroblastotic infants was reported by Bevis[15] and by Walker and Jenimson.[16] This is a reflection of intravascular hemolysis. It correlates well with the level of cord hemoglobin. This pigment is not excreted by the mother but apparently is acquired during circulation of the amniotic fluid through the fetal gastrointestinal tract. It shows a distinct spectrophotometric peak at 450 nm (Fig. 9-4).

In cases in which fetal death is anticipated before 31 weeks, Freda initiates amniocentesis in the early weeks of the second trimester, as early as 16 weeks. Freda believes that one should be prepared to transfuse the fetus in utero if indicated; otherwise, there is no point in initiating amniocentesis before 31 weeks, since premature delivery before that age is not safe for the baby.

Information on performing amniocentesis is readily available in the literature. After centrifuging the amniotic fluid to remove particles that may render it cloudy, it is examined in a continuous recording spectrophotometer at wavelengths between 350 and 700 nm on a linear scale. The optical density (O.D.) may be recorded on other instruments, preferably at intervals of 10 nm in the critical range between 350 and 525 nm. If the curve shows that the fetus is likely to die in utero, early delivery or intrauterine transfusion of the fetus is indicated. If the infant is not in serious jeopardy, studies may be repeated at a later date.

The **normal tracing** is a smooth, curved line that always sweeps upward in the lower wavelength range, due to turbidity caused by vernix, uric acid, and other substances normally present in amniotic fluid. The term "normal" refers to the tracings

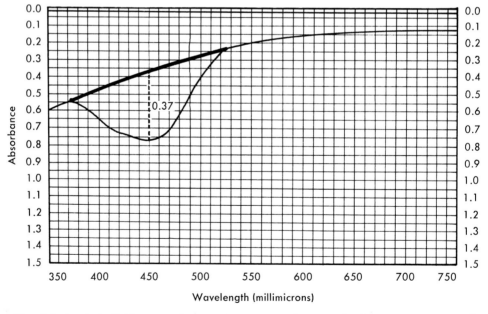

Fig. 9-4. Amniotic fluid spectrophotometric scan on a linear scale demonstrating a typical "bilirubin hump." Heavy line projected from 375-525 nm demonstrates approximate course of amniotic fluid scan in absence of bilirubin. Upright (broken) line drawn at 450 nm shows deviation of this bilirubin peak from normal, in this case 0.37. (From Queenan, J. T.: Clin. Obstet. Gynecol. **9:**491, 1966.)

and not to the clinical condition of the fetus.

In the presence of bile pigments the fluid becomes pale yellowish. Each related bile pigment absorbs monochromatic light somewhere in the wavelength between 375 and 525 nm. The summation of their respective light absorptions produces a characteristic abnormality in the tracing between 375 and 525 nm, identified as a "broad hump," or an elevation above the expected normal slope of the curve. As the concentration of pigments increases, the hump effect becomes more pronounced. The width is constant and does not change, but the height above the expected slope of the curve increases in amplitude as the concentration of the bile pigments increases. The amplitude is an arbitrary measurement at 450 nm of the difference in O.D. on a linear scale between the measured and expected curves.

If even a small amount of fetal or maternal blood contaminates the fluid, there could be a large oxyhemoglobin peak, 405 to 415 nm, that could tend to obscure the 450 nm peak, especially when plotted on a straight graph. In such cases, a logarithmic graph should be used.

The **amniotic fluid bilirubin concentration** can be measured, and in laboratories without a scanning spectrophotometer it is necessary to determine the bilirubin content by chemical means. Amniotic fluid bilirubin levels of 0.27 mg/100 ml or higher are probably abnormal, whereas between 0.10 and 0.27 mg/100 ml there is a possibly affected fetus. The degree of bilirubin elevation correlates with fetal vitality. Above 0.47 mg/100 ml the fetus is usually distressed, and some degree of circulatory failure is probably present. Above 0.95 mg/100 ml death of the fetus is almost inevitable unless immediate delivery can be effected. The method of Gambino and Freda[19] or of Bower and Swale[20] may be used for the test.

Intrauterine transfusion of the fetus is dangerous and is therefore indicated only when the expectant Rh-negative mother is very strongly sensitized and the fetus in utero is certainly Rh positive and severely affected. This procedure, introduced by Liley,[17,18] is based on the principle that the baby will absorb enough of the Rh-negative blood injected into its peritoneal cavity to be rendered temporarily Rh negative, in which case it would no longer be vulnerable to the Rh antibodies passively acquired from the mother. The procedure is dangerous to the mother as well as to the fetus and therefore remains experimental. Further research is necessary.

INCIDENCE OF EBF

The mating of an Rh-negative woman to an Rh-positive man occurs in one out of every ten marriages. Congenital hemolytic disease, however, affects only one out of 250 newborn infants, which suggests that only about one in twenty-five Rh-negative women becomes sensitized when bearing an Rh-positive fetus. The firstborn child is only rarely affected, which differs from EBF resulting from A-B-O incompatibility.

If the mother forms *only* 19S agglutinating antibodies, which seldom if ever occurs, the infant is not in danger because such antibodies cannot traverse the placenta and so do not enter the fetal circulation.

PREVENTION OF EBF

In many cases isosensitization of the mother and subsequent erythroblastosis of the infant can be prevented. Levine[21,22] first noted in families with erythroblastotic infants that the husband's A-B-O blood group was compatible with that of the mother more often than in the general population. Where the A-B-O factors in the mother and fetus were incompatible, as, for example, when the mother was group A and the fetus was group B or the mother group B and the fetus group A, the presence of either or both anti-**A** or anti-**B** antibodies in the mother could cause removal of group A and B Rh-positive fetal red cells from the maternal circulation without initiating an immune response to the Rh factor. It is extremely difficult to immunize Rh-negative volunteers by using A-B-O incompatible Rh-positive cells.

According to the observations of Theobald Smith[23] as early as 1909, in the presence of passive antibody the corresponding antigen will not immunize. Gorman and Freda,[24] and Gorman et al.,[25] in 1965, utilized the latter principle of completely suppressing active immunity by administering **passive antibody.** Passive antibody can cause specific immunosuppression of the active immunity that follows injection of an antigen. These authors also found that specific IgG antibody is 100 to 200 times more immunosuppressive than specific IgM antibody. Rh-positive cells that are coated in vitro with IgG 7S anti-Rh antibodies are nonantigenic.

Freda et al.[26] used anti-Rh_o–containing gamma G globulin rather than plasma to provide passive immunity for reasons of safety. They used fraction II gamma globulin from a pool of high-titered IgG anti-Rh_o donor plasma. This was designated Rh_o immunoglobulin, and it had to be administered intramuscularly. In their experiments with male volunteers, they found that 5 ml intramuscularly gave an artificial antiglobulin titer up to 1:128 in the volunteers who received it, 1 ml gave a titer up to 1:32, and 0.1 ml up to 1:2. No side effects were produced in their experiments, and no hepatitis developed in any of the subjects. Their series of experimental trials of anti-Rh_o gamma globulin was performed in Rh-negative male volunteers. All failed to develop immune anti-Rh_o antibodies, and even as late as 24 weeks after the last injection of Rh-positive blood there was no indication of antibody formation. This demonstrates that suppression of antibody formation was complete. However, when eight of the original fourteen volunteers later received a fourth and a fifth antigenic stimulus of 10 ml of Rh-positive blood that *did not* contain the gamma globulin, two of them became actively immunized to Rh_o.

The experiments provided complete suppression of immunization to Rh_o in subjects who had previously been heavily stimulated with Rh-positive cells. It was found that anti-Rh_o gamma G globulin could be given up to 72 hours after the red cell challenge and still provide complete suppression.[27,28]

RhoGAM* is a concentrated anti-Rh_o IgG immunoglobulin. It is administered intramuscularly to an Rh_o-negative woman immediately after delivery of an Rh_o-positive or an $\mathfrak{R}h_o$-positive infant to suppress the mother's antibody response to Rh_o-positive fetal cells. It is not given to women who have been previously immunized against Rh_o through a prior pregnancy or transfusion. It is also administered to nonimmunized Rh_o-negative women following abortion, miscarriage, or ectopic pregnancy. It is kept in a refrigerator at 2° to 8° C.

Anti-Rh_o IgM does not have the protective action of anti-Rh_o IgG.

Certain criteria must be met for the use of RhoGAM:

1. The mother must be both Rh_o and $\mathfrak{R}h_o$ negative.

2. She must not be already immunized to the Rh_o factor.

3. The baby must be Rh_o or $\mathfrak{R}h_o$ positive.

4. The baby must have a negative direct reaction in the Coombs test because a positive Coombs test indicates that the mother has already produced antibodies which have coated the infant's cells which would contraindicate the use of RhoGAM.

Prophylaxis against production of immune Rh antibodies is obtained by giving Rh-negative pregnant women at risk an injection of 4.5 ml of anti-Rh_o gamma G globulin intramuscularly within 72 hours after delivery. The globulin should be administered as soon as possible after delivery, at least within 72 hours to be effective. The passively administered antibody apparently completely disappears; that is, it is not detectable by any laboratory method

---

*Ortho Diagnostics, Raritan, N.J.

—saline agglutination, antiglobulin test, or use of enzyme-treated cells—and when the protected mothers again become pregnant, they remain nonsensitized.

Hyperimmune gamma G globulin, developed by Pollack, Freda, and Gorman and available commercially as RhoGAM,[29] is important as a partial but not complete answer to the prevention of EBF resulting from natural sensitization of the mother through leakage of fetal blood into her circulation at delivery. No one, however, has been able to prevent the mother from becoming sensitized by leakages of fetal blood into her circulation at any time *during* the pregnancy. In addition, EBF is partly an iatrogenic disease; the incidence is remarkably lower now than it was before the Rh factor was discovered because now there is no indiscriminate injection of Rh-positive blood into Rh-negative patients, at least not in well-organized hospitals. Fewer women therefore are already sensitized to the Rh factor at the time they become pregnant.

In some countries hyperimmune untreated plasma is injected in place of anti-Rh$_o$ gamma G globulin.

SENSITIZATION TO OTHER BLOOD GROUP FACTORS

Other blood group incompatibilities leading to EBF are possible, although the vast majority of cases are due to isosensitization to the **Rh$_o$** factor. The following blood group factors have also been implicated in some cases of hemolytic disease of the newborn: **rh′, rh″, hr′, hr″, hr^s**, and probably all the other factors in the Rh-Hr system, although **Rh$_o$** is the most antigenic, followed by **hr′, rh″**, and the **Rh$_o$** variants; antigens of the A-B-O system when the mothers are group O, usually because of their **C** factor; **U** of the M-N-S system; **S** or **s** of the M-N-S system; **K** and **k** of the Kell-Cellano system, as well as **Ku; Jk** of the Kidd system; and rarely **Fy^a, Di,** and others. There have also been some rare instances of isosensitization to the factor **M.**

Erythroblastosis fetalis due to the A-B-O factors

Mild cases of erythroblastosis fetalis (hemolytic disease) due to A-B-O incompatibility are rather common and are often overlooked. Although most infants recover spontaneously, in some cases the manifestations are severe and warrant treatment. In A-B-O sensitization, firstborn infants are affected in 50% of the cases, in contrast to those cases due to Rh-Hr incompatibility, in which almost invariably the firstborn infant is not affected (unless the mother has previously received an Rh-positive transfusion and she is Rh negative).

The red count and hemoglobin are usually normal, but the hemoglobin may be as low as 10 gm/100 ml or even lower. Spherocytes are the characteristic feature in the blood film, with smaller diameters than the accompanying macrocytes of newborn infant's blood. There may be reticulocytosis, polychromatic cells, and an increased number of nucleated red cells, indicating a compensated hemolytic anemia. The indirect bilirubin level is higher than normal. The direct antiglobulin test of the cord or infant's cells is generally negative or at most only weakly positive.

The clinical, hematologic, and serologic abnormalities in A-B-O hemolytic disease are not consistent in appearance. Kaplan et al.[30] gave their criteria for diagnosis as clinical icterus appearing in the first 24 hours of life, bilirubin in serum exceeding 12 mg/100 ml, or A-B-O incompatibility with resulting hemolytic disease diagnosed in prior siblings. Suspicion of the disease is strengthened if the blood film shows microspherocytosis or elevated reticulocytosis (more than 12% reticulocytes) in the infant's blood. The diagnosis is made more probable if the direct antiglobulin test is negative and the indirect antiglobulin test is positive after incubation of infant serum with adult erythrocytes of the same A-B-O blood group as the infant or if there is a positive test with similar adult erythrocytes incubated with eluate from the infant's

blood. These authors demonstrated reduced stromal acetylcholinesterase (AChE)
activity in the red cells of the infants with
proved A-B-O hemolytic disease and normal AChE activity in the blood cells of
infants with Rh-Hr erythroblastosis fetalis.
The reduction in AChE in A-B-O hemolytic disease was significant. The normal
range is 76-105, mean 89, S.D. ±11. In
A-B-O hemolytic disease it was 47-82,
mean 65, S.D. ± 13. In Rh-Hr hemolytic disease it was 68-128, mean 93, S.D. ±17.

Rosenfield[31] was the first to notice that
EBF due to A-B-O incompatibility is almost always confined to babies having
group O mothers, and it occurs in about
20% to 25% of all pregnancies. Wiener and
Unger[32] showed that group O babies of
group O mothers acquire by placental
transfer about sixteen times as much isoantibody as do babies whose mothers are
group A or group B. They concluded that
this was adequate to account for the excess
of group O mothers whose babies have
A-B-O hemolytic disease. Wiener proposed another explanation. As noted elsewhere, agglutinogens A and B are characterized by a specificity **C** that they share
with one another, so that erythrocytes of
groups A and B have this factor, but group
O cells do not. Group O individuals therefore are the only ones in the A-B-O system
who can become sensitized to specificity **C**
and can form anti-**C** antibodies. Such antibodies are usually 7S IgG and thus can
readily traverse the placenta. Anti-**C** antibodies are normally present in most group
O sera. Such antibodies rise in titer when
confronted with the proper antigenic stimulus such as group A or B cells (there could be
no group AB fetus if the mother is group
O). Anti-**A** and anti-**B**, on the other hand,
are usually of the 19S variety and therefore
do not readily cross the placenta. (See
Table 9-3.)

As an example, if the mother is group O
and the fetus is group A, and if some of the
fetal group A cells pass into the mother's
circulation, the **C** specificity of these cells
stimulates formation of or increase in titer

Table 9-3. Homospecific and heterospecific
mother-child combinations[*]

Homospecific		Heterospecific	
Mother	**Child**	**Mother**	**Child**
O	O	O	A or B
A	A or O	A	B or AB
B	B or O	B	A or AB
AB	A, B, or AB	AB	None

[*]From Wiener, A., S., and Socha, W., W.: A-B-O blood
groups and Lewis types, New York, 1976; with permission
of Stratton Intercontinental Book Corporation.

of her anti-**C** antibody (as well as anti-**A**),
and this antibody is usually of the 7S variety. These anti-**C** antibodies now pass
through the placenta and attach themselves to the fetal red cells, and A-B-O
hemolytic disease can result. Immune isoantibodies of the anti-**C** variety seem to
be more dangerous to the fetus than are
the natural isoagglutinins because they are
more likely to be of high titer and can
readily pass through the placenta.[33]

As previously stated, in A-B-O hemolytic
disease the firstborn may be affected,
whereas in Rh-Hr incompatibilities the
firstborn child is usually spared. Anti-**C** of
the A-B-O system also exists as a naturally
occurring antibody, which may explain the
occurrence of A-B-O hemolytic disease in
firstborn babies.

Blood selected for the exchange transfusion must be compatible with the antibody
in the mother's serum. It is suggested therefore that group O red cells be used.

The mother's serum should be titrated by
the acacia method (p. 269), which will distinguish between IgM and IgG antibodies.
IgM antibodies cannot traverse the placenta, whereas IgG can. When a baby of
a group A mother has A-B-O hemolytic
disease, the mother has proved to be subgroup A_2 rather than subgroup A_1.

Hemolytic disease due to other blood group factors

There are many other blood group specificities that are antigenic and that have
been involved in EBF (p. 145). An example of isosensitization of this kind in

the Rh-Hr system would be formation of anti-**hr'** antibodies by an Rh-positive, type Rh₁Rh₁ woman mated to an Rh-negative man or one of type Rh₁rh or Rh₁Rh₂, in which cases the mother lacks **hr'** specificity and the father's cells have this factor. Rh-negative individuals (type rh) are homozygous for factors **hr'**, **hr''**, and **hr**. Factor **hr'** is the most antigenic of the Hr factors. It can cause formation of anti-**hr'** antibodies in an individual who lacks it and has been noted as the etiologic agent in certain cases of EBF.

In any of the blood group systems, for example, K-k, the individual who lacks the specificity can form antibodies against it; since the antibodies are usually of the 7S variety, they can cross the placenta and affect the infant if they are present in high enough concentration and are of sufficiently great avidity. In this example, an individual of type k, who lacks the **K** specificity, can form anti-**K** antibodies, which then pass through the placenta and affect the **K**-positive fetus.

If the specificities of a blood group system are known to have been found in cases of EBF, this fact is mentioned in the part of this book where the particular blood group system is discussed.

TESTS OF MOTHER'S BLOOD AFTER DELIVERY

The following tests should be made on mother's blood after delivery: (1) the Kleihauer test to determine presence of fetal cells in the mother's circulation (pp. 294 and 295); (2) test of her serum for presence of anti-**Rh₀** (or other) antibodies (p. 284ff); and (3) test of her cells in the Rho-GAM cross match (pp. 309 and 310).

TESTS OF NEWBORN INFANT'S BLOOD

(1) The infant's or cord blood should be tested by the direct antiglobulin method (Coombs test) (p. 252); (2) elution tests may also be applied to the cells to separate and identify the antibodies that might coat the red cells (pp. 248 to 250).

FETOMATERNAL BLEEDING

In fetomaternal bleeding, the Kleihauer stain of maternal blood shows two erythrocyte populations: the maternal cells with no fetal hemoglobin, and the fetal cells with almost nothing but fetal hemoglobin. The **fetal red cell loss** can be roughly estimated on the basis of the following formula:

$$\text{ml fetal blood} = \%\text{ Hb F cells} \times 50$$

The maximal release of fetal cells into the maternal circulation occurs at the time of delivery. In Rh incompatibility, fetal Rh-positive red cells may be released into the Rh-negative mother's circulation. If the fetal red cells are eliminated from the maternal circulation by the administration of anti-**Rh₀** gamma G globulin (RhoGAM), sensitization of the mother will not occur as a rule. If only a very few fetal red cells are released into the mother's circulation, isosensitization to the Rh specificity is not likely to occur. If the fetal cells that are released into her circulation are rapidly destroyed within the maternal organism because of A-B-O fetomaternal incompatibility, the mother is not likely to be sensitized, as already pointed out. (See Fig. 19-5.)

The Kleihauer technic permits evaluation of the extent to which fetal cells have escaped into the maternal circulation.

REFERENCES

1. Wiener, A. S., and Wexler, I. B.: Bull. Jewish Hosp. 3:5, 1961.
2. Darrow, R. R.: Arch. Pathol. 24:378, 1938.
3. Pieri, R. J., and Schwartz, R. C.: N.Y. State J. Med. 46:387, 1946.
4. Freese, U. E.: Lab. Digest 20(1):18, 1965.
5. Levine, P., and Stetson, R. E.: J.A.M.A. 113:126, 1939.
6. Freda, V. J., Gorman, J. G., Galen, R. S., and Treacey, N.: Lancet 2:147, 1970.
7. Weiner, W., and Wingham, J.: Lancet 2:85, 1966.
8. Wiener, A. S.: Exp. Med. Surg. 7:200, 1944.
9. Wiener, A. S., Wexler, I. B., and Gamrin, E. L.: Am. J. Dis. Child. 68:317, 1944.
10. Wiener, A. S., and Wexler, I. B.: J. Lab. Clin. Med. 31:1016, 1946.
11. Wiener, A. S., Wexler, I. B., and Brancato, G. J.: J. Pediatr. 45:546, 1954.

12. Wiener, A. S.: J. Exp. Med. **94:**213, 1951.
13. Freda, V. J. In Brown, E. B., and Moore, C. V., editors: Progress in hematology, vol. 5, New York, 1966, Grune & Stratton, Inc.; see references 25 to 33 in that volume.
14. Wiener, A. S., Nappi, R., and Gordon, E. B.: Blood **6:**789, 1951.
15. Bevis, D. C. A.: J. Obstet. Gynaecol. Br. Commw. **63:**68, 1956.
16. Walker, A. H. C., and Jenimson, R. F.: Br. Med. J. **2:**1152, 1962.
17. Liley, A. W.: Br. Med. J. **2:**1107, 1963.
18. Liley, A. W.: Aust. N.Z. Obstet. Gynaecol. **4:**145, 1964.
19. Gambino, S. R., and Freda, V. J., Am. J. Clin. Pathol. **46:**198, 1966.
20. Bower, D., and Swale, J.: Lancet **1:**1009, 1966.
21. Levine, P.: J. Hered. **34:**71, 1943.
22. Levine, P.: Hum. Biol. **30:**14, 1958.
23. Smith, T.: J. Exp. Med. **11:**24, 1909.
24. Gorman, J. G., and Freda, V. J.: Lancet **1:**1311, 1965.
25. Gorman, J. G., Freda, V. J., and Pollack, W.: Lancet **2:**1965; letter to editor.
26. Freda, V. J., Gorman, J. G., Pollack, W., Robertson, J. G., Jennings, E. R., and Sullivan, J. F.: J.A.M.A. **199:**390, 1967.
27. Gorman, J. G., Freda, V. J., and Pollack, W.: Fed. Proc. **23:**238, 1964.
28. Gorman, J. G., Freda, V. J., and Pollack, W.: Proceedings of the 10th Congress International Society of Hematology **3:**12, 1964.
29. Pollack, W., Freda, V. J., and Gorman, J. G.: Lab. Digest **32**(2):8, 1968.
30. Kaplan, E., Herz, F., and Hsu, K. S.: Pediatrics **33:**205, 1964.
31. Rosenfield, R. E.: Proc. Am. Assoc. Blood Banks, 1953; cited in Wiener, A. S., Samwick, A. A., Morrison, H., and Cohen, L.: Exp. Med. Surg. **11:**276, 1953.
32. Wiener, A. S., and Unger, L. J.: Exp. Med. Surg. **13:**204, 1955.
33. Socha, W. W., and Wiener, A. S.: State J. Med. **73:**2144, 1973.

RECOMMENDED READINGS

Charles, A. G., editor: Rh immunization and erythroblastosis fetalis, New York, 1969, Meridith Corporation.

Clarke, C. A., editor: Rhesus haemolytic disease. Selected papers and extracts, Lancaster, England, 1975, Medical & Technical Publishing Co.

Woodrow, J. R.: Rh immunization and its prevention, Series Haematologica, vol. 3, Munksgaard, Copenhagen; Baltimore, 1970, The Williams & Wilkins Co.

10 □ Other important blood group systems

THE K-k (KELL-CELLANO) SYSTEM
Specificities K and k

The discovery of blocking, or incomplete, antibodies, now known as IgG, and production of antiglobulin serum to test for such antibodies gave impetus to the finding of other blood group antigens and thus other blood group systems. In 1946 Coombs et al.[1] found in the serum of a mother of an erythroblastotic infant an antibody that gave reactions not related to the Rh-Hr system. The patient's name was Kell, and so the antibody was designated anti-**Kell** and the specificity it detected was called **Kell.** The Kell antigen has been found in 7% to 12.9% of all persons tested.

At about the same time, Wiener and Sonn-Gordon,[2] working independently and using the conglutination test, found an abnormal isoantibody in the serum of a patient who had had a hemolytic transfusion reaction, and they named it **Si,** after the patient, Singer. When **Si** proved to be the same as **Kell,** Wiener discarded the symbol **Si.** The symbol K for the Kell antigen had been suggested by the British investigators. Wiener and Sonn-Gordon showed that the **Si (K)** specificity is inherited as a simple mendelian dominant.

In 1949 Levine et al.[3] found in the serum of a woman who had delivered an erythroblastotic infant an antibody that gave reactions reciprocal to the anti-**K.** Since the patient's name was Cellano, the antibody was originally designated anti-**Cellano** and the specificity it detected was called the Cel-

lano factor. Later this was changed to anti-k for the antibody and k for the specificity and the antigen. The **incidence** of k is 99.8% among Caucasoids.

Simultaneous tests with anti-K and anti-k distinguished three blood types—K, Kk, and k—entirely comparable to the three M-N types. Heredity has been proved, by family studies and methods of population genetics, to be due to allelic genes *K* and *k* so that there are three genotypes corresponding to the three phenotypes—type K, genotype *KK;* type Kk, genotype *Kk;* and type k, genotype *kk.* (See Table 10-1.)

In a study of 500 Caucasoids, 500 Negroids, and 400 Chinese in New York City, Wiener found the frequencies of the *K* and *k* genes to be as in Table 10-2.

The K-k types are of clinical importance because isosensitization can give rise to hemolytic transfusion reactions and the birth of erythroblastotic babies. The Kell antigen is evidently less antigenic than the Rh antigen because, although opportunities for sensitization are frequent, this occurs far less often than Rh sensitization. The K-k types are not usually tested for routinely when selecting donors for transfusion. Such tests are made as a rule only when selecting donors for patients already sensitized (pp. 298 and 299).

Sensitization to the k specificity is even rarer, which is not surprising, considering the low frequency (only one in 500) of individuals of genotype *KK,* the only ones who can be sensitized to the k factor.

The K-k types are inherited indepen-

149

Table 10-1. Results possible using anti-**K** and anti-k sera with unknown cells

Reaction with		Phenotype	Corresponding genotype
Anti-K	**Anti-k**		
+	−	KK	*KK*
−	+	kk	*kk*
+	+	Kk	*Kk*
−	−	Error or atypical blood (see K₀)	

Table 10-2. Distribution of the Kell types in the New York City metropolitan area*

Population	Kell types (%)		Total number persons tested	Gene frequencies (%)	
	Negative	**Positive**		**k**	**K**
Caucasians	91.6	8.4	500	95.7	4.3
Negroids	99.0	1.0	500	99.5	0.5
Chinese	99.5	0.5	400	99.7	0.3

*Modified from Wiener, A. S.: Am. J. Clin. Pathol. **51**:9, 1969.

dently of the A-B-O, M-N, Rh-Hr, and P types and thus constitute a separate blood group system.

Tests for the **Kell** factor (**K**) have been applied not infrequently in cases of disputed parentage, but tests for the **Cellano** (**k**) specificity are not done often because of the scarcity of the anti-k reagent and the rarity of control blood of genotype *KK*, which must be included when such tests are made. Tests for the **K** specificity increase the chances of excluding paternity only slightly. However, the simultaneous presence of the **K** specificity in the blood of the putative father and child when absent in the mother has been useful as circumstantial evidence, not proof, that the accused man is actually the father.

The K-k blood group system at first appeared to be simple, but related factors have been discovered, making it no longer a simple system. The **K** specificity is most common in Caucasians, much less common among Negroids, and rare in Chinese, as seen in Table 10-2.

Specificities Kpᵃ and Kpᵇ (Penney)

In 1957 Allen and Lewis[4] described a "new" antigen in the Kell blood group sys-

tem, which they named Kpᵃ after the individual, Penney, in whose blood the antibody had been detected. This person had never been exposed to the antigen, either through pregnancy or by transfusion. The original anti-Kpᵃ reacted with the red cells of only about 2% of random unrelated Caucasoids tested in Boston, where the factor had been discovered.

The specificity **Kpᵃ** is shown by family studies to be inherited as a simple mendelian dominant. That the antigen is part of the K-k system was shown by family studies. In eighteen families, one parent had both **K** and **Kpᵃ**, and no child had both factors or neither factor. In these families therefore the **Kpᵃ** specificity was associated with the *k* gene of the heterozygous K-positive parent.

Two kinds of gene *k* were distinguished in this way—*k* proper, determining an antigen k that lacks the specificity **Kpᵃ**, and *kᵖ*, determining an antigen kᵖ, so designated because it also has the specificity **Kpᵃ**. The reaction of the k specificity to antisera is not as sharp when k is associated with **Kpᵃ**, which is comparable to the weakness of the **rh′** specificity when associated with **rhʷ**. Heterozygous blood *Kkᵖ*, which is **Kpᵃ**

Table 10-3. Expanded scheme of the Kell blood types

Allelic gene	Corresponding agglutinogen	Gene frequency in Caucasians (%)	K	k	Kp^a	Kp^b	Ku	Binary code number
K	K	4.3	+	−	−	+	+	10011
k	k	94.7	−	+	−	+	+	01011
k^p	k^p	1.0	−	+	+	−	+	01101
K^o	K$_o$	Extremely rare	−	−	−	−	−	00000

positive, may react only weakly with anti-k; this proved to be a source of difficulty during the early investigations.

The Kp^a antigen has not so far been found in Negroids (1977).

The possibility that **Kp^a** might be transmitted also in association with gene *K* appears to be refuted because to date no genetic evidence has been found of a Kell agglutinogen having the two specificities **K** and **Kp^a** together.

An antigen reciprocal to Kp^a and therefore designated Kp^b was found by tests with the serum of a patient, Rautenberg, whose serum also contained antibodies for the **Kell** factor. Among 5500 Caucasians, Allen et al.[5] found only two individuals negative for **Kp^b** who were subsequently proved to be homozygous for **Kp^a**, whereas Cleghorn found only one Kp^b-negative person among 7251 Caucasians. Anti-Kp^a reacts best in the laboratory by the antiglobulin method. The two specificities **Kp^a** and **Kp^b** are already demonstrable at birth. The relationship of the specificities **Kp^a** and **Kp^b** to the K-k system is summarized in Table 10-3.

Specificity Ku and blood type K$_o$ (Peltz)

Chown et al.[6] in 1957 described a new antibody, anti-**Ku**, originally called anti-**Peltz**, in the blood serum of two patients from two unrelated families. This antibody agglutinated the red cells of all individuals except their own, and were mutually compatible. Both patients proved to react as K− k− Kp^a− Kp^b−, a very rare combination, lacking all the four known K-k specificities.

Such blood, not previously described, was designated K$_o$ because of absence of all **Kell** specificities and had been proved to be related to the K-k system. Since the antibodies in the patient's serum could not be fractionated by absorption, they were evidently detecting a very high frequency factor, later given the symbol **Ku** (Table 10-3). The very rare homozygous phenotype K$_o$ appears to be associated with very rare granulomatous disease.

The anti-**Ku** antibody was separated by elution from three bloods and caused the agglutination of 525 bloods chosen at random; it failed to agglutinate only the very rare bloods of type K$_o$ and some other highly unusual K types. The frequency of K$_o$ is 0.006%.

The propositus in the first family had antibodies that caused erythroblastosis fetalis in her fetus. The antibody, detecting a factor related to the Kell system, was named anti-**Ku**; the u represents the almost universal occurrence of the antigen,[7,8] just as the factor **U** of the M-N-S system was given that designation because it occurs almost universally.

Specificity Ul^a (Karjula)

In 1967 Furuhjelm et al.[9] found in the serum of a transfused man an antibody they called anti-Ul^a and the antigen it defines, Ul^a. With the anti-Ul^a serum they found 2.6% of the 2620 Helsinki blood donors to be Ul(a+), and a frequency as high as 5% among certain Finnish people. Only one Ul(a+) person was detected in 501 Swedish people and none in 140 Lapps, 314 non-Scandinavian whites, 66 Negroids, and 5000 Oxford donors. *Ul*[a] proved to be transmitted as a dominant characteristic and appears to belong to the Kell complex.

Specificities Wk[a] (Weeks) and Côté (K11)

Wk[a] is a low frequency antigen transmitted as a dominant characteristic. It is not associated with A-B-O, M-N-S-s, Rh-Hr, Lu, Jk, and secretor types but is now known to be part of the Kell system. It was first described by Strange et al.[10] in 1974.

Anti-**Côté,** described in 1971 by Guévein et al.,[11] reacts with all cells tested except K₀, the patient's own cells, and those of two of her eight sibs. The antigen was later called K11 and was at first designated a para-Kell antigen. (Wiener considered K11 to be a cognate of Ku in the same sense that Rh[A], Rh[B], etc., are cognates of Rh₀). It was later found that Wk[a] and K11 are antithetical antigens and that Wk[a] and Côté (K11) are part of the Kell system proper.

Specificities Js[a] and Js[b] (Sutter)

In 1958 Giblett[12] found in the serum of a white male patient an antibody that reacted with the red cells of 20% of Negroid donors but with none of the 240 Caucasian donors tested. The new antibody therefore appeared to be defining a specificity peculiar to Negroids, especially when it was later found that the specificity did not occur among Asiatics, American Indians, or Eskimos.[13] The new antibody was originally called **Sutter** after the donor who had provided the original antiserum, but was later changed to anti-Js[a].

Type Js[a] was found to have a frequency ranging from 4.8% in African Pigmies and 16% in other tribes of Negroids in the Congo to 19.6% in Negroids in the United States. The Js[a] antigen was shown to be inherited as a simple mendelian dominant and to be independent of all known systems except P, Kell, and Lutheran.

Walker et al.[14] found an antibody antithetical to anti-Js[a] and therefore designated anti-Js[b] in the serum of a Negroid woman whose family studies indicated that she was probably homozygous *Js*[a]*Js*[a]. That the specificity was really that of anti-Js[b] was proved when, among 1269 Negroid, thirteen Js[b]-negative individuals were found and all were shown to be Js[a] positive. Further evidence was provided by tests on blood from Caucasians who were all Js[b] positive, as was to be expected, since Caucasians lack the Js[a] specificity. The only exceptions were the two type K₀ persons who were shown by Stroup et al.[15] to be Js(a–b–). This strange coincidence provided convincing evidence that Js[a] and Js[b] are part of the K-k blood group system. With the discovery of this rare type, it is now agreed that there are four possible Js types: Js(a+b–), Js(a–b+), Js(a+b+), and Js(a–b–). (See Table 10-4.)

The McLeod phenotype

The McLeod phenotype was described in 1961 by Allen et al.[16] It is an X-linked characteristic that, when present, results in weak antigenicity of the red cells in the Kell group. Individuals with this phenotype lack Kx, a precursor-like substance that seems to be necessary for proper biosynthesis of Kell antigens and is also required for establishment of normal cell morphology, according to Wimer et al.[17] When Kx is absent, an abnormal erythrocytic membrane results in acanthocytosis, and a compensated hemolytic state exists.

Table 10-4. Reaction of cells with Anti-Js serum

Anti-Js[a]	Anti-Js[b]	Type
+	+	Js (a+b+)
+	–	Js (a+b–)
–	+	Js (a–b+)
–	–	Js (a–b–) (rare in Caucasians; see K₀)

The weak antigenicity occurs in the Kell blood group only, with other blood group antigens unaffected. It is considered a variant. It has an X-link mode of inheritance, although the *Kell* gene is autosomal. Some young male subjects with X-linked chronic granulomatous disease (CGD) have the McLeod phenotype.[18] Marsh et al.[19] have concluded that the McLeod phenotype and CGD have a common cause. Patients with CGD and the McLeod phenotype may produce an anti-**KL** antibody when transfused with blood of the common Kell type. Anti-**KL** is compatible only with blood containing the McLeod phenotype.

The X-linked gene is designated X^1k. Inheritance of a variant allele at the *Xk* locus results in lack of Kx synthesis and thus the McLeod phenotype. The *Xk* locus is inactivated by the Lyon effect (inactivation of the X chromosome). Female carriers of the variant gene exhibit blood group mosaicism in the Kell system and have a double red cell population of acanthocytes and discocytes.

Medicolegal aspects of the K-k system

For medicolegal purposes, the Kell system has some limited usefulness, according to Sussman.[89] The tests must be performed only by specially qualified persons. At present, the principal practical application of the system in medicolegal cases is the unequivocal exclusion of paternity when a child who is Kell positive has a Kell-negative mother and the putative father is also Kell negative. Since the **K** blood specificity cannot appear in the blood of an offspring unless present in at least one parent, this finding would exclude such a man as the father of the child.

Importance of the K-k factors

Although **K** and **k** are far less antigenic than the **Rh**$_o$ factor, they nevertheless are antigenic, ranking with factor **hr'** in importance, especially in cases of erythroblastosis fetalis. The tests for the antibodies are delicate and require special care in performance. When two antisera, anti-**K** and anti-**k**, are employed in these tests, the results are as shown in Table 10-1.

Many of the panel cells include the K and k antigens for testing unknown serum, and the battery of antisera for testing unknown cells also contains anti-**K** and anti-**k**. Some blood banks test for **K-k** factors routinely, whereas others restrict their tests to routine searching for anti-**K** or anti-**k** antibodies in donor's blood only. A person who is known to have anti-**K** antibodies must be transfused with K-negative blood only.

Combining sites in the K-k system

When Wiener and Gordon[20] titrated anti-human globulin serum against Kell-positive cells maximally coated with anti-**K** antibodies, they found the titer on the average to be only about one fourth or one fifth as high as the titers of the same antiglobulin sera for Rh-positive red cells maximally coated with anti-**Rh**$_o$. They believed this indicates that there are only one fifth to one fourth as many K antigenic sites on the red cell envelope as there are Rh-Hr antigenic combining sites.

THE Fy (DUFFY) SYSTEM

The Duffy system of blood groups was discovered in 1950 independently by Cutbush et al.[21,22] and by van Logham and van der Hart[23] who both reported a blood specificity that could not be placed in any of the known blood group systems: A-B-O, M-N, P, Rh-Hr, or K-k. The antibody was present in the blood serum of a hemophiliac patient who had had a long series of blood transfusions over a period of 20 years and who had sustained a mild transfusion reaction after the last injection of blood. The antibody was named for the patient, Duffy, and designated anti-**Duffy**, and the specificity it identified was called **Duffy**. Cutbush and Mollison introduced the symbol Fy to indicate the **Duffy** factor. Those individuals whose blood had the **Duffy** specificity were called Fy(a+), and those who lacked it were Fy(a−). The antibody was renamed anti-**Fy**^{a}.

Cutbush and Mollison found the antigen in 64.9% of 205 blood samples from unrelated English adults. It was apparently inherited through the gene *Fy*[a]. The Fy[b] antigen had not as yet been discovered, but it was postulated that an allelic gene *Fy*[b] existed.

Other examples of **Fy**[a] sensitization were later found. The antibody was discovered as a cause of hemolytic disease of the newborn in only some rare cases. Usually **Fy**[a] is associated only with incompatible transfusion reactions.

The first example of anti-**Fy**[b] was reported in 1951 in the blood serum of a woman after the birth of her third child.[24] She had had no transfusion history, and none of her children had hemolytic disease. The second example was discovered by Levine et al.,[25] and since that time there have been additional examples.

The **Fy** factors are **inherited as simple mendelian dominants** by a pair of allelic genes, *Fy*[a] and *Fy*[b], giving rise, respectively, to agglutinogens Fy[a] and Fy[b]. In 1955 Sanger et al.[26] found that the majority of

Negroids lack both Fy[a] and Fy[b] and therefore are of the phenotype Fy(a–b–), a type not found in Caucasians. It is therefore necessary to involve a third allelic gene *fy*.

With the use of anti-**Fy**[a] and anti-**Fy**[b] antisera, four phenotypes in this system can be found: Fy(a+b+), Fy(a+b–), Fy(a–b+), and Fy(a–b–) (Table 10-5). According to Allen,[27] the null *Duffy* gene is a recessive at the *Duffy* locus on chromosome No. 1.

One of the most interesting features of the Duffy types is their marked difference in distribution among Caucasians and Negroids, as shown in Table 10-6. In Caucasians there are only three types, analogous to the three M-N types, whereas in Negroids there are four types, analogous to the four A-B-O blood groups. The reason for this is that the amorph gene *fy* has a high frequency in Negroids (77.8%) but so far has not been found in Caucasians. Therefore, if a blood specimen reacts as Fy(a–b–), this can be taken as strong evidence that it was derived from a Negroid subject. The phenotype Fy(a–b–), however, seems to be common also among

Table 10-5. Results possible in Fy[a] and Fy[b] tests

Reactions of cells with		Phenotype	Genotype	Binary code number
Anti-Fy[a]	Anti-Fy[b]			
+	+	Fy(a+b+)	*Fy*[a]*Fy*[b]	11
+	–	Fy(a+b–)	*Fy*[a]*Fy*[a] or *Fy*[a]*fy*	10
–	+	Fy(a–b+)	*Fy*[b]*Fy*[b] or *Fy*[b]*fy*	01
–	–	Fy(a–b–)	*fyfy*	00

Table 10-6. Comparison of distribution of the Duffy types in Caucasians and Negroids

Population	Totals	Distribution of type				Gene frequencies (%)		
		Fy(a+b–)	Fy(a–b+)	Fy(a+b+)	Fy(a–b–)	*Fy*[a]	*Fy*[b]	*fy*
Caucasians*								
Number	1286	230	435	621	0			
Percent		17.9	33.7	48.4	0	42.1	57.9	0
Negroids†								
Number	179	19	43	9	108			
Percent		10.6	24.0	5.0	60.4	6.4	14.0	77.8

*Data from Chown, B., Lewis, M., and Kaita, H.: Am. J. Hum. Genet. 17:384, 1965.
†Data from Pfizer Diagnostics; cited by Race, R. R., and Sanger, R.: Blood groups in man, ed. 4, Oxford, 1962, Blackwell Scientific Publications Ltd.

Yemenite Jews, according to Race and Sanger.[28] The Fy(a+) type was found by Won et al.[29] in all but one out of 145 Japanese tested and by Speiser[30] in all but one out of 394 Koreans tested.

Wiener and Gordon[20] titrated anti-human globulin serum against Fy(a+) red cells maximally coated with anti-Fy^a and compared this with the titer of the same anti-globulin serum against Rh$_o$-positive cells maximally coated with anti-Rh$_o$. They found that on the average the titer of anti-globulin sera was 9.3 times as high for the red cells coated with anti-Rh$_o$. This indicates that there are only about one tenth as many antigenic combining sites for the Fy antigen on the red cell surface as for the Rh antigen, which may account for some of the peculiarities of the tests for Fy^a and Fy^b.

Nature of the Fy antibody

Anti-Fy^a is usually of the Ig (7S) type and requires antiglobulin to react. A few anti-Fy^a sera, however, have been found that react with saline-suspended cells. **The antibody does not react with trypsinated cells.**

Anti-Fy^b does not react in the direct test with trypsinated cells nor with cells treated with papain. However, by using the trypsinated cell anti-globulin method of testing, the anti-Fy^a serum will react with Fy(a+) cells, but the papain-antiglobulin method is always neg-ative. With trypsinated cells plus the anti-globulin test, the Fy^b antibody will react with Fy(b+) cells.

The Fy^a antigen is well developed at birth.

Renwick and Lawler[31,32] presented evidence in 1963, based on family studies, of a close linkage between the genes for Duffy and the genes for a form of congenital cataract called zonular cataract, and 5 years later, in 1968, it was found to be linked to a deformity of the long arm of No. 1 autosome.[33] Thus it was the first locus in man to be assigned to a particu-lar autosome. Later, in 1971, the assigning

to chromosome No. 1 was confirmed by the linkage of *Duffy* locus to the loci for pancreatic and salivary amylase.[34]

Duffy antigen and Plasmodium vivax malaria

Approximately 70% of American Ne-groids, as well as West Africans, are re-sistant to infection by *P. vivax*, although they are susceptible to the other three species of human malarial parasites (*ovale, malariae, falciparum*). The *vivax* resistance factor completely blocks infection. Sickle cell trait decreases mortality from *P. falci-parum* infection but does not block infec-tion. Miller et al.,[35] in looking for erythro-cyte receptors for malarial parasites (merozoites), tested red cells lacking various antigenic determinants for suscepti-bility to invasion by *P. knowlesi*, a simian malarial parasite.

P. knowlesi invades human red cells in culture and can infect man. Miller and his colleagues prepared cultures of a mixture of human and parasitized red cells from infected rhesus monkeys to determine the invasion frequency of both Duffy-positive and Duffy-negative red cells. The invasion frequency for Duffy-positive cells was 53 to 99 (mean, 80.3) per 1000 erythrocytes, whereas that for Duffy-negative cells was 0 to 5 (mean, 2.2). The one type—Duffy negative, Fy(a–b–), genotype *fyfy*—was resistant to invasion. Both the Fy^a and Fy^b antigens are absent from these cells. *P. knowlesi* merozoites can attach to and interact with both Duffy-positive and Duf-fy-negative red cells, but the complete in-vasion process is possible only with Duffy-positive erythrocytes. This may account for the failure of some Negroids to develop a patent infection after intravenous inocula-tion of *P. knowlesi* infected blood for the former accepted treatment of neurosyphilis with malaria.

Genotype *fyfy* is present in approxi-mately 90% of West Africans, but is ex-tremely rare in other racial groups who are susceptible to *P. vivax*. The suscepti-bility of other negative and null erythrocytes from the collection of frozen cells (Blood Bank, NIH) was studied. Rh_{null}, Le(a–b–), and Lu(a–b–) cells were invaded normally. Red cells of the Bombay type, K_o, and Jk(a–b–) could not be evaluated because the freezing process apparently damaged the cells and no fresh cells were available for testing.

Among other findings, it was shown that the resistance of West Africans and some American Negroids to *P. vivax* corresponds to the unique distribution of Duffy-negative red cells, type Fy(a–b–), in the world.

THE Jk (KIDD) BLOOD GROUP SYSTEM

A different antibody from those which had previously been found was identified by Allen et al.[36] in the blood serum of a woman who had delivered an erythroblastotic infant. The patient's name was Kidd, and the antibody was given the designation anti-**Kidd**. The antigen it identified was at that time called Kidd. The capital K could not be utilized because it was already in use in the Kell-Cellano types, so that a different designation was needed. The Kidd designation was therefore changed to **Jk**^{a}, and when the reciprocal factor was later found, it was designated as **Jk**^{b}.

The reciprocal antibody, anti-**Jk**^{b}, was found in 1953 by Plaut et al.,[37] after which other examples were reported.

When tests with anti-**Jk**^{a} and anti-**Jk**^{b} are made together, three types of blood can be distinguished among Europeans: Jk-(a+b–), Jk(a+b+), and Jk(a–b+). Among the 1296 native Caucasians examined, Chown et al.[38] found these three types to be distributed as in Table 10-7.

If one assumes heredity by a pair of al-

lelic genes *Jk*^{a} and *Jk*^{b}, as in the case of the three M-N types, there are three genotypes corresponding to the three phenotypes, and the gene frequencies can be estimated by direct count (p. 351) as follows: *Jk*^{a} = 51.16% and *Jk*^{b} = 48.84%.

When the expected three phenotype numbers, or frequencies, are calculated from these gene frequencies, there is excellent agreement between the findings and the genetic expectations.

The most extensive family studies on the Jk types were carried out by Chown et al., who examined 500 Canadian families without encountering a single contradiction to the genetic theory.

Lewis et al.[39] also found that the theory held true in fifty-five Eskimo families and at the same time observed that the distribution of the Kidd type among the Eskimos was very close to that in Europeans.

As stated, blood lacking both factors **Jk**^{a} and **Jk**^{b} has not been found among Europeans. In 1959, however, Pinkerton et al.[40] encountered a Philippine woman whose red cells gave such reactions. This patient was tested because she had an antibody in her serum that agglutinated all red cells except her own. Because the patient was Jk(a–b–), the antibody was named anti-**Jk**^{a}**Jk**^{b}. Jk null type Jk(a–b–) lacks a common antigen, **Jk**^{a}**Jk**^{b}. A recessive gene at the Kidd locus is responsible.

Since the antibody apparently cannot be fractionated by absorption, a more appropriate name would appear to be anti-**Jk**, since it appears to detect a serologic specificity shared by all persons having either **Jk**^{a} or **Jk**^{b}, or both. Later, three more Jk(a–b–) persons were found because they had formed anti-**Jk** in response to blood

Table 10-7. Distribution of the Jk types

Type	Number	Percent	Gene frequency
Jk(a+b–)	337	26.00	
Jk(a+b+)	652	50.31	*Jk*^{a}—51.16%
Jk(a–b+)	307	23.69	*Jk*^{b}—48.84%
Totals	1296	100.00	100.00%

transfusions. The first was a Chinese, the second of Hawaiian-Chinese-European descent, and the third was a Maori woman. Presumably the type Jk(a–b–) is due to homozygosity for an **amorphic gene,** *jk.* The gene *jk* appears to be rare in Europeans, but Crawford et al.[41] described a family in which the gene was evidently transmitted through three generations.

The **incidence** of factor **Jk**[a] has been found to be 75% to 77% among Caucasoids 90% among Negroids, and 50% to 100% among Asiatic Mongolians.

Not infrequently it is found that the sera initially will agglutinate cells suspended in saline, but within a short time, even when stored in a refrigerator, they lose their ability to produce agglutination. The antiglobulin method must then be used for such sera to react. Even then the sera may fail to react, although the titer originally may have been high. The explanation appears to be that these antibodies require the use of **complement** to bring about agglutination, even when the antiglobulin technic is used. Therefore Stratton[42] has recommended the addition of human complement to the test mixtures in the form of fresh group AB serum. Ficination of the red cells sometimes appears to help, but the most consistent results are obtained by the antiglobulin test with red cells treated with trypsin as first recommended by Unger.[43]

Because there is need for extra careful, complicated, and repeated testing technics before conclusions can be drawn about blood in the Jk (Kidd) system, this blood group system is not of as much practical value for serologic testing and genetic studies as are the other systems. It is imperative that tests for the Jk specificities

be performed only by those who are especially trained in this field.

THE P-p BLOOD GROUP SYSTEM (INCLUDING P[k], Tj[a], AND "Luke")

At the same time that Landsteiner and Levine[44] produced the first anti-**M** and anti-**N** sera, they obtained from a different rabbit an antiserum that defined another specificity they designated anti-**P**. The agglutinogen P proved to be inherited as a simple mendelian dominant independent of A-B-O and M-N and was therefore evidently defining another blood group system. Further attempts to produce anti-**P** reagents by immunization of rabbits have not been as successful so that these reagents are presently derived mostly from other sources. Later attempts of Landsteiner and Levine[45] showed that the same antibody, anti-**P**, occurs naturally, occasionally in normal humans and in animals (horse, pig, rabbit),[46] and it has since been found that the antibody can also be produced by isoimmunization and can even give rise to hemolytic transfusion reactions.[47,48]

In 1936 Japanese workers[49] described a blood factor, **Q**, detected with absorbed pig sera, but parallel tests by Wiener showed that **P** and **Q** were the same or were closely related. The initial failure of the Japanese workers to recognize that **P** and **Q** were the same appears to have been due to differences in distribution in various races— 30% in Japan as compared with 79% in New York City Caucasians and 98% in Negroids (Table 10-8).

Family studies show **P** to be inherited as a simple mendelian dominant, and its application to medicolegal cases of disputed paternity has been suggested. How-

Table 10-8. Frequencies of phenotypes and genes in the P-p system*

	P+ (%)	P− (%)	Gene frequencies (approximate)	
			P (%)	p (%)
Caucasians	79	21	54	46
Negroids	98	2	86	14
Chinese	30	70	16	84

*Based on data from Wiener, A. S., and Wexler, I. B.: Heredity of the blood groups, New York, 1958, Grune & Stratton, Inc.

ever, the majority of anti-**P** reagents have proved to be cold agglutinins, and the reactions are often not readily reproducible. The distinction between P+ and P– bloods is not always sharp, and absorption of anti-**P** reagents with P– blood to purify them weakens or even destroys their activity. For these reasons, the forensic application of P tests is not recommended.

Anti-**P** sera, when fresh, may produce hemolysis with the aid of complement. Because of the similarity between the reactions of anti-**P**, irregularly occurring cold isoagglutinins and the natural anti-**A** and anti-**B** isoagglutinins, Wiener[50] suggested that the irregular cold anti-**P** agglutinin might likewise be due to inapparent immunization by organisms having P-like antigens, comparable to the case of the naturally occurring anti-**A** and anti-**B** isoagglutinins. This idea was confirmed when, among 132 cases of hydatid disease, Cameron and Stavely[51] found two with strong anti-**P** agglutinins. The cyst fluids inhibited the anti-**P** serum, except when the scolices were absent; these fluids were evidently the source of sensitization.

In 1968 Reimann[52] discovered a P-like substance in the leaves and flowers of certain mucilaginous plants, notably *Tilia* and *Tussilago farfara*. Reimann et al.[53] in 1972 reported on further experiments with the extracts. From the manner in which the carrier molecule influenced the immunogenicity, it was to be expected that this plant material could serve as an immunogen. This plant material is, of course, heterologous with respect to the experimental animal, the rabbit. To clarify the problem, immunization attempts were initiated on rabbits.

The antigen was prepared by extracting the leaves and flowers of two plants, *Tilia* and *Tussilago farfara*, for 2 hours at 37° C, using physiologic salt solution. The concentration was in the nature of 1 part of plant material to 10 parts of saline. The scheme of immunization of the rabbits was as follows:

1. For the first 3 weeks there were six injections of 2 ml each, intravenously. Then there was a waiting period of 2 weeks, making a total of 5 weeks.

2. During the sixth to eighth weeks, there were also six injections of 2 ml intravenously.

3. A waiting period of 1 month was instituted.

4. The same regimen was repeated once more, making twenty-four injections in all.

The injections led to the formation of anti-**P** antibodies in high titer in the blood serum of the rabbits, but unfortunately, anti-**H** was also produced, although in low titer. Since there was an undesired rise in anti-**H** titer without a further increase in anti-**P** during the second immunization course, the second course should be omitted.

The serum was absorbed with equal volumes of group O and group A_1 P-negative erythrocytes for 60 minutes. At first this did not produce satisfactory strong P-specific serum, since the residual titers were too low. When smaller volumes of cells were used for absorption, weak anti-**H** titers remained behind. Raw sera of goats turned out to be a little more acceptable in this regard.[52]

One may visualize the surface of immunogenic proteins as a mosaic of amino acids that determine the specificity of the immune response. However, the remainder of the molecule also has an influence on the formation of antibodies, qualitatively as well as quantitatively. Since the present experiments deal with blood group–*like* substances, such an adjuvant effect of the carrier molecule is to be expected. If a hapten is coupled to a heterologous (the experimental animal) carrier molecule, it provokes a stronger hapten-specific antibody formation than it would on an isologous species-specific carrier protein. The heterology of the plant materials therefore represented a potent adjuvant in the immunization attempts. The results show that the plant P-like substances tried by the authors on rabbits did induce anti-**P** formation. Whether the preparation of usable anti-**P** testing sera can be developed from this remains to be seen, however. One complication was that persistence in the injections did *not* improve the anti-**P** titer but did lead to increase in the undesired anti-**H**.

This is easily explained from the simultaneous presence of a lesser H activity in *Tilia* and *Tussilago farfara*. The authors concluded that the plant substances examined are suitable as immunogens for producing anti-**P** in rabbits. Further experiments with extracts of plant material having P substance activity alone without the undesired H activity (succulents and fungi) are in process.

Lehmann[53] described the results by oral immunization in rabbits using a P_1-like substance found in mucilaginous plants. The plants were ground (leaves of *Tussilago farfara* and of *Tilia*), and the fine particles were fed orally, in 100 ml suspensions, in the morning. Four hours later the rabbits were given their usual food. The serum was tested for anti-**P** and anti-**H** antibodies. The results indicated that minute particulate materials evidently can penetrate the intact intestinal mucosa and reach the bloodstream and then act as immunogens.

Four animals were given the extracts daily for 14 days; then 30 days later they were bled and the serum inactivated and titrated. The titers were then considerably higher, and it was concluded that oral introduction of particulate P-like substance containing mucilaginosa can produce high anti-**P** titers in rabbits. After a longer feeding period (47 days), a low anti-**H** titer

was found, which increased noticeably on further feeding, with little or no increase in the anti-**P** titer.

In 1968 Prokop and Schlesinger[54,55] showed that saline extracts of *Lumbricus terrestris* exhibited anti-P_1, anti-**B**, and anti-**H** characteristics, as do extracts of *Ascaris suum*. These authors suggested that the anti-**P** in P_2 people and anti-**PP₁P**[k] in p people may be due to previous immunization by *Ascaris* and other helminths. Bevan et al.[56] found that five patients who were P_2 had powerful anti-P_1 in their serum during an outbreak of *Fasciola hepatica* (liver fluke) disease.

Further development of the P system resulted from the discovery of the very high-frequency **Tj** factor by Levine et al.[57] This antibody, found in the serum of a blood donor named Jay, agglutinated the red cells of 3000 random group O persons but not the donor's own cells. Later, when additional Tj-negative individuals were found, Sanger[58] noted that they were all P negative, which suggested that **Tj** belonged to the P system. Further studies proved that indeed anti-**Tj** is related to anti-**P**, as anti-**A** is related to anti-A_1. Therefore anti-**Tj** was renamed anti-**P**, and the original anti-**P** of Landsteiner and Levine was renamed anti-P_1. In this way, the P system became a system of three blood types, the third of which was extremely rare, all inherited by triple allelic genes, as shown in Table 10-9.

It was then found that anti-**Tj** sera could be fractionated by absorption with type P_2 red cells (the original P-negative type of

Table 10-9. Expanded P system (after Sanger)

Blood type (phenotype)	Approximate frequency in Caucasians (%)	Reactions of red cells with		Agglutinogen present	Specificities detected	Corresponding genotypes
		Anti-P (Anti-Tj)	Anti-P_1 (Anti-P)			
P_1	79	+	+	P_1	P_1 and **P**	P^1P^1, P^1P^2, and P^1p
P_2	21	+	−	P_2	**P**	P^2P^2 and P^2p
p (extremely rare)		−	−	None	None	pp

Landsteiner and Levine). It can be seen that anti-**Tj** serum therefore is actually a mixture of anti-**P** and anti-**P₁**, just as group B (anti-**A**) serum contains a mixture of anti-**A** and anti-**A₁**.

The occasionally occurring natural anti-**P** sometimes found in human serum, now designated anti-**P₁**, is an irregular cold iso-agglutinin occurring in P₂ persons, just as anti-**A₁** occurs as an irregular cold isoag-glutinin in individuals of subgroups A₂ and A₂B.

As stated previously, Sanger postulated that the specificities **Tj** and **P** are related like **A** and **A₁**, thus giving rise to three P blood types. Wiener directed attention to the fact that if one assumes instead that **Tj** and **P** are related like **Rh₀** and **rh′** of the Rh-Hr system, *four* blood types could occur, as shown in Table 10-10, two of which are extremely rare. As can be seen from the table, the fourth blood type, p′, according to this concept, would be ex-

pected to be extremely rare, like type p. Moreover, the antibody in the serum, anti-P, would react with all bloods except those of type p and of its own type, p′, and therefore would simulate the original anti-**Tj** of Levine et al. However, the red cells would be agglutinable by the sera from type p persons. As a matter of fact, Matson et al. soon found a rare sample of blood that contained an anti-**Tj**–like antibody whose red cells did not give the expected negative reactions characteristic of type p persons. Since this concept did not fit into their concept of three blood types, they postulated that the blood in question had a special P-like antigen, called Pᵏ by them, and that the sera from type p persons had, in addition to anti-**P** and anti-**P₁**, also anti-**Pᵏ**; they claimed to be able to fractionate the antibody from the anti-**P** sera of type p persons by absorption with type P₂ cells.

The genetic theory to account for the four P types including the concept of a Pᵏ

Table 10-10. The four blood types in the P-p system*

Blood type	Frequencies New York Caucasians (%)	Reactions with Anti-P (Anti-P₀)	Anti-P₁† (Anti-p′)	Red cells Agglutinogens	Specificity	Serum natural isoagglutinins
P₁	79	+	+	P₁	**P** and **p′**	None
P₂	21	+	−	P₂	**P₀**	Anti-**p′** (irregularly occurring)
p′	Extremely rare	−	+	p′	**p′**	Anti-**P₀** (regularly occurring)
p	Extremely rare	−	−	None	None	Anti-**P₀**+**p′** (regularly occurring)

*From Wiener, A. S.: Personal communication, Aug., 1971.
†Alternative designation.

Table 10-11. Comparison of genetic theories for P types of Matson and of Wiener

	Theory of Matson Phenotypes	Corresponding genotypes	Theory of Wiener Phenotypes	Corresponding genotypes
1	P₁	P^1P^1, P^1p, P^1P^k	P₁	P^1P^1, P^1p', P^1p, and P^op'
2	P₂	P^2P^2, P^2P^k, P^2p	P₀	P^oP^o and P^op
3	Pᵏ	P^kP^k and P^kp	p′	$p'p'$ and $p'p$
4	p	pp	p	pp

Note that for phenotype 1 Matson postulates three genotypes and Wiener four, whereas for phenotype 2 Matson postulates three genotypes and Wiener only two.

antigen and involving four allelic genes has been proposed by Matson, and an alternative genetic theory modeled after that for the Rh system was suggested by Wiener. The latter would obviate the assumption of a P^k antigen. The two theories are compared in Table 10-11.

The situation has been further complicated by the postulation by Race and Sanger of two kinds of P^k bloods, designated by them as P_1^k and P_2^k, respectively.[59,60]

Crawford et al.[61] found in 1974 that the rare dominant inhibitor of the antigens Lu^a, Lu^b, and Au^a also inhibits P_1. The antigen P is not involved in the inhibition.

The Tj null type is Tj(a−), determined by homozygosity for a recessive gene. It is extremely rare. Everyone who has Tj(a−) lacks P_1 as well as Tj^a, and has a hemolytic type of antibody, anti-**Tj**^{a} (anti-**PP**$_1$), which is very dangerous.

Blood factor "Luke"

Another antibody, called anti-**Luke**, was found in the serum of a Negroid male, Luke P., who had never been transfused but who had Hodgkin's disease.[62] It appears to be like anti-**P** in that it does not react with cells of types p and P^k but differs from anti-**P** in that it does not react with cells of about 2% of types P_1 and P_2 persons. Two types are described, Luke(+) and Luke(−).

Biochemistry

Although the P substance has not as yet been isolated from human red cells, as has been indicated, a substance of similar specificity appears to be present in **hydatid cyst fluid.** Cameron and Stavely[51] provided evidence that the substance of such a specificity isolated from the fluid of a sheep hydatid cyst had a carbohydrate structure. According to Watkins and Morgan[63] D-galactose, in alpha linkage, appears to be the most important part of the determinant group.

Naiki and Marcus[64] identified the P antigen as the glycosphingolipid globoside

βGalNac$(1{\rightarrow}3)\alpha$Gal$(1{\rightarrow}4)$Glc-cer and the P^k antigen as ceramide trihexoside αGal $(1{\rightarrow}4)\beta$Gal$(1{\rightarrow}4)$Glc-cer. Their results were based on their work with red cell extracts. In 1974 Cory et al.[65] worked with sheep hydatid cyst fluid and found P_1 to be D-galactosyl-$\alpha(1{\rightarrow}4)$-D-galactosyl-$\beta(1{\rightarrow}4)$-N-acetyl-D-glucosamine.

The P^k phenotype is subdivided into P_1^k and P_2^k.[66] Individuals who belong to the P_1^k phenotype have P_1 and P_2^k activity. Those belonging to P_2^k have P_2^k activity but lack P_1. Watkins and Morgan[67] believe that for this situation to occur with a single enzyme responsible for the formation of both P_1 and P^k structures, it is necessary to postulate that the acceptor substrate for the formation of the P_1 structure βGal$(1{\rightarrow}4)$ βGlcNac$(1{\rightarrow}3)\beta$Gal$(1{\rightarrow}4)$Glc-cer (paragloboside) is missing in P_2^k persons.

Importance of the P system

The P system has not been of great value in medicolegal studies because the line between weak positive and negative reactions is indistinct and the antisera are generally weak. The P_1 specificity rarely causes clinical symptoms, but anti-P_1 has been found after P_1-positive tranfusions, and it was also reported as the cause of a fatal transfusion reaction.[68]

THE LUTHERAN BLOOD GROUP SYSTEM AND FACTOR Lu

The first report of an antibody later designated as anti-**Lu**^{a} was made by Callender et al.[69] in 1945, later detailed by Callender and Race[70] in 1946. It was found in the serum of a patient with disseminated lupus erythematosus who had received numerous blood transfusions and had produced various isoimmune antibodies, including the one described. Because the patient's name was Lutheran, the antibody was designated anti-**Lutheran,** later changed to anti-**L,** and the antigen it defined was termed L. This designation caused confusion with the terms used for the Lewis antigen, so that the name was again changed, this time to Lu^a, and this designation remains.

The reciprocal antibody was found by Cutbush and Chanarin[71] in 1956 and by Greenwalt and Sasaki[72] in 1957 and was designated anti-**Lu**[b]. This is an exceedingly rare antibody because the percentage of Lu(b−) individuals is low. Therefore once such a person becomes isoimmunized with blood having the **Lu**[b] factor, it is difficult to find a compatible donor; the **frequency** of phenotype Lu(a+b−) is only 0.15%.

The antigens and blood factors are **Lu**[a] and **Lu**[b], the antibodies anti-**Lu**[a] and anti-**Lu**[b], and the genes *Lu*[a] and *Lu*[b]. *Lu*[a] was shown by Callender and Race to be inherited as a mendelian dominant.

In 1961 Crawford et al.[73] found the rare type Lu(a−b−). Four **phenotypes** in the Lu system are designated as Lu(a+b+), Lu(a+b−), Lu(a−b+), and Lu(a−b−). Darnborough et al.[74] found that when Lu(a−b−) persons are isoimmunized with the **Lu** specificity, they form antibodies designated anti-**Lu**[a]**Lu**[b] because they react with both Lu(a+b−) and Lu(a−b+) bloods. However, since the antisera cannot be fractionated by absorption, the simpler designation anti-**Lu** appears to be preferable, to indicate that they detect another specificity, **Lu,** and thus are comparable to anti-C of the A-B-O system, anti-**M**[e] and anti-**U** of the M-N-S system, and anti-**rh**[G] of the Rh-Hr system, etc.

The Lutheran null type is Lu(a−b−). It lacks many common antigens. Persons of type Lu(a−b−) can be immunized against any of the specificities they lack. The type may be due to a rare recessive gene at the Lutheran locus,[74] but commonly it is also caused by a dominant modifier at a different locus.[73]

If the **inheritance** of the Lu blood types were to follow the ordinary rules that hold for other blood group systems, one would expect that the Lu(a−b−) type would be due to homozygosity for an amorph recessive gene *lu,* that is, genotype *lulu.* In fact, in some families Lu(a−b−) type does behave as a recessive.[73] In many families, however, the very rare Lu(a−b−) type appears to be transmitted as a dominant characteristic, as in the family described by Crawford et al.,[73] in which she herself was the propositus. According to Race and Sanger, the postulation of a **suppressor gene** closely linked to or as a part of the *Lu* locus does not provide a satisfactory explanation. Race and Sanger postulated instead **another locus,** spatially independent of the *Lu* locus, where a dominant rare allele converts the Lu precursor substance into a form such that it cannot be used for the production of normal Lu antigens. The inhibitors, or suppressor genes, in the Lutheran system are called by Race and Sanger *In(Lu)* and *in(Lu)*[76]; *in(Lu)* is not part of the Lutheran locus and is not part of *P.* It is not situated at the loci of *A-B-O, M-N-S-s, Rh, Kell, Duffy, Kidd,* or *Yt,* and it is not carried on the X or Y chromosome.

The **distribution** of the Lu genes among 1456 white Canadians was as follows[77]: for *Lu*[a], 3.53%; for *Lu*[b], 96.47%. This makes no allowance for a possible amorphic gene, *lu.* Nevertheless, recalculation of the estimated number of each of the three types on the assumption of only two alleles shows an excellent fit between the expected and actually found numbers.

In 1951 Mohr[78,79] described results of family studies that provided the first convincing evidence of **autosomal linkage** in man. He presented what appeared to be convincing evidence of a linkage between the Lewis and Lutheran blood types. As will be recalled (pp. 84 and 85), the red cell reactions with anti-**Lewis** sera are affected by the A-B-H secretor type, and it is now believed that Mohr's findings actually establish a linkage between the Lutheran and A-B-H secretor genes. The linkage between *Lu* and *Se* genes was not complete, and the recombination frequency was estimated as 0.15.

In another chapter, reference is made to the **Auberger groups** (Au). Tippett[80] found that in Crawford's family, already cited, the seven Lu(a−b−) individuals were all Au(a−), whereas the other six members were all Au(a+), and the same happened in the second family. Thus the Au groups appear to be closely related in some way to the dominantly transmitted Lu(a–b–) phenotype. (See p. 170.)

Frequency

The incidence of Lu(a+) was found to be 6.93%. Wiener and Wexler[81] stated that if heredity by a pair of allelic genes, Lu^a and Lu^b, is postulated, the genotype frequencies calculated from these data are Lu^aLu^a, 0.12%; Lu^aLu^b, 6.81%; and Lu^bLu^b, 93.07%. This does not provide for the rare possible third allelic gene *lu* responsible for part of type Lu(a–b–).

Lu^a has not been found in Asians, Eskimos, or Australian aborigines.

Antibody type

Most of the **Lu**^{a} antibodies are of the 19S IgM type and react by saline agglutination method at 12° to 18° C. The antibody may be naturally occurring or isoimmune.

Laboratory tests

In tests for the **Lu** factors there appear to be large agglutinates with many unagglutinated cells. Tests with anti-**Lu**^{b} exhibit the same phenomenon, but the picture is not as striking. The tests for **Lu**^{b} may be difficult, and most anti-**Lu**^{b} sera react best by the antiglobulin tests. Most anti-**Lu**^{b} sera therefore seem to be of the 7S, IgG type.

Development

The **Lu**^{a} antigen is well developed in cord blood; **Lu**^{b} reactions, however, are weaker.

Complexities

There are other complexities in the Lu system. Bove, at Yale–New Haven Hospital, and Marsh,[82] at The New York Blood Center, have described an antibody formed by Lu(a–b+) persons that reacts with all cells, except those of type Lu(a–b–) and the Lu(a–b+) cells of the individual who formed the antibodies. All other examples of the Lu(a–b+), Lu(a+b+), and Lu(a+b–)

bloods react with these antibodies. There seem to be three other high-incidence antigens in the Lu system detected by antibodies like these.

A series of antibodies related to the Lutheran system has been found and given numbers such as anti-**Lu4**, anti-**Lu5**, and so on, up to anti-**Lu20**. Except for Lu9 and Lu6, Race and Sanger refer to the antigens as para-Lutherans. Wiener classified them as *cognates* of Lu, comparable to Rh^A, Rh^B, Rh^C, Rh^D, which are cognates of Rh$_o$.

An antibody, anti-**Lu8**, which recognizes another Lutheran-related antigen, was described by MacIlroy et al.[83] Anti-**Lu3**, or anti-**Lu**^{a}**Lu**^{b}, preferably called simply anti-**Lu**, clumps all human red cells except those of the type Lu(a–b–). Lu(a–b–) is rare and, as stated previously, in some families is due to a corresponding recessive gene (genotype *lulu*), whereas in other families it is due to a suppressor gene for individuals of all Lu genotypes. This is comparable to the situation for Rh$_{null}$, except that the Lutheran suppressor is a dominant rather than a recessive gene. The antibodies anti-**Lu4,5,6,7,8** can occur in individuals of any Lu type and have the peculiarity that they react with all bloods except those of the patient and Lu(a–b–) of both kinds. They are thus **cognates of the Lu factor** (shared by **Lu**^{a} and **Lu**^{b}), comparable in this respect to the cognates of the **Rh**$_o$ factor of the Rh-Hr system. In this case of Lu8, a family study showed that the blood of two siblings failed to react with the antiserum, whereas that of two siblings and both parents and of two children of the propositus did react, indicating that the rare blood type is hereditary.

Antigens Lu9 and Lu6 are comparable in the Lutheran system to Kp^a and Kp^b in the Kell system. An antibody was found in the serum of Mrs. Mull in Philadelphia by Molthan et al.[84] Mrs. Mull was Lu(a–b+). The antigen was given the number Lu9. It proved to be transmitted as a dominant characteristic.

The gene *Lu9* is linked to the *Lutheran* locus. In a random sample of 521 people tested, the frequency proved to be 1.7%, with a significantly higher proportion of Lu9 in Lu(a+b+) than in Lu(a–b+) persons.

Lu6 was shown to be part of the *Lutheran* complex locus when two unrelated individuals of the very rare phenotype Lu6 and a relative of one of these all proved to be Lu9. Anti-**Lu6** was described in 1972 by Marsh[85] and by Wrobel et al.[86] in the same year. Wrobel et al. noted that the reaction of anti-**Lu6** is weaker with cord cells than with adult cells.

Much. antigen

The Much. antigen, Lu12, was described in 1973 by Sinclair et al.[87] The antibody did not react with Lu(a–b–) cells nor with the individual's own cells. The Much. phenotype was Lu(a–bw), that is, her Lu^b antigen was more weakly reactive than that of homozygous Lu(a+b+) people.

The Lutheran system provides, with the secretor system, the first example in man of autosomal linkage and of autosomal crossing over. It also demonstrates that crossing over in humans can be more common in females than in males.

Clinical significance

In 1966 three examples of anti-**Lu**^{b} were described by Moltham and Crawford[88]— one patient with repeated hemolytic transfusion reactions and two in whom the antibody was associated with pregnancy. However, the antibody was not responsible for a clinical problem.

REFERENCES

1. Coombs, R. R., Mourant, A. E., and Race, R. R.: Lancet 1:264, 1946.
2. Wiener, A. S., and Sonn-Gordon, E. B.: Rev. Hematol. 2:3, 1947.
3. Levine, P., Wigod, W., Backer, A. M., and Ponder, R.: Blood 7:869, 1949.
4. Allen, F. H., and Lewis, S. J.: Vox Sang. 2:81, 1957.
5. Allen, F. H., Lewis, S. J., and Sudenberg, H.: Vox Sang. 3:1, 1958.
6. Chown, B., Lewis, M., and Kaita, H.: Nature (Lond.) 180:711, 1957.
7. Kaita, H., Lewis, M., Chown, B., and Gard, F.: Nature (Lond.) 183:1586, 1959.
8. Corcoran, P. A., Allen, F. H., Jr., Lewis, M., and Chown, B.: Transfusion 1:181, 1961.
9. Furuhjelm, U., Nevanlinna, H. R., Nurkka, R., Gavin, J., Tippett, P., Gooch, A., and Sanger, R.: Vox Sang. 15:118, 1968.
10. Strange, J. J., Kenworthy, R. J., Webb, A. J., and Giles, C. M.: Vox Sang. 27:81, 1974.
11. Guévin, R. M., Taliano, V., and Waldmann, O.: American Association of Blood Banks Program, 24th Annual Meeting, p. 100, 1971.
12. Giblett, E. R.: Nature (Lond.) 181:1221, 1958.
13. Giblett, E. R., and Chase, J.: Br. J. Haematol. 5:319, 1959.
14. Walker, R. J., Argall, C. I., Steane, E. A., Sasaki, T. T., and Greenwalt, T. J.: Transfusion 3:94, 1963.
15. Stroup, M., MacIlroy, M., Walker, R., and Aydelotte, J. V.: Transfusion 5:309, 1965.
16. Allen, F. H., Jr., Krabbe, S. M. R., and Corcoran, P. A.: Vox Sang. 6:555, 1961.
17. Wimer, B. M., Marsh, W. L., Taswell, H. F., and Galey, W. R.: Br. J. Haematol. 36:219, 1977.
18. Giblett, E. R., Klebanoff, S. J., Pinous, S. H., Swanson, J., Park, B. H., and McCullough, J.: Lancet 1:1235, 1971.
19. Marsh, W. L., Øyen, R., Nichols, M. E., and Allen, F. H.: Br. J. Haematol. 29:247, 1975.
20. Wiener, A. S., and Gordon, E. B.: Am. J. Clin. Pathol. 23:708, 1955.
21. Cutbush, M., Mollison, P. L., and Parkin, D. M.: Nature (Lond.) 165:188, 1950.
22. Cutbush, M., and Mollison, P. L.: Heredity 4:383, 1950.
23. van Loghem, J. J., and van der Hart, M.: Ned. Tijdschr. Geneeskd. 11:148, 1950.
24. Ikin, E. W., Mourant, A. E., Pettenkofer, J. J., and Blumenthal, G.: Nature (Lond.) 168:1077, 1951.
25. Levine, P., Sneath, J. S., Robinson, E. A., and Huntington, P. W.: Blood 10:941, 1955.
26. Sanger, R., Race, R. R., and Jack, J.: Br. J. Haematol. 1:370, 1955.
27. Allen, F. H., Jr.: Am. J. Clin. Pathol. 66:467, 1976.
28. Race, R. R., and Sanger, R.: Blood groups in man, ed. 4, Oxford, England, 1962, Blackwell Scientific Publications, Ltd.
29. Won, C. D., Shin, H. S., Kim, S. W., Swanson, J., and Matson, G. A.: Am. J. Phys. Anthropol. 18:115, 1960.
30. Speiser, P.: Wien. Klin. Wochenschr. 71:549, 1959.
31. Renwick, J. H., and Lawler, S. D.: Am. J. Hum. Genet. 27:67, 1962.

32. Renwick, J. H., and Lawler, S. D.: Ann. Hum. Genet. **27**:67, 1963.
33. Donahue, R. P., Bias, W. B., Renwick, J. H., and McKusick, V. A.: Proc. Natl. Acad. Sci. U.S.A. **61**:949, 1968.
34. Kamarýt, J., Adamék, R., and Vrba, M.: Humangenetik **11**:213, 1971.
35. Miller, L. H., Mason, S. J., Dvorak, J. A., McGinniss, M. H., and Rothman, I. K.: Science **189**:561, 1975.
36. Allen, F. H., Diamond, I. K., and Niedziela, B.: Nature (Lond.) **167**:482, 1951.
37. Plaut, G., Ikin, E. W., Mourant, A. E., Sanger, R., and Race, R. R.: Nature (Lond.) **168**:207, 1953.
38. Chown, B., Lewis, M., and Kaita, H.: Transfusion **5**:506, 1965.
39. Lewis, M., Chown, B., and Kaita, H.: Am. J. Hum. Genet. **15**:203, 1963.
40. Pinkerton, F. J., Mermod, L. E., Liles, B. A., Jack, J. A., and Noades, J.: Vox Sang. **5**:155, 1959.
41. Crawford, M. N., Greenwalt, T. J., Sasaki, T., Tippett, P., Sanger, R., and Race, R. R.: Transfusion **1**:228, 1961.
42. Stratton, F.: Vox Sang. **1**:160, 1956.
43. Unger, L. J.: J. Lab. Clin. Med. **37**:825, 1951.
44. Landsteiner, K., and Levine, P.: Proc. Soc. Exp. Biol. Med. **24**:941, 1927.
45. Landsteiner, K., and Levine, P.: J. Exp. Med. **47**:757, 1928.
46. Landsteiner, K., and Levine, P.: J. Immunol. **17**:1, 1929.
47. Wiener, A. S., and Peters, H. R.: Ann. Intern. Med. **13**:2306, 1940.
48. Wiener, A. S.: Am. J. Clin. Pathol. **12**:302, 1942.
49. Furuhata, T., and Imamura, I.: Jpn. J. Hum. Genet. **12**:50, 1936.
50. Wiener, A. S.: J. Immunol. **66**:287, 1951.
51. Cameron, G. L., and Stavely, G. M.: Nature (Lond.) **179**:147, 1957.
52. Reimann, W.: Blutgruppenaktive Substanzen aus Mucilaginosa, Berthold Mueller zum 70. Geburtstag gewidmet, Wiss. A. Univ. Halle XVII, 1968, H.A.S. 531-534.
53. Reimann, W., Lehmann, K., and Schulze, M.: Immun-Information 2. Jahrgang, Heft 6, 1972.
54. Prokop, O., and Schlesinger, D.: Z. Immunitätsforsch. **129**:344, 1965.
55. Prokop, O., and Schlesinger, D.: Dtsch. Gesundh. Ves. **34**:1584, 1965.
56. Bevan, B., Hammond, W., and Clarke, R. L.: Vox Sang. **18**:188, 1970.
57. Levine, P., Bobbitt, O. B., Waller, R. K., and Kuhmichel, A.: Proc. Soc. Exp. Biol. Med. **77**:403, 1951.
58. Sanger, G.: Nature (Lond.) **176**:1163, 1955.
59. Matson, G. A., Swanson, J., Noades, J., Sanger, R., and Race, R. R.: Am. J. Hum. Genet. **11**:26, 1959.
60. Wiener, A. S.: Lab Digest **31**(4):6, 1968.
61. Crawford, M. N., Tippett, P., and Sanger, R.: Vox Sang. **26**:283, 1974.
62. Tippett, P., Sanger, R., Race, R. R., Swanson, J., and Busch, S.: Vox Sang. **10**:269, 1965.
63. Watkins, W. M., and Morgan, W. T. J.: Science **152**:172, 1966.
64. Naiki, M., and Marcus, D. M.: Biochem. Biophys. Res. Commun. **60**:1105, 1974.
65. Cory, H. T., Yates, A. D., Donald, A. S., Watkins, W. M., and Morgan, W. T. J.: Biochem. Biophys. Res. Commun. **61**:1289, 1974.
66. Race, R. R., and Sanger, R.: Blood groups in man, ed. 6, Oxford, England, 1975, Blackwell Scientific Publications.
67. Watkins, W. M., and Morgan, W. T. J.: J. Immunogenet. **3**:15, 1976.
68. Moureau, P.: Rev. Belge. Sci. Med. **16**:258, 1945.
69. Callender, S. T., Race, R. R., and Pavkoc, A.: Br. Med. J. **2**:83, 1945.
70. Callender, S. T., and Race, R. R.: Ann. Eugen. **13**:102, 1946.
71. Cutbush, M., and Chanarin, I.: Nature (Lond.) **178**:855, 1956.
72. Greenwalt, T. J., and Sasaki, T.: Blood **12**:998, 1957.
73. Crawford, M. N., Greenwalt, T. S., Sasaki, T., Tippett, P., Sanger, R., and Race, R. R.: Transfusion **1**:228, 1961.
74. Darnborough, J., Firth, R., Giles, C. M., Goldsmith, K. L. G., and Crawford, M. N.: Nature (Lond.) **198**:796, 1963.
75. Brown, F. N. H., Simpson, S. L., and Read, H. C.; cited by Race, R. R., and Sanger, R.: Blood groups in man, ed. 5, Oxford, England, 1968, Blackwell Scientific Publications.
76. Crawford, M. N., Tippett, P., and Sanger, R.: Vox Sang. **26**:283, 1974.
77. Chown, B., Lewis, M., Kaita, H.: Vox Sang. **11**:108, 1966.
78. Mohr, J.: Acta Pathol. Microbiol. Scand. **28**:61, 1951; **29**:339, 1951.
79. Mohr, J.: A study of linkage in man, Copenhagen, 1954, Einar Munksgaard Forlag.
80. Tippett, P.: Serological studies of the inheritance of unusual Rh and other blood group phenotypes, Ph.D. thesis, University of London; cited by Race, R. R., and Sanger, R., 1963.
81. Wiener, A. S., and Wexler, I. B.: Heredity of the blood groups, New York, 1958, Grune & Stratton, Inc.
82. Bove, J. R., and Marsh, W. L.; cited by

Issitt, P. D.: Applied blood group serology, Oxnard, Calif., 1970, Spectra Biologicals.

83. MacIlroy, M., McGreary, J., and Stroup, M.: Vox Sang. **23**:455, 1972.
84. Molthan, L., Crawford, M. N., Marsh, W. L., and Allen, F. H.: Vox Sang. **24**:468, 1973.
85. Marsh, W. L.: Transfusion **12**:27, 1972.
86. Wrobel, D. M., Moore, B. P. L., Cornwall, S., Wray, E., Øyen, R., and Marsh, W. L.: Vox Sang. **23**:205, 1972.

87. Sinclair, M., Buchanan, D. I., Tippett, P., and Sanger, R.: Vox Sang. **25**:256, 1973.
88. Molthan, L., and Crawford, M. N.: Transfusion **6**:584, 1966.
89. Sussman, L. N.: Paternity testing by blood grouping, ed. 2, Springfield, Ill., 1976, Charles C Thomas, Publisher.

11 □ High- and low-frequency blood group factors (specificities)

THE DIEGO BLOOD GROUP SYSTEM—SPECIFICITY Di

An antibody, later identified as anti-**Di**[a], was found in Venezuela in 1955 by Layrisse et al.[1] in the blood serum of the mother of an erythroblastotic baby. This antibody identified a specificity different from those of other known blood group systems. It derives its name, **Diego**, from the family in which the antibody was found. The antigen was present in four generations and was shown by Levine et al.[2] to behave like a dominant characteristic. It has been identified in as many as 36% of members of some South American Indian tribes, but it is very rare in Caucasians, if present at all; it was not found in 2600 Caucasoids examined. It is common among Chinese, Japanese, pure-blooded Negroes, and South American Indians, in whom the incidence ranges from 2% to 45%. According to some authors, it is also found among Eskimos and Polynesians, although others assert that it is virtually absent in Eskimos. The incidence among the Carib Indians of Cachama is 36%.

Originally the phenotypes in the Di system were written Di(a+) and Di(a−), but, since the antithetical anti-**Di**[b] was found by Thompson et al.[3] in 1967, there are actually three phenotypes: Di(a+b−), Di(a−b+), and Di(a+b+). No phenotype Di(a−b−) has been reported, which indicates that heredity is probably by a pair of allelic genes *Di*[a] and *Di*[b].

Lewis et al.[4] in tests on fifty Japanese families, nine of which had the antigen, showed that in the mating Di(a+) × Di(a−) there could be Di(a−) children, but in the mating Di(a−) × Di(a−) there are no Di(a+) children. The Di[a] antigen is apparently developed at birth. It has been known to cause erythroblastosis fetalis. Di[b] is also well developed at birth.

Clinically and medically the Diego blood group is not of great significance because antibodies to the **Di** factor are so rarely found. It is important, however, as an anthropologic marker, since it is so often present primarily in the Mongolian races (Orientals) and the South American Indians.

At a symposium before the American Association for the Advancement of Science in Boston on February 18, 1976, it was stated that "The predominant presence in the Amerindian of the O group, the Diego group, D$_{Chi}$, and various types of albumin, and the absence of Rh-negative and hemoglobin variants show not only the presence of very well-defined genetic factors but also the fact of having been subjected to very different environmental conditions than other Mongoloid branches." Of 816 Indians belonging to six different tribes, 76% were lactase deficient. The authors found a high incidence of mixtures of Caucasian and Negro in the Indians studied. *Di* is considered a genetic marker of extremely ancient Asiatic populations.

BLOOD FACTOR Vel (Ve^a) AND THE Vel BLOOD GROUP SYSTEM

In 1952 Sussman and Miller[5] found in the serum of a patient named Vel an antibody that, when tested against 10,000 samples of group O blood cells, agglutinated all but four. This patient had had a transfusion reaction. The antibody that caused the reaction was designated anti-**Vel**, and the specificity that it identified was named **Vel.** The antibody did not agglutinate the patient's own red cells and so was not an autoantibody. When the siblings of the five Vel-negative persons were tested, no other Vel-negative individuals were found, although it was assumed and later proved correct that Vel is inherited. The Vel-negative type presumably resulted from homozygosity for a rare, recessive gene, *ve*.

The antibody clumped saline-suspended cells to a titer of only 4 units, but when the cells were suspended in plasma, the titer was 32 units. The patient had had previous pregnancies and transfusions that could have sensitized her.

A second example of sensitization to the **Vel** factor was reported in 1955 by Levine et al.[6] The antibody reported by these workers had hemolytic as well as agglutinating properties. Whereas this ability to cause hemolysis has not been found for all anti-**Vel** sera, when hemolysis involving a high-frequency factor is observed, the possibility of **Vel** sensitization should be borne in mind. The antibody found by Levine et al. was shown to be different from anti-**Tj^a**, anti-**U**, and anti-**H**. Levine's patient was a woman who had had previous pregnancies and transfusions that could have sensitized her. Cross-matching tests with the blood of 1000 donors showed all to be incompatible. When her red cells were tested with the original anti-**Vel** serum, they proved to be Vel negative.

The third case of **Vel** sensitization was reported in 1959 by Bradish and Shields.[7] This was a male patient who had been sensitized by transfusions. The serum reacted like that of Levine's patient; that is, it hemolyzed the cells when the serum was freshly drawn and agglutinated the cells after the serum was inactivated. Higher titers were obtained when the cells were suspended in plasma than in saline. The serum also reacted by the indirect antiglobulin technic.

Another **Vel**-sensitized patient was found by Levine et al.[8] in 1961. This patient had had a hemolytic transfusion reaction. Her antibody caused both hemolysis and agglutination. There were seven Vel-negative persons in three generations of her family.

In 1961 Wiener et al.[9] described still another case of **Vel** sensitization that was discovered during routine cross-matching tests preliminary to transfusion. The patient was group O MN k Rh$_2$rh. Every group O Rh-positive blood tried was incompatible with her serum. This patient's serum hemolyzed the cells but only to the extent of about 5% to 50%. The titer for hemolysins against saline-suspended cells, with the dilutions of the serum being carried out in saline, was up to 4 units. After the unlysed cells had been washed in saline three times, an antiglobulin test was made and clumping occurred. The antibody titer by the antiglobulin technic was 30 units. Ficinated cells were also lysed by the patient's fresh serum, and this was more pronounced than with the unmodified cells. Her serum did not agglutinate or lyse her own cells. The direct antiglobulin test was negative. No compatible bloods were found in tests on 200 donors. Since the patient was type k and hr″ positive, the possibility of sensitization with **k** or **hr″** was ruled out, especially because the antibody did not have the serologic characteristics of **hr″** or **Kell.** The patient was U and I positive, as well as H positive, but she was Vel negative according to tests with the original anti-**Vel** serum. She showed no evidence of autosensitization by any laboratory method tried. Family studies found that three of her siblings were also Vel negative.

The **Vel** specificity has thus been shown to have a frequency of 99.96%, which is why it is referred to as a high-frequency blood factor. Negatively reacting bloods are extremely rare. No naturally occurring anti-**Vel** antibodies have been reported, and because of the low frequency of the Vel-negative type, isoimmune antibodies have only rarely been found. Apparently, however, Vel-negative individuals readily become sensitized by transfusions of Vel-positive blood.

With the results of the examinations of all these patients and the investigations of a family by van Loghem and van der Hart[10] in 1958, it is well established that the Vel characteristic is inherited. Two **genes,** *Ve* and *ve,* have been postulated, giving rise to three **genotypes,** *VeVe, Veve,* and *veve,* having the frequencies 97.20%, 2.78%, and 0.02%, respectively.

The **Vel** specificity is important primarily in transfusions and in some family studies. The **problem of transfusing** a sensitized Vel-negative person is very difficult to resolve because of the rarity of Vel-negative donors. It would perhaps be simpler to prevent sensitization by conducting tests for Vel routinely and maintaining a list of Vel-negative persons and at the same time not transfusing them with Vel-positive blood. Vel-negative persons are probably homozygous for a rare recessive gene. Whenever such a person is found, all siblings should be tested. If any of these are Vel negative, they should be so informed and given suitable identification, as well as a warning to refuse all transfusions except in extreme emergency unless Vel-negative donors are used.

If transfusions are essential and if there is sufficient time for testing, a sibling known to be Vel negative and compatible should be selected as a donor to avoid sensitizing the patient. Once sensitization has occurred, transfusion is unsafe unless a Vel-negative donor can be found.

There are central clearinghouses where the names and addresses of donors with rare blood types are kept on file, and these could supply the blood. As an example, the central clearinghouse of the American Association of Blood Banks lists a number of Vel-negative donors.

The Vel-negative patient may be a donor for himself, provided he has contemplated the possibility of a transfusion and made suitable arrangements. Some types of surgery—cardiac, for example—are often scheduled months in advance. The patient can therefore be bled periodically and his blood stored in the frozen state or in ACD solution in a refrigerator. Since it is now known how to preserve red cells frozen at extremely low temperatures over long periods of time, this is no longer an insurmountable problem. When the patient needs blood, his own could then be used for the transfusion.

There are individuals whose red cells give weak reaction with anti-Vel sera. Unless powerful antisera are used for testing, false negative reactions could be obtained with such blood specimens. The anti-**Vel** sera are often difficult to use; therefore any blood that appears to be Vel-negative should be retested with as many anti-**Vel** reagents as possible before drawing any final conclusions as to the presence or absence of the Vel specificity. The anti-**Vel** sera react best by the antiglobulin method using **anti-nongamma globulin reagents.** All anti-**Vel** sera react strongly with fresh Vel-positive cells at room temperature if the serum is added to a small volume of packed cells and the mixture is incubated for 30 minutes, then centrifuged lightly for 2 minutes, provided that the cells are fresh.

The antibody is usually of the IgM type. It has been postulated that a high-titered maternal IgG anti-**Vel** may occur in a pregnancy in which the Vel antigen in the fetus is strong and the mother is Vel negative. This could give rise to erythroblastosis fetalis.

Whereas some anti-**Vel** sera react in saline, the reaction is better by albumin, enzyme, or antiglobulin tests. As already stated, fresh cells must be used for testing purposes.

The Vel antigen is well developed in cord blood, although it reacts more weakly than in adult blood.

A number of articles have been written

purportedly showing some relationship between **Vel** and **P**, but no such relationship has been established, and the consensus is that Vel is a distinct antigen defining a separate blood group system.

THE DOMBROCK BLOOD GROUP SYSTEM—ANTIGEN Do

In 1965 Swanson et al.[11] found an antibody in the serum of a woman named Dombrock after transfusion. They called it anti-**Do**[a]; the specificity it identifies is designated **Do**[a]. Tippett et al.,[12] in 1965, and Polesky and Swanson,[13] in 1966, gave further information on the Do[a] antigen, including its distribution among certain races, as well as the variation in amount of antigen produced by different Do(a+) individuals.

The **antibody** reacts best by the antiglobulin method using papainized red cells after incubation of the mixture of cells and antiserum at 37° C for an hour in a water bath. Reactions with unmodified red cells are also clear-cut but weaker. If human gamma globulin, fraction II, is added to the antiglobulin serum, it will inhibit agglutination of cells sensitized by anti-**Do**[a].

The Do[a] antigen is present on cord cells. Complement is not needed for the reaction between **Do**[a] and its antiserum, and the antibody is not inhibited by secretor or nonsecretor saliva or by hydatid cyst fluid.

Serum containing the antibody can be stored at –20° C for at least a year without the antibody losing its potency.

Two **types** have been reported—Do(a+), having a frequency of 64%, and Do(a–) with a frequency of 36%. Polesky and Swanson noted a lower frequency of Do(a+) in American Indians and in Negroids.

In 1973 Molthan, Crawford, and Tippett[14] reported finding the antithetical antibody, anti-**Do**[b]. The inheritance of Dombrock blood groups is supposed to be by two corresponding genes, *Do*[a] and *Do*[b], the former being a dominant one. Three genotypes are proposed: *Do*[a]*Do*[a], *Do*[a]*Do*[b], and

Do[b]*Do*[b]. The old symbol *Do* is now used to denote Dombrock *locus*. No Do(a–b–) phenotype has been found to date.

The Dombrock blood groups seem to constitute an independent blood group system, since, as shown by Tippett,[15] the gene *Do*[a] is not sited at the loci for any of the established red cell systems: A-B-O, M-N-S-s, P, Rh-Hr, Lutheran, Kell, Lewis, Duffy, Kidd, or Yt or for the secretor system and it is not X- nor Y-linked.

The antigen is well developed at birth.

THE AUBERGER BLOOD GROUP SYSTEM AND ANTIGEN Au[a]

In 1961 Salmon et al.[16] found in the serum of a French woman who had had many transfusions an antibody they named anti-**Au**[a], since her name was Auberger, and the specificity it defines was named **Au**[a]. In addition to anti-**Au**[a] and the natural anti-**A** and anti-**B** antibodies, the patient's serum also contained anti-**rh''**, anti-**K**, and anti-**Fy**[b]. In 1971 a second anti-**Au**[a] was found in a serum that contained additionally anti-**A**, anti-**Lu**[a], anti-**K**, anti-**Fy**[b], and anti-**Yt**[b].

The antibody reacts best by the antiglobulin method with anti–gamma globulin serum added or by using the papain method of pretreatment of cells.

The antigen is well developed at birth.

Two **genes** have been proposed—*Au*[a] and *au*, giving rise to **genotypes** *Au*[a]*Au*[a], *Au*[a]*au*, and *auau*, with **frequencies** of 33.13%, 48.86%, and 18.01%, respectively. Family studies show that the gene responsible for the Au[a] antigen has segregated independently of the genes for A-B-O, M-N-S, P, Rh-Hr, Fy, Jk, and Le and it is not sex-linked.

There has been some controversy as to whether the Auberger groups are related to the rare type Lu(a–b–) (p. 162), but there has not been enough anti-**Au**[a] serum for a sufficient number of family studies. However, in 1974 Salmon et al. (cited in Race and Sanger, l.c.) found that Au[a] is controlled from a locus independent of the *Lu* locus. There apparently is a rare allele at an inhibitor locus for *In(Lu)* (inhibitor gene for Lu), which inhibits the Au^a, Lu^a, and Lu^b antigens as well as P$_1$ and i.[17] It has been suggested that the gene *Au^a* competes with the *Lu* genes for a common hypothetical precursor substance.

About 18% of Caucasoids have been found to be Au(a–), the remaining being Au(a+). Gene frequencies in Negroids are about the same as for Caucasoids. The fact that the frequencies of the Au-positive type and the Rh-positive type are both about 85% is probably only an interesting coincidence.

THE Yt BLOOD GROUP SYSTEM

In 1956 Eaton et al.[18] described an antibody that reacted with the great majority of blood cells tested. The antibody was called anti-**Yt^a** and the specificity it defined **Yt^a**. The antibody was discovered in the blood serum of a patient who had had several transfusions before its presence was noted during an incompatible cross-matching test. It reacted in a modification of the indirect antiglobulin test and with the trypsin antiglobulin test.

In 1964 Giles and Metaxas[19] found the predicted anti-**Yt^b**, which defines the contrasting factor **Yt^b**. Whereas **Yt^a** is a high-frequency blood group factor, **Yt^b** is classified as a low-frequency specificity.

Two **genes** for the specificities, *Yt^a* and *Yt^b*, determine three possible **phenotypes**, Yt(a+b+), Yt(a+b–), and Yt(a–b+), with calculated frequencies of 7.91%, 91.92%, and 0.17%, respectively. No example of phenotype Yt(a–b–) has so far been found.

Yt is most likely an independent blood group system. It has been excluded from A-B-O, M-N-S, Rh-Hr, P, K-k, Le, secretor, Fy, Jk, and Do systems. It has not been excluded from the *Diego* locus.

It must be pointed out that only those who lack the factor can form the antibodies and the scarcity of clinical cases of isosensitization is most likely due to the almost universal incidence of factor **Yt^a**.

The Yt^a antigen is present at birth but

is more weakly reactive than in adults. Yt^b also appears to be fully developed at birth.

THE En BLOOD GROUP SYSTEM— SPECIFICITY En^a

In 1969 Darnborough et al.[20] reported an antibody they had found in the blood serum of a patient in England, which had resulted from a blood transfusion. The antibody was designated anti-**En^a**, and the specificity it defined was named **En^a**. The antigen was given the name En(a+) in accordance with custom. The patient who had formed the antibody was designated as En(a–). Another example of En(a–) was later described in Finland. The En(a+) antigen is common, occurring in almost every person examined. Cells that lack the antigen, or type En(a–), are the result of a rare recessive gene. These cells have only about 33% of the normal amount of sialic acid, and they exhibit an electrophoretic mobility of only about 50% normal. The red cells are also characterized by their weak M-N antigens, their positive agglutination with anti-**Rh$_o$** IgG, 7S (blocking), sera even when the cells are suspended in saline, and their preferential agglutination by certain seed extracts and nonimmune animal sera in contrast to red cells in other systems that react preferentially with human or animal antisera. The En designation refers to envelope, since apparently the red cell envelope is modified.

The specificity **En^a** is antigenic in rabbits and in man. The locus for the gene that is responsible for En^a (called *En^a*) is genetically independent of the loci for the genes of the A-B-O, M-N-S, Rh-Hr, and Fy systems and for the haptoglobins, and it is not sex-linked. En(a+) heterozygous cells have the same characteristics as the homozygous ones but to a modified degree.

The specificity **H** is much enhanced in En(a–) cells, especially when they are tested with *Ulex europeus* and *Lotus tetrangonolobus* seed extracts and with eel serum. It has been proved that the reaction is due to anti-**H** itself and not to some other effect of the lectin. The reaction is inhibited by secretor saliva but not by non-secretor saliva. When the *Ulex* extract is absorbed with group O En(a+) cells, it loses its reactivity for En(a−) cells. The En(a−) cells also exhibit a high Le^b content.[21]

The **role of variations in sialic acid** has been studied in the En^a system. In addition to the effect of sialic acid on the surface charge of red blood cells, sialic acid and variations in its content contribute to certain reactivities of red cells, as follows: (1) sialic acid is an integral part of the M and N antigens and is itself the myxovirus receptor; (2) splitting off sialic acid from the surface of normal red cells uncovers the so-called T or Friedenreich agglutinogen (p. 230ff). The greatly reduced reactivity of En(a−) red cells with rabbit or human anti-**M** and anti-**N** sera can be explained on the basis of a deficiency in the terminal sialic acid of M-N-active carbohydrate chains. Likewise, a reduced myxovirus-receptor content of En(a−) red cells could explain the increased elution rate of viruses from their surface, whereas the slightly increased agglutination by mumps and NDV viruses is most likely due to the reduced surface charge density.[20]

En(a−) red cells have a decreased amount of T antigen for anti-**T** agglutinin in normal human sera but a normal T agglutinogen for peanut anti-**T**. The T agglutinogens for the two **T** agglutinins seem to be different, and there most likely is some additional defect rather than sialic acid in the chains involving the T antigen for **T** agglutinin of normal human sera. The En(a−) red cells may perhaps also lack some M-N precursor substance and thus would be comparable to the Bombay phenotype of the A-B-O system if En^a actually belonged to the M-N system. Apparently it does not.

S-s antigens apparently are not affected in the En(a−) cells.

En(a−) red cells have a reduced surface charge density, as stated previously. The En^a antigen is not destroyed by treatment with proteolytic enzymes and neuraminidase. It is not located in the M-N mucoprotein.

Anti-En^a was found in the serum of an untreated woman.[20] It is active in saline media at room temperature and at 37° C, as well as in albumin, pepsin, and antiglobulin serum at 37° C. It is not active against the cells of the woman in whom the antibody was found and therefore is not an autoagglutinin. It reacts, however, with all red cells that are negative for several of the high-incidence antigens. Apparently it is immune in origin.

Out of 12,509 donors tested with the anti-En^a antibody, only three siblings were found to be En(a−).

The genes postulated for the En^a system are *En^a* and *En^b*. The *En^b* gene is exceedingly rare. The following genotypes are possible: *En^{a}En^a*, the normal genotype; *En^{a}En^b*, representing a single gene dose modified; *En^{b}En^b*, representing a double gene dose modified.

THE I-i BLOOD GROUP SYSTEM

It has been known for a long time that some patients with acquired hemolytic anemia have high titers of cold agglutinins in their sera. When the sera from patients with hemolytic anemia of the cold autoantibody type were tested, Wiener[22] showed that cold autoagglutinins also have a special type specificity and assigned the symbol I to it. Probably the first observation on antibodies of this and related specificities was that made by Unger et al.[23] in 1952. These investigators found two contrasting cold agglutinating sera—one in an adult and one in a newborn infant with hemolytic anemia. In 1956 Wiener et al.[24] reported finding a cold autoantibody of extremely high titer in the serum of a group A$_1$B woman with acquired hemolytic anemia.

At refrigerator temperature a titer exceeding 100,000 units was obtained, and the antibodies produced a high, wide peak in the globulin region on serum electrophoresis. However, in tests conducted at room temperature the antibody agglutinated the cells of almost all other humans tested but not those of the patient. The factor that was detected by the patient's serum was a high-frequency specificity, different from all others known to that date. Because of the high degree of **individuality of blood specimens** that failed to react with the patient's antibody at room temperature, the antibody was designated anti-**I**, and the specificity it defined was called **I**. Out of 22,964 random donors tested, only five proved to be compatible—that is, they were **I** negative—and four of these five were Negroids. The designation i was given to indicate absence of the I antigen or factor. The I antigen is not developed at birth so that the red cells of newborn babies react as I negative. Jenkins et al.[25] and Marsh and Jenkins[26,27] then found a **cold antibody** called anti-i by them, since it agglutinated cord blood that was I negative but not blood from adults except those of the rare type i.

Further examples of the anti-I antibody were soon reported: (1) anti-**I** in the serum of patients with acquired hemolytic anemia of the cold antibody type, (2) anti-**I** in sera that in the past had been said to contain a nonspecific, 19S, IgM cold auto-agglutinin, and (3) anti-**I** in the sera of normal persons whose red cells are type i or have abnormally little I antigen. Shapiro[28] found an example of anti-**I** in South Africa.

Because of the markedly different titers obtained against different cells, ranging from 25 to 5000 units, Wiener suggested that there are **variants of the I agglutinogen** —I_1, I_2, I_3, etc. and i. According to Marsh and Jenkins, there are also three **types of the i antigen:** (1) those in umbilical cord blood, called i; (2) the rare i of adult Caucasians, or i_1; and (3) the i of adult Negroids, or i_2. As stated previously, the **I** specificity is not developed at birth, and all cord blood is I negative and i positive.

In 1959 W. Weiner et al.[29] demonstrated that two of their patients with acquired hemolytic anemia of the cold antibody type had the antigen I on their red cells and

anti-**I** in their serum. It is now known that some but not all patients with acquired hemolytic anemia of the cold antibody type have the I antigen on their cells and anti-**I** in their sera.

As has been pointed out, practically all newborn babies are I negative and i positive. A **fundamental gene enzyme system** working through the first year of life apparently results in the development of the I antigen at the expense of the i. Antigen i progressively decreases while antigen I increases on the red cells up to 18 months and 2 years of age.

Because of the extremely low frequency of the type i in adults, there have been scarcely any family studies on the **heredity** of the antigen I, especially since this specificity is not demonstrable in newborn babies. However, there seems to be no doubt that the type is hereditarily determined, since families have been found with several type i siblings: for example, a family of Claflin,[30] with three type i and three type I sibs, and another family of Jacobowicz,[31] with three type i sibs. The occurrence of multiple type **i** individuals among siblings of a family with normal type I parents supports the recessive character of the i phenotype in adults.

The agglutinin that reacts with the I antigen is a **cold agglutinin.** It is a 19S, IgM globulin that does not traverse the placenta and therefore is not a factor in erythroblastosis fetalis. It may, however, cause a transfusion reaction.

All adult red cells, with almost no exception, are **I** positive and are therefore agglutinated by anti-**I.** On the other hand, anti-**i** agglutinates cord cells and essentially no adult cells, with the exception of a few i-positive adults. Only one out of 25,000 adults in New York was found to have the i antigen. It has been reported that anti-**i** agglutinin occurs not infrequently in infectious mononucleosis.[32]

In choosing donors for transfusions, most blood banks will ignore the cold autoantibody anti-**I** when found in a patient's serum. Mollison[33] considers that anti-**I** with a titer of 64 units by microscopic reading or 10 units by macroscopic reading, up to about 15° C, is harmless in normal cases. When anti-**I** is present, there may be other clinically more significant antibodies in the same serum, and these may be masked by the anti-**I**. It is therefore advisable, when anti-**I** is found in a serum, to absorb it out with the subject's own enzyme-treated cells and then retest the absorbed serum for other isoantibodies.

It is also necessary, when testing serum for anti-**I**, that cord cells be included in the controls. If the serum fails to agglutinate adult red cells (group O) and does agglutinate cord cells, it presumably contains anti-**i**; if it agglutinates adult cells but not cord cells, it is assumed to contain anti-**I**.

When a patient's blood has anti-**i** antibodies, ordinary adult I-positive blood is used for the transfusion, since it will be i negative.

In **summary**, anti-**I** antibodies react in high titer with red cells from almost all human adults and in low titer or not at all with red cells from newborn infants. Anti-**i** antibodies react in high titer with red cells from newborn infants and weakly or not at all with red cells of human adults. Red cells of adults in general have specificity **I** and lack **i**. Very rare adults who lack blood specificity **I** have specificity **i** and are called type i. Blood specificity **i** is present in infants and cord bloods, where **I** is still undeveloped.

Distribution in animals

The distribution of blood factors **I** and **i** in apes, monkeys, and lower mammals was reported by Wiener et al.[34] as part of their investigations on blood groups of nonhuman primates. They found that chimpanzees lack blood factor **I** but have **i**, gibbons lack both factors, and orangutans are intermediate. Some monkeys have **I** and lack **i**, others have **i** and lack **I**, and some lack both factors. See Chapter 15.

Among the nonprimate animals tested, sheep, goats, deer, cats, and South Ameri-

can agouti lack both factors; dogs and rats lack **I** but have a weak factor **i**; and rabbits have a very strong factor **I** but lack **i**. The distribution of the **I-i** specificities thus indicates a heterophil behavior, since it cuts across taxonomic lines.

Costea et al.[35] confirmed the **heterogenetic nature** of the I-i antigens by producing high-titered, anti-**I** cold agglutinins in rabbits as a response to injections of heat-killed *Listeria monocytogenes*. Serotype 4b of these bacteria produced high-titered anti-**I** and moderately strong 4a, but serotypes 1, 2, and 3 had no discernible effect.

OTHER HIGH- AND LOW-FREQUENCY BLOOD GROUP SPECIFICITIES

Some blood group specificities have been found in almost 100% of the world's population, others only in very rare individuals, and still others seem to be limited mostly to particular families. Those that are present in very high percentages are called **high-frequency**, or **public**, **antigens**, and the others **low-frequency**, or **private**, **antigens**. Some of the high-frequency factors already discussed are **H**, related to the A-B-O system; **U** of the M-N-S system; **hr″** of the Rh-Hr system; **Tj**[a] of the P system; **k** and **Kp**[b] of the K-k system; **Vel**; **Yt**[a]; and **I**. Others are **Sc1** (formerly **Sm**), **Ge, Lan, Co**[a], **At**[a], and **LW**.

That an antigen may be labeled public in one population but not in another is dramatically illustrated by Ge (Gerbich). This antigen was found to be absent from the blood of only one white person in over 44,000 tested, but in some parts of New Guinea, Booth et al.[36] found that up to half the people lacked it.

Some of the private antigens may eventually be shown to be part of an established system; a recent example (1975) is Be[a] which, after 20 years, has been found to belong to the Rh-Hr system.[37]

High-frequency blood factors

Specificities Sm and Bu[a]. An antibody was reported by Schmidt et al.[38] in 1962, which they designated anti-**Sm.** It was found in the serum of a mother who apparently had been isosensitized by pregnancy. Her serum agglutinated all cells tested except her own. The antibody was designated anti-**Sm** and the corresponding specificity and antigen Sm. Three of the patient's siblings were Sm negative, which provides strong evidence of the recessive nature of the Sm-negative type.

In 1963 Anderson et al.[39] described an antibody, which they called anti-**Bu**[a], that reacted with the cells of only a small number of people. It was noted that a member of the original family with Sm-negative persons was Bu(a+), which seemed to indicate that the two specificities, **Sm** and **Bu**[a], might be controlled either by allelic genes or by genes in closely linked loci. No relationship with any other blood group antigens was found.

Both Sm and Bu[a] have been shown to be genetically independent of all the established red cell antigen systems except Di and Yt, which will probably also be excluded when enough antisera are obtained for further studies.

The Sm antigen is well developed in cord blood, which reacts as Bu(a+).

The anti-**Sm** antibody reacts by the antiglobulin method and apparently is stimulated by pregnancy. Anti-**Bu**[a] serum has been produced in Bu(a−) individuals by injection of Bu(a+) blood.

The antibodies appear to be of the IgG type.

Sc, the Scianna blood groups. The specificity formerly called **Sm** is now called **Sc1,** and **Bu**[a] is now **Sc2** because the allelic relationship of the two antigens has become clear. The null type is Bu(a−)Sm−.[40]

Specificity Ge (Gerbich). An antibody, designated anti-**Ge,** was found almost simultaneously in sera from three mothers, all of whose babies gave positive direct antiglobulin reactions but did not develop frank hemolytic disease. The mothers were, respectively, an American of Italian extraction, a Mexican, and a Dane. The antigen identified by the antibody is termed "Ge."

A fourth example of anti-**Ge** was found later in a woman from Turkish Cyprus.[41] The antibody appears to be of the IgG type.

The **Ge** specificity has been shown to be inherited. The antigen is well developed at birth. **Ge** is another high-frequency blood group factor; it has been found in all of more than 34,000 randomly selected persons tested.

Two **Ge types** are identifiable by the present antisera: Ge(−) and Ge(+). The antibody behaves like an immune antibody and reacts best by the antiglobulin technic. Only one example of naturally occurring anti-**Ge** has been found. It caused agglutination of red cells in saline suspension at 37° C by all the methods tested. The direct antiglobulin test on the baby's cells was negative even though the antibody was present in the mother's serum, indicating that the baby's cells were not coated by antibody.

Specificity Jo[a].[42] An antibody was found in the serum of a patient, Mrs. Jo, after her two pregnancies and a blood transfusion. The antibody was also found in the serum of Mr. Be after a blood transfusion when undergoing surgery for cancer of the prostate. No autoagglutinins were present in either case. The direct antiglobulin test was negative. Mrs. Jo's serum reacted by the antiglobulin test with thirty-six red blood samples and with cells considered null phenotypes in the A-B-O, Kell, Rh, Lu, and Jk blood group systems, which are therefore Jo(a+). No compatible siblings were found. Mrs. Jo and Mr. Be are Negroids and are Jo(a−). The antigen is named Jo. Those having it are Jo(a+) and those lacking it are Jo(a−). The antigen is developed at birth. There is no evidence of its causing hemolytic disease of infants.

Specificity Lan. Anti-**Lan** was found by van der Veer and van Loghem[43] in 1961 in the serum of a man who had reacted adversely to his third transfusion. The antibody is of the IgG type and reacts only by the antiglobulin method. The antigen is called Lan. Only one Lan-negative person was found among 4000 randomly selected individuals tested. It is believed that the Lan-negative condition is a recessive characteristic. The antigen is well developed in cord cells.

Specificity Co^a (Colton).[44] The frequency of specificity **Co^a**, for which the antibody anti-**Co^a** was found simultaneously in Oslo, Minneapolis, and Oxford, England, in 1965, has been estimated as 99.7%. Those who lack the factor therefore constitute only 0.3% of all individuals tested to date. The symbol Co(a+) has been used to indicate the presence of the factor and Co(a−) its absence.

Co(a+) appears to be part of a separate blood group system, although its genetic independence of Lu, K-k, Di, and Yt has not as yet been established. The Co^a antigen seems to be fully developed at birth.

Of the four known examples of anti-Co^a, three occurred as a result of transfusion. The four anti-Co^a sera react well by the antiglobulin method, but the reactions are better by the papain-treated antiglobulin technic.

Two genes, *Co^a* and *co*, have been postulated, producing three possible genotypes— *Co^{a}Co^a*, *Co^{a}co*, and *coco*.

Co^b was reported by Giles et al.[45] in 1970. In 1974[46] anti-**Co^a** was found in the serum of the null type Co(a-b-) patient.

According to de La Chapelle et al.[47] monosomy-7 in the bone marrow is the rare chromosomal disorder of which five examples are known in Finland. Blood group tests show two of the five to have the Colton system phenotype Co(a-b-), which had previously been observed only in a French-Canadian family. This conjunction of two such rarities could hardly be due to chance.

Specificity El. Anti-El was described in 1970 by Frank et al.[48] It had been found in the serum of a nontransfused Negro woman (Mrs. El) during her seventh pregnancy. It reacted by both the antiglobulin and enzyme tests. *El* is an inherited dominant characteristic. The *El* gene is independent of the secretor locus and is not X-borne. All seven children of the propositus were positive. One of her three sisters was El negative.

Specificity Dp. Anti-**Dp** was also found by Frank et al.[48] in the serum of a white woman whose parents were first cousins. It reacts by the antiglobulin and enzyme methods. No Dp-negative person was found in 600 unrelated donors.

Specificity Gn^a (Gonsowski). Anti-**Gn^a** was found by Fox and Taswell[49] in the serum of a nontransfused mother of six children. It reacts best by the antiglobulin method. No Gn(a−) persons were found among 2600 Rh-negative donors, although both living sibs of the propositus and one of the five children of a deceased brother proved to be Gn(a−). *Gn^a* is believed to be a dominant characteristic.

Specificity Gy^a (Gregory). Swanson et al.[50] in 1966 and 1967, reported an antibody, anti-**Gy^a**, that they had found in the serum of a patient named Gregory. This antibody reacted with red cells from the patient's parents, her husband, her five children, and three of her six sibs. Two of the three compatible sibs were male and did not have anti-**Gy^a**, but the antibody was found in the serum of the female sib, the mother of two children. The anti-**Gy^a** antibody was found during routine antenatal testing. It reacted positively with all random bloods tested. It was proved to be related to an antibody called anti-**Hy**, reported by Schmidt et al.[51] in 1967.

Anti-**Gy^a** is an IgG antibody. The antigen is developed at birth and is best detected by the antiglobulin method.

Specificity At^a (August).[52] Anti-**At^a** was found for the first time in the serum of a Negroid mother after the birth of her third child. She had apparently been sensitized by pregnancy, since she had never been transfused. The specificity that this antibody identifies has been named **At^a**.

The infant's cells gave a weak positive reaction by the direct antiglobulin method, although the mother's antibody reacted powerfully with random bloods. No person lacking antigen At^a has been found in random tests, although the brother of the patient is also At(a–). The At^a antigen is well developed in cord cells.

Although the antibody was found in the blood of an At(a–) Negroid, absence of the At^a factor is very rare in Negroids. In 6600 bloods tested from the New York area, 2200 were from Negroids, all of which had the At^a specificity.

Specificity Yk^a (York). The blood group specificity **York**, now designated **Yk^a**, was first reported by Molthan, of Temple University, at the meeting of the American Association of Blood Banks in 1970. If a sensitized Yk(a–) patient is given Yk(a+) blood in a transfusion, only a mild reaction results. It is estimated that 95% of the population are Yk(a+), although some authors believe the frequency to be only 88%. To date there are no records of erythroblastosis fetalis due to this factor.

Specificity Cs^a (Stirling). Three examples of anti-Cs^a were found almost simultaneously by Giles et al.[53] The antigen Cs^a has been found in 97.5% of randomly selected European Caucasians. It appears to be serologically distinct from practically every known blood group antigen. From family studies of two Cs(a–) individuals, it seems that Cs^a is most probably a dominant mendelian characteristic. Cs^a is not controlled by genes at the loci for Rh-Hr, M-N-S, Fy, or Jk. The antigen is developed at birth.

There is a marked variation in the strength of the antigen.

Specificity Jr^a. In 1970 Stroup and MacIlroy[54] reported an antigen, Jr^a, that can stimulate production of anti-Jr^a by pregnancy, but so far no case of erythroblastosis fetalis has been reported as due to this antibody. Anti-Jr^a can cause a cross-matching problem in a patient who has previously been transfused. No random white or Asiatic person has yet been found to be Jr(a–).

Specificities D-B-G (Donna-Bennett-Goodspeed). Specificities known as **D-B-G** have been described, along with others designated **Ho, Ot,** and **Stobo.** Space does not permit detailing the complexities of these factors. Perhaps more information will be forthcoming in the future. At present, these are not important for transfusions, nor have they given rise to any clinical conditions. They serve only to add more general knowledge about the blood groups and their genetics.

The LW factor. In 1961 Levine et al.[55] were able to confirm the early findings of Landsteiner and Wiener that sera from guinea pigs immunized with rhesus monkey red cells preferentially agglutinate human Rh-positive red cells. They pointed out that absorption of the anti-rhesus guinea pig sera with Rh-negative human red cells, if repeated with large enough amounts of cells, could remove the reactivity of the reagent also for Rh-positive cells. This is, of course, comparable to the ability of type M cells to absorb anti-**N** agglutinins and of A$_2$ cells to absorb anti-**A$_1$** agglutinins when an excessive amount of red cells is used for the absorptions. Pursuing their experiment further, Levine and Celano[56] found that the anti-rhesus guinea pig sera, when absorbed in an appropriate manner, continued to agglutinate all but a very low percentage of human red cells. The reagent prepared in this manner was therefore evidently defining a hitherto undescribed high-frequency (over 99%) blood factor. Because the new antibody had been produced by the same method that Landsteiner and Wiener had used to produce their first anti-Rh sera, Levine[57] named the new antibody anti-**LW** and the corresponding agglutinogen LW in honor of Landsteiner and Wiener. That the factor in question was different from the original Rh factor of Landsteiner and Wiener was obvious, especially since Rh-positive as well as Rh-negative individuals were found who lacked the factor. Unfortunately, the symbol LW has led many workers to confuse the newly-found LW factor of Levine with the Rh factor of Landsteiner and Wiener; some workers believe that LW and Rh are identical or that, if LW is different from Rh, it nevertheless is part of the Rh system. Both ideas are incorrect, however, as Wiener and others have shown.[58,59]

To understand the serologic properties of the anti-rhesus guinea pig sera produced first by Landsteiner and Wiener and later by Levine et al., one must bear in mind the fact that all immune sera contain an entire spectrum of antibodies of different and related specificities. For example, anti-**A** and anti-**B** sera of human origin are not monospecific, even though they behave so in routine blood grouping tests. Absorption of anti-**A** serum with A_2 cells removes a fraction of the spectrum of antibodies in such serum, leaving behind those antibodies that react with A_1 cells, but not with A_2 cells. Moreover, absorption of anti-**A** serum with different kinds of A cells, e.g. $A_{1,2}$ or A_3 cells, will fractionate the spectrum of antibodies differently. One would have no way of determining that anti-**A** sera are not monospecific if human red cells of different subtypes of A were not available for such absorption experiments. The same is true for the serum of guinea pigs injected with rhesus monkey blood. As pointed out by Wiener et al.,[58] by using different kinds of absorbing red cells, more than six different antibody fractions have so far been separated from the sera of rabbits and guinea pigs injected with red cells of rhesus monkeys (and, more recently, also with red cells of baboons):

1. Antibodies reactive with rhesus monkey or baboon red cells alone and not with human red cells
2. Antibodies cross-reactive with all rhesus monkey or baboon red cells, as well as with all human red cells[60,61]
3. Antibodies cross-reactive with rhesus monkey or baboon red cells and human cord cells but not with human adult cells[62]
4. Antibodies cross-reactive with rhesus monkey and baboon red cells and human Rh-positive but not human Rh-negative cells, that is, anti-Rh of Landsteiner and Wiener[63]

5. Antibodies cross-reactive with rhesus monkey or baboon red cells and human LW-positive cells but not with the rare LW-negative red cells, that is, anti-**LW** of Levine and Celano[56]
6. Antibodies cross-reactive with rhesus monkey and baboon red cells and human red cells having agglutinogen M but not type N (This could be fractionated from the rabbit anti-rhesus sera but not from guinea pig anti-rhesus sera.)

It is reasonable to expect that still more fractions of antibodies could be separated from anti-rhesus guinea pig or rabbit sera by using appropriate red cells for absorption and testing. Comparable fractionation of human anti-**Rh₀** sera is described on p. 215.

From these observations it becomes obvious that the misinterpretation of the nature of the **LW** factor results from the *false assumption* that an antiserum to a particular kind of blood could contain only a single kind of antibody: the antibodies found by Levine and Celano and those found by Landsteiner and Wiener in the serum of guinea pigs injected with rhesus monkey blood had to be one and the same. To be sure, Levine and Celano found their antibody in a serum produced in the same way that Landsteiner and Wiener had produced their first anti-Rh serum, but this immune serum, like human anti-**Rh₀** serum, contained multiple fractions of antibodies with this important difference: the antibodies in human anti-**Rh₀** serum are all directed against one and the same agglutinogen molecule or combining group, whereas the antibodies found in the guinea pig and rabbit anti-rhesus monkey sera are directed against many different agglutinogens, including some that are species specific, others specific for the red cells of newborns, others specific for the M-N system, still others specific for the agglutinogen Rh of Landsteiner and Wiener, and now, finally, an antibody specific for the agglutinogen LW of Levine. No convincing evidence has been offered that might lead one to believe that the specificity detected by the serum anti-**LW** is in any way related to the Rh factor of Landsteiner and Wiener any more than are the other factors such as factor **M** also detected by antibodies present in anti-rhesus monkey rabbit sera. Moreover, the **LW** factor appears in the blood of more than 99% of whites of both Rh-positive and Rh-negative types, whereas the Rh factor is present in only 85% of whites.

In conclusion, we support Wiener's opinion that the **LW** factor is merely another high-frequency blood factor unrelated to the Rh-Hr blood group system.

Low-frequency blood group factors

Low-frequency blood group factors are also called **private factors** by some authors because they seem to occur only in particular families and not in others. Race and Sanger[64] have established rules governing the possibility that such antigens should be designated "private." These antigens must conform to the following rules:

1. They must be shown to be hereditarily transmitted as dominant characteristics.
2. They must be known not to be controlled by previously established blood group loci.
3. They must show an incidence of less than one in 400 among individuals randomly selected from the general population.
4. They must be defined by a specific antibody.
5. They must not duplicate others already on the list, and this must be determined by parallel testing.
6. They must be available. Donors having the antigen must be available, or some of the antiserum must exist at least in vitro.

A number of low-frequency specificities in established blood group systems have been found, such as **Mi** and **Gr** of the M-N-S system: **rh**[w1], **rh**[w2], and **rh**[x] of the Rh-Hr system; and **Kp**[a] of the K-k system. The following additional low-frequency

blood group specificities have been reported* : **Bi** (Biles), **Bp**[a] (Bishop), **Bx**[a] (Box), **By** (Batty), **Chr**[a], **Evans, Gf** (Griffiths), **Good, Heibel, Hey, Hov, Ht**[a] (Hunt), **Je**[a] (Jensen), **Jn**[a], **Levay, Ls**[a] (Lewis II), **Mo**[a] (Moen), **Or, Raddon, Rd** (Radin), **Re**[a] (Reid), **Rl**[a] (Rosenlund), **Sw**[a] (Swann), **To**[a] (Torkildsen), **Tr**[a] (Traversu), **Wb** (Webb), **Wu** (Wulfsberg), and a factor called **Ca** (or **Wr**[a]).[65] Most of these have been found in the sera of mothers of babies with hemolytic disease. The various antigens are distinguishable by specific antisera, and all are independent of the other known blood group systems.

There are few positively reacting bloods of the above factors so that isoimmune antibodies are rare, and there have been no reports of any naturally occurring antibodies to any of these specificities.

Be[a] (Berrens). In 1953 Davidsohn et al.[66] described a powerful antibody that they termed anti-**Be**[a], since it had been found in the serum of a patient named Mrs. Berrens. The antibody in this case had been the cause of hemolytic disease of the newborn and of stillbirth in a later pregnancy of Mrs. Be. By injecting the father's red cells into two volunteer Be(a–) men, anti-**Be**[a] was formed in their serum. **Be**[a] is a strong antigen that seems to be part of the Rh system. Many thousands of people (25,000) have been tested since 1953 when the original antigen was detected, and all proved to be Be(a–). Not until 1973 were other Be(a+) people found. The antigen has been found in one East German family (Berrens) and in two Polish families (Klep and Koz). It is therefore classified as a private, or low-frequency, antigen.

An[a]. The systemic name for **An**[a] is Ahonen. Anti-**An**[a] was found in the serum of Mr. A. L., 66 years of age, in Helsinki.[65]

*For details concerning investigators, unrelated people tested (population, total, positive), and notes about the antibody, consult Table 75, in Race, R. R., and Sanger, R.: Blood groups in man, ed. 6, Oxford, England, 1975, Blackwell Scientific Publications.

An^a is rare. Out of 10,000 Finnish and 3266 Swedish individuals, only 8 were found to be positive. Anti-**An**^{a} reacts weakly against An(a+) cells in saline at 37° C, more strongly at room temperature, well by antiglobulin methods and routine antiglobulin sera, but best by anti-**IgG**. The reaction is inhibited by papain but not by ficin and not by saliva of An(a+) people, either secretors or nonsecretors of A-B-H substance. Anti-**An**^{a} is readily adsorbed by An(a+) cells. An^a has been found to be genetically transmitted as a dominant. The antibody is naturally occurring. Pregnancy is not known to have stimulated it, nor is it stimulated by transfusion. The first example of anti-**An**^{a} was found during cross matching. The antigen has been shown not to belong to the A-B-O, M-N-S-s, P, Rh-Hr, Fy, Kidd, or Do systems, and it is not sex-linked. It is genetically independent of the Lu, Kell, Yt, Di, and Co blood group systems. Anti-**An**^{a} occurs in the serum of about one in 1000 normal persons.

Specificity Ca, or Wr^a. Wiener and Brancato[67] described an agglutinogen discovered during a study of a puzzling case of erythroblastosis fetalis, that proved to be a rare heritable human agglutinogen. That same year Holman[68] found an antigen that proved to be the same as the one described by Wiener and Brancato. Wiener and Brancato called the factor **Ca**, and Holman described the specificity he had found as **Wr^a**. Many textbooks used the terminology **Wr^a** to describe the factor.

Wiener and Brancato's case was of a baby and her mother, both Rh negative and with no A-B-O blood group incompatibility. The problem of the specificity of the antibody remained unsolved for 8 years until newer and more sensitive methods of detecting antibodies were devised—the antiglobulin and enzyme technics. At that time it was possible to demonstrate that the mother's serum, in addition to having anti-**Rh**$_o$ antibody, had an antibody for a second blood specificity present on the cells of the child. Since the family name was Cavaliere, the factor was designated **Ca**.

The **Ca** specificity was not found in blood cells of forty-eight consecutive type rh bloods taken at random. It was present in four out of seven type rh individuals in the patient's own family. No **Rh**$_o$ variant was demonstrable on the patient's cells.

The **Ca** (**Wr^a**) specificity therefore appears to be a rare heritable blood factor that is probably independent of the Rh-Hr types.

Holman showed the antigen to be present in three generations of a family and that inheritance is by means of a dominant gene. Cleghorn found only thirty unrelated Ca (**Wr^a**)-positive persons among 45,631 London blood donors—a frequency of one in 1500.

Wr^b was reported in 1971 by Adams et al.[69] In 1975 Issitt et al.[70] showed that En(a−) people are the null type Wr(a−b−).

Sd(a+) and Sd(a−), the Sid blood groups. A vaguely defined antigen-antibody system that had been under investigation for a number of years was found[71] in 1967 to delineate a blood group system separate from A-B-O, M-N-S-s, P, Rh-Hr, Lu, K-k, Le, Fy, Kidd (Jk), Yt, Do, and Xg. The system has been called Sid after Mr. Sidney Smith of the Lister Institute because for years his cells had been used to study the antibodies. The antibodies, called anti-**Sd^a**, detect agglutinogen Sd^a present on the red cells of about 91% of people tested. In addition, the Sd^a antigen was found by Morton et al.[72] to be present in saliva (particularly of newborn infants), in urine, in meconium, and in milk. It is also widely distributed in the tissues and body fluids of various mammals, but it is not present in birds.

In tests on the red cells, the anti-**Sd^a** antibodies behave somewhat similarly to anti-**Lu^a** in that only a portion of cells are agglutinated. There are grades of strength of agglutination of Sd^a-positive red cells. The most common, weakly agglutinating red cells are designated Sd(a+), whereas the symbol Sd(a++) is used to designate the so-called super Sid variety or strongly reacting Sd^a-positive red cells. Both types, Sd(a+) and Sd(a++), are supposedly inherited as dominant characteristics. The super Sid, or Sd(a++) type, proved to be identical to the so-called Cad antigen described in 1968 by Cazal et al.[73] The Sd(a++) type is considered to be a private antigen, its frequency being cited by different sources as between 0.02% and 0.2%.

An interesting observation by Cazal et al. was that, in the Cad family, cells of *Dolichos biflorus*-positive, non-A_1 members were polyagglutinable. Polyagglutinability of red cells had never before been found to be an inherited trait. Sanger and Race[74] believe that the polyagglutinability in the Cad family is in reality not true polyagglutinability but is due rather to the presence of anti-**Sd**^{a} antibodies in the sera of

a majority of people. When cells of super Sid type are used for testing, almost all the normal sera tested seem to have traces of anti-**Sd**^{a} activity. In tests with type Sd(a+) cells, only 1% of all donors tested were found to have "natural" anti-**Sd**^{a} agglutinins in their sera. Despite the seemingly ubiquitous nature of anti-**Sd**^{a} antibodies, they do not cause any serious transfusion troubles, although they may make cross matching difficult under some circumstances.

Although *Dolichos biflorus* lectin reacts with Sd(a++) cells, other anti-A_1 lectins fail to react; on the other hand, most snail anti-**A** reagents, like *Helix pomatia* and *H. aspersa*, agglutinate Sd(a++) cells. As Sang-

Table 11-1. The null types of human blood*

| System | Designation | Responsible gene | | | Erythrocytic abnormalities |
		Designation	Frequency in Caucasoids	Inheritance	
A-B-O	Group O	*O*	0.67	Recessive at A-B-O locus	None
	Bombay	*h*	Extremely rare	Recessive at separate locus	None
Rh-Hr	$\overline{R}h_o$	$\overline{R}^{\circ}$	Rare	Recessive at Rh locus	None
	$\overline{R}h_1$	$\overline{R}^1$	Rare	Recessive at Rh locus	None
	$\overline{R}h^w$	$\overline{R}^w$	Rare	Recessive at Rh locus	None
	Rh$_{null}$ $\overline{\overline{r}}h$	$\overline{r}$	Rare	Recessive at Rh-Hr locus	Stomatocytosis
	Rh$_{null}$ $\overset{\circ}{r}h$	$X^{\circ}r$	Rare	Recessive at separate locus	Stomatocytosis
M-N	S-s-U-	*u*	Rare	Recessive at M-N locus	None
	Null (heterozygote)	*null*	Rare	Recessive at M-N locus	None
Kell	K$_o$	K°	Rare	Recessive at Kell locus	None
	McLeod		Rare	Recessive on X chromosome	Acanthocytosis
Lutheran	Lu(a-b-)	*InLu*	Rare	Dominant at separate locus	None†
	Lu(a-b-)	*Lu*	Rare	Recessive at Lutheran locus	None
Duffy	Fy(a-b-)	*fy*	Rare‡	Recessive at Duffy locus	None§
Kidd	Jk(a-b-)	*jk*	Rare	Recessive at Kidd locus	
P	Tj(a-)	*p*	Rare	Recessive	
Wright	Wr(a-b-)	*en*	Rare	Recessive	‖
Colton	Co(a-b-)	*co*	Rare	Recessive	
Lewis	Le(a-b-)	*le*	Rare	Recessive	
Scianna	Sc:-1,-2	$Sc^{-1,-2}$	Rare	Recessive	‖

*Modified from Allen, F. H., Jr.: Am. J. Clin. Pathol. **66**:467, 1976.
†Au^a (Auberger) is usually suppressed, P^1 is often suppressed entirely, and *i* is also suppressed. (Crawford et al.: Vox Sang. **26**:283, 1974.)
‡Common in Africa.
§Resistant to *Plasmodium knowlesi* and *P. vivax*.
‖Sialic acid deficiency of erythrocyte membrane; M and N weakened.

er et al.[75] pointed out, reaction of *D. bi-florus* lectins with Sd(a++) cells is due to the presence of terminal N-acetyl-D-galactosamine both in Sd(a++) cells and in A_1 cells. This view is supported by observations that papain or ficin treatment of group O Sid(a++) and A_1 cells results in mutual enhancement of their reaction with *Dolichos*, whereas trypsin treatment leaves the reactions of both unaltered.

Other low-frequency factors. Many other blood group specificities have been reported, but information on these and their places in the various systems or in systems of their own is incomplete, and they will not be included in this text.

The Null types

The null types are called by Allen[76] "the jewels of the blood groups." With the exception of group O of the A-B-O blood group system, for the most part they are very rare and are usually discovered by accidental immunization. Some are associated with disorders of erythrocytic structure and function. Many of the blood group systems are now known to have null types, which is reason to believe that the genes for null types are normal components of all blood group systems. Several genetic mechanisms are involved in the inheritance of the null types. Most often they are inherited by autosomal recessives that are independent of the genes of the blood group system itself. At least one is known to be inherited by a dominant suppressor gene, and one probably depends on a gene on the sex chromosome X.

A panel of null type cells is invaluable to any blood bank laboratory, to be used as negative controls.

Table 11-1 is a compilation of the null types of human blood.

REFERENCES

1. Layrisse, M., Arends, T., and Dominguez, S. R.: Acta Med. Venez. 3:132, 1955.
2. Levine, P., Robinson, E. A., Layrisse, M., Arends, T., and Dominguez, S. R.: Nature (Lond.) 177:40, 1956.
3. Thompson, P. R., Childers, D. M., and Hatcher, D. E.: Vox Sang. 13:314, 1967.
4. Lewis, M., Kaita, H., and Chown, B.: Am. J. Hum. Genet. 9:274, 1957.
5. Sussman, L. N., and Miller, E. B.: Rev. Hématol. 7:368, 1952.
6. Levine, P., Robinson, E. W., Harrington, L. B., and Sussman, L. N.: Am. J. Clin. Pathol. 25:751, 1955.
7. Bradish, E. B., and Shields, W. F.: Am. J. Clin. Pathol. 31:104, 1959.
8. Levine, P., White, J. A., and Stroup, M.: Transfusion 1:111, 1961.
9. Wiener, A. S., Gordon, E. B., and Unger, L. J.: Bull. Jewish Hosp. 3:46, 1961.
10. van Loghem, J. J., and van der Hart, M.; cited in Race, R. R., and Sanger, R.: Blood groups in man, ed. 5, Philadelphia, 1968, F. A. Davis Co.
11. Swanson, J., Polesky, H. F., Tippett, P., and Sanger, R.: Nature (Lond.) 206:313, 1965.
12. Tippett, P., Sanger, R., Swanson, J. L., and Polesky, H. F.: Proceedings of the 10th Congress of the European Societies of Haematology, 1965.
13. Polesky, H. F., and Swanson, J. L.: Transfusion 6:268, 1966.
14. Molthan, L., Crawford, M. N., and Tippett, P.: Vox Sang. 24:382, 1973.
15. Tippett, P.: J. Med. Genet. 4:7, 1967.
16. Salmon, C., Salmon, D., Liberge, G., André, R., Tippett, P., and Sanger, R.: Nouv. Rev. Fr. Hématol. 1:649, 1961.
17. Crawford, M. N., Tippett, P., Sanger, R.: Vox Sang. 26:283, 1974.
18. Eaton, B. R., Morton, J. A., Pickles, M. M., and White, K. E.: Br. J. Haematol. 2:333, 1956.
19. Giles, C. M., and Metaxas, M. N.: Nature (Lond.) 202:1122, 1964.
20. Darnborough, J., Dunsford, I., Wallace, J. A.: Vox Sang. 17:241, 1969.
21. Furuhjelm, U., Myllylä, G., Nevanlinna, R., Nordling, S., Pirkola, A., Gavin, J., Gooch, A., Sanger, R., and Tippett, P.: Vox Sang. 17:256, 1969.
22. Wiener, A. S., Unger, L. J., Cohen, L., and Feldman, J.: Ann. Intern. Med. 44:221, 1956.
23. Unger, L. J., Wiener, A. S., and Dolan, D.: Rev. Hématol. 7:495, 1952.
24. Wiener, A. S., Briggs, D. K., Weiner, L., and Burnett, L.: J. Lab. Clin. Med. 51:539, 1958.
25. Jenkins, W. J., Marsh, W. L., Noades, J., Tippett, P., Sanger, R., and Race, R. R.: Vox Sang. 5:97, 1960.
26. Marsh, W. L., and Jenkins, W. J.: Nature (Lond.) 188:753, 1960.
27. Marsh, W. L.: Br. J. Haematol. 2:321, 1956.
28. Shapiro, M.; cited in Wiener, A. S., and

Wexler, I. B.: Heredity of blood groups, New York, 1958, Grune & Stratton, Inc.

29. Weiner, W., Shinton, N. K., and Gray, J. R.; cited in Tippett et al.: Vox Sang. **5**:97, 108, 1960.

30. Claflin, A. F.: Transfusion **3**:216, 1963.

31. Jacobowicz, R., and Simmons, R. T.: Med. J. Aust. **1**:194, 1964.

32. Rosenfield, R. E., Schmidt, P. J., Calvo, R. C., and McGinniss, M. H.: Vox Sang. **10**:631, 1965.

33. Mollison, P. L.: Blood transfusion in clinical medicine, ed. 4, Philadelphia, 1967, F. A. Davis Co.

34. Wiener, A. S., Moor-Jankowski, J., and Gordon, E. B.: Am. J. Phys. Anthropol. **23**:389, 1965.

35. Costea, N. L., Yakulis, V., and Heller, P.: Blood **25**:323, 1965; **35**:583, 1970.

36. Booth, P. D., Albrey, G. A., Whittaker, J., and Sanger, R.: Nature (Lond.) **228**:462, 1970.

37. Ducos, J., Marty, Y., Furre, J., Gavin, J., Teesdale, P., and Tippett, P., 1975. (In preparation.)

38. Schmidt, R. P., Griffitts, J. J., and Northman, F. F.: Transfusion **2**:338, 1962.

39. Anderson, C., Hunter, J., Zipursky, A., Lewis, M., and Chown, B.: Transfusion **3**:30, 1963.

40. McCreary, J., Vogler, A. L., Sabo, B., et al.: Transfusion **13**:350, 1973.

41. Rosenfield, R. E., Haber, G. V., Kiemeyer-Nielsen, F., Jack, J. A., Sanger, R., and Race, R. R.: Br. J. Haematol. **6**:344, 1960.

42. Jensen, L., Scott, E. B., Marsh, W. L., MacIlroy, M., Rosenfield, R. E., Rancato, P., and Fay A. B.: Transfusion **12**:322, 1974.

43. van der Hart, M., Mose, M., van der Veer, M., and van Loghem, J. J.: Paper read at the 8th Congress of the European Societies of Haematology, 1961.

44. Heistö, H., van der Hart, M., Madsen, G., Mose, M., Noades, J., Pickles, M. M., Race, R. R., Sanger, R., and Swanson, J.: Vox Sang. **12**:18, 1968.

45. Giles, C. M., Darnborough, J., Aspinall, P., et al.: Br. J. Haematol. **19**:267, 1970.

46. Rogers, M. J., Stiles, P. A., and Wright, J.: Transfusion **14**:508, 1974.

47. de la Chapelle, A., Vuopio, P., Sanger, R., and Teesdale, P.: Lancet, p. 817, 1975.

48. Frank, S., Schmidt, R. P., and Baugh, N.: Transfusion **10**:254, 1970.

49. Fox, J. A., and Taswell, H. I.: Transfusion **9**:265, 1969.

50. Swanson, J. L., Zweber, M., and Polesky, H. F.: Transfusion **7**:304, 1967.

51. Schmidt, R. P., Frank, S., and Baugh, M.: Transfusion **7**:386, 1967.

52. Appelwhaite, F., Ginsberg, V., Gerena, J., Cunningham, C. A., and Gavin, J.: Vox Sang. **13**:444, 1967.

53. Giles, C. M., Huth, M. C., Wilson, T. E., Lewis, H. B. M., and Grove, G. E. B.: Vox Sang. **10**:405, 1965.

54. Stroup, M., and MacIlroy, M.: Proceedings of the 23rd Annual Meeting of the American Association of Blood Banks, San Francisco, 1970, p. 86.

55. Levine, P., Celano, O. M., Fenichel, R., Pollack, W., and Singer, H.: J. Immunol. **87**: 747, 1961.

56. Levine, P., and Celano, M. J.: Nature (Lond.) **193**:184, 1962.

57. Levine, P., and Celano, M. J.: Science **156**: 1744, 1967.

58. Wiener, A. S., Moor-Jankowski, J., and Brancato, G. J.: Haematologia (Budap.) **3**:385, 1969.

59. Wiener, A. S., Socha, W. W., and Gordon, E. B.: Haematologia (Budap.) **5**:227, 1971.

60. Landsteiner, K., and Miller, C. P., Jr.: J. Exp. Med. **42**:841, 1925.

61. Buchbinder, L.: J. Immunol. **25**:33, 1933.

62. Fisk, R. T., and Foord, M. J.: Nature (Lond.) **193**:184, 1962.

63. Landsteiner, K., and Wiener, A. S.: J. Immunol. **33**:19, 1937.

64. Race, R. R., and Sanger, R.: Blood groups in man, ed. 6, Philadelphia, 1975, F. A. Davis Co.

65. Furuhjelm, H. R., Nevanlinna, H. R., Gavin, J., and Sanger, R.: J. Med. Genet. **9**:385, 1972.

66. Davidsohn, I., Stern, K., Strauser, E. R., and Spurrier, W.: Blood **8**:747, 1953.

67. Wiener, A. S., and Brancato, G. J.: Am. J. Hum. Genet. **5**:4, 1953.

68. Holman, C. A.: Lancet **2**:119, 1953.

69. Adams, J., Broviac, M., Brooks, W., et al.: Transfusion **11**:290, 1971.

70. Issitt, P. D., Powone, B. G., Goldfinger, et al.: Transfusion **15**:523, 1975.

71. Macvie, S. I., Morton, J. A., and Pickles, M. M.: Vox Sang. **13**:485, 1967.

72. Morton, J. A., Pickles, M. M., and Terry, A. M.: Vox Sang. **19**:472, 1970.

73. Cazal, P., Monis, M., Caubel, J., and Brives, J.: Rev. Fr. Transfus. **11**:209, 1968.

74. Sanger, R., and Race, R. R.: Nouv. Rev. Fr. Hématol. **11**:878, 1971.

75. Sanger, R., Gavin, J., Tippett, P., Teesdale, P., and Eldon, K.: Lancet **1**:1130, 1971.

76. Allen, F. H., Jr.: Am. J. Clin. Pathol. **66**: 467, 1976.

12 □ The sex-linked blood group system—Xg

The human sex chromosomes are XY in the male and XX in the female. This means that every ovum must carry an X chromosome, whereas half the spermatozoa carry an X and the other half a Y chromosome. The following conclusions can be noted as a result of mating:

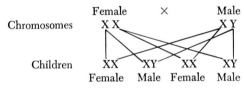

In other words, if the X-carrying ovum is fertilized by an X-carrying sperm, the offspring will be XX, with a resultant female child. If, however, the X-carrying ovum is fertilized by a Y-carrying sperm, the offspring will be XY, and a male child results.

Until 1962 no sex linkage of any of the human blood groups had been demonstrated. In 1962, however, Mann et al.[1] found a new blood group antibody and showed that the corresponding antigen was controlled by an X-linked gene locus. To indicate the presence of the gene on the X chromosome, the antigen was called Xg^a and the corresponding antibody, anti-**Xg^a**. This discovery opened a new chapter in the study of human genetics.

The antibody was found during cross-matching tests on a Mr. A., who had been transfused many times. The statistical proof that the antigen was determined by a sex-linked gene provided an important marker for mapping the X chromosome.

The gene responsible for the antigen is Xg^a, the phenotypes are Xg(a+) and Xg(a–), and the gene for the "silent" allele may be designated xg.

Since the genes for hemophilia, red-green color blindness, glucose-6-phosphate dehydrogenase (G6PD) deficiency, ocular albinism, and others are on the X chromosomes—that is, are sex-linked—families in which these abnormalities occurred were tested for Xg^a to determine the frequency of crossing over between the abnormal structural gene and the marker Xg^a gene on the X chromosome. In this way, theoretically, the mapping of the X chromosomes should be possible. A large number of articles describing studies along these lines has been published, but so far there has been only limited success in determining the frequency of crossing over.

The **genotype** for an Xg(a+) male would be Xg^aY; for an Xg(a–) male it is xgY. The genotype for a homozygous female who is Xg(a+) is Xg^aXg^a; for a heterozygous Xg(a+) female it is Xg^axg. An Xg(a–) female would be genotype $xgxg$.

The following matings and children are possible in the Xg system:

1. Mating Xg(a+) male × Xg(a+) homozygous female:

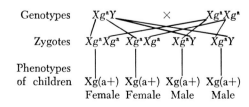

In this mating, all the offspring, both female and male, will be Xg(a+).

2. Mating Xg(a+) male × Xg(a+) heterozygous female:

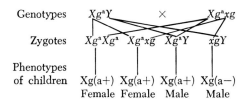

Genotypes Xg^aY × Xg^axg

Zygotes Xg^aXg^a Xg^axg Xg^aY xgY

Phenotypes
of children   Xg(a+) Xg(a+) Xg(a+) Xg(a−)
               Female Female Male   Male

In this mating, all the female offspring would be Xg(a+), half the males would be Xg(a+), and the other half would be Xg(a−). Of the females, half would be homozygous for the **Xg** specificity, the other half heterozygous.

3. Mating Xg(a+) male × Xg(a−) female:

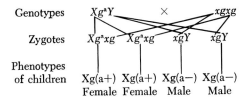

Genotypes Xg^aY × $xgxg$

Zygotes Xg^axg Xg^axg xgY xgY

Phenotypes
of children   Xg(a+) Xg(a+) Xg(a−) Xg(a−)
               Female Female Male   Male

In this mating, all the female offspring will be heterozygous for the **Xg** specificity; the males would all be Xg(a−).

4. Mating Xg(a−) male × Xg(a+) homozygous female:

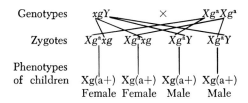

Genotypes xgY × Xg^aXg^a

Zygotes Xg^axg Xg^axg Xg^aY Xg^aY

Phenotypes
of children   Xg(a+) Xg(a+) Xg(a+) Xg(a+)
               Female Female Male   Male

All the offspring will be Xg(a+), whether male or female, but the Xg(a+) females are all heterozygous.

5. Mating Xg(a−) male × Xg(a+) heterozygous female:

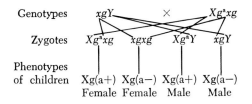

Genotypes xgY × Xg^axg

Zygotes Xg^axg $xgxg$ Xg^aY xgY

Phenotypes
of children   Xg(a+) Xg(a−) Xg(a+) Xg(a−)
               Female Female Male   Male

Of the offspring, half the females are Xg(a+) heterozygous, the other half Xg(a−). Of the male offspring, half will be Xg(a+), and half will be Xg(a−).

6. Mating Xg(a−) male × Xg(a−) female:

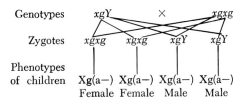

Genotypes xgY × $xgxg$

Zygotes $xgxg$ $xgxg$ xgY xgY

Phenotypes
of children   Xg(a−) Xg(a−) Xg(a−) Xg(a−)
               Female Female Male   Male

All the offspring will be Xg(a−).

Random tests of 342 Caucasoids showed the following **distribution:** females, 88.83% positive; males, 61.69% positive. The difference is overwhelmingly significant (χ^2 = 34.8 for 1 d.f.). The females have two X chromosomes and the males only one, so that the incidence for the Xg(a+) phenotype would necessarily be higher in the female, and this has proved to be the case. Xg(a+) females comprise two genotypes— Xg^aXg^a and Xg^axg—whereas Xg(a+) males are all genotype Xg^aY.

Blood group antigen Xg^a is hereditarily transmitted as a dominant characteristic.

Mann et al. compared the theoretically expected distribution of the Xg groups in Caucasian parents and offspring with those actually observed in fifty Caucasian families with 104 children. Studies of these families confirmed the genetic theory and illustrated clearly certain **rules** that may be laid down **for any X-borne dominant antigen:**

1. From the mating in which the father is positive for Xg^a there can be no negative daughters; only sons can be negative, which is the most striking feature in this situation.

2. From the mating of a positive male with a negative female, all sons have to be negative and all daughters positive. The findings for Xg^a conformed with this pattern.

3. From the mating of a negative male with a positive female, all types of children are possible, and all types have been found.

4. Mothers and daughters of positive men must be positive.
5. Fathers and sons of negative women must be negative.

The above rules apply to normal males and females and do not necessarily apply to those with Turner's syndrome (XO) or with Klinefelter's syndrome (XXY).

Since innumerable Xg(a−) people have been transfused with Xg(a+) blood without becoming isosensitized, it seemed that another example of sensitization through transfusion of an Xg(a−) person with the **Xg**^{a} specificity might not be found for years, but a second example of anti-**Xg**^{a} was reported in 1963 by Cook et al.[2] This antibody, like the first, could be detected only by the antiglobulin method, and the antiglobulin serum must contain either an adequate amount of anti-β_1 (complement) globulin or an exceptionally large amount of anti-7S gamma globulin.

The Xg^a antigen is well developed at birth. Bloods of two fetuses tested were Xg(a+) and two others were Xg(a−). Eight of the twelve cord samples tested in this experiment were Xg(a+). It is possible that the Xg^a antigen of babies with the trisomies of Down, Edwards, and Patau may be weaker than that of normal babies.

Sanger et al.[3] reported observations on two families tested with anti-**Xg**^{a}, which did not fit the genetic theory. Thus of more than 1000 normal families examined, only two did not conform to the rules of X-linked inheritance.

The Xg^a antigen has not been found in serum, in saliva, or on spermatozoa.

Xg^a was detected by Fellous et al.[4] on cultured fibroblasts up to the twelfth passage and in man-man, man-mouse, and man-hamster hybrid lines. Some cultured lymphoid cell lines also showed the antigen expressed. Fresh peripheral lymphocytes did not show the Xg^a antigen.

The distribution of the *Xg*^{a} gene among Negroids so far tested is the same as in Caucasians. The Chinese people seem to have the lowest frequency of *Xg*^{a} genes; the New Guineans have the highest.

Xg^a has been found in gibbons, *Hylobates lar lar.* None of the following has shown the antigen: *H. lar pileatus,* chimpanzees, gorillas, orangutans, baboons, Celebes black apes, and various monkeys, mice, dogs, and one Coelacanth *Latimeria chalumnae.*

REFERENCES

1. Mann, J. D., Cahan, A., Gelb, A. B., Fisher, N., Hamper, J., Tippett, P., Sanger, R., and Race, R. R.: Lancet 1:8, 1962.
2. Cook, I. A., Polley, M. J., and Mollison, P. L.: Lancet 1:857, 1963.
3. Sanger, R., Race, R. R., Tippett, P., Gavin, R. M., Hardisty, R. M., and Dubowitz, V.: Lancet 1:955, 1964.
4. Fellous, M., Bengston, B., Finnegan, D., and Bodmer, W. F.: Ann. Hum. Genet. 37:421, 1974.

13 □ Heredity of the blood groups

HISTORY

Early tests for the A-B-O blood groups were plagued by numerous technical errors. These might have delayed the development of knowledge of heredity indefinitely had it not been for the help provided by mathematics and the introduction by Felix Bernstein of the method of **population genetics.** When von Dungern and Hirszfeld conducted some of the first studies on the heredity of the A-B-O groups in 1910, they postulated that agglutinogens A and B were inherited as mendelian dominants independently of one another by corresponding pairs of genes, *A-a* and *B-b,* with loci on separate pairs of chromosomes. According to Mendel's second law, the **law of independent assortment,** corresponding to the four A-B-O blood groups nine genotypes were implied, as in Table 13-1.

Numerous family studies appeared to support this theory of independent inheritance. In 1923, however, applying the methods of population genetics, Bernstein pointed out that if agglutinogens A and B

□ Additional and more complete data on heredity in the different blood group systems are presented in their respective chapters.

were inherited independently of one another, they should also be distributed independently of one another in the general population; for example, the frequency of agglutinogen A should be the same among persons having agglutinogen B as among those lacking it. Thus:

$$\frac{\overline{AB}}{\overline{B} + \overline{AB}} = \frac{\overline{A}}{\overline{O} + \overline{A}}$$

Therefore $\overline{A} \times \overline{B} + \overline{A} \times \overline{AB} = \overline{O} \times \overline{AB} + \overline{A} \times \overline{AB}$, or $\overline{A} \times \overline{B} = \overline{O} \times \overline{AB}$. (The bar is used to indicate the frequency of the group in the population.)

However, analysis of the results of population studies by the Hirszfelds during World War I on the Macedonian front showed that $\overline{A} \times \overline{B}$ was invariably much larger than $\overline{O} \times \overline{AB}$. Obviously therefore the theory of independent inheritance of A × B was incorrect, and Bernstein proposed in its place his own **theory of triple allelic genes.**

According to Bernstein's theory (Table 13-2), instead of nine genotypes there were only six; the difference between the two theories was mainly in blood group AB. According to Bernstein, group AB individuals could be only of the single genotype *AB* and so had to transmit to half their children

Table 13-1. Von Dungern and Hirszfeld's theory of heredity of the A-B-O groups

Phenotypes	Genotypes
O	*aabb*
A	*AAbb* and *Aabb*
B	*aaBB* and *aaBb*
AB	*AABB, AABb, AaBB,* and *AaBb*

Table 13-2. Heredity of the A-B-O blood groups according to Bernstein

Phenotypes	Genotypes
O	*OO*
A	*AA* and *AO*
B	*BB* and *BO*
AB	*AB*

the gene *A* and to the other half the gene *B*, and they themselves must have acquired their gene *A* from one parent and their gene *B* from the other. No group AB person therefore could theoretically be the parent of a group O child, nor could a group O person be the parent of a group AB child. According to the theory of von Dungern and Hirszfeld, however, group AB individuals could belong to any of the four genotypes and could even be heterozygous for both A and B. Their theory thus asserted that group AB persons could be parents of group O children and that group O people could be parents of group AB children. Analysis of the numerous family studies that had accumulated by 1925 gave results compatible with the theory of von Dungern and Hirszfeld but conflicted with the Bernstein theory.

This presented a paradox. The results of family studies supported the idea of independent inheritance, but the methods of population genetics showed that *A* and *B* were not independent of one another. As shown in Chapter 23, gene frequency analysis supports the Bernstein theory.

The controversy that arose was resolved when it was realized that the earlier family studies had included hundreds of technical errors in simple A-B-O blood grouping. The population studies, however, had been made by the careful workers Hirszfeld and Hirszfeld and therefore were relatively free of errors. By this time, too, the technics of blood grouping had somewhat improved, and when new family studies were carried out, the contradictions to Bernstein's theory suddenly disappeared. No longer were families reported having parents of group AB and children of group O, nor were there families of group O having group AB children.

More recently, there has been reported an unusual case of transmission of blood group AB in a family as if by means of a single chromosome, in a very rare blood group called cis AB. This is described on p. 76.

When blood grouping tests were introduced in legal medicine to resolve problems of disputed paternity, only the theory of von Dungern and Hirszfeld was known so that only the dominance rule was used as evidence of nonpaternity; that is, paternity was considered excluded when the mother and putative father were both group O and the child group A but not if the father was group AB and the child group O. In those early days of forensic application of blood grouping, many men no doubt were convicted or acquitted of the paternity charge when they should not have been.

The history is presented here as a caution, especially to neophytes in the field, to avoid applying every newly discovered blood factor to resolve forensic problems until the methods of testing have been perfected and enough family studies have been made to establish the correctness of the genetic theory.

The general principles of heredity are given in Chapter 4.

In 1910 von Dungern and Hirszfeld established the fact that the blood groups are inherited as mendelian dominant characteristics, and this eventually led to family studies to determine the genotypes and the existence of blood group systems. The original work on inheritance of the blood groups was done in the A-B-O system, since it was the only blood group system known at that time. Later, when Landsteiner and Levine found the M-N and P systems, and especially when Landsteiner and Wiener discovered the Rh factor and Wiener developed the Rh-Hr system, immunogenetics entered its present, scientific period. Because of the knowledge of the role of genetics in the Rh-Hr system, hemolytic disease of the newborn (erythroblastosis fetalis) can be anticipated before birth and in many instances prevented.

Correct genetic study of blood group systems is possible only when accurate laboratory tests are performed. Development of sophisticated methods of detecting antibodies and recognition that all antibodies do not react by all methods have contributed to this field of investigation. This, along with family studies, has produced the present knowledge of genotypes and phenotypes in most of the blood group systems.

THEORY OF TRANSMISSION OF THE BLOOD GROUPS THROUGH ALLELIC GENES

This text will follow the theory of transmission of blood groups through allelic genes. There is a difference of opinion among those who follow the Wiener theory of allelic genes and those who believe in the linked gene theory, in the Rh-Hr system especially. In the Wiener theory, the **serologic specificities** of the agglutinogens are called **blood group factors,** or **specificities,** and these are hereditarily transmitted through the agglutinogen as a **block** or in **sets.** In the linked gene theory of the British workers, each of the blood factors is considered a gene; such genes appear closely linked on the chromosome and are inherited in that manner.

There are some excellent books on the fundamentals of genetics. Some are listed in the recommended readings at the end of this chapter.

PHENOTYPES AND GENOTYPES OF THE BLOOD GROUPS

The special terms used in the study of genetics are defined in the Glossary and will not be repeated here.

The characteristics of an individual that can be detected by observation are said to be his **phenotypes.** These occur as a result of the inheritance of two allelic **genes** for each characteristic, each gene occupying a particular site, or **locus,** on a particular pair of chromosomes. The various genes in the different blood group systems occupy different loci on different chromosomes. When fertilization occurs, one gene for a characteristic is transmitted from the male parent and one from the female parent so that the offspring inherits two genes—one from each parent. **No characteristic therefore can appear in an offspring unless it is present in at least one of the parents.** This is the **first law of inheritance.** Likewise, it is also true that if a characteristic appears in the offspring, it must have been present in at least one parent.

When both genes for a characteristic are alike, the individual is **homozygous** for that characteristic; if they are different, he is **heterozygous.** An individual must pass to each offspring one but not both of the two genes he has inherited.

Although the loci for almost all the blood group factors are **autosomal,** there is also a **sex-linked gene,** the Xg, located on the X chromosome.

The **genotype** is the makeup of an individual according to his two genes for any given characteristic. Genotypes are expressed in italics with superscripts. The genotypes determine the agglutinogens of the blood or blood group. Genotypes can be identified directly in some instances, for example, in blood group O, genotype OO; blood group AB, genotype AB (not including the subgroups); blood group M, genotype MM; blood group N, genotype NN; blood group MN, genotype MN; blood group rh, genotype rr; and so on. In most cases, however, there is more than one genotype corresponding to a given **phenotype.** For example, phenotype A_1 has three corresponding genotypes: A^1A^1, A^1A^2, and A^1O. Similarly, at least three genotypes correspond to the phenotype Rh_1Rh_2: R^1R^2, R^1r'', and R^2r'. Phenotypes and genotypes may be expressed differently, for example, phenotype Lu^a and genotype Lu^a would preferably be designated phenotype Lu (a+) or Lu(a+b−) and genotype Lu^aLu^a.

It must be kept in mind that every individual has but a single genotype for any given characteristic. Blood grouping tests for parentage are mostly valuable in a "negative" way; that is, it can be stated that a person could not be the parent of a particular child. In cases of extremely rare genotypes, such tests can also provide strong circumstantial evidence of parentage.

The blood group genes are considered

dominant characteristics. However, when two genes for a given characteristic are different and present laboratory methods will distinguish only the product of one of the genes, the other is at times referred to as a **recessive** characteristic. An example is group A_1, genotype A^1A^2, in which the individual is presumably of phenotype A_1A_2, but laboratory tests show the subgroup simply as A_1. The exact genotype in such a case can be determined only by **family studies** and not by laboratory serologic methods alone.

In general, once the blood group of an individual is established, it remains substantially unaltered for life. Exceptions are I-i, Le, etc. This is one of the principles on which all studies of heredity in the blood groups are based. This principle and the evidence of the blood groups are accepted in most courts. New York was the first state in the United States to adopt a blood test law, March 22, 1935. The reliability of blood group tests is so great that no other type of evidence can approach it, and certainly none can equal it. All blood group tests, however, must be performed by experts. A person who is capable of testing blood in a blood bank or for transfusion does not necessarily qualify as an expert in performing some of the delicate tests on which court decisions are based.

Before any conclusions can be drawn concerning inheritance of any of the blood groups, it is necessary that the genotypes of each blood group be known. Tables 13-3 through 13-15 give the blood group, or phenotype, as well as specificities, or blood group factors, and possible genotypes in the various systems, but they do not include many of the rare factors or phenotypes.

The A-B-O system

Tables 13-3 and 13-4 give the blood groups and subgroups in the A-B-O system along with the blood specificities and possible genotypes.

Blood factor **C** (of the A-B-O groups) is shared by agglutinogens A and B, and since it is simply a specificity, it does not have a corresponding gene.

The H substance is determined by the gene *H*, which competes with the genes for the A-B-O groups for the same substrate. It is considered that almost all individuals must be homozygous for the **H** factor.

It must be emphasized that the agglutinogens are not the direct products of the corresponding genes. Instead, there is evidence that the genes give rise to enzymes that determine the corresponding agglutinogen; for example, gene *A* gives rise to an α-N-acetylgalactosaminyl transferase that transfers the determinant sugar α-N-acetylgalactosamine from a donor molecule to the appropriate substrate to produce the A blood group substance.[1]

Table 13-3. The A-B-O blood group system (subgroups not included)*

Blood group (phenotype)	Specificities (blood group factors)	Possible genotypes
O	None	*OO*
A	**A** and **C**	*AA* or *AO*
B	**B** and **C**	*BB* or *BO*
AB	**A** and **B** and **C**	*AB*

*See cis AB, p. 76.

Table 13-4. The A-B-O blood group system (subgroups of A included)

Blood groups (phenotypes)	Specificities (blood factors)	Possible genotypes
O	None	*OO*
A_1	A_1, **A**, and **C**	A^1A^1, A^1A^2, or A^1O
A_2	**A** and **C**	A^2A^2 or A^2O
B	**B** and **C**	*BB* or *BO*
A_1B	A_1, **A**, **B**, and **C**	A^1B
A_2B	**A**, **B**, and **C**	A^2B

The Lewis and secretor systems

In the Lewis system (Table 13-5), which differs from the usual blood groups, there is no agglutinogen as such but rather a water-soluble Lewis substance, present in body fluids and secretions such as saliva, semen, and vaginal fluids secondarily adsorbed onto the blood cells. These cells are then reactive with anti-**Lewis** sera. Another substance, H, is present in the saliva of A-B-H secretors, genetically independent of the A-B-O groups, and substance H can be detected in the secretions of the body. Lewis and A-B-H substances are thought to be derived from the same substrate and are of related chemical structure (pp. 67 to 69). When the Lewis gene, *Le,* and the secretor gene, *Se,* occur together, they compete for the same substrate. This is explained in the section on the Lewis type. Genotypes in the Lewis system are determined not only by testing the **cells** of the individual with the various anti-**Lewis** sera but also by testing the **saliva** for A-B-H and Lewis substances. Table 6-3 gives the presently used symbols for the Lewis types in blood, the previous symbols, the Le substance in saliva, the A-B-H substance in saliva, and the possible genotypes, according to the theory of R. Ceppellini.[2]

The M-N-S system

Consult Tables 13-6 and 13-7 for phenotypes and possible genotypes in the M-N-S system.

The P system

Tables 13-8 and 13-9 give the phenotypes and possible genotypes for the P blood group system in the Wiener and the Matson nomenclatures and theories.

Table 13-5. Lewis blood types in man (after Wiener)*

Red blood cells		Saliva		Possible genotypes
Present symbol	**Previous symbol**	**Le**	**A-B-H**	
Le₁	*Lewis positive* Le(a+) Le(a+b−)	*Present* (type Les)	*Absent* (type nS)	*Le Le se se* *Le le se se*
Le₂	*Lewis negative* Le(a−) Le(a−b+)	*Present* (type Les)	*Present* (type Sec)	*Le Le Se Se* *Le le Se Se* *Le Le Se se* *Le le Se se*
le	*Lewis negative* Le(a−) Le(a−b−)	*Absent* (type nL)	*Present* (type Sec) *Absent* (type nS)	*le le* { *Se Se* *Se se* *le le se se*

*Modified from Erskine, A. G. In Frankel, S., Reitman, S., and Sonnenwirth, A. C., editors: Gradwohl's clinical laboratory methods and diagnosis, ed. 7, St. Louis, 1970, The C. V. Mosby Co.

Table 13-6. Blood types M, N, and MN

Phenotype	Possible genotypes
M	*MM*
N	*NN*
MN	*MN*

Table 13-7. Blood types M, N, and MN, including S

Phenotype	Possible genotypes
M.S	*M.S/M.S* or *M.S/M.s*
M.s	*M.s/M.s*
N.S	*N.S/N.S* or *N.S/N.s*
N.s	*N.s/N.s*
MN.S	*M.S/N.S* or *M.S/N.s* or *M.s/N.S*
MN.s	*M.s/N.s*

Table 13-8. P-p system—Wiener theory and nomenclature[*]

Blood groups (phenotypes)	Possible genotypes
P_1	P^1P^1, P^1P, P^1p', or Pp'
P	PP or Pp
p′	$p'p'$ or $p'p$
p	pp

[*]From Wiener, A. S.: Lab. Digest **31**(4): 6, 1968.

Table 13-9. P-p system—Matson nomenclature[*]

Blood groups (phenotypes)	Possible genotypes
P_1	P_1P_1, P_1P_2, P_1P^k, or P_1p
P_2	P_2P_2, P_2P^k, or P_2p
P^k	P^kP^k or P^kp
p	pp

[*]From Matson, G. S., Swanson, J., Noades, J., Sanger, R., and Race, R. R.: Am. J. Hum. Genet. **11**:26, 1959; copyrighted by The University of Chicago Press.

The Rh-Hr system

The Rh-Hr blood group system is probably the most complex of all the blood group systems. The genotypes have been derived from extensive family studies, many of which are by A .S. Wiener and his colleagues. (See Table 13-10.)

The K-k (Kell-Cellano) system

The phenotypes and possible genotypes in the Kell-Cellano blood group system are given in Table 13-11.

The **Kp** and **Js** specificities of the K-k system have not been included in the table because more studies are indicated before conclusions can be drawn as to the genetic mechanism.

The Lu (Lutheran) system

Table 13-12 lists the phenotypes and possible genotypes in the Lu system.

It must be stressed that (as explained on p. 161ff) the problem of inheritance of the Lutheran blood types remains unsolved in

Table 13-10. The Rh-Hr system (after Wiener)[*]

Blood type	Phenotypes	Possible genotypes
rh	rh	rr
rh′	rh′rh	$r'r$
	rh′rh′	$r'r'$
rh′w	rh′wrh	r'^wr
	rh′wrh′	r'^wr' or $r'^wr'^w$
rh″	rh″rh	$r''r$
	rh″rh″	$r''r''$
rhy	rh′rh″	$r'r''$
	rhyrh	r^yr
	rhyrh′	r^yr'
	rhyrh″	r^yr''
	rhyrhy	r^yr^y
rh$_y^w$	rh′wrh″	r'^wr''
	rh$_y^w$′rh′	r'^wr^y
Rh_o	Rh_o	R^oR^o or R^or
Rh_1	Rh_1rh	R^1r, R^1R^o, or R^or'
	Rh_1Rh_1	R^1R^1 or R^1r'
Rh_1^w	Rh_1^wrh	$R^{1w}r$, $R^{1w}R^o$, or $R^or'^w$
	$Rh_1^wRh_1$	$R^{1w}R^1$, $R^1r'^w$, $R^{1w}r'$, $R^{1w}R^{1w}$, or $R^{1w}r'^w$
Rh_2	Rh_2rh	R^2r, R^2R^o, or R^or''
	Rh_2Rh_2	R^2R^2 or R^2r''
Rh_z	Rh_1Rh_2	R^1R^2, R^1r'', or R^2r'
	Rh_zrh	R^zr, R^zR^o, or R^or^y
	Rh_zRh_1	R^zR^1, R^zr', or R^1r^y
	Rh_zRh_2	R^zR^2, R^zr'', or R^2r^y
	Rh_zRh_z	R^zR^z or R^zr^y
Rh_z^w	$Rh_1^wRh_2$	$R^{1w}R^2$, $R^{1w}r''$, or $R^2r'^w$
	$Rh_z^wRh_1$	$R^{1w}R^z$, $R^{1w}r^y$, or $R^zr'^w$

[*]Modified from Erskine, A. G. In Frankel, S., Reitman, S., and Sonnenwirth, A. C., editors: Gradwohl's clinical laboratory methods and diagnosis, ed. 7, St. Louis, 1970, The C. V. Mosby Co.

Hypothetical genes are not included in the table nor are the variants of the Rh and Hr factors.

The genotypes for these phenotypes, with the C-D-E notations or the Rosenfield numbers, are not given, since this text follows the Rh-Hr nomenclature only.

Table 13-11. The K-k system

Phenotypes	Possible genotypes
K	KK or Kk
k	kk

Table 13-12. The Lu system

Phenotypes		Possible genotypes
Lu(a+)	{Lu(a+b−)	Lu^aLu^a or Lu^alu
	Lu(a+b+)}	Lu^aLu^b
Lu(a−)	{Lu(a−b+)	Lu^bLu^b or Lu^blu
	Lu(a−b−)}	$lu\ lu$

Table 13-13. The Fy system

Phenotypes		Possible genotypes
Fy(a+)	{Fy(a+b−)	Fy^aFy^a or Fy^afy
	Fy(a+b+)}	Fy^aFy^b
Fy(a−)	{Fy(a−b+)	Fy^bFy^b or Fy^bfy
	Fy(a−b−)}	$fyfy$

Table 13-14. The Jk system

Phenotypes		Possible genotypes
Jk(a+)	{Jk(a+b−)	Jk^aJk^a or Jk^ajk
	Jk(a+b+)}	Jk^aJk^b
Jk(a−)	{Jk(a−b+)	Jk^bJk^b or Jk^bjk
	Jk(a−b−)}	$jkjk$

Table 13-15. The I-i system

Phenotypes	Possible genotypes
I or I+i−	II or Ii
i or I−i+	ii

that the existence of recessive gene *lu* has not as yet been proved conclusively. It is known, moreover, that in some families the rare Lu(a–b–) type appears to be transmitted as a dominant characteristic.

The Fy (Duffy) system

The phenotypes and possible genotypes of the Fy system are listed in Table 13-13.

The Jk (Kidd) system

Consult Table 13-14 for the phenotypes and possible genotypes in the Jk system.

The I-i system

As stated in the discussion of the I-i system (p. 173), hardly any family studies have been possible because of the extremely low frequency of type i in adults. In addition, there are many subgroups in the I groups such as $I_1, I_2 \ldots , i_1, i_2 \ldots ,$ so that studies of the genetics in the I-i system must await the discovery of further facts. Table 13-15 gives a simplified scheme of the inheritance of the I-i blood groups.

The Xg (sex-linked) system

The Xg system differs from the other blood group systems in that the Xg characteristic is sex-linked. The heredity of the Xg characteristic is discussed in detail in Chapter 12 and will not be repeated here.

METHOD OF DETERMINING POSSIBLE PHENOTYPES OF CHILDREN IN VARIOUS MATINGS

In most cases the exact genotype of an individual cannot be determined by any laboratory test known to date. The genotypes must therefore be worked out by family studies, except in such groups where they are self-evident. In determining what phenotypes would be possible in the children of certain matings, every conceivable combination of genotypes of the parents must be considered, even though it is true that every person has only a single genotype for any one characteristic. In the examples that follow, it will be shown that even though in some combinations (mating a group O person with an AB individual) there can be only one possible combination of parental genotypes, in other matings (two group A_1 parents) as many as six different genotype combinations must be considered.

Each allelic gene for a blood group or type characteristic occurs on a different chromosome from all other allelic genes for other blood group characteristics.* For this reason, the genetics for each system must

---

*An exception is blood group cis AB, p. 76, in which AB seems to be transmitted as if by a single chromosome or gene.

be worked out separately. In other words, to determine the children possible to the mating of group O MN Rh negative × group AB M Rh negative, one would have three sets of diagrams: O × AB, MN × M, and rh × rh. This is given as an example of simple combinations.

To determine the phenotypes possible to the offspring, first put down the possible combinations of genotypes of the parents. Next, determine what the zygotes might be for this combination by combining the first gene of the genotype of parent 1 with the first gene of the genotype of parent 2; then combine the first gene of parent 1 with the second gene of parent 2; next combine the second gene of parent 1 with the first gene of parent 2; last combine the second gene of parent 1 with the second gene of parent 2. From the zygotes, determine the phenotypes of the children by consulting the previous tables. In the following example the groups and types of the parents are O MN rh × A_1B M rh.

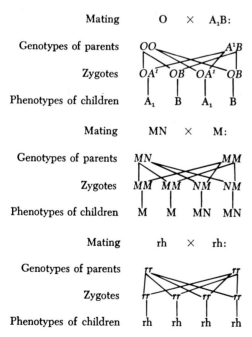

Mating	O × A_1B:
Genotypes of parents	OO A^1B
Zygotes	OA^1 OB OA^1 OB
Phenotypes of children	A_1 B A_1 B

Mating	MN × M:
Genotypes of parents	MN MM
Zygotes	MM MM NM NM
Phenotypes of children	M M MN MN

Mating	rh × rh:
Genotypes of parents	rr rr
Zygotes	rr rr rr rr
Phenotypes of children	rh rh rh rh

Summarizing, children possible to this mating are A_1 and B, M and MN, and rh; children not possible are O, A_2, A_1B, A_2B; N; rh′, rh″, rh_y, and any of the Rh_o-positive types.

In this example the genotypes of the parents are known, since in each instance there can be but one genotype for the specific blood group or type. In some cases, however, several possible genotypes must be considered. Again it must be emphasized that an individual can have only a single genotype for any one characteristic, so that the persons involved in the next example would have to be in just one category. However, because, as stated, there are no laboratory tests available at present to identify all genotypes, several possibilities may have to be included in heredity tests.

The following example is about as complicated as is possible using only the three principal blood group systems: A-B-O, M-N, and Rh-Hr.

Mating A_1 M Rh_1Rh_2 × A_1 N Rh_zrh

The possible genotypes of the first parent are A^1A^1, A^1A^2, or A^1O; MM; and R^1R^2, $R^1r″$, or $R^2r′$.

The possible genotypes of the second parent are A^1A^1, A^1A^2, or A^1O; NN; and R^Zr, R^ZR^o, or R^or^y.

The following diagrams need to be made:

1. In the A-B-O system:

A^1A^1	×	A^1A^1	A^1A^2	×	A^1A^2
A^1A^1	×	A^1A^2	A^1A^2	×	A^1O
A^1A^1	×	A^1O	A^1O	×	A^1O

2. In the M-N system:

MM	×	NN

3. In the Rh-Hr system:

R^1R^2	×	R^Zr	$R^1r″$	×	R^or^y
R^1R^2	×	R^ZR^o	$R^2r′$	×	R^Zr
R^1R^2	×	R^or^y	$R^2r′$	×	R^ZR^o
$R^1r″$	×	R^Zr	$R^2r′$	×	R^or^y
$R^1r″$	×	R^ZR^o			

Having determined what the combinations of genotypes in the different systems are for this mating, the next step is to prepare the diagrams, using the following outline:

Mating
Genotypes of parents
Zygotes
Phenotypes of children

One such diagram must be prepared for each possible mating in all the systems. Combine the various genes as directed previously. For purposes of illustration, only one diagram for the six possible combinations of genotypes in the A-B-O system, one for the M-N system (the only one), and one for the Rh-Hr system will be given. The other five in the A-B-O system and the other eight in the Rh-Hr system possible for this mating would be prepared in a like manner. Consult tables of genotypes in each system, pp. 191 to 193. This is the fifth possible combination as listed on p. 194 and will be the only one diagrammed here.

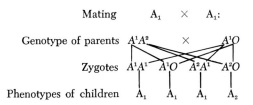

In all, a total of sixteen diagrams would have to be prepared for this mating. The diagrams and the possible phenotypes of the offspring will be as in Tables 13-16 and 13-17. For the M-N types (Table 13-18) there will be only one diagram. The children possible to various matings in the Rh-Hr system are given in Table 13-17. That table, however, does not include the Rh_0

Table 13-16. The six possibilities of genotype combinations of group $A_1 \times A_1$ parents, resulting zygotes, and children possible

Genotypes of parents	Genotypes of zygotes	Children possible
$A^1A^1 \times A^1A^1$	$A^1A^1, A^1A^1, A^1A^1, A^1A^1$	All group A_1
$A^1A^1 \times A^1A^2$	$A^1A^1, A^1A^2, A^1A^1, A^1A^2$	All group A_1
$A^1A^1 \times A^1O$	$A^1A^1, A^1O, A^1A^1, A^1O$	All group A_1
$A^1A^2 \times A^1A^2$	$A^1A^1, A^1A^2, A^2A^1, A^2A^2$	A_1, A_2
$A^1A^2 \times A^1O$	$A^1A^1, A^1O, A^2A^1, A^2O$	A_1, A_2
$A^1O \times A^1O$	A^1A^1, A^1O, OA^1, OO	A_1, O

Table 13-17. The nine possibilities of genotype combinations of types $Rh_1Rh_2 \times Rh_Zrh$ parents, resulting zygotes, and children possible (phenotypes)*

Genotypes of parents	Genotypes of zygotes†	Children possible (phenotypes)* (see Table 13-7)
$R^1R^2 \times R^Zr$	$R^1R^Z, R^1r, R^2R^Z, R^2r$	$Rh_ZRh_1, Rh_1rh, Rh_ZRh_2, Rh_2rh$
$R^1R^2 \times R^ZR^0$	$R^1R^Z, R^1R^0, R^2R^Z, R^2R^0$	$Rh_ZRh_1, Rh_1rh, Rh_ZRh_2, Rh_2rh$
$R^1R^2 \times R^0r^y$	$R^1R^0, R^1r^y, R^2R^0, R^2r^y$	$Rh_1rh, Rh_ZRh_1, Rh_2rh, Rh_ZRh_2$
$R^1r'' \times R^Zr$	$R^1R^Z, R^1r, r''R^Z, r''r$	$Rh_ZRh_1, Rh_1rh, Rh_ZRh_2, rh''rh$
$R^1r'' \times R^ZR^0$	$R^1R^Z, R^1R^0, r''R^Z, r''R^0$	$Rh_ZRh_1, Rh_1rh, Rh_ZRh_2, Rh_2rh$
$R^1r'' \times R^0r^y$	$R^1R^0, R^1r^y, r''R^0, r''r^y$	$Rh_1rh, Rh_ZRh_1, Rh_2rh, rh_yrh''$
$R^2r' \times R^Zr$	$R^2R^Z, R^2r, r'R^Z, r'r$	$Rh_ZRh_2, Rh_2rh, Rh_ZRh_1, rh'rh$
$R^2r' \times R^ZR^0$	$R^2R^Z, R^2R^0, r'R^Z, r'R^0$	$Rh_ZRh_2, Rh_2rh, Rh_ZRh_1, Rh_1rh$
$R^2r' \times R^0r^y$	$R^2R^0, R^2r^y, r'R^0, r'r^y$	$Rh_2rh, Rh_ZRh_2, Rh_1rh, rh_yrh'$

*Eliminating duplicates and rearranging the phenotypes in a more logical order—rh'rh, rh''rh, rh$_y$rh′, rh$_y$rh″, Rh$_1$rh, Rh$_2$rh, Rh$_Z$Rh$_1$, and Rh$_Z$Rh$_2$.
†Arranged as they would fall in the diagrams.

Table 13-18. Possibilities of genotype combinations of parents in the M-N system, with resulting zygotes and children possible (phenotypes)

Mating	Genotypes of parents	Zygotes	Phenotypes of children	Children not possible
M × M	*MM* × *MM*	All *MM*	M	N, MN
M × N	*MM* × *NN*	All *MN*	MN	M, N
N × N	*NN* × *NN*	All *NN*	N	M, MN
M × MN	*MM* × *MN*	*MM* and *MN*	M and MN	N
N × MN	*NN* × *MN*	*NN* and *MN*	N and MN	M
MN × MN	*MN* × *MN*	*MM, NN, MN*	M, N, and MN	—

Note: Tables 7-3 and 7-4 list the genotypes and possible phenotypes in the M-N-S system, which are not repeated here.

Table 13-19. Possibilities of children's Rh-Hr types in mating of individuals lacking Rh$_o$*

Mating	Children possible	Children not possible
rh × rh	rh	rh′, rh″, rh$_y$, Rh$_o$, Rh$_1$, Rh$_2$, Rh$_z$
rh × rh′	rh, rh′	rh″, rh$_y$, Rh$_o$, Rh$_1$, Rh$_2$, Rh$_z$
rh × rh″	rh, rh″	rh′, rh$_y$, Rh$_o$, Rh$_1$, Rh$_2$, Rh$_z$
rh × rh$_y$	rh, rh′, rh″, rh$_y$	Rh$_o$, Rh$_1$, Rh$_2$, Rh$_z$
rh′ × rh′	rh, rh′	rh″, rh$_y$, Rh$_o$, Rh$_1$, Rh$_2$, Rh$_z$
rh′ × rh″	rh, rh′, rh″, rh$_y$	Rh$_o$, Rh$_1$, Rh$_2$, Rh$_z$
rh′ × rh$_y$	rh, rh′, rh″, rh$_y$	Rh$_o$, Rh$_1$, Rh$_2$, Rh$_z$
rh″ × rh″	rh, rh″	rh′, rh$_y$, Rh$_o$, Rh$_1$, Rh$_2$, Rh$_z$
rh″ × rh$_y$	rh, rh′, rh″, rh$_y$	Rh$_o$, Rh$_1$, Rh$_2$, Rh$_z$
rh$_y$ × rh$_y$	rh, rh′, rh″, rh$_y$	Rh$_o$, Rh$_1$, Rh$_2$, Rh$_z$

*This table is useful only when Rh types lacking Rh$_o$ are considered without tests for the Hr factors.

variants or any of the other variants in the Rh-Hr system.

In summary, children of groups A$_1$, A$_2$, O are possible; those not possible to this mating are B, A$_1$B, A$_2$B.

If there are two or more children in a family, additional exclusions are possible; for example, in the mating A$_1$ × A$_1$, if one child is group O there can be no children of subgroup A$_2$. On the other hand, if one child is subgroup A$_2$, there can be no children of group O.

In the Rh-Hr system the first combination of possible Rh-Hr genotypes in this mating is as follows (consult Table 13-10):

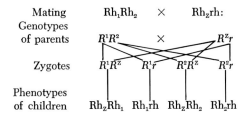

Altogether there are nine different possible combinations of parents' Rh-Hr genotypes, as stated previously. Using diagrams similar to the example in the Rh-Hr system, results obtained are as shown in Table 13-17. Note that the phenotypes are those shown in Table 13-10, which represents the results of family studies.

Table 13-20. Exclusion of paternity or maternity by the Rh-Hr blood types*

Phenotype of putative mother	1 rh Rh_o	2 rh'rh Rh_1rh	3 rh'rh' Rh_1Rh_1	4 rh"rh Rh_2rh	5 rh"rh" Rh_2Rh_2	6a rh'rh" Rh_1Rh_2	6b rh_yrh Rh_zrh	7 rh_yrh' Rh_zRh_1	8 rh_yrh'' Rh_zRh_2	9 rh_yrh_y Rh_zRh_z
1 rh Rh_o	2, 3, 4, 5, **6a,** 6b, **7, 8, 9**	3, 4, **5, 6a,** 6b, **7, 8, 9**	1, 3, 4, 5, **6a,** 6b, **7, 8, 9**	2, 3, 5, **6a,** 6b, **7, 8, 9**	1, 2, 3, 5, **6a,** 6b, **7, 8, 9**	1, 3, 5, **6a,** 6b, **7, 8, 9**	2, 3, 4, 5, **6a,** 6b, **7, 8, 9**	1, 3, 4, 5, **6a,** **7, 8, 9**	1, 2, 3, 5, **6a,** **7, 8, 9**	1, 2, **3, 4, 5, 6a,** **7, 8, 9**
2 rh'rh Rh_1rh	3, 4, **5, 6a,** 6b, **7, 8, 9**	4, 5, 6a, 6b, **7, 8, 9**	1, 4, 5, 6a, 6b, **7, 8, 9**	3, 5, 6b, 7, **8, 9**	1, 2, 3, 5, **6b, 7, 8, 9**	1, 5, **6b, 7, 8, 9**	4, 5, 6a, **7, 8, 9**	1, 4, 5, 6a, **8, 9**	1, 2, 3, 5, **9**	1, 2, 3, 4, 5, **6a,** 8, 9
3 rh'rh' Rh_1Rh_1	1, 3, **4, 5, 6a,** **6b,** 7, 8, 9	1, 4, 5, 6a, **6b,** 7, 8, 9	1, 2, 4, 5, 6a, **6b,** 7, 8, 9	1, 3, 4, 5, 6b, 7, **8, 9**	1, 2, 3, 4, 5, **6b,** 7, 8, 9	1, 2, 4, 5, 6b, 7, **8, 9**	1, 3, 4, 5, 6a, **6b, 8, 9**	1, 2, 4, 5, 6a, **6b, 8, 9**	1, 2, 3, 4, 5, **5, 6b, 8, 9**	1, 2, 3, 4, 5, **6a, 6b, 8, 9**
4 rh"rh Rh_2rh	2, 3, 5, 6a, 6b, **7, 8, 9**	3, 5, 6b, **7, 8, 9**	1, 3, 4, 5, 6b, **7, 8, 9**	2, 3, 6a, 6b, **7, 8, 9**	1, 2, 3, 6a, 6b, **7, 8, 9**	1, 3, 6b, **7, 8, 9**	2, 3, 5, 6a, 7, **9**	1, 3, 4, 5, **7, 9**	1, 2, 3, 6a, **7, 9**	1, 2, **3, 4, 5,** 6a, **7, 9**
5 rh"rh" Rh_2Rh_2	1, 2, 3, 5, 6a, **6b, 7, 8, 9**	1, 2, 3, 5, **6b,** 7, 8, 9	1, 2, 3, 4, 5, **6b, 7, 8, 9**	1, 2, 3, 6a, **6b, 7, 8, 9**	1, 2, 3, 4, 6a, **6b, 7, 8, 9**	1, 2, 3, 4, **6b, 7, 8, 9**	1, 2, 3, 5, 6a, **6b, 7, 9**	1, 2, 3, 4, 5, **6b, 7, 9**	1, 2, 3, 4, 6a, **6b, 7, 9**	1, 2, **3, 4, 5,** 6a, **6b, 7, 9**
6a rh'rh" Rh_1Rh_2	1, 3, 5, 6a, **6b, 7, 8, 9**	1, 5, **6b, 7,** 8, 9	1, 2, 4, 5, 6b, **7, 8, 9**	1, 3, 6b, 7, **8, 9**	1, 2, 3, 4, **6b,** 7, 8, 9	1, 2, 4, **6b,** 7, 8, 9	1, 3, 5, 6a, **6b, 9**	1, 2, 4, 5, **6b, 9**	1, 2, 3, 4, **6b, 9**	1, 2, **3, 4, 5, 6a, 6b, 9**
6b rh_yrh Rh_zrh	2, 3, 4, 5, **6a,** 7, 8, 9	3, 4, 5, **6a,** 8, 9	1, 3, 4, 5, **6a,** 6b, 8, 9	2, 3, 5, 6a, 7, **9**	1, 2, 3, 5, 6b, **7, 9**	1, 3, 5, 6a, **6b, 9**	2, 3, 4, 5, **6a,** 7, 8	1, 3, 4, 5, **6a,** 8	1, 2, **3, 5, 6a,** 7	1, 2, **3, 4, 5, 6a,** 7, 8
7 rh_yrh' Rh_zRh_1	1, 3, 4, 5, **6a,** 7, 8, 9	1, 4, 5, 6a, 8, 9	1, 2, 4, 5, 6a, 6b, 8, 9	1, 3, 4, 5, 7, **9**	1, 2, 3, 4, 5, 6b, **7, 9**	1, 2, 4, 5, 6a, 6b, 9	1, 3, 4, 5, 6a, 8	1, 2, **4, 5,** 6a, 6b, 8	1, 2, **3, 4, 5,** 6b	1, 2, **3, 4, 5,** 6a, 6b, 8
8 rh_yrh'' Rh_zRh_2	1, 2, 3, 5, 6a, **7, 8, 9**	1, 2, 3, 5, 8, **9**	1, 2, 3, 4, 5, 6b, 8, 9	1, 2, 3, 6a, 7, **9**	1, 2, 3, 4, 6a, 6b, 7, 9	1, 2, 3, 4, 6b, **9**	1, 2, 3, 5, 6a, 7	1, 2, **3, 4,** 5, 6b	1, 2, **3, 4,** 6a, 6b, 7	1, 2, **3, 4, 5,** 6a, 6b, 7
9 rh_yrh_y Rh_zRh_z	1, 2, 3, 4, 5, **6a,** 7, 8, 9	1, 2, 3, 4, 5, **6a,** 8, 9	1, 2, 3, 4, 5, **6a,** 6b, 8, 9	1, 2, 3, 4, 5, **6a,** 7, 9	1, 2, 3, 4, 5, **6a,** 6b, 7, 9	1, 2, 3, 4, 5, **6a,** 6b, 9	1, 2, 3, 4, 5, **6a,** 7, 8	1, 2, **3, 4, 5, 6a,** 6b, 8	1, 2, **3, 4, 5, 6a,** 6b, 7	1, 2, **3, 4, 5, 6a,** 6b, 7, 8

*From Wiener, A. S., and Nieberg, K. C.: J. Forensic Med. 10:608, Jan.-Mar., 1963.
Boldface figures represent phenotypes of children for whom maternity is excluded.
This table is to be applied only to matings in which at least one of the parents is Rh_o positive. Where both parents are Rh_o negative, necessarily all Rh_o-positive children are also excluded.
The phenotypes corresponding to the code numbers are given in the marginal headings; e.g., 1 is the code number for phenotypes rh and Rh_o.

Children not possible, by elimination, are rh, rh′rh′, rh″rh″, rh′rh″, rh$_y$rh, rh$_y$rh$_y$, Rh$_o$, Rh$_1$Rh$_1$, Rh$_2$Rh$_2$, Rh$_1$Rh$_2$, Rh$_z$rh, Rh$_z$Rh$_z$. For more complete information on heredity of the Rh-Hr specificities and exclusion of paternity and maternity, refer to Tables 13-19 and 13-20.

The next step in determining the phenotypes of children possible to a mating is to combine the results of all the diagrams. In this example, the children possible to the mating A$_1$ M Rh$_1$Rh$_2$ × A$_1$ N Rh$_z$rh would be as follows:

Children possible:
  O, A$_1$, or A$_2$
  MN
  rh′rh, rh″rh, rh$_y$rh′, rh$_y$rh″, Rh$_1$rh, Rh$_2$rh, Rh$_z$Rh$_1$, or Rh$_z$Rh$_2$

The laboratory reports are written in a like manner, except that many include a list of phenotypes of children not possible to the mating, as:

Children not possible:
  B, A$_1$B, or A$_2$B
  M or N
  rh, rh′rh′, rh″rh″, rh′rh″, rh$_y$rh, rh$_y$rh$_y$, Rh$_o$, Rh$_1$Rh$_1$, Rh$_2$Rh$_2$, Rh$_1$Rh$_2$, Rh$_z$rh, or Rh$_z$Rh$_z$

In the A-B-O system, if only the subgroups A$_1$, A$_2$, A$_1$B, and A$_2$B and groups O and B are utilized, Table 13-21 may be consulted to determine phenotypes of offspring in the various matings in the A-B-O system.

For phenotypes of children possible in the various matings in the Rh-Hr system, consult Table 13-20 only if at least one of the parents is Rh$_o$ positive. Matings between Rh-positive individuals lacking Rh$_o$ or between these and Rh-negative individuals are shown in Table 13-19.

LAWS OF HEREDITY OF THE BLOOD GROUPS

A study of Tables 13-3 through 13-21 in the three blood group systems, A-B-O, Rh-Hr, and M-N, will demonstrate the following **laws of heredity with respect to the blood groups:**

1. No blood group factor can appear in the blood of a child unless it is present in at least one of the parents.

Table 13-21. Possibility of children in various matings in the A-B-O blood group system

Mating	Children possible	Children not possible
O × O	O	A$_1$, A$_2$, B, A$_1$B, A$_2$B
O × A$_1$	O, A$_1$, A$_2$	B, A$_1$B, A$_2$B
O × A$_2$	O, A$_2$	A$_1$, B, A$_1$B, A$_2$B
O × B	O, B	A$_1$, A$_2$, A$_1$B, A$_2$B
O × A$_1$B	A$_1$, B	O, A$_2$, A$_1$B, A$_2$B
O × A$_2$B	A$_2$, B	O, A$_1$, A$_1$B, A$_2$B
A$_1$ × A$_1$	O, A$_1$, A$_2$	B, A$_1$B, A$_2$B
A$_1$ × A$_2$	O, A$_1$, A$_2$	B, A$_1$B, A$_2$B
A$_1$ × B	O, A$_1$, A$_2$, B, A$_1$B, A$_2$B	—
A$_1$ × A$_1$B	A$_1$, B, A$_1$B, A$_2$B	O, A$_2$
A$_1$ × A$_2$B	A$_1$, A$_2$, B, A$_1$B, A$_2$B	O
A$_2$ × A$_2$	O, A$_2$	A$_1$, B, A$_1$B, A$_2$B
A$_2$ × B	O, A$_2$, B, A$_2$B	A$_1$, A$_1$B
A$_2$ × A$_1$B	A$_1$, B, A$_2$B	O, A$_2$, A$_1$B
A$_2$ × A$_2$B	A$_2$, B, A$_2$B	O, A$_1$, A$_1$B
B × B	O, B	A$_1$, A$_2$, A$_1$B, A$_2$B
B × A$_1$B	A$_1$, B, A$_1$B	O, A$_2$, A$_2$B
B × A$_2$B	A$_2$, B, A$_2$B	O, A$_1$, A$_1$B
A$_1$B × A$_1$B	A$_1$, B, A$_1$B	O, A$_2$, A$_2$B
A$_1$B × A$_2$B	A$_1$, B, A$_1$B, A$_2$B	O, A$_2$
A$_2$B × A$_2$B	A$_2$, B, A$_2$B	O, A$_1$, A$_1$B

2. A group O person cannot be the parent of a group AB child.*

3. Similarly, a group AB person cannot be the parent of a group O child.*

4. A group M person cannot be the parent of a group N child.

5. A group N person cannot be the parent of a group M child.

6. If both parents are type M, all the children will be type M.

7. If both parents are type N, all the children will be type N.

8. If both parents are type MN, the children can be type M, N, or MN.

9. If both parents are group O, all the children must be group O.

10. If one parent is group A_1 and the other is group B, the children may belong to any of the A-B-O blood groups or subgroups.

11. A child of type M has parents of M × M or of M × MN or of MN × MN; the **M** specificity must be present in both parents.

12. A child of type N has parents of N × N or N × MN or MN × MN; the **N** specificity must be present in both parents.

13. If both parents are Rh negative (type rh), all the children will be Rh negative.

14. If both parents are Rh_0 positive and either or both are homozygous for the Rh factor, all the children will be Rh positive.

15. If one parent is Rh positive and homozygous for the Rh factor and the other parent is Rh negative, all the children will be Rh positive.

16. If both parents are Rh positive and heterozygous for the Rh factor, there may be both Rh-positive and Rh-negative children.

17. If one parent is Rh positive and heterozygous for the Rh factor and the other parent is Rh negative, there may be both Rh-positive and Rh-negative children.

---

*For an exception, see blood group cis AB, p. 76.

Heredity of the specificities in the other blood group systems is explained in the chapters dealing with those factors. Since most medicolegal cases involving heredity of the blood groups are concerned only with the Rh-Hr blood group system and the A-B-O and M-N types, these are the only ones under discussion in this chapter.

The preceding laws may be stated in a more general fashion[3]:

1. An agglutinogen cannot appear in the blood of a child unless it is present in one or both parents.

2. A parent who is homozygous for an agglutinogen must transmit a gene for the agglutinogen to every child.

3. A child who is homozygous for an agglutinogen must have inherited a gene for this agglutinogen from each of his parents.

CLINICAL IMPORTANCE

In addition to its value in anthropologic investigations, a study of the genetics in the blood group systems is important clinically. An example is in the Rh-Hr types, to predict the Rh type of the fetus in matings of Rh-negative women with Rh-positive men. If the mother is Rh negative, her genotype must be *rr*. If the father is Rh positive, he may be homozygous or heterozygous for the Rh factor. Assuming only one Rh-positive type with genotypes *RR* for homozygous and *Rr* for heterozygous persons, the offspring for the mating Rh negative with homozygous Rh positive would be *rr* × *RR*, and the offspring of this union would all inherit one Rh-negative and one Rh-positive characteristic and would develop as Rh positive (by laboratory tests). On the other hand, if one of the parents is Rh positive heterozygous, the mating would be *rr* × *Rr*, and the children would be *Rr* or *rr*, 50% Rh positive and 50% Rh negative. This explains why an Rh-negative woman mated to an Rh-positive man may give birth to an Rh-negative baby, and in such a case she could not be isosensitized to the Rh factor.

If the exact phenotype of the Rh-positive individual is determined, using not only the standard anti-Rh sera but also the anti-Hr sera, one can go still farther in predicting the Rh type of the offspring.

OTHER USES
Medicolegal applications

Blood grouping tests to establish hereditary characteristics are useful in exclusion of paternity and in cases of disputed maternity as well. This is the subject of a separate chapter (Chapter 22).

Although some cases of baby mixing may unfortunately still occur in hospitals, they are rare. In such cases the blood groups and types of the babies, mothers, fathers, and in some instances also the siblings, must be determined. Facts about the heredity of the blood groups and their specificities may be the only means to right such an accident.

Kidnapping cases have been reported in which a woman insists that a certain child is her natural-born child. A study of the blood groups of the suspect, the child, and the parents of the missing child should be made, and if there are any siblings, their blood groups should also be determined. This is discussed in Chapter 22 on medicolegal applications, along with other aspects of the application of genetics of blood grouping in forensic problems.

Linkage

The tests for blood group antigens are relatively simple and reliable, and the heredity of blood groups is well established; the red cell antigens still remain one of the most useful tools for linkage investigations. **Linkage** is an association of two or more genes in inheritance due to the fact that they are located in the same chromosome pair. By tracing the appearance of two or more pairs of allelic genes in the parents and in the offspring, the frequency of cross-over can be determined and then is used as a measure of the distance separating the loci for two alleles. The recombination frequency is a direct index of the distance between the genes. Special mathematical methods for detection and measurement of linkage in man have been devised, among others those by Bernstein, Wiener, Haldane, and Fisher. For details, the reader is referred to articles by Smith.[4,5]

The first example of autosomal linkage involving blood groups was discovered in man in 1951 by Mohr.[6,7] It dealt with the *Lutheran* genes and with what then seemed to be the *Lewis* genes but which later proved to be *secretor* genes. During the next 25 years several other linkages were found between autosomal blood group loci and other hereditary characteristics (isozymes, white cell antigens, serum groups, certain congenital malformations, etc.). A detailed review of the subject can be found in the book by Race and Sanger.[8]

Mapping of the chromosomes

The knowledge of genetic markers, such as blood groups, serum groups, and isozymes, and the development of statistical methods for detection and measurement of linkage between chromosomal markers opened the doors to the possibility of locating particular genes on numbered pairs of human autosomes. This was first observed in 1968 when the *Duffy* locus was shown to be on autosome No. 1.

More recent additions to the knowledge of the location of blood group genes were the finding of the A-B-O loci on the ninth pair of autosomes, and of the Rh loci on the first pair of autosomal chromosomes. The most complete (1977) presentation of the status of the gene map of the human chromosomes is that by McKusick and Ruddle.[9]

Particularly promising are studies concerning loci situated on the X-chromosome because of the characteristic inheritance of these alleles. It is not surprising that more is known about the relative positions of X-chromosome genes than about autosomal ones, even though the latter are more numerous. Particular attention has been paid in recent years to the Xg blood group locus (p. 184ff) and to the traits and conditions linked to the Xg group. The problem of linkage with *Xg* and of mapping of X-chromosomes is discussed at length by Race and Sanger[8] and by Levitan and Montagu.[10]

Determination of zygosity of twins

Blood groups are of practical importance for discriminating between identical (monovular) and fraternal (biovular) twins. If the blood groups or the sex of twins are different, it is obvious that the twins are biovular. If the twins are of the same sex and their blood groups are identical, the problem of zygosity is not automatically solved, but the chances that the twins are biovular can be calculated on the basis of blood grouping tests. Two sets of formulas have been derived for calculating the chances that a pair of presumably fraternal twins is actually biovular. One set deals with cases in which parental blood groups are known; the other concerns cases in which parental groups are not known. For details, see Wiener and Socha[11] or Wiener and Leff.[12]

Identity

Except for identical (monovular) twins, it is estimated that no two individuals have identical blood groups and types, but until and unless all the blood group specificities possible to man can be found and identified, cataloguing people by their blood group factors will not be as precise as identifying them by their fingerprints. Such a goal has been established. Research continues not only in the realm of human blood groups but also in the study of the blood of nonhuman primates and other animals.

More than 50 million combinations of blood group factors can be clearly differentiated by blood typing today, assuming that the antisera employed to identify each specificity are available and usable. Some are exceedingly difficult to use or to read once they have reacted, and they are therefore worthless, except in the hands of specially trained and experienced experts. Some are in such short supply that

they are unavailable to many serologists. It is fortunate that only a few of the blood group specificities play a significant role in blood transfusion and in the development of erythroblastosis fetalis.

It must be constantly stressed that only an expert with his systems of checks and counterchecks, controls, blind tests, and reliable reagents should be permitted to make and report results of examinations involving parentage.

REFERENCES

1. Watkins, W. M. In Wiener, A. S., editor: Advances in blood grouping, vol. 3, New York, 1970, Grune & Stratton, Inc.
2. Ceppellini, R. In International Society of Blood Transfusion: Proceedings of the 5th Congress, Paris, 1955.
3. Sussman, L. N.: Am. J. Med. Technol., p. 87, March-April, 1965.
4. Smith, C. A. B.: J. R. Stat. Soc. [B] **15**:153, 1953.
5. Smith, C. A. B.: Am. J. Hum. Genet. **11**: 289, 1959.
6. Mohr, J.: Acta Pathol. Microbiol. Scand. **29**: 339, 1951.
7. Mohr, J.: A study of linkage in man, Copenhagen, 1954, Einar Munksgaard Forlag.
8. Race, R. R., and Sanger, R.: Blood groups in man, ed. 6, Oxford, England, 1975, Blackwell Scientific Publications.
9. McKusick, V. A., and Ruddle, F. H.: Science **196**:390, 1977.
10. Levitan, M., and Montagu, A.: Textbook of human genetics, ed. 2, New York, 1977, Oxford University Press.
11. Wiener, A. S., and Socha, W. W.: A-B-O blood groups and Lewis types, New York, 1976, Stratton Intercontinental Medical Book Corporation.
12. Wiener, A. S., and Leff, I. L.: Genetics **25**: 187, 1940.

RECOMMENDED READINGS

Prokop, O., and Uhlenbruck, G.: Human blood and serum groups, New York, 1969, John Wiley & Sons, Inc.

Stern, C.: Principles of human genetics, ed. 3, San Francisco, 1973, W. H. Freeman & Co.

Wiener, A. S., and Wexler, I. B.: Heredity of the blood groups, New York, 1958, Grune & Stratton, Inc.

Refer also to the list in Chapter 4.

14 □ Blood groups and disease

Hemolytic disease due to serologic incompatibility between the mother and the fetus constitutes the best-known example of an association between blood groups and disease. This association has been proved in many ways—by statistical analysis, by serologic investigations, and by clinical evidence, among others. In 1968 the Duffy locus was found to be linked to deformity of the long arm of No. 1 autosome (p. 155), and more recently (1975) direct proof was obtained of an association between Duffy (Fy) genotypes and susceptibility to invasion by the simian malarial parasite *Plasmodium knowlesi* (p. 155). Some other associations also appear to be irrefutable; for example, a relationship has been discovered between concentration and kind of plasma alkaline phosphatase isozymes and the A-B-O blood groups and secretor status.[1] A similar association has been found in cattle. In pigs an association has been established[2] between the red cell antigen I_b and the serum amylase enzymes, and in sheep there is a close association between M red cell antigen and serum potassium concentration.[3] So far no satisfactory explanation for these associations has been demonstrated. They are, however, reminiscent of the negative association in man between the A-B-H secretor types and the Lewis blood types, which has been explained by competition between the *Se* and *Le* genes for a common substrate. A similar plausible explanation for the association between the blood types and isozymes could be that the products of the blood group genes are somehow involved in the biosynthesis of the isozymes.[4] At any rate, the association between blood groups and isozymes constitutes a new field of research that promises to yield important results once the biochemical basis for the association has been discovered.

Biochemical studies of the human blood group antigens have recently (1974, 1975) resulted in discovery[5,6] of an association between M and N agglutinogens and their precursors and the tumor antigens on the surface of the human breast cancer cells. The importance of this discovery, which, for the first time, has shown a direct link between red cell antigens and malignancy, may be far reaching. Another important discovery links a very rare homozygous Kell phenotype, K_o, with so-called chronic granulomatous disease[7,8] (p. 152), and the McCleod phenotype (KL) with certain hematologic changes (pp. 152 and 153).

In contrast to these associations, which can be either experimentally reproduced or at least theoretically explained, a very large number of controversial reports have claimed the existence of an association between blood groups and disease merely on the basis of statistical comparison of the distribution of blood groups among patients with various diseases and that among healthy controls. The purpose of such studies was to determine whether the blood group to which a person belongs has any effect on his susceptibility to disease. In the case of the A-B-O blood groups, such studies appeared reasonable because the ubiquitous nature of A and B blood group substances and of anti-**A** and anti-**B** agglutinins suggested their fundamental importance.

During the past 25 years, hundreds of

Table 14-1. A-B-O blood groups of patients with carcinoma of the stomach[*]

Source		Total	Group O		Group A		Group B		Group AB	
			Number	Percent	Number	Percent	Number	Percent	Number	Percent
Austria										
Vienna	Carcinoma	1,146	415	36.2	505	44.1	143	12.5	83	7.2
	Control	10,000	3,631	36.3	4,422	44.2	1,343	13.4	604	6.0
Italy										
Cremona	Carcinoma	300	31	10.3	254	84.7	10	3.3	5	1.7
	Control	1,762	671	38.1	826	46.9	183	10.4	82	4.7

[*]Modified by Wiener[4] from McConnell, R. B.: The genetics of gastro-intestinal disorders, London, 1966, Oxford University Press.

reports have been published on distributions of blood groups among patients with such conditions as schizophrenia (dementia precox), general paresis, rheumatic fever, epilepsy, longevity, arteriosclerosis, poliomyelitis, hypertension, gastric and duodenal ulcers, stomach cancer, pernicious anemia, and many others. In many cases the investigations have disclosed no evidence of any association; in other cases in which an association was reported, this could not be confirmed in subsequent studies. Often, as pointed out by Wiener,[9] the fallacious conclusions and claims of association between blood groups and disease are due to fundamental errors. For instance, in some cases the technic of blood typing is suspect, as in the report that claimed every one of twenty-eight patients with Dupuytren's contracture belonged to type Rh_1Rh_2. Among many examples of gross errors in blood grouping, the article claiming association between type N and rheumatic fever has been shown by Wiener[10] to have a great excess of type MN (more than 56%, as opposed to the theoretical maximum of 50%).

Another frequent error is the failure to take into account the *a priori* likelihood of an association. Maternofetal incompatibility is a reasonable explanation, but there is no plausible mechanism by which one's blood group could affect one's personality or the occurrence of pituitary adenomas, for which, therefore, the *a priori* probabilities of an association are minute. To illustrate this point, Wiener[11] quoted Mc-

Connell's book, *The Genetics of Gastrointestinal Disorders,* in which an association between group A and carcinoma of the stomach is claimed on the basis of large numbers of independent studies. Wiener selected two of the seventy-one series on which this conclusion was based; they are shown in Table 14-1.

As can be seen, the larger Vienna series shows no evidence of association, whereas the smaller Cremona series shows almost twice as many group A individuals among patients with carcinoma as among healthy controls. Obviously, the series for Vienna and for Cremona cannot both be correct. Based on *a priori* probabilities, the Vienna series, which shows no association, is almost surely the correct one, and it seems likely that bias in collecting the data was responsible for the contrasting results observed in the Cremona series.

A further serious pitfall is the danger of bias when selecting cases for inclusion in a series, especially when criteria for diagnosis of a disease are not sharply defined. For example, Billington[12] could not confirm his cases according to anatomic location and concluded that the association existed only for lesions in the body of the stomach. When challenged by Wiener, Billington forthrightly acknowledged that he might have been influenced in borderline cases by knowledge of the patient's blood group.

"Stratification" is another pitfall when one compares the distribution of the blood groups in a series of patients with that of a control series. Few populations in large cities are homogenous; most consist of individuals of more than one ethnic origin. Very often the control series has consisted of tens of thousands of blood donors typed within a short period of time in blood donor centers, whereas the experimental group was pulled from the records of many hospitals over a period of several years. As shown by Socha,[13] this difference in the method of compiling the data in the two series may introduce a serious bias into the results.

It is obvious that reliability of conclusions based on statistical analysis, as in the case of studies of blood groups in various diseases, depends largely on careful elimination of all possible sources of errors and bias. When such conditions are met, the evidences indicating possible relationship of blood groups to disease cannot all be dismissed lightly. When so many independent workers report an association between group O, secretor status, and duodenal ulcer, for example, the matter cannot be considered closed, even though no plausible mechanism for such association has been proposed. As with other research problems, what is needed here is not more statistical data, but rather new ideas and insight.

REFERENCES

1. Arfors, K. E., Beckman, L., and Lundin, L. K.: Acta Genet. Statis. Med. (Basel) **13**: 366, 1963.
2. Andresen, E.: Science **153**:1660, 1966.
3. Rasmussen, B. A., and Hall, J. G.: Science **151**:1551, 1966.
4. Wiener, A. S.: Am. J. Hum. Genet. **22**:476, 1970.
5. Springer, G. F., and Desai, P. R.: Ann. Clin. Lab. Sci. **4**:294, 1974.
6. Springer, G. F., Desai, P. R., and Scanlon, E. F.: In Cellular membranes and tumor cell behavior, Baltimore, 1975, The Williams & Wilkins Co.
7. Marsh, W. L., Øyen, R., Nichols, M. E., and Allen, F. H.: Br. J. Haematol. **29**:247, 1975.
8. Marsh, W. L., Øyen, R., and Nichols, M. E.: Vox Sang. **31**:356, 1976.
9. Wiener, A. S.: Advances in blood grouping, vol. II, New York, 1965, Grune & Stratton, Inc.
10. Wiener, A. S., and Wexler, I. B.: J.A.M.A., p. 1474, Dec. 15, 1956.
11. Wiener, A. S.: Med. Opinion Rev. **3**:148, 1967.
12. Billington, B. R.: Lancet **2**:859, 1956.
13. Socha, W. W.: Problems of serological differentiation of human populations, Warsaw, 1966, Polish State Medical Publication.

PART TWO □ **Blood groups of nonhuman primates**

15 □ Human-type blood groups in nonhuman primates

The study of blood groups in nonhuman primates is of interest not only as an end in itself but especially because of the close relationship of their groups to those of man. Such studies have contributed insight into the human blood groups that could not otherwise have been obtained short of unacceptable human experimentation.

The first systematic studies of the blood group of apes and monkeys were those of Landsteiner and Miller,[1] but these were principally limited to the A-B-O groups, and only relatively few animals were tested. Intensive studies have more recently been carried out, notably by Wiener and Gordon and by Wiener, Moor-Jankowski, and their team of workers. From these investigations has come a good deal of knowledge about the blood groups of the nonhuman primates.

Wiener and Moor-Jankowski[2,3] classified their studies under two broad categories: (1) tests for human-type blood factors, which are made with reagents originally prepared for typing human blood and therefore detect homologues of the human blood groups in apes and monkeys, and (2) tests for simian-type blood factors, which are made with reagents produced by immunizing experimental animals with the blood of apes and monkeys or, preferably, by isoimmunization or cross-immunization of these animals. The results are presented in this chapter and Chapter 16 and are classified under these two main categories —human-type and simian-type blood groups. Methodology of blood grouping in apes and monkeys is discussed in Chapter 24.

A-B-O GROUPS

Some of the early workers used human anti-**A** and anti-**B** sera directly for typing the blood of apes and monkeys, which resulted in errors, since these reagents usually contain nonspecific heteroagglutinins. Consequently, some chimpanzees were incorrectly grouped as AB, a blood group that does not occur in this species. Wiener showed that this problem could be avoided by using potent reagents diluted beyond the point of activity of the nonspecific heteroagglutinins or by absorbing the reagents with chimpanzee group O red cells. This obviates preparation of eluates as used by Landsteiner and Miller in their earlier work. Lectins and snail agglutinins are advantageous because they do not require purification by absorption.

When red blood cells and sera of primate animals are cross matched, isoagglutination is observed in the case of chimpanzees, gibbons, and orangutans among the anthropoid apes but not in gorillas. Isoagglutination does not usually occur when red cells and sera of animals of Old World and New World monkeys of the same species are cross matched. Wiener was the first to call attention to the fact that, despite the absence of isoagglutinins in gorillas and monkeys, they do have A-B-O blood groups homologous to the human A-B-O blood groups. It is true that the red cells fail to agglutinate even with the most potent anti-**A**, anti-**B**, or anti-**H** reagents, but the blood group substances are present in the body fluids and secretions, notably in the saliva. In fact, among hundreds of apes and monkeys tested by Wiener and Moor-Jankowski and their team, all proved to be A-B-H secretors, except for a single orangutan. Thus the A-B-O blood groups of gorillas and monkeys can be determined by **testing their saliva for the blood group substances** by the inhibition method and the **serum for anti-A and anti-B agglutinins** by absorbing it first with human group O blood cells to remove nonspecific heteroagglutinins, then testing the absorbed serum against human A and B cells.

Landsteiner's rule* holds in general, except that in gorillas and monkeys the reciprocal relationship is between agglutinins in serum and blood group substances in saliva or other secretions, whereas in man, chimpanzees, gibbons, and orangutans it is between serum agglutinins and red cell agglutinogens.

Table 15-1 gives the results obtained in the studies of A. S. Wiener and his collaborators[4] on the human-type A-B-O blood groups of apes and monkeys.

All the chimpanzees of the common species *Pan troglodytes* tested so far were found to be group A or group O, the frequency of group O ranging in different subspecies of *P. troglodytes* from as low as 9% in *P. troglodytes verus* to as high as 40% in *P. troglodytes schweinfurthi*. This is comparable to the situation in various populations of man.

The very rare pigmy chimpanzee, *P. paniscus*, is considered to be a distinct species rather than a subspecies of chimpanzees. All nine pigmy chimpanzees tested so far were group A, and their red cells gave reactions indistinguishable from human subgroup A_1 with various anti-A_1 reagents. In contrast, the red cells of *P.*

troglodytes give weaker reactions with anti-A_1 than do human subgroup A_1 cells. Moreover, in chimpanzees of the common species *P. troglodytes,* subgroups of A appear to exist, since the red cells of about one tenth of group A chimpanzees give still weaker reactions with anti-A_1 although they are not negative as are human subgroup A_2 cells. Thus the relative reactivity of the human and chimpanzee group A red cells may be arranged as follows[5]:

Human A_1
P. paniscus $>$ *P. troglodytes* A_1 $>$
$\qquad$ *P. troglodytes* A_2 $>$ Human A_2

Another difference between human and chimpanzee group A red cells is that, in contrast to man, red cells from chimpanzees of group A, irrespective of subgroup, almost invariably fail to agglutinate with anti-**H** lectin. However, salivas from group A as well as group O chimpanzees generally strongly inhibit anti-**H** lectin. Group O chimpanzee red cells are, with few exceptions, agglutinated by anti-**H** lectins.

In gibbons, isoagglutination defines three blood groups homologous to the human groups A, B, and AB; group O was not found among 140 animals tested to date. Although the subspecies *Hylobates lar lar* makes up the bulk of the gibbons tested so far, there are enough data to indicate significant racial differences in the distributions of A-B-O blood groups in gibbons. For example, all four *Hylobates lar pileatus* tested were group B.

Tests for subgroups of A reveal the presence of subgroups A_1, A_2, A_1B, and A_2B in gibbons whose red cells give reactions with anti-**A** reagents comparable to those of human red cells of the corresponding subgroups. Gibbon red cells differ from human red cells, however, in that group B gibbon red cells are strongly agglutinated by anti-**H** lectin, the intensity and titer of the reactions being comparable to those of human group O cells. On the other hand, gibbon red cells of groups A and AB give negative or only weakly positive reactions with anti-**H.**

---

*When an isoagglutinogen is lacking in the blood cells, the corresponding isoagglutinin is present in the serum of the same blood.

Table 15-1. A-B-O blood groups of apes and monkeys[*]

Species	Blood groups				Totals	Remarks
	O	**A**	**B**	**AB**		
Anthropoid apes						
Chimpanzees						
Common type	50	483	0	0	533	Subgroups A_1 and A_2 present
Pigmy	0	9	0	0	9	All of type A_1
Gibbons (various species)	0	27	59	54	140	Subgroups A_1, A_2, A_1B and A_2B present
Siamangs	0	0	2	0	2	
Orangutans	0	41	14	16	71	Subgroups A_1, A_2, A_1B, and A_2B observed
Gorillas						
Lowland	0	0	23	0	23	Subgroups B_1 and B_2 present
Mountain	0	0	4	0	4	
Old World monkeys						
Baboons						
Olive	0	5	133	56	194	
Hamadryas	0	15	107	50	172	
Hybrids	0	5	81	43	129	
Yellow	0	18	20	22	60	
Chacma	0	4	59	26	89	
Guinea	2	27	93	66	188	
Species unknown	1	42	65	65	173	
Macaques						Subgroups of B possible
Rhesus	0	0	150	0	150	
Bonnet	0	18	12	15	45	
Crab-eating	1	23	19	19	62	
Stump-tailed	0	0	14	0	14	
Pig-tailed	87	18	10	3	118	
Geladas	18	0	0	0	18	Anti-**A** and anti-**B** not always present
Drills	0	4	0	0	4	
Celebes black apes	1	23	2	0	26	Expected isoagglutinins often lacking
Patas monkeys	0	26	0	0	26	Subgroups A_1 and A_2 present
Vervet monkeys						
Jolley et al.[†]	0	126	1	1	128	Ethiopia
Downing et al.[‡]	0	39	10	10	59	South Africa
New World monkeys						
Spider monkeys, various species	1	10	4	0	15	
Squirrel monkeys	1	3	0	0	4	
Capuchins						
White-fronted	1	0	3	0	4	
Black-capped	0	5	0	0	5	
Howler monkeys	0	0	52	0	52	
Marmosets (various species)	0	45	0	0	45	

[*]Modified from Wiener, A. S., Socha, W. W., and Moor-Jankowski, J.: Haematologia (Budap.) **8**:195, 1974.
[†]Modified from Jolley, C. J., Turner, T. R., Socha, W. W., and Wiener, A. S.: J. Med. Primatol. **6**:54, 1977.
[‡]Downing, H. J., Benimadho, S., Bolstridge, M.C., et al.: J. Med. Primatol. **2**:290, 1973.

Salivas from fifty-seven gibbons have been tested, and all the animals were found to be A-B-H secretors. All secreted the H substance in high titer, together with the A-B blood group substances corresponding to their blood group.

In orangutans, as in gibbons, isoagglutination shows the presence of only three blood groups homologous to the human blood groups A, B, and AB, with group O absent or very rare. When tested with anti-A_1 reagent, the red cells of groups A and AB orangutans gave reactions corresponding to human subgroups A_1, A_2, A_1B, or A_2B. In contrast to gibbon red cells, the red cells of all orangutans, irrespective of blood group, fail to react with anti-**H** lectin.

The reactions of gorilla blood resemble those of Old World monkeys more closely than those of other anthropoid apes and man in that the red cells fail to react with anti-**A,** anti-**B,** and anti-**H** reagents. The A-B-O groups can nevertheless be determined easily by testing the saliva for the A-B-H group substances, as in monkeys, and by testing the serum, after absorption with human group O cells, for anti-**A** and anti-**B** agglutinins. With these methods, all twenty-seven gorillas tested so far were found to be group B. In inhibition tests on their salivas carried out by titration methods, differences in inhibition titer for anti-**B** were observed, indicating the existence of subgroups B_1 and B_2. Two species of gorilla exist, the lowland gorilla, *Gorilla gorilla gorilla*, and the mountain gorilla, *G. gorilla beringei,* but unlike the situation with common and pigmy chimpanzees, no serologic differences have been detected that could distinguish between two kinds of gorillas.[6]

The fact that gorilla blood, with respect to the A-B-O groups, sharply differs from that of other great apes and resembles more closely that of monkeys does not allow for any conclusions as to the taxonomic position of this species, since it was found that in other blood group systems such as M-N and Rh-Hr, gorillas more closely resemble man than the other apes.[7]

Of the Old World monkeys, the most intensively studied have been baboons because of their use in surgical experimentation, for which blood grouping is important. As can be seen in Table 15-1, various species of baboons have been tested, each showing different distribution of the A-B-O blood groups. In general, groups B and AB are the most common, whereas group O is either absent or is extremely rare, a fact that must be considered when using these animals for transplantation or cross-circulation experiments.

Since not a single animal among more than a thousand baboons tested so far has proved to be a nonsecretor of A-B-H substance, it has always been possible up to now to determine the A-B-O blood groups of baboons from tests on the saliva. In most cases, Landsteiner's rule holds in baboons; however, a certain number of animals have been found with anti-A in the serum despite the presence of the blood group substance A in their saliva. The anti-A in these group A and AB animals is peculiar in that it is not inhibitable by secretor saliva from group A baboons and group A human beings, in contrast to the anti-A from group B baboons and group B humans. These results establish the existence of anti-A agglutinins of two kinds: one designated anti-A^c because it is reactive exclusively with the A substance on the red cells and not in secretions, and the other, designated anti-A^s, which is reactive for the group substances both in secretions and on red cells. Obviously, a group A baboon would hardly be likely to form anti-A^s agglutinins but could produce anti-A^c, which would not react with soluble group A substance in its own secretions and therefore would not be inhibitable by group A secretor saliva.

It is of interest to mention that whereas baboon red cells fail to agglutinate in tests with human anti-**A** serum, human anti-**B** serum, and anti-**H** lectin *(Ulex europeus),* even when reagents of the highest titers and avidity are used, it is possible to bring about the agglutination of baboon red cells with anti-**A** lectin lima bean. Although the reactivity of baboon red cells with that lectin is about the same for animals of groups A, B, and AB, it has been proved that the reaction is due to an A-like specificity, since agglutination of baboon red cells can be inhibited by group A and group AB secretor saliva but not by saliva of group O, group B, or saliva from human nonsecretors. Thus all baboons have on their red cells an agglutinogen with a weak A-like specificity separate from their human-type A-B-O groups. The A-like agglutinogen on the red cells of all baboons evidently does not interfere with the production of anti-**A** agglutinins in the serum of animals that lack A substance in their saliva.

Unlike baboons, all geladas tested so far have seemed to belong to group O, since their salivas inhibited anti-**H** but not anti-**A** or anti-**B**. However, most of the animals did not have the expected anti-**A** and anti-**B** agglutinins in their sera; instead, some animals had anti-**B** alone, others had anti-**A** alone, and still others had neither anti-**A** nor anti-**B**. This suggests that the geladas tested actually had the blood groups A, B, and AB, but for some still undetermined reason, the group substances A and B could not be detected in their saliva.

As many as twelve species of macaques are known. Among these, only a few have so far been studied systematically for their A-B-O blood groups. The results obtained indicate the existence of striking differences in the distribution of the A-B-O blood groups, even between closely related species of macaques. As shown in Table 15-1, all rhesus monkeys and stump-tailed macaques reacted as group B; that is, their saliva gave positive inhibition for B and H but not for A, whereas the serum regularly contained anti-**A** but not anti-**B**. Differences in inhibition titer for anti-**B** may indicate the presence of subgroups of B. In contrast, crab-eating macaques have all four A-B-O blood groups, although, as in baboons, group O is rare. In bonnet macaques, on the other hand, only groups A, B, and AB have been found, but not group O; nevertheless, the

presence of gene O can be inferred from population genetic studies.[8] Pig-tailed macaques, on the other hand, have all four A-B-O blood groups, with group O being the most common.

Two sets of vervet monkeys presented in Table 15-1 offer an example of striking geographic differences in the distribution of the A-B-O blood groups within one and the same primate species. Similar differences have been observed among troops of feral Ethiopian baboons. Observations of these and similar differences in frequencies of blood groups in various populations of primates are the object of **sero-primatology**. The term "sero-primatology" was coined by A. S. Wiener in analogy to "sero-anthropology," to define the characterization of simian populations by differences in the distribution of their serologic properties.

Studies on New World monkeys have been less intensive than on Old World monkeys. Nevertheless, by testing their saliva and serum, it has been possible to demonstrate that they also have homologues of the human type A-B-O blood groups, for which some of the species were shown to be polymorphic. As early as 1925, Landsteiner and Miller[1] pointed out that the red cells of all New World monkeys have a B-like agglutinogen. This occurs irrespective of their "true" A-B-O blood group (as determined by saliva inhibition and serum tests). An outstanding example is provided by the marmosets, which are all human-type group A despite the presence of the B-like agglutinogen on their red cells. This kind of B-like agglutinogen is not limited to New World monkeys but occurs also in lower mammals such as rabbits and guinea pigs and in many species of microorganisms. This is comparable to the Forssman antigen, the distribution of which cuts across taxonomic lines in nature.

The differences among the B agglutinogen of human group B red cells and B-like agglutinogens of the New World monkeys and of rabbits have been shown to be readily demonstrable by successful fractionation experiments of the anti-**B** sera, using the red cells that possess B-like antigen.[9] This has not been possible with the B agglutinogen of ape bloods such as gibbons and orangutans. This is further evidence that whereas the B agglutinogen of apes is truly a homologue of the human agglutinogen B, the B-like agglutinogen of the red cells of New World monkeys has a different significance.

It is noteworthy that parallel studies with anti-**A** reagents gave analogous results, and an A-like antigen could be demonstrated on the red cells of certain mammals, notably sheep and pigs. Again, whereas absorption of human anti-**A** sera with red cells of chimpanzees, orangutans, or gibbons removed the reactivity for sheep red cells as well as for human and ape group A red cells, absorption with sheep red cells left behind a considerable fraction reactive for human or ape group A red cells.[10]

AGGLUTINOGENS M AND N IN APES AND MONKEYS

In early studies on the agglutinogen M in rhesus monkeys, conflicting results were obtained, since some investigators reported its presence and others its absence. Wiener demonstrated the presence on the red cells of rhesus monkeys of an agglutinogen similar but not identical to the human agglutinogen M. Using a panel of six different anti-**M** reagents prepared by immunization of rabbits with human blood, he extended his studies to other monkeys and to the apes and published his findings in collaboration with Landsteiner in 1937.[11] The principles involved are most simply explained by citing Wiener's studies on chimpanzees,[12] as in Table 15-2.

Wiener found that most anti-**M** reagents agglutinate the red cells of all chimpanzees, but a few anti-**M** sera fail to react. That the positively reacting reagents were detecting an M-like agglutinogen on the red cells of chimpanzees was clear, since absorption of the active anti-**M** reagents by human M cells removed the reactivity also for chimpanzee red cells. When the active anti-**M** reagents were absorbed by chimpanzee red cells, however, in some cases the reactivity for human M blood cells was also removed, but in other cases a fraction of the agglutinins still reactive for human type M blood remained behind. Thus at least two fractions of antibodies could be separated from anti-**M** sera, one of which was reactive for chimpanzee red cells as

Table 15-2. Reactions of red cells of apes and monkeys with anti-**M** reagents*

	Anti-M reagents					
Red cells	**1**	**2**	**3**	**4**	**5**	**6**
Human M	+++	+++	++±	++±	++±	++±
Human N	−	−	−	−	−	−
Human MN	+++	+++	++±	++±	++±	++±
Chimpanzee						
(*Pan troglodytes*)	+++	+++	++±	++±	++±	−
Rhesus monkey						
(*Macaca mulatta*)	++±	++±	++	+	−	−
Green monkey						
(*Cercopithecus pygerythrus*)	+++	+++	−	−	−	−
Black spider monkey						
(*Ateles ater*)	+++	−	−	−	−	−
White spider monkey						
(*Ateles*)	+	−	−	−	−	−
Capuchin monkey						
(*Cebus capucinus*)	−	−	−	−	−	−

*Modified from Moor-Jankowski, J., and Wiener, A. S. In Fiennes, R. N., editor: Pathology of simian primates, Basel, 1972, S. Karger AG.

well as for human M red cells, the other reactive for human M red cells alone. (This is comparable to the two fractions of agglutinin that can be separated from anti-**A** serum by absorption—one reactive for both A₁ and A₂ human red cells, the other reactive for human A₁ cells alone.)

Similarly, in tests with anti-**N** reagents, two analogous fractions of antibodies could be separated by absorption experiments using chimpanzee red cells.

When Wiener and Landsteiner extended the experiments to other species of apes and to monkeys, the situation was found to be far more complicated, as shown in Table 15-2. From the cross-reactions of anti-**M** reagents with simian red cells, at least five different kinds of anti-**M** specificities were demonstrated in these early experiments, even though these five different kinds of anti-**M** reagents gave parallel reaction in tests on human blood.

As expected, Landsteiner and Wiener found that when rabbits were immunized with red cells of rhesus monkeys the resulting immune rabbit sera, after absorption with human type N cells, yielded anti-**M** reagents suitable for typing human blood. Of course, the specificity of anti-**M** reagents produced by immunization with rhesus

monkey blood could hardly be identical to that of anti-**M** reagents produced by immunization with human type M blood. Nevertheless, the two kinds of reagents gave indistinguishable reactions when the tests were limited to human blood alone. These findings were important especially because continuation of the immunization experiments with rhesus monkey blood led to the discovery of the Rh factor by Landsteiner and Wiener. Moreover, they showed again the fallacy of the concept of a 1:1 correspondence between antigen and antibody, as well as the fundamental importance of Wiener's concept of the difference between an agglutinogen and its serologic specificities (blood factors), without which these findings would be totally unintelligible.

The studies on agglutinogen N yielded results similar in principle but not as complex, though this was only because of the lack of a great enough variety of potent anti-**N** reagents. For their studies on the N agglutinogens in apes, Wiener et al.[13] found anti-**N** lectin *(Vicia graminea)*, first described by Ottensooser and Silberschmidt,[14] extremely useful (Table 15-3).

In Table 15-3 are summarized the findings to date of Wiener and his collabora-

Table 15-3. Human-type **M** and **N** blood factors in apes*

Species	M-like factors		
	Present	Absent	Totals
Chimpanzees *(Pan troglodytes)*	130	0	130
Gibbons			
Hylobates lar lar	21	31	52
Hylobates lar pileatus	4	0	4
Orangutans *(Pongo pygmaeus)*	12	12	24
Gorillas *(Gorilla gorilla gorilla)*	9	3	12
	Nᵛ factor *(Vicia graminea)*		
Chimpanzees *(Pan troglodytes)*	42	62	104
Gibbons			
Hylobates lar lar	43	9	52
Hylobates lar pileatus	0	4	4
Orangutans *(Pongo pygmaeus)*	0	24	24
Gorillas *(Gorilla gorilla gorilla)*	12	0	12

*Modified from Moor-Jankowski J., and Wiener, A. S. In Fiennes, R. N., editor: Pathology of simian primates, Basel, 1972, S. Karger AG.

tors in their studies on homologues of the human M-N types in apes. The most interesting results were obtained in gibbons. Some anti-**M** reagents clumped the red cells of all gibbons, other anti-**M** reagents failed to react at all with red cells of any gibbons, and still others showed individual blood differences among gibbons; the same was true for anti-**N** reagents. Using selected anti-**M** reagents together with anti-**N** lectin, three types of gibbon blood could be defined homologous but not identical, of course, to the three human M-N types. These three types were found in the subspecies *Hylobates lar lar;* the distribution of the types satisfied the Hardy-Weinberg law under the assumption that heredity is by a mechanism similar to that in man.

Because of the limited space in this book, the reader is referred to original sources at the end of the chapter for further details regarding this subject.

Rh-Hr BLOOD TYPES IN APES AND MONKEYS

In the initial tests on chimpanzee red cells, Wiener and Wade found all the animals tested to be Rh negative. This report was confirmed by British investigators. However, as Wiener and his associates soon found, all chimpanzees are actually Rh positive, but the Rh agglutinogen in chimpanzees is not the same as the Rh agglutinogen of human blood, although it is homologous. For the original experiments, Wiener had used anti-rhesus monkey guinea pig serum and saline agglutinating anti-Rh_0 serum to test the cells, but neither of these agglutinates chimpanzee red cells. However, when chimpanzee red cells are ficinated or treated with other proteolytic enzymes, they are strongly agglutinated by human anti-Rh_0 sera and to almost the same titer as are human Rh_0-positive cells.[15] Likewise, when the chimpanzee red cells are maximally coated with anti-Rh_0 sera, they are clumped by anti-human globulin sera to almost the same titer as maximally sensitized human Rh_0-positive red cells. All chimpanzees, therefore, have an Rh agglutinogen

homologous but not identical to the human Rh_0 agglutinogen. In addition, Wiener et al.[16] found that ficinated chimpanzee red cells are also agglutinated by anti-**hr′** sera to almost the same titer as are human **hr′**-positive red cells, but they fail to react with anti-**rh′**, anti-**rh″**, or anti-**hr″** reagents. Since the red cells lack both members of the contrasting pair, **rh″-hr″**, the chimpanzee Rh type has been assigned the symbol $\overline{Rh}_0^{Ch}$.

Absorption of human anti-Rh_0 sera by human Rh-positive red cells eliminates the reactivity also for chimpanzee red cells, as expected, but absorption with chimpanzee red cells leaves behind a fraction of Rh_0 antibodies still having a considerable titer for human Rh-positive red cells. These experiments show that, as in the case of the anti-**M** reagents, anti-Rh_0 sera can be fractionated into antibodies reactive with chimpanzee red cells, as well as with human Rh_0-positive red cells, and into other antibodies reactive with human Rh_0-positive red cells alone. Moreover, absorption of the human anti-Rh_0 sera with appropriately selected chimpanzee red cells leaves behind at least two other fractions, each detecting a different simian-type specificity on the chimpanzee red cells, namely c^c [17] and L^c [18] (see section on simian-type blood groups). Thus human anti-Rh_0 reagents detect, in chimpanzee blood, types somewhat analogous to the human Rh-positive and Rh-negative types. Recent discovery of a chimpanzee isoimmune serum capable of distinguishing between human Rh-positive and Rh-negative red cells constitutes further evidence of the intimate relationship between human and chimpanzee Rh agglutinogens.[18]

Gorilla red cells react with human Rh-Hr antisera much like the chimpanzee red cells do; that is, they give positive reactions for Rh_0 and **hr′** but negative reactions for **rh′**, **rh″**, and **hr″**. Some gorilla red cells give only weak reactions with anti-Rh_0 sera, however, and these, as well as the strong reactions, can be eliminated by absorption with the human Rh_0-positive red cells. Among gorillas, therefore, most react as type $\bar{R}h_o$, with a minority reacting as type $\bar{r}h$ or $\bar{\Re}h_o$. By absorption experiments on ape red cells, Wiener, Socha, and Gordon[19] have separated so far the following fractions of antibodies, among others, from human anti-Rh_o sera.*

1. Antibodies reactive for red cells of chimpanzees and gorillas as well as for human Rh_o-positive red cells
2. Antibodies reactive with the red cells of gorillas and with human Rh_o-positive red cells but not with the red cells of the chimpanzee
3. Antibodies reactive with the red cells of all chimpanzees and Rh-positive gorillas but not with the red cells of "Rh-negative" gorillas
4. Antibodies reactive with human Rh_o-positive red cells alone but not with the red cells of *any* chimpanzees or gorillas

It would seem that the possibilities for fractionation of antibodies of human anti-Rh_o sera are virtually limitless.

The red cells of gibbons have also been tested; they fail to react with anti-Rh_o reagents. They do react with anti-hr' reagents but not with anti-rh', anti-rh'', or anti-hr''. Gibbons therefore are all type $\bar{r}h$.

Orangutans have red cells giving reactions comparable to human Rh_{null} blood.[20]

OTHER HUMAN-TYPE BLOOD FACTORS OF APES AND MONKEYS

Tests for human-type blood factors of other blood group systems have also been carried out, but because of the low titer of the reagents and the presence in them of interfering nonspecific heteroagglutinating substances, in most cases the results have been inconclusive. Among the most convincing results were those observed with anti-P reagents. The red cells of all chimpanzees tested gave negative reactions for this blood factor. The most interesting re-

sults were those obtained in tests for the **I-i** blood factors.

BLOOD FACTORS I AND i IN NONHUMAN PRIMATES AND OTHER ANIMALS

The tests for blood specificities **I** and **i** in nonhuman primates have been made with anti-**I** serum of human origin, the antiserum having been derived from the same source as that with which the factor **I** was discovered by Wiener et al.[21] The anti-i serum came from a patient with severe idiopathic hemolytic anemia. In humans, adults in general have blood factor **I** but lack **i**, and those rare adults who lack **I** have blood factor **i**. Blood factor **i** is found, however, in cord blood and in the blood of newborn infants, whereas **I** is not yet developed. (See p. 173.)

All chimpanzees and orangutans tested have lacked blood factor **I** but have had blood factor **i**. Gibbons lack both blood factors **I** and **i**.[22]

All species of Old World monkeys tested lacked factor **I** and had factor **i** well developed (Table 15-4), but the findings in New World monkeys varied from one species to another. For example, the red cells of two species of *Cercocebus* reacted weakly with anti-**I** serum but strongly with anti-**i**. Squirrel monkeys and white-whiskered spider monkeys also had **i** but little or no **I**. On the other hand, capuchin monkeys' red cells reacted strongly with anti-**I** but hardly at all with anti-**i**.

Sheep, goats, deer, cats, and South American agouti all lacked specificities **I** and **i**. Dogs and rats lacked **I** but reacted distinctly, although in low titer, for blood factor **i**. Rabbit red cells reacted strongly and in high titer with anti-**I** but did not react with anti-**i**.

Wiener has pointed out that chimpanzee red cells resemble those of newborn human beings in their reactions not only with anti-**I** and anti-**i** but also with anti-A_1 and anti-**H** reagents.

There is no discernible, consistent pattern in the distribution of blood factors **I**

---

*See p. 178 for antibodies fractionated from guinea pig anti-rhesus monkey sera.

Table 15-4. Human-type blood factors **I** and **i** in primates and lower animals[*]

Species	Titers† with		Species	Titers† with	
	Anti-I	Anti-i		Anti-I	Anti-i
Man			New World monkeys		
Newborn	0	64	Capuchin monkeys (various		
Adult, typical	32	0	species)	128	1
Adult, type i	0	16	Squirrel monkeys (*Saimiri*		
Apes			*sciureus*)	0	16
Chimpanzees (*Pan troglodytes*)	0	16	Spider monkeys (various species)	2	32
Gibbons (*Hylobates lar lar* and			Marmosets (various species)	32	64
Hylobates lar pileatus)	0	0	Prosimians		
Orangutans (*Pongo pygmaeus*)	0	4	Potto (*Perodicticus potto*)	0	0
Old World monkeys			Slow loris (*Nycticebus coucang*)	0	32
Baboons (*Papio cynocephalus*			Lower mammals		
and *Papio anubis*)	0	64	Sheep	0	0
Geladas (*Theropithecus gelada*)	0	64	Goats	0	0
Patas monkeys (*Erythrocebus*			Cats	0	0
patas)	1	32	Dogs	0	0
Vervet monkeys			Rabbits	512	0
(*Cercopithecus pygerythrus*)	1	32	Rats	0	8
Sykes monkeys (*Cercopithecus*			Deer	0	0
albogularus)	0	32			
Mangabeys (various species)	2	64			

[*]Modified from Moor-Jankowski J., and Wiener, A. S. In Fiennes, R. N., editor: Pathology of simian primates, Basel, 1972, S. Karger AG.

†Titers are the reciprocals of the highest dilution of the antiserum giving a positive reaction; for example, a titer of 64 means that clumping occurs with the reagent in dilutions up to 1:64, whereas a titer of 1 means that clumping occurs only with undiluted reagent.

and **i** among the nonhuman primates other than those already listed. In many cases, blood factors **I** and **i** behave as though they were reciprocally related, but since both occur in the cells of marmosets and both are absent in gibbons and in most of the lower mammals, this relationship is certainly not absolute. Both factors **I** and **i** behave like heterophile antigens in that their distribution cuts across taxonomic lines.

The work of Costea et al. in producing anti-**I** cold agglutinins of high titer in rabbits by injection of heat-killed *Listeria monocytogenes* has already been mentioned on p. 174.

Table 15-4 is a résumé of the findings of Wiener et al. on the blood factors **I** and **i** in primates and lower animals.

REFERENCES

1. Landsteiner, K., and Miller, C. P.: J. Exp. Med. **42**:841, 1925.
2. Wiener, A. S.: Advances in blood grouping, vols. I, II, and III, New York, 1961, 1965, 1970, Grune & Stratton, Inc.
3. Moor-Jankowski, J., and Wiener, A. S.: In Fiennes, R. N., editor: Pathology of primates, Basel, 1971, S. Karger AG.
4. Wiener, A. S., Socha, W. W., and Moor-Jankowski, J.: Haematologia (Budap.) **8**:195, 1974.
5. Wiener, A. S., and Socha, W. W.: Int. Arch. Allergy **47**:946, 1974.
6. Socha, W. W., Wiener, A. S., Moor-Jankowski, and Mortelmans, J.: J. Med. Primatol. **2**:364, 1973.
7. Wiener, A. S., Socha, W. W., Arons, E. B., Mortelmans, J., and Moor-Jankowski, J.: J. Med. Primatol. **5**:317, 1976.
8. Socha, W. W., Moor-Jankowski, J., Wiener, A. S., Risser, D. R., and Plonski, H.: Am. J. Phys. Anthropol. **45**:485-491, 1976.
9. Wiener, A. S., and Socha, W. W.: Int. Arch. Allergy **44**:547, 1974.
10. Wiener, A. S., and Socha, W. W.: A-B-O blood groups and Lewis types, New York 1976, Stratton Intercontinental Medical Book Corporation.

11. Landsteiner, K., and Wiener, A. S.: J. Immunol. **33**:19, 1937.
12. Wiener, A. S.: J. Immunol. **34**:11, 1938.
13. Wiener, A. S., Gordon, E. B., Moor-Jankowski, J., and Socha, W. W.: Haematologia (Budap.) **6**:419, 1972.
14. Ottensooser, F., and Silberschmidt, K.: Nature (Lond.) **172**:914, 1953.
15. Wiener, A. S.: Am. J. Phys. Anthropol. **10**:372, 1952.
16. Wiener, A. S., Gavan, J. A., and Gordon, E. B.: Am. J. Phys. Anthropol. **11**:38, 1951.
17. Wiener, A. S., Moor-Jankowski, J., Gordon, E. B., and Kratochvil, C. L.: Proc. Natl. Acad. Sci. U.S.A. **56**:458, 1966.
18. Socha, W. W., and Moor-Jankowski, J.: Int. Arch. Allergy **56**:30-38, 1978.
19. Wiener, A. S., Socha, W. W., and Gordon, E. B.: Haematologia (Budap.) **5**:227, 1971.
20. Moor-Jankowski, J., Wiener, A. S., Socha, W. W., Gordon, E. B., and Kaczera, Z.: Folia Primatol. **19**:360, 1973.
21. Wiener, A. S., Unger, L. J., Cohen, L., and Feldman, J.: Ann. Intern. Med. **44**:221, 1956.
22. Wiener, A. S., Moor-Jankowski, J., Gordon, E. B., and Davis, J.: Am. J. Phys. Anthropol. **23**:239, 1965.

16 □ Simian-type blood groups

In the last 15 years significant progress has been made in the knowledge of the simian-type blood groups of apes and monkeys, thanks primarily to the work of Wiener, Moor-Jankowski, and their collaborators. By isoimmunization or cross-immunization, reagents were produced that were capable of identifying various blood factors on the red cells of anthropoid apes and Old World monkeys. Using the method of population genetics, it has been possible to group a number of factors into blood group systems, some of which were later confirmed by family studies. Table 16-1 presents the current status of knowledge of the simian-type blood groups.

The most thoroughly studied of nonhuman primates have been chimpanzees because of their close relationship to man. To date three blood group systems have been defined, of which the so-called V-A-B[1] and the C-E-F[2] systems are the best known.

THE V-A-B BLOOD GROUP SYSTEM

The V-A-B system appears to be a homologue of the human M-N-S system. The **V** specificity is identified by three different kinds of reagents that give parallel reactions: anti-N^v lectin *(Vicia graminea)*, anti-V^c serum produced by cross immunizing chimpanzees with human red cells, and anti-V^c serum produced by isoimmunizing chimpanzees with red cells of another chimpanzee. The remaining three specificities of the same system, A^c, B^c, and D^c, are defined by isoimmune chimpanzee sera.

That the V-A-B system is a counterpart of the human M-N-S system follows from two facts: (1) anti-N^v, which detects chimpanzee blood specificity V^c, also detects the human blood factor **N** and (2) when chimpanzee red cells are treated with proteolytic enzymes like ficin, they no longer are agglutinable by V-A-B-D reagents, just as human red cells lose their reactivity for M-N-S reagents after proteolytic enzyme treatment.

As a link between the chimpanzee blood group system and the human M-N-S system, the specificity V^c occupies a special position in the V-A-B system, and that is indicated in the symbols for the phenotypes. The four standard sera, anti-V^c, anti-A^c, anti-B^c, and anti-D^c, can theoretically determine eleven phenotypes within the V-A-B system: namely, v.O, v.A, v.B, v.D, v.AB, v.AD, v.BD, V.O, V.A, V.B, and V.D. To account for the eleven blood groups supposed to exist, of which all but one (type v.O) have actually been observed, five allelic genes must be postulated: the codominant alleles V, v^A, v^B, and v^D and the amorph (silent) gene v. Statistical analysis of large populations of chimpanzees strongly supports the validity of the five allele theory of inheritance of the V-A-B blood groups. It also explains why no animal of the theoretically expected type v.O has so far been observed; only one would be expected to occur among a total of 500 animals, whereas only about 350 animals have been tested to date with the complete battery of V-A-B-D reagents.

THE C-E-F BLOOD GROUP SYSTEM

The other important blood system in chimpanzees, the C-E-F system, is a counterpart of the human Rh-Hr system. So

Table 16-1. Simian-type blood groups of apes and monkeys

Species	Blood group system	Specificities	Remarks
Anthropoid apes			
Chimpanzees (common type and pigmy)	V-A-B	V^c, A^c, B^c, D^c	Types observed in common chimpanzee —v.O, v.A, v.B, v.D, v.AB, v.AD, v.BD, V.O, V.A, V.B, V.D; in pigmy chimpanzee only v.D observed
	C-E-F	C^c, c^c, E^c, F^c	Types observed in common chimpanzee —cef, Ccef, CCEf, CcEf, CCeF, Ccef, CCEF, CcEF; in pigmy only CCEf observed
	L-P	L^c, P^c	Types observed—1p, Lp, 1P, LP
		G^c, H^c, I^c, K^c, N^c, O^c, X^c, Y^c	Unrelated factors
Gorillas			Specific reagents not produced; red cells known to react selectively with some chimpanzee isoimmune sera—anti-C^c and anti-F^c
Gibbons		A^g, B^g, C^g	Unrelated factors
Orangutans		Specific reagents unknown	
Old World monkeys			
Baboons		A^p, B^p, C^p, G^p, N^p, hu, ca	G^p and B^p possibly belong to one system; hu and ca possibly related to one another
Rhesus monkeys	Graded D^{rh} system	D_1, D_2, D_3	
		A^{rh}, B^{rh}, C^{rh}, E^{rh}, F^{rh}, G^{rh}, H^{rh}, I^{rh}, J^{rh}	Unrelated factors
Pig-tailed macaques		Share several red cell specificities, including D^{rh} graded system, with rhesus monkeys	
Crab-eating macaques		Share some red cell specificities with rhesus monkeys	

far, by use of isoimmune sera, four blood factors have been identified in this system, C^c, c^c, E^c, and F^c, of which C^c and c^c behave as though inherited by contrasting allelic genes. All chimpanzee red cells having blood factor E^c or F^c or both also have blood specificity C^c, but anti-C^c is not merely a mixture of anti-E^c and F^c, as proved by absorption experiments and the fact that a few chimpanzees have been found having specificity C^c, although lacking both E^c and F^c. Thus the relationship of chimpanzee factor C^c to E^c and F^c is comparable to the relationship of blood factor C of the human A-B-O blood group system to the blood factors A and B.

That the C-E-F system is the counterpart of the human Rh-Hr system follows from two observations: (1) Anti-C^c, anti-c^c, anti-E^c, and anti-F^c reagents react well with chimpanzee red cells by the anti-globulin method but give their strongest reactions with ficinated red cells, just as do human red cells with Rh-Hr antisera, and (2) human anti-Rh_0 sera absorbed with chimpanzee c^c-negative red cells give reactions with red cells of chimpanzees paralleling those of anti-c^c isoimmune serum.

Theoretically, the following nine C-E-F types are possible: cef, CCef, Ccef, CCEf, CcEf, CCeF, CceF, CCEF, and CcEF. Of these, only one has not actually been observed—CCef. Based on analysis by the method of population genetics and using observations on the distribution of the C-E-F types, Wiener et al.[2] postulated the existence of the following five alleles: c, C, C^E, C^F, and C^{EF}. When tested on several chimpanzee populations, the theory of multiple allelic genes gave a good fit. Considering the very low frequency of gene C

(less than 1%), it is not surprising that not a single animal of the homozygous type CCef has been encountered so far.

Quite recently, a third chimpanzee blood group system has emerged,[3] defined by two simian-type specificities, L^c and P^c, which, in turn, determine four types: $l^c p^c$, $L^c p^c$, $l^c P^c$, and $L^c P^c$. Heredity of the L^c-P^c system seems to be by multiple allelic genes, L^c and P^c and the amorph r^c. The importance of the newly discovered chimpanzee blood group system stems from its intimate relationship to the human Rh-Hr blood group system. On the one hand, the isoimmune chimpanzee serum of anti-L^c specificity distinguishes sharply between human Rh-positive and Rh-negative red cells; on the other hand, human anti-Rh_o sera absorbed with chimpanzee L^c-negative red cells give reactions with chimpanzee red cells paralleling those of anti-L^c reagents of chimpanzee origin. That this reciprocal relationship between human and chimpanzee isoimmune sera does not result from serologic identity of the L^c and Rh_o combining sites on the surface of chimpanzee and human red cells follows from the results of cross-absorption experiments.[3]

As shown in Table 16-1, additional simian-type blood specificities of chimpanzee red cells have been identified, some, like H^c or N^c, possibly related to one or another chimpanzee blood group system, whereas others, like G^c or K^c, appear to be independent.

Except for chimpanzees, the studies on simian-type blood factors of apes have been limited almost entirely to gibbons, in which three unrelated factors, A^g, B^g, and C^g, were identified by isoimmunization.[4,5] In other species of anthropoid apes the studies have been hampered by unavailability of animals for immunization. Attempts have been made to test gorilla red cells for simian-type blood factors by using reagents prepared in chimpanzees. The gorillas were found to be polymorphic for the factors C^c and F^c of the chimpanzee blood group system C-E-F, whereas all animals were proved to have homologues of the chimpanzee V^c, G^c, and H^c agglutinogens.[6]

Extensive immunization programs have been conducted in Old World monkeys because of the increasing use of these animals in medical experiments. As a result, reagents have been produced that are capable of recognizing various simian-type specificities on the red cells of baboons, rhesus monkeys, and pig-tailed and crab-eating macaques. Some of those specificities are listed in Table 16-1.

In baboons, of special interest are blood group specificities **hu** and **ca**, believed to be species specific in that they seem to define serologic differences among the red cells of baboons of various subspecies[7] (yellow, olive, chacma, etc.).

At least twenty-five different simian-type specificities have been found on the red cells of rhesus monkeys,[8] and some of these are shown in Table 16-1. Particularly interesting are specificities D^{rh}, of which three kinds have been identified—D_1^{rh}, D_2^{rh}, and D_3^{rh}. These antigens, which give graded reactions comparable to those of human A_1 and A_2 subgroups, constitute a graded blood group system.[9]

Reagents produced by isoimmunization of rhesus monkeys have been found to be useful for typing red cells of another species of macaques—crab-eating and pig-tailed macaques—which were found to share with rhesus monkeys, among other specificities, also the graded variants of the D^{rh} specificity.

SPONTANEOUSLY OCCURRING AGGLUTININS IN PRIMATE SERA

Besides the anti-**A** and anti-**B** agglutinins normally present in the sera of apes and monkeys as part of their A-B-O phenotype, cross matching of the sera and the red cells of nonimmunized animals of one and the same species may not infrequently reveal the presence of agglutinating antibodies of other specificities.[10] Some of these could be identified as specific for the known simian-type blood factors, for example, **G**^{P} or **B**^{P} of baboons. The origin of these spontaneously occurring antibodies in the sera of animals not known to have been previously exposed to immunogenic factors is not clear. Recent observations on maternofetal incompatibility in primate animals due to differences in simian-type antigens suggest that some of the antibodies observed may be the result of isoimmunization in pregnancy. The occurrence of such "spontaneous" antibodies is of prime importance for the use of primate animals in experiments involving transfusion, cross-circulation, and transplantation, as well as in the breeding of primates.

REFERENCES

1. Wiener, A. S., Moor-Jankowski, J., Socha, W. W., and Gordon, E. B.: Am. J. Hum. Genet. **26**:35, 1974.
2. Wiener, A. S., Gordon, E. B., Socha, W. W., and Moor-Jankowski, J.: Am. J. Phys. Anthropol. **37**:301, 1972.
3. Socha, W. W., and Moor-Jankowski, J.: Int. Arch. Allergy. (In press.)
4. Moor-Jankowski, J., Wiener, A. S., and Gordon, E. B.: Transfusion **5**:235, 1965.
5. Wiener, A. S., Moor-Jankowski, J., Gordon, E. B., Daumy, O. M., and Davis, J. H.: Int. Arch. Allergy **30**:466, 1966.
6. Wiener, A. S., Socha, W. W., Arons, E. B., Mortelmans, J., and Moor-Jankowski, J.: J. Med. Primatol. **5**:317, 1976.
7. Moor-Jankowski, J., Wiener, A. S., Socha, W. W., Gordon, E. B., and Davis, J. H.: J. Med. Primatol. **2**:71, 1973.
8. Wiener, A. S., Socha, W. W., Moor-Jankowski, J., Gordon, E. B., and Kaczera, Z.: Int. Arch. Allergy **44**:140, 1973.
9. Socha, W. W., Wiener, A. S., Moor-Jankowski, J., and Valerio, D.: Int. Arch. Allergy **52**:355, 1976.
10. Socha, W. W., Wiener, A. S., Moor-Jankowski, J., Scheffrahn, W., and Wolfson, S. K., Jr.: Int. Arch. Allergy **51**:656, 1976.

PART THREE □ **Methods**

17 □ Technics in blood grouping

In all laboratory investigations, thorough and strict adherence to technic is a prerequisite for accuracy and reproducibility of results. In the field of blood grouping, improper or sloppy methods, failure to use adequate controls, lack of knowledge and insight in judging results, or absence of constant awareness of possible errors can lead to mistakes and result in severe and even fatal reactions in transfusions, as well as tragic miscarriage of justice in medicolegal cases.

Blood groups are identified by **agglutination reactions,** that is, by the clumping of red blood cells due to the specific action of antibodies. Some tests also make use of **hemolysis** (dissolving) of the red cells, in which **complement** plays a role. The **antigens** are on the red cell surface, the **antibody** in the serum. The antibody combines with its corresponding antigen, or combining group, to bring about a visible reaction. If, therefore, the type of antigen is known but the antibody is unknown, the reaction can be used to identify the antibody; conversely, if the specificity of the antibody is known and the antigen is unknown, the type of antigen can be determined. If both the antigen and the antibody are known and if they correspond in specificity, the combination serves as a **control,** since a certain reaction, positive or negative, is expected; if such a reaction does not take place, something is amiss in the technic or with the reagents.

By convention, antibodies are designated by the prefix "anti-", followed by the symbol for the specificity that they detect. Thus anti-A reacts with specificity **A,** anti-**B** with **B,** anti-**rh'** with **rh',** anti-**K** with **K,** anti-**M** with **M,** etc.

To avoid false positive reports, it is necessary to recognize the appearances of **agglutination, partial agglutination,** and **pseudoagglutination** and to be aware of the possibilities of **autoagglutination, panagglutination, polyagglutination,** etc. when performing tests.

SPECIFIC AGGLUTINATION

When red blood cells are suspended in an isotonic or physiologic solution, for example, in 0.85% sodium chloride or in **compatible** plasma or serum, they remain separated from one another but eventually settle to the bottom of the container or slide. If, however, they are mixed with **incompatible** serum or plasma, that is, serum or plasma containing an antibody with which they can react, the cells come together in clumps and are said to have agglutinated.

The term **agglutinate** is both a transitive and intransitive verb, as well as a noun used to designate the specific clumps of cells formed in a reaction. It can be said that red cells agglutinate, which means that they clump together, but it can also be said that the serum agglutinates the red cells, which means that the serum causes agglutination of the cells. This can lead to misunderstanding on the part of the beginning student.

In **true agglutination,** resulting from the action of an agglutinin, the red cells clump together and cannot be separated by shaking or stirring. When the clumps are large, they are usually brick red and clearly visible to the naked eye. They may vary in size, with tiny "star-shaped" clumps, which more often are brownish and usually cannot be seen except under a microscope. Complete clumping with few if any free

225

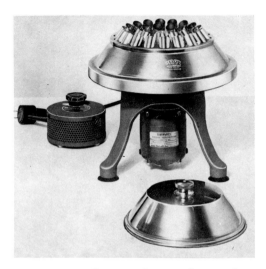

Fig. 17-1. Servall M, medium angle centrifuge. (Courtesy Ivan Sorvall, Inc., Norwalk, Conn.)

cells occurs when the antibody titer is high and the number of combining sites on the red cells is high. Incomplete clumping occurs when the antibody titer is low or when the number of combining sites on the red cells is low. A scanning lens is recommended for examining material in small tubes, but with slides it is best to use the 10×, or low power, objective with the 10× eyepiece, with or without the condenser.

There are **false appearances of agglutination**. In addition, certain interfering substances at times make reading a positive reaction difficult or impossible, but false negative reactions can also occur.

Time and **temperature** of reactions are important. Certain antibodies react only at low temperature, 4° C; others react best at body temperature, 37° C; and still others are adversely affected by heat and react best at room temperature, 22° C. Antibodies that react best at 4° C are referred to as **cold antibodies**. **Warm antibodies** react best at 37° C. The time allowed for reaction between antibodies and antigens can be varied in some instances, but it is usually best to follow the manufacturers' suggestions when using commercially prepared antisera or when employing panels of cells against an unknown serum. Some

antibodies may dissociate if left in contact with their antigens too long.

The **serum** used for testing should be fresh. If both hemolytic and agglutinating antibodies are believed to be present, the serum may be tested fresh and again after inactivation, which destroys the natural complement. Complement is needed to complete a hemolytic reaction.

Centrifugation (Fig. 17-1) is important in certain tests. Time and speed are critical, especially with the antiglobulin tests. Fixed speed centrifuges are available for exclusive use in the blood grouping tests.* Speed and centrifugal force are more significant than revolutions per minute (rpm), although many methods still refer to rpm. The following equation may be used to determine **centrifugal force**, or **gravities**, expressed as g.

$$RFC = 0.00001118 \times N^2 \times r;$$ RFC = centrifugal force (gravities, or g), N = revolutions per minute, and r = rotating radius in centimeters from the center of the centrifuge head to the outer tip of the tube.

If centrifugation proceeds at too rapid a rate for too long a time, the cells are packed together so tightly that they may **sludge**, which could be mistaken for agglutination. Centrifugation, especially of enzyme-treated cells or of cells suspended in a high-protein medium like albumin or plasma, must be carried out with great care to prevent false readings. Inadequate centrifugation, on the other hand, may result in weak, unclear clumping.

The result of centrifugation should be a clear supernatant fluid with a clearly visible "button" of cells at the bottom of the tube. The cells should be easily removable and easily dispersed in a suspending medium by employing only gentle shaking. Positive reactions, even when weak, should be clearly visible. *Always use the least centrifugal force necessary to produce a button of cells at the bottom of the tube.*

Fixed-speed centrifuges have been standardized by the manufacturers, but they

*Clay-Adams Co., New York, as Sero-fuge.

should be reevaluated periodically and re-standardized. The manufacturers' directions give the methods in detail with each centrifuge. The period and time of centrifugation may be varied after studying the results of centrifuging mixtures of different dilutions of serum added to the cells. Select the time of centrifugation as that in which the strongest reaction is obtained with positive cells but which still gives a clear-cut negative reaction with negative cells and which likewise identifies weakly positive reactions.

Degree of positive reaction is reported differently by different individuals. The **American Association of Blood Banks** (**AABB**) recommends the following:

4+ = One solid aggregate of red cells
3+ = Several large aggregates
2+ = Medium-sized aggregates, clear background
1+ = Small aggregates, turbid reddish background
+w = Tiny aggregates, turbid reddish background, or microscopic aggregates only
Complete or partial hemolysis = positive reaction

Unger used the following scheme:

3+s = One solid aggregate
3+w = Large red clumps, no unagglutinated cells
2+s = Smaller red clumps, about one fourth of the cells not clumped
2+w = Smaller red clumps than 2+s, but still visible macroscopically, about one fourth of the cells not clumped
1+s = Clearly visible clumps microscopically, about one half of the cells not clumped
1+w = Scattered clumps visible only microscopically, brownish and star shaped, about three fourths of the cells not clumped
± = Doubtful reaction, occasional small clump
- = No clumps at all microscopically
NOTE: s means strong; w means weak

QUALITY CONTROL OF AGGLUTINATION METHODS
Slide tests

Slide tests are excellent methods because they are rapid and can be performed almost immediately on blood taken in an anticoagulant. In addition, they are the best means of demonstrating mixed agglutination such as occurs in blood group A_3, in patients transfused with a different blood group such as group O blood into a group A individual, in erythroblastosis fetalis when there has been an intrauterine transfusion, in blood group chimeras, and in cases in which there is extensive fetal bleeding into the maternal circulation. In these tests, most inaccuracies can be traced to poor technic.

Small clots must not be mistaken for agglutinates. When slides stand too long, they dry along the edges, and this might be misinterpreted as agglutination.

The cells must be mixed before use, but the fingers must not be placed over the tops of the tubes to mix the cells.

It is imperative that the correct specimen be used in the correct quantity and concentration and that the mixture cover a large enough reaction area. The proper temperature for the reaction must be rigidly adhered to, and the mixture of cells and serum must be stirred sufficiently. Timing is extremely important.

Tube tests

In tube tests mixed agglutination reactions are difficult or impossible to determine. One advantage over the slide method is that once completed, the reactions do not have to be read immediately. In addition, there is less chance of drying, and the tests are protected from air currents.

In performing the tests, the tip of the pipet must not be allowed to contact the glass or the serum or cells previously added. The drop should fall into the *bottom* of the tube and not on the side. The test must be checked to make certain that the serum is in the bottom of the tube. The serum is placed in the tube first. Cells are added in the same manner as the serum, making sure that they, too, go to the bottom of the tube. This is also true of enzymes, albumin, etc. The technologist must be absolutely sure that the reactants are placed in each tube, since omitting reagents can mean a false result. The correct time and temperature must be observed for each reaction, as well as proper centrifugal force. The button of cells must not be packed too hard.

After centrifugation, the supernate should be examined for hemolysis. If there is no hemolysis in the original specimen and there is hemolysis after centrifugation, this is usually interpreted as a positive reaction and is regarded the same as a strong agglutination. In dislodging cells from the tube after centrifuging, one must be as gentle as possible so that weakly agglutinated cells are not broken loose and disrupted. The tube must not be banged against the table or flicked with the fingers; it should be shaken gently or rolled until all the cells are removed from the bottom. Then the reactions can be read and recorded.

FALSE NEGATIVE REACTIONS

If antisera of low titer and avidity are used to test cells, there might be no reaction or an extremely weak one. This is a false negative reaction. The commercial testing sera should give strong, clear-cut reactions that are not easily mistaken, even by a beginner. The Division of Biologic Standards requires these antisera to have standardized antibody content. When working with an unknown serum from a patient, however, the antibody content may be high, moderate, or low. It is important, therefore, in using an unknown serum in which the antibody content might be low, to use a larger volume of serum and avoid an excess of red cells. If the suspension of cells is too dilute, however, it may be difficult to read a reaction, even though it is positive. The relative proportion of cells and serum is important in antibody-antigen reactions. Too few cells may form only small agglutinates difficult to read, whereas a high concentration of cells may absorb the antibodies in a weak serum without agglutinating.

There is no control over the antibody content in an unknown serum, which must

be kept in mind during cross matching. Tests using unknown serum must be examined diligently so as not to overlook any clumps of cells that might be present.

In the A-B-O system if the anti-A is weak, it could fail to detect the specificity A, especially of blood group A_2B, and such group AB blood would be erroneously recorded as group B, as in Table 17-1. Controls are mandatory in all blood grouping tests.

Some agglutinogens are poorly developed or expressed, as in the blood of **newborn infants** or certain preserved blood cell suspensions. One of the most common errors is to mistake group A_2B blood for group B because of the weak reactivity of A_2 when in combination with B. (See Table 17-1.) High-titered anti-A sera will detect this subgroup. Although commercial antisera for testing purposes are under strict government supervision and license, nevertheless they should not be used without proper controls because antibodies can deteriorate even when antisera are refrigerated. They should not be used past the expiration date on the label unless they have been retested and their activity confirmed.

Difficulty is encountered not just in the A-B-O system because of the use of weakly

Table 17-1. Results of using weak anti-**A** sera for blood grouping tests

Cells	High-titered anti-A serum	High-titered anti-B serum	Group reported
O	−	−	O
A_1	+	−	A
A_2	+	−	A
B	−	+	B
A_1B	+	+	AB
A_2B	+	+	AB

Cells	Low-titered anti-A serum	Low-titered anti-B serum	Group reported
O	−	−	O
A_1	+	−	A
A_2	+ or ±	−	A
B	−	+	B
A_1B	+	+	AB
A_2B	−	+	B

reacting antisera. In the Rh-Hr system **hr″** is often difficult to detect, probably because of the variations in the strength of anti-**hr″** testing sera. Blood specificities in other systems can also react weakly, and if such reactions are incorrectly read or interpreted, false negative reports will be made. Tests should be run at least in duplicate, using the "blind" technic (p. 233). False negative reactions when the antiglobulin test is used will be discussed in the part of this chapter dealing with the antiglobulin test.

NONSPECIFIC AGGLUTINATION
False positive reactions

Pseudoagglutination. Pseudoagglutination is false appearance of clumping but not true serologic agglutination. It is usually due to **rouleaux formation** of the red cells, a formation in which the cells resemble a stack of coins that has been pushed over. Pseudoagglutination is due to high concentration of globulins in serum or fibrinogen in plasma and has been noted when tests are made at higher temperatures on open slides in an air current, where such exposure causes surface drying and thus concentration of the globulins or proteins in the serum or plasma. In some patients with **rapid sedimentation rates** the serum propels the red cells to the bottom of the tube or slide, giving a false appearance of agglutination, especially when the sedimented red cells separate into clusters on the slide. Microscopically this does not look like agglutination, especially when the slide has been properly rotated or after a drop of saline has been added and the slide has been rotated again and reexamined.

Patients with **multiple myeloma** and those with **high globulin content** or abnormal globulins in their sera, as well as those who have received **dextran** as a plasma expander, frequently show pseudoagglutination in blood grouping tests.

Some **gums** and other substances give a false appearance of agglutination unless the tests in which they are used are correctly handled before reading the results; these substances are gum acacia, gum tragacanth, and gelatin. **Trypsin** and **ficin** also render reactions difficult to read, and inexperienced persons sometimes report these as positive reactions, when the cells have simply stuck together and are not serologically agglutinated. Negative controls for comparison in reading, which are prepared and handled exactly like the tests, are essential when using gums or the enzymes.

Adding a few drops of saline to the reaction and then mixing will usually break up rouleaux. Saline is added *after* and *not before* the reaction. If it is added before a reaction has had sufficient time to occur, it dilutes the antibody before the antibody can react. If added after the reaction, the antibody has already reacted and dilution will not affect true agglutination.

If pseudoagglutination occurs in crossmatching tests, it may require much extra effort on the part of the laboratory worker unless it is of the type that can be dispersed simply by adding saline.

Umbilical cord serum and false agglutination. Some cord sera produce a reaction that simulates true agglutination. If the slide containing cord serum mixed with red cell suspensions is tilted back and forth, the cells clump but separate again when the slide is allowed to rest on the table. The process can be repeated indefinitely. Wharton's jelly from the umbilical cord contaminating the cord serum is responsible for the phenomenon.

MIXED-FIELD ERYTHROCYTIC AGGLUTINATION

Mixed-field red cell agglutination appears in blood grouping tests as red cell agglutinates in a field of nonagglutinated red cells. There are five different classes of true mixtures: (1) artificial mixtures; (2) incomplete agglutination due to low numbers of blood group antigen sites; (3) chimeras; (4) mixtures seen in malignant diseases of lymphoreticular tissue, in somatic mutation, or in monosomy without apparent disease; and (5) polyagglutination.

Artificial mixtures

Artificial mixtures may be accidental, or they may occur after a transfusion, in feto-maternal or maternofetal transfer, or in transfer of a therapeutic marrow graft.

Low density of blood group antigen sites

Forms of A and B agglutinogens such as A_3 and B_3 have been reported[1] that are characterized by incomplete agglutination. In addition, weakening of A, B, and other antigens in old age and in such diseases as leukemia may be responsible for this reaction. The antigens Lu and Sd^a also may give weak reactions.

Chimeras

Chimeras are discussed on pp. 79 and 80. In chimerism, more than one kind of blood may be present in an individual, for example, two different A and B agglutinogens on separate cells. There are two classes of chimeras—twin and di-spermic (two sperms). In twin chimeras, the mixture of blood apparently takes place in utero by exchange of marrow cells from one fraternal twin to another, or possibly from primary accident of gametogenesis.

Malignant diseases of lymphoreticular tissue, somatic mutation, or monosomy without apparent disease

This category includes mosaics associated with myeloproliferative disease, polycythemia vera, erythroleukemia, and a case in which the two red cell populations differed in both rhesus and Duffy groups.[2] In a case reported by Bird et al.,[3] the mixture appeared at first to be of group O and B cells, but further investigation showed it to be normal B and weak B cells.

Polyagglutinability of red blood cells[4]

Polyagglutination is a condition in which red blood cells are agglutinated by most normal human sera regardless of blood group, and often including the individual's own serum. It creates many problems in blood grouping and cross matching. It is often associated with infection by certain microorganisms and can occur in vivo and in vitro. It results at times from adsorption of bacterial antigens onto the red cell surface; such cells are then agglutinated by *antibacterial* antibody and not by the blood group agglutinins. Certain in vivo infections, such as with vibrios and corynebacteria, can alter the red cells so as to cause them to be agglutinated by many sera. This is due to the enzymes produced by these organisms. Polyagglutination also occurs when certain red blood cell membrane receptors are exposed to the red cell surface or are present de novo on it.

Three receptors of this nature have been described: T, Tn, and Cad. T was the first one discovered and was designated T after Thomsen, who first described it. Red cells with such receptors are polyagglutinable because the corresponding IgM antibodies, anti-**T**, anti-**Tn**, and anti-**Cad**, are usually present in normal human sera and react with red cells containing their specific factor (anti-**T** with **T**, etc.). These agglutinins react best at low temperatures.

T is a latent receptor concealed in normal red blood cells, which is exposed by the action of neuraminidase (sialidase), a receptor-destroying enzyme (RDE) that is produced by some bacteria and viruses. T-polyagglutinability can also occur in vitro when stored blood specimens have been contaminated by neuraminidase-producing bacteria and can often be recognized by purplish discoloration of the red blood cells. When T polyagglutinability occurs, the physician should be alerted to make a careful search for a source of infection, as pointed out by Greenwalt and Steane.[5] If an infection is found to exist, a direct relationship may in this way be established between the infection and the transfusion problem. As a rule, T-polyagglutinability disappears from the blood on the patient's recovery.

Infusion of *donor* whole blood or plasma should be avoided under these circumstances because the donor's plasma contains anti-T and could therefore destroy the recipient's red cells that have the T antigen.

Tn polyagglutinability occurs only in vivo, seems to be acquired, and is persistent. It usually is called to the attention of the technologist when there is difficulty in blood grouping or cross matching. The polyagglutination is characterized by mixed-field reaction pattern. In some very rare instances there is no mixed-field reaction pattern because all the cells have been altered. This is known as **persistent mixed-field polyagglutinability.** It has been reported in healthy blood donors, antenatal patients, hemolytic anemias, myeloproliferative disease (with aplasia), pancytopenia with ringed sideroblasts, and myeloid leukemia undergoing blast cell metamorphosis. Tn polyagglutinability has also been associated with *Proteus mirabilis* wound infection that persisted after the infection had been cured. In determining if the cross-matching problem is due to Tn agglutination, it should be established whether there is an associated hemolytic anemia, thrombocytopenia, or leukopenia.

T and Tn cryptantigens may also be present on leukocytes and platelets, and such cells may also be polyagglutinable. Tn cells seem to have an affinity for sera containing anti-**A.**

T polyagglutinability has been called **panagglutination, bacteriogenic agglutination,** and the **Huebener-Thomsen phenomenon.**[6]

Most normal sera have anti-**T,** which is absent from the blood serum of newborn babies and infants. It can be removed from serum by absorption with cells containing activated T antigen. A closely related agglutinin is also found in and can be extracted from peanuts.

Cad is a rare characteristic inherited as a mendelian dominant. Cad polyagglutination is permanent. It derives its name from the donor in whom the antigen was first found. The group B red cells of this donor and of his mother, and the group O red cells of a sibling, were strongly clumped by extracts of *Dolichos biflorus,* a source of potent anti-A_1 lectin.

There is a relationship between **Cad** and **Sd**[a], a red cell antigen that is expressed in varying strength on red cells of more than 90% of persons tested and is secreted in soluble form in saliva. A sample of the original Cad cells reacted strongly with anti-**Sd**[a]. It is suggested that the phenomenon occurs only in persons in whom Sd[a] antigen is strongly expressed. The two have been shown to be the same antigen. See p. 181.

Extracts of certain seeds have long been used as laboratory reagents in blood grouping. Anti-**T** occurs in peanuts (*Arachis hypogaea);* both anti-**Cad** and anti-**Tn** are present in the seeds of *Dolichos biflorus.* Hexamethrine bromide (Polybrene) is used to differentiate types of polyagglutination. It does not agglutinate neuraminidase-treated (T-transformed) red blood cells, nor does protamine. In other words, loss of sialic acid from the red cell membrane reduces or abolishes the ability of red cells to be agglutinated by polybrene or protamine.

Since *Dolichos biflorus* extracts contain an anti-A_1 agglutinin, the results in Table 17-2 cannot be applied to group A or AB cells.

Tk. In 1972 Bird and Wingham[7] reported transient agglutinability associated with severe infection in which the patient's cells were agglutinated by sera from which anti-**T** had been removed. The antigen was

Table 17-2. Simple differentiation of T, Tn, and Cad polyagglutinability*

	Arachis hypogaea	Dolichos biflorus	Polybrene	Effect of papain on receptor
T	+	–	–	None
Tn	–	+	Mixed field	Destroyed
Cad	–	+	+	Enhanced

*Modified from Bird, G. W. G., Shinton, N. K., and Wingham, J.: Br. J. Haematol. **21:**443, 1971.

named Tk and the antibody anti-**Tk**.[7]

The use of still other lectins for identification of red blood cell polyagglutination is shown in Table 17-3. General discussion of lactins can be found on p. 237ff.

Laboratory applications

When blood that seems to be group AB has anti-**A**, anti-**B**, or both antibodies in the serum, polyagglutinability should be suspected. When testing group AB serum, which has neither anti-**A** nor anti-**B**, against the suspected cells in saline suspension at room temperature, if agglutination occurs it is due to anti-**T**, anti-**Tn**, or anti-**Cad** in the serum, since all normal adult sera contain these antibodies. This would prove the presence of agglutinogen T, Tn, or Cad on the red cells.

A history of infection in individuals whose red cells are agglutinated by almost all adult sera suggests the possibility of T polyagglutinability.

To obtain correct blood grouping results, such red cells should be pre-warmed and maintained at 37° C when testing with all reagents, and the results should be read directly from the water bath while the tests are still warm. Eluates made of the antibodies anti-**T**, anti-**B**, and anti-**Rh**$_0$, etc., eluted from specially prepared normal red cells, may be used for testing, since these do not contain anti-**T**, anti-**Tn**, or anti-**Cad**.

If blood serum is contaminated by bacteria in the laboratory or if it has become contaminated before submission to the laboratory for testing, it can cause agglutination of all red cells. This is true also of the antisera used for testing purposes. Contamination can be avoided by aseptic handling of blood serum and cells in the laboratory and during withdrawal of blood from the patient or donor.

Pretreatment of the cells with papain destroys the Tn receptors and makes it possible to type Tn-activated red cells for blood groups other than those of the M-N-S and Duffy systems, in which groups the antibodies do not react with enzyme-treated red cells. Adequate controls must always be run.

It must be kept in mind that the transfusion problem lies in the *donor* plasma and not in that of the patient. Destruction of the recipient's cells may occur if sufficient quantities of the donor antibody are transfused. A hemolytic reaction was reported by van Loghem et al.[9] after infusion of whole blood containing anti-**T** into an infant with T-activated red cells. If packed or washed red cells are used for the transfusion, the problems are avoided, since no antibodies are present in cells.

For classification of erythrocytic polyagglutinability, see Table 17-4.

Chemistry

Tn is a cryptic determinant of periodate oxidized Smith-degraded desialized human erythrocyte determinant of an alkali-labile tetrasaccharide in which *N*-acetyl-D-galactosamine is α-glysodically linked to serine

Table 17-3. Identification of red blood cell polyagglutination using seed agglutinins*

	Arachis hypogaea	Salvia sclarea	Salvia horminum Saline	Salvia horminum Papain
T or Tk	+	−	−	−
Tn	−	+	+	−†
Cad	−	−	+	+

*Modified from Bird, G. W. G.: Rev. Fr. Transfus. Immunohématol. 19:231, 1976.
†Tn is inactivated by papain.

Table 17-4. Classification of erythrocytic polyagglutinability*

Acquired	Passenger antigens such as bacterial products and drugs
	T
	Tk
	Acquired B
	Tn
	Artificial; for example, periodate
Inherited	Cad
	HEMPAS†

*Modified from Bird, G. W. G.: Rev. Fr. Transfus. Immunohématol. 19:247, 1976.
†Hereditary erythroblastic multinuclearity with positive acidified serum test, an uncommon recessive type of anemia by which the cells are agglutinated and lysed by an antibody present in the serum of most adults.[11, 12]

or threonine.[7] According to Springer and Desai,[10] T and Tn are precursors in the M-N biosynthetic pathway. Tn is α-linked to a precursor (serine or threonine) and is itself the precursor of T, which is the precursor of N (one N-acetylneuraminic acid, or NANA) and M (two NANAs). Since Tn cells can be T-transformed, the T receptor must also be present elsewhere. Tn cells are sialic acid (NANA)-deficient but serologically distinguishable from other NANA-deficient cells, such as T, En(a–), M^k, and M^g.

AUTOAGGLUTINATION (PANAGGLUTININS)

In autoagglutination the serum agglutinates its own red cells due to an adsorbable agglutinin in the serum and a corresponding agglutinogen on the red cells. Autoagglutinins usually act not only on a person's own red cells but also on the red cells of all other humans, regardless of their blood group. Such agglutinins are therefore called **panagglutinins.** Autoagglutination reactions generally occur at low temperatures, disappear on warming, then reappear when chilled. Frequently cold agglutinins have a specificity for the high-frequency blood factor **I** and less commonly for blood factor **i.**

Some conditions are characterized by the presence of **cold autoagglutinins** in greatly increased titer so that the reaction takes place also at room temperature. These conditions are mycoplasmal pneumonia, paroxysmal hemoglobinuria, trypanosomiasis of man and animals, syphilitic or hypertrophic cirrhosis of the liver, hemolytic icterus, Raynaud's syndrome, severe anemias, and others. Even at room temperature cold agglutination may become a source of error in blood grouping. Some patients with Hodgkin's disease, lymphoma, or febrile tuberculosis have a markedly elevated autoagglutinin titer to such an extent that it may become impossible to perform a red count or to determine the blood group because of spontaneous clumping of the patient's red cells.

Autoagglutinins can be removed from the serum by separating the serum from the cells at $0°$ to $5°$ C, at which temperature the blood cells adsorb the autoagglutinins. If the red cells are then washed in warm saline ($37°$ C), the agglutinin is removed and the cells can be used for blood grouping and cross matching.

COLD AGGLUTINATION

In cold agglutination, for example with anti-**P** serum, the cells take up the adsorbable antibodies in the cooled state. These cold agglutinins are active in human bloods exposed to temperatures of $0°$ to $15°$ C. They become inactive if higher temperatures are used in testing. This must be kept in mind when conducting laboratory tests.

SECONDARY COAGULATION SIMULATING AGGLUTINATION

When unwashed cells are used for testing, secondary coagulation or formation of a clot from fibrinogen in the residual plasma may occur. Washing the cells with saline removes the proteins in which they are suspended so that there can be no secondary clot when cells are properly washed. If heat-inactivated sera are used to test the unwashed cells, secondary coagulation does not occur, since heating destroys thrombin as well as complement present in fresh serum.

BLIND TEST

The blind test and its advantages were first demonstrated by Wiener[13] in 1952. It is often difficult to be objective when reading weak reactions, because of a subconscious tendency to shake the tubes a little harder when anticipating a negative reaction or to handle them more gently when expecting a positive reaction. Such inaccuracies can be avoided if the readings are taken blind, that is, if one investigator sets up the tests and a different person reads the reactions without knowing the identity of the mixture being examined. If the observations are truly objective, they should be reproducible when the tests are made on a different day with the tubes arranged in a different order.

CONTROLS

All laboratory tests require a system of controls. Controls are tests in which the content and reactions of all reagents and substances are known so that certain specific results are to be expected. If the expected results do not materalize, one or all of the reagents could be at fault, or some environmental factor(s) may be playing a part in producing the errors. The controls obviously must be made at the same time that the tests are run, and all reagents, glassware, etc. used for the controls must be the same as those employed in the tests proper.

As an example of one type of control, if the anti-**A** reagent serum is to be used for blood grouping unknown cells, it must not only strongly agglutinate group A cells, but also it must *not* clump group B cells; likewise, anti-**B** serum must agglutinate group B but not group A cells, and neither antiserum must agglutinate group O cells. Anti-**A** must also be effective in clumping subgroups A_2 and A_2B cells as well as subgroups A_1 and A_1B.

Even when all precautions are taken—performing the blind test, using the best possible technic and the cleanest possible glassware, controlling temperature and air currents, regulating the centrifuge and the incubator, etc.—errors can creep in that would not be detected except for the controls. If the controls show false results, the tests are unreliable and must be discarded and new tests must be run, using a new battery of reagents. Controls are run simultaneously with the tests.

At times it is not possible to control either the serum or the cells, as when testing an unknown serum against known cells or unknown cells against known serum. The blind test is helpful in such cases; performing multiple tests also helps.

QUALITY CONTROLS IN BLOOD GROUPING

Various methods are used in laboratory studies of the different antigens and antibodies with which blood grouping deals. Many are simple but all require rigid ad-herence to technic, along with suitable quality controls, and these must be applied to each method. Records of the quality control procedures must be retained for scrutiny at a later date if needed to demonstrate that the procedures have been properly followed and that the methods were operative.[14] The following are important: The specimen must be obtained from the correct patient (p. 235). Reading of labels must be stressed. The specimens must be processed in a proper manner. The reagents must be added in optimal amounts and in the correct order. The tests must be performed so that they react maximally. The reactions must be read correctly and the results accurately recorded for the correct patient or donor. The protocols of laboratory reactions should follow a standard arrangement—for example, in the A-B-O system, results with anti-**A**, anti-**B**, anti-**A**$_1$, and group O sera, and in the Rh-Hr system anti-**Rh**$_o$, anti-**rh′**, anti-**rh″**, anti-**hr′**, anti-**hr″**, anti-**hr** sera, and so on—when these tests are made.

Patient identification is all important, since there are instances in which the blood was removed from the wrong subject. Mistakes in patient or donor identification are preventable and inexcusable.

After determining which tests are to be made, the type of specimen needed, and the number of samples required, the sample tubes are labeled, then the venepuncture performed. The labels must include the name of the subject, hospital number, and date. A record of age, sex, and room or ward number is usually made. Only nonremovable labels are indicated. The label should be initialed after the specimen has been procured.

In the patient's room, the name and hospital number should be checked by asking the patient to spell his name. If the name on the wristband and the patient's stated name agree, this should be checked with the name on the prelabeled tube, then the blood withdrawn. The name on the wristband and the name on the label should be checked again, then the label initialed. An unconscious patient is another problem.

The patient must always be identified by both name and number.

According to Medart,[15] the hospital computer can be programmed to prepare a daily list of patients' names that are similar to one another, or even identical. This will help prevent some errors such as obtaining blood from the wrong patient.

When it is necessary to divide the blood in the laboratory or to remove the serum, the tubes that receive the blood or serum should be identified with the proper label containing the patient's name and hospital number. Wax pencil labels are absolutely forbidden because they can easily rub off. The original tube is kept refrigerated with a portion of the original sample still in it for future reference if needed. All specimens must be handled in an aseptic manner, stored at 1° to 10° C, and removed from the refrigerator only when needed.

If a patient requires more than one transfusion, a fresh specimen should be obtained for testing within 48 hours after the first transfusion. The reasons for this are (1) if the antibodies in the serum are complement-dependent, the complement in the serum may have deteriorated in the old laboratory specimen; (2) the previous transfusion may have caused an anamnestic response, and an antibody that was formerly not detected may now react.

The donor(s) should also be identified by some means such as social security number, driver's license number, or a photograph. The pilot tube should be attached to the blood container in a nonremovable fashion. The number used to identify the donor and blood unit should be attached to the pilot tube, as well as to the donor container and the donor's history card. These numbers should be checked during blood withdrawal. For cross matching, blood should be aspirated from the pilot tube, but the pilot tube should not be removed during such withdrawal. Myhre[14] prefers using a syringe and needle to insert through the rubber stopper if a Vacutainer tube has been used. It is not necessary to remove the rubber stopper, and in fact such practice is not condoned. However, if the pilot tube contains clotted blood, it may be necessary to remove the stopper.

Many blood banks use segments of the remaining donor tubing as pilot samples so that there is no problem with a pilot tube. This requires additional care in identification.

Specimens of the patient's and all donors' bloods should be stored at least 7 days at 1° to 10° C after the transfusion so that they may be retested if necessary. Specimens taken in anticoagulants are preferred to clotted blood. Nonrefrigerated specimens may have become contaminated with bacteria, which will grow at room temperature and render the blood or serum unfit for use. There must be some serum or plasma on top of clotted blood when it is stored. If the serum has been used up in the tests, group AB plasma or albumin can be added to cover the clot.

Saline-washed cells should not be kept in saline for storage, but instead should be packed and the supernate removed; otherwise, they might hemolyze. They should then be covered with group AB serum or albumin, taking care that the group AB serum does not contain unexpected antibodies and that it was derived from a nonsecretor of Lewis substance. The tubes must be corked before refrigeration. To use, the cells are washed adequately with saline to remove excess hemoglobin, red cell stroma, and serum. Such cells may be stored for 3 or 4 days.

GLASSWARE

Strict adherence to technic is mandatory in blood grouping. All glassware must be scrupulously clean and dry; it must not have any residue of soap or detergent or remnants of serum or other substances. When possible, it is best to use the glassware only once and then discard it, that is, to use **disposable glassware,** which is available from a number of manufacturers. Ceramic ring slides (Fig. 17-2) may be used over and over if properly washed. Welled slides (Fig. 17-3) should first be washed by hand, then in running water, and then

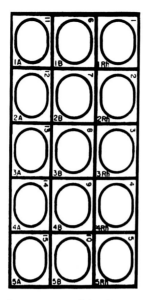

Fig. 17-2. Ceramic ring slide that permits large numbers of blood grouping tests at one time. This is the type of slide used in blood banks or in laboratories where a large number of such tests are performed simultaneously. (Courtesy Behring Diagnostics, Woodbury, N.Y.)

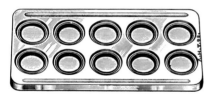

Fig. 17-3. Ten-welled slide for blood grouping. (Courtesy Arthur H. Thomas Co., Philadelphia, Pa.)

thoroughly dried. It is important to rinse all glassware in distilled water before drying. A large container of tap water should be available into which the slides and tubes can be dropped immediately after use, if they are to be cleaned and used again.

It is difficult to remove all traces of blood or serum from droppers, and so these should be soaked in water immediately after use. They must be rinsed many times in tap water and finally in distilled water before being dried in a hot-air oven.

Pipets are preferably washed in an au-

tomatic pipet washer, but they, too, can be washed by hand, using large quantities of tap water, then distilled water, and then drying in an oven. Cylinders that are long enough to hold the pipets and wash water are available.

One of the best cleansers for glassware is **Super Edisonite.*** The glassware is first soaked in a weak solution, washed in running tap water to remove the cleanser, rinsed in distilled water, and finally dried in an oven. The solution may be used more than once, depending on the quantity of glassware cleaned in it. It is a good general cleaner for any glassware that has contained blood or blood products.

ANTISERA (REAGENTS) FOR BLOOD GROUPING

To determine the presence or absence of a particular agglutinogen, it is necessary to have an antiserum that contains an antibody which will react with cells having that particular antigen. An entire battery of antisera is needed if the laboratory performs many tests besides the routine ones, but for routine purposes such as grouping cells prior to transfusion, testing for Rh-Hr factors, or for some of the other more common factors like those of the K-k system, it is not necessary to have all the antisera that are available.

All antisera used for testing purposes should be kept refrigerated at $2°$ to $5°$ C when not in use. As soon as the tests have been completed, the antisera should be returned to the refrigerator. They should be allowed to warm to room temperature before use.

The following **antisera** and reagents are recommended especially **for routine use:**

1. Anti-**A** serum
2. Anti-**B** serum
3. Anti-**A**$_1$ serum or anti-**A**$_1$ lectin, or both
4. Anti-**Rh**$_0$ conglutinating serum for slide test
5. Anti-**Rh**$_0$ serum for saline agglutination test in a tube
6. Anti-**rh**′ saline agglutinating serum for tube test

---

*Manufactured by S. M. Edison Co., Inc., Chicago, Ill.

7. Anti-rh" saline agglutinating serum for tube test
8. Anti-hr' saline agglutinating serum for tube test
9. Anti-hr" saline agglutinating serum for tube test
10. Anti-Rh'$_0$ conglutinating serum for the slide screening test
11. Anti-human globulin for the antiglobulin test
12. Witebsky group A– and group B–specific substances for inhibition test titrations in A-B-O erythroblastosis fetalis
13. Anti-M serum
14. Anti-N serum or anti-N lectin, or both.

Some laboratories also keep anti-Rh"$_0$ and anti-Rh'$_0$" slide sera at hand. Numbers 13 and 14 are useful for differential agglutination tests of transfused red cells, and they are also necessary in disputed parentage tests and in genetic studies.

All blood sera for testing purposes that are not prepared for private use, as well as whole blood and other fractions, are biologics under the Biologic Products Law of the United States. They must be licensed, prior to commercial distribution, by the National Institutes of Health (NIH), U.S. Public Health Service. There are similar laws in other countries to regulate the specificity and potency of antisera.

Methods of preparing these antisera are available in other texts and will not be repeated here.[16]

LECTINS

Lectins are plant agglutinins prepared primarily from certain seeds, leaves, roots, or branches. The term "phytoagglutinins" has also been applied to such extracts. However, lectins implies specificity of reaction, whereas phytoagglutinins does not. These lectins are useful in blood grouping tests to detect antigens or blood group factors not found with the use of ordinary blood grouping sera. As a rule, the reactions are strong, rapid, clear-cut, and easy to read.

Anti-A lectin. The first lectin with blood group specificity was *Vicia cracca*, which had anti-A activity. *Phaseolus limensis*, derived from lima beans, also proved useful,

as has *P. lunatus*. Other anti-A lectins are derived from nonleguminous seeds, *Hyptis suaveoleus* and *Moluccella laevis*. *M. leavis* reacts also as an anti-N reagent against O and B cells. It apparently has the specificity anti-(A+N), since the agglutinin so far has been "unsplittable."

Anti-A from snails. Extracts produced from the snails *Helix hortensis*, *H. pomatia*, *H. aspersa*, and *Cepea nemoralis* are good anti-A reagents. Snail lectins identify the specificity designated A$_{hel}$ by Prokop et al.,[38] who first described them.

Anti-A$_1$ lectin. Of major importance in blood grouping was the preparation and use of extracts of *Dolichos biflorus*, an anti-A$_1$ lectin. It is used to differentiate between the subgroups of A and AB, namely A$_1$ and A$_2$, and A$_1$B and A$_2$B. It is an excellent anti-A$_1$ reagent. It will agglutinate A$_1$ and A$_1$B cells, but not A$_2$ or A$_2$B. The extract is available commercially. Anti-A$_1$ lectin is used in saliva tests on A-B-H secretors. It does not react with the Forssman antigen or with altered T antigen, but it agglutinates cells of the rare phenotype Sd(a++) in groups O and B individuals. It reacts strongly with unaltered T cells and with Cad cells.

Anti-B lectin. Anti-B lectins have been prepared from the mushroom *Morasmius oreades* and the fungus *Fomes fomentarius*, but these have not proved to be useful.

Anti-A+B (anti-C) lectins. Seeds of *Sophora japonica* (predominantly B-specific), *Crotolaria striata*, *C. mucronata*, *Banderiaea simplicifolia*, *Calpurnia aurea*, and *Phlomis fructiosa* have yielded extracts that agglutinate A and B cells more strongly than they do O cells. It is believed that the anti-A and anti-B properties in these lectins are one agglutinin that reacts with a specificity shared by A and B cells but absent from O, probably the C specificity of the A-B-O groups.

Anti-B,H lectin. A valuable lectin of the specificity anti-B,H can be extracted from the arils (seed covers) of *Evonymus europeus*. In inhibition tests it has anti-B specificity when group B red cells are used as indicator, but it has anti-**H** specificity when group O cells are used as indicator.

Anti-H lectins. The most useful of the anti-**H** lectins is that made from *Ulex europeus.* Other lectins of anti-**H** specificity are *Laburnum alpinum, Cerastium tomentosum,* the roots of *Ononis spinosa,* and the fruit pulp of *Clerodendron viscosum.* The extract of *Lotus tetragonolobus* was the lectin used by Bird[17] to theorize the relationship of anti-**Le**[b] to anti-**H**. Extract of *Cytisus sessilifolius* is also an anti-**H** reagent.

Anti-M lectin. Despite claims to the contrary, no anti-**M** lectins have so far been produced that can be useful in blood grouping tests.

Anti-N lectins. A major contribution to blood grouping was made by Ottensooser and Silberschmidt[18] when they described the anti-**N** qualities of a lectin produced from extracts of the South American plant *Vicia graminea.* There are other less satisfactory sources of anti-**N** lectin, such as *Bouhinia variegata* and *B. purpurea.* Another source of a potent anti-**N** lectin is that prepared from the leaves of the Korean plant *Vicia unijuga.* This is described on pp. 77 and 296.

Anti-A+N lectin. Extracts of the seeds of the plant known as Belles of Ireland, *Moluccella laevis,* have an apparently unsplittable agglutinin that reacts with all A cells having the N antigen. It acts as exclusively anti-**N** only against groups O and B cells.

Anti-Cl lectin. A lectin that detects the blood factor **Cl** is derived from *Clerodendron trichotomum.* The specificity **Cl** is described on p. 64.

Anti-T lectin. Lectins that react with T are made from the peanut *Arachis hypogaea.* See the discussion on polyagglutinability, p. 230ff.

Anti-Tn lectins. Anti-**Tn** lectins from *Salvia sclarea* and other species of *Salvia* react with Tn. See the discussion on polyagglutinability, p. 230ff.

Anti-Tn and anti-Cad lectins. The *Salvia horminum* contains a lectin that is reactive with both Tn and Cad. See p. 231 for methods of differentiation.

In the case of lectins used in testing for the H substance in the A-B-O system and in saliva tests and blood stain identification, as well as the anti-**N** tests and tests for the subgroups of A, the directions of the manufacturer must be followed; otherwise, the results may not be accurate.

Antisera of specificities other than those listed on p. 236 are available.*

QUALITY CONTROL OF SERUM REAGENTS

When using commercially prepared serum reagents, as soon as the sera are received, they should be checked to make certain that the expiration date has not been passed. Next the lot number(s) and expiration dates should be recorded. The sera should then be tested to determine if they meet requirements not only for a positive but also for a negative reaction. They may then be placed in the laboratory refrigerator.

In using such sera, always follow the manufacturer's instructions to the letter.

Daily controls on grouping sera are included in the technics that follow and will not be repeated here.

If using frozen serum, do not refreeze after thawing.

Avidity of a serum is the speed at which a standardized end point is reached. This must be measured with each serum reagent. Anti-A should react with A_1 cells in 15 seconds, with A_2 and A_1B cells in 30 seconds, and with A_2B cells in 45 seconds.

---

*Ortho Diagnostic Division, Rt. 202, Raritan, N.J. 08869.
Pfizer, Inc., 235 E. 42nd St., New York, N.Y. 10036.
Dade Pharmaceuticals, Inc., 420 S.W. 11th St., Hallandale, Fla. 33009.
Hyland Laboratories, 3300 Hyland Ave., Costa Mesa, Calif. 92626.
Biological Corporation of America, 40 Markley St., Port Reading, N.J. 07064.
Gamma Biologicals, 3925 Dacoma, Houston, Texas 77018.

Anti-**B** should agglutinate B cells in 15 seconds.

CELL SUSPENSIONS FOR BLOOD GROUPING

Cells are suspended in physiologic (isotonic) saline made by dissolving 8.5 gm NaCl in a liter of distilled water, filtering to clarify, and storing in moderate quantities, 500 to 1000 ml per bottle, for short periods of time. It is best to keep a week's supply on hand. This is 0.85% saline. Sterility is not essential unless the cells are to be injected into an animal or kept for a long time. Chemical cleanliness is all important. If blood is to be kept for some time, the saline used to suspend the cells must be sterile, and the container in which the suspension is stored should also be sterile and should be stoppered.

At times cells are treated with enzymes, then suspended in saline. In other methods the cells are suspended in a high-protein medium like plasma. Group AB plasma (or serum) is used because it has neither anti-**A** nor anti-**B** agglutinins and is therefore neutral.

When test cells are needed for injecting animals, ordinarily the choice is group O because such cells have neither A nor B agglutinogen that could stimulate production of anti-**A** or anti-**B**, respectively, in the animal and possibly mask the other antibody that the animal is expected to produce. Group O cells containing specific antigen(s) are also used in panel cells, etc. when testing a serum for antibodies.

Preparation of cells for reagent purposes

Reagent cell suspensions* containing the various blood group factors are available commercially, or they may be prepared in one's own laboratory. The commercial cell panels often contain a formula that prevents hemolysis. The cell suspensions may be used either for controls or as testing reagents to detect antibodies in a blood serum. Since the cells have a hemolysis-preventing reagent, the serum under test need not be inactivated before use. These panel cells remain maximally active under refrigeration for at least 3 weeks. Control tests should be included, however, to determine that they have remained active.

Cell panels* are sets of vials of group O red cells, some with and others without blood group specificities such as rh', rh^w, Rh_o, rh'', hr', hr'', rh_i, hr, hr^v, **K**, **k**, Fy^a, Fy^b, Le^a, Le^b, **M, N, U, S, s, P,** Lu^a, Jk^a, and Jk^b. This is a list of factors in one type of red cell panel from one manufacturer. See p. 289 for methods of using cell panels to identify antibodies in serum.

When testing only for A-B-O and Rh-Hr types, however, complete cell panels are not necessary. There should be suspensions of cells of groups O, A_1, A_2, and B in the A-B-O system and others, both positive and negative, for Rh_o, rh', rh'', hr', and hr'' in the Rh-Hr system. A small laboratory might find it difficult to obtain blood specimens with the various Rh-Hr factors singly, and for that reason the following types of blood should be kept at hand:

> Group O Rh_zRh_o—cells clumped by all five standard Rh-Hr antisera, anti-Rh_o, anti-rh', anti-rh'', anti-hr', and anti-hr''
> Group O Rh_1Rh_1—cells clumped only by anti-Rh_o, anti-rh', and anti-hr''
> Group O Rh_2rh—cells clumped by anti-Rh_o, anti-rh'', anti-hr', anti-hr'', and anti-hr
> Group O rh—cells clumped only by anti-hr', anti-hr'', and anti-hr

and, if available:

> Group O Rh_2Rh_2—cells clumped only by anti-Rh_o, anti-rh'', and anti-hr'
> Group O $rh'rh$—cells clumped only by anti-rh', anti-hr', and anti-hr''

---

*Cell panels (including mixed antigen cells) are available from many manufacturers, including Pan-O-Cell prepared by Ortho, Raritan, N.Y.; Accucell by Hyland Laboratories, Costa Mesa, Calif.; and Data Cyte by Dade Pharmaceuticals, Inc., 420 S.W. 11th St., Hallandale, Fla. 33009.

*Cell panels (including mixed antigen cells) are available from many manufacturers, including Pan-O-Cell prepared by Ortho, Raritan, N.Y.; Accucell by Hyland Laboratories, Costa Mesa, Calif.; and Data Cyte by Dade Pharmaceuticals, Inc., Hallandale, Fla.

Group O rh″rh—cells clumped only by anti-**rh″**, anti-**hr′**, and anti-**hr″**

These last three are rare and therefore not easily obtained.

Panel cells that are purchased may be saline suspensions or enzyme-treated cells, and they are ready for use after thorough but gentle mixing.

Quality control of reagent red cells

As already stated, panels of red cells containing certain antigens are available commercially for identifying antibodies. These may be obtained with or without enzyme alteration. There is an information sheet with each new supply of panel cells, prepared by the manufacturer. This sheet must be used only for those cells included in the package and for no others. The old sheet must be discarded when new cells are purchased. No two donors whose cells are included in the panels should have all the same antigens on their red cells.

The cells should be kept refrigerated when not in use and exposed to room temperature only as they are needed. The red cell antigen content must be accepted on faith, since the entire supply could be used up in trying to check them. Only such antigens as P and Le^a, which deteriorate easily on storage, have to be tested using weak antisera to see if they are still reactive. If such antigens are reactive, it can be assumed that the remainder of the panel of cells is also reactive.

Each day each red cell reagent bottle should be scrutinized for bacteria or hemolysis.

After establishing the identity of an antibody using cell panels, it is best to check the serum with the subject's own red cells. A negative reaction is the rule, except in cases in which an intervening transfusion has taken place or in patients with autoimmune hemolytic anemia. Identification of the antibody can be confirmed by testing it with three known positive and three known negative suspensions of cells that are specific for that antibody.

For long-term preservation of reagent red cells, especially those containing rare antigens, the best method is freezing at –30° C after mixing with glycerin. Another method entails addition of sucrose to the cells, spraying with liquid nitrogen with a droplet-forming apparatus, and storing in a liquid nitrogen freezer.

After thawing, the cells are stored in 0.15M saline at 2° to 6° C as 2% suspensions. Such suspensions do not keep well overnight. They may, however, be packed by centrifugation and decantation, and the red cell mass stored in an equal volume of group AB serum free of irregular antibodies and derived from a nonsecretor of Lewis substance, or in bovine albumin. They must be washed three times in saline and reconstituted to a 2% suspension before use, after which they can be kept in a refrigerator for 3 to 4 days before deteriorating.

Preparation of cells for reagent purposes or for use as unknowns

SALINE-SUSPENDED UNTREATED CELLS

Preparation of blood in anticoagulant

Dry double oxalate anticoagulant. The formula for this anticoagulant includes the following:

Ammonium oxalate	3 gm
Potassium oxalate	2 gm
Distilled water	100 ml

1. Pipet 0.2 ml of the anticoagulant into the *bottom* of each tube, then dry the tubes in an oven, being careful not to use excessive heat.
2. For use, add 5.0 ml of venous blood and mix by inverting about twenty times to keep the blood from clotting. Excess oxalate interferes with the tests, at times resulting in false negative results.
3. For **smaller amounts of blood,** use the following formula:

Ammonium oxalate	1.2 gm
Potassium oxalate	0.8 gm
Distilled water	100 ml

Put 0.1 ml in the *bottom* of each tube, then dry by gentle heat in a hot-air oven. Add 1.0 ml of blood and proceed as above.

EDTA anticoagulant. The sodium and potassium salts of ethylenediamine tetra-acetic acid, EDTA-S or EDTA-P, respectively, form nonionized calcium salts and prevent coagulation in that manner. The dipotassium salt is recommended. EDTA is also known as **Versene** or **Sequestrene.**

1. Prepare a 0.5% aqueous solution by dissolving 0.5 gm in 100 ml of distilled water. The solution contains 5 mg of EDTA per ml.
2. For use, place 0.2 ml or 4 drops of the 0.5% solution in a small tube and dry in an oven at 90° to 100° C. For certain other laboratory tests the anticoagulant may be used in liquid form, but for blood grouping the dry anticoagulant is mandatory.
3. Add 1 ml of blood to the tube containing 1 mg of dry anticoagulant and mix by inverting five or six times. Use proportionately larger amounts of EDTA for greater quantities of blood.

EDTA-P* is available in 5 mg tablets. Place 1 tablet in a small tube with 1 drop of distilled water, then add 5 ml of venous blood and mix by inverting five or six times.

Preparation of saline suspension of cells

1. Place about 1 ml of saline in a Kahn tube 75 × 12 mm.
2. Using a straw or glass dropper, transfer some cells from blood taken in an anticoagulant to the saline until a 3% concentration is attained (the color of tomato juice). If an accurate 3% suspension is needed, centrifuge the cells to pack them, remove all the supernate, and use 1 drop of packed cells for 32 drops of saline, taking care to hold the pipet or straw at the same angle when measuring all the drops.
3. If clotted blood is used, loosen the clot with a wooden applicator, centrifuge, and remove the serum. Shake some of the cells loose from the clot and transfer them to another tube, then add enough saline to make a 3% suspension. Do not let clots enter the suspension. These could be mistaken for clumps of agglutinated red cells.
4. Some laboratories recommend dipping several wooden applicator sticks into the clot, twisting them around, then transferring the cells adhering to the sticks to saline in a small tube, taking care that no clots are carried along.

Washing the cells

Cells may be used as soon as the suspensions are made, or they may be washed once in saline. Centrifuge to pack the cells, decant all the supernate, and resuspend the cells in fresh saline to a 3% concentration. The quantity of saline used for washing should be larger than that needed for the final suspension. Heavier suspensions may be desirable for some tests.

---

*Cambridge Chemical Products, Inc., Dearborn, Mich.

Reagents

1. *Glycerol-citrate freezing solution:* Mix 4 vol of glycerin CP with 8 vol of citrate-phosphate solution.
2. *Citrate-phosphate solution*

K_3 citrate	3.25 gm
K_2HPO_4	0.6 gm
KH_2PO_4	0.47 gm
Distilled water to make	100 ml

3. *3% citrate for washing:* Dissolve 3 gm of sodium citrate in sufficient water to make 100 ml.
4. *Citrate-glycerin solution for washing*
   16% glycerin (v/v) in 3% citrate solution
   8% glycerin (v/v) in 3% citrate solution
   4% glycerin (v/v) in 3% citrate solution
   2% glycerin (v/v) in 3% citrate solution

Freezing method

1. Take blood in citrate, NIH formula A, or heparin anticoagulant.
2. Centrifuge and remove the plasma.
3. Add slowly and with constant agitation a volume of glycerol-citrate freezing solution equal to the volume of packed red cells.
4. Dispense the cells in small vials and freeze at -20° C or lower.

The cells may be kept at this temperature for 1 year or longer. They may be thawed once or twice but not more because they may begin to hemolyze.

Thawing method

1. Place the vial in a water bath at 37° C. When thawed, transfer the cells to a test tube.
2. Centrifuge and remove as much glycerol-citrate as possible.
3. Transfer 2 ml of the packed cells to a 15 × 100 mm test tube. Smaller quantities may be used.
4. Fill the tube with 16% glycerin-citrate wash solution, mix, and centrifuge, then remove as much supernate as possible.
5. Repeat the washing with 8%, then 4%, then 2% glycerol-citrate solution.
6. Wash the cells with 1% (0.165M) saline solution.
7. Resuspend the cells in saline to the proper concentration. Store reconstituted cells at refrigerator temperatures.

After the cells have been thawed, washed, and resuspended, they may be used during that day, but they must be stirred to be resuspended. To store them overnight, centrifuge, remove the supernatant saline, and add an equal volume of group AB plasma with no irregular antibodies and coming from a nonsecretor of Lewis substance. Before use, wash three times in 0.165M saline, then reconstitute in 0.15M saline. The red cells usually tolerate the procedure for 2 or 3 days before they begin to hemolyze. They cannot be used if there is hemolysis.

METHODS OF FREEZING RED CELLS IN LIQUID NITROGEN[19]

Droplet freezing method[20,21]

Freezing solution: 0.3M glucose and 0.45M sodium chloride.

Thawing solution: 0.3M glucose, 0.45M sucrose, and 0.05M sodium chloride. A solution of normal saline (0.15M sodium chloride) can be used, but this results in slightly higher hemolysis.

1. Remove the plasma from the blood and add a volume of freezing solution equal to that of the remaining packed red cells. Mix.
2. Allow to stand for 15 to 30 minutes, take up the cell-additive mixture in a syringe, and spray manually through a 25-gauge needle onto a moving film of liquid nitrogen in a rotating drum of a droplet freezer. (Some of the droplet freezers* automatically form the blood droplets.)
3. Collect the droplets and retrieve them from the bottom of the conical drum of the droplet freezer.
4. Place in a liquid nitrogen refrigerator for storage.
5. To thaw: Suspend the frozen droplets on the end of a precooled spatula and sprinkle into a flask containing 10 ml of thawing solution. Approximately 85% to 95% of the cells can be recovered after droplet freezing and thawing.
6. Wash the red cells three times with saline and either leave in the saline or resuspend in their original plasma.

The droplet freezing technic is especially advantageous for **preserving small quantities of blood.**

Low-glycerol rapid-freeze procedure[22]

Glycerol freezing solution: 28% v/v glycerol, 3% mannitol, and 0.65% sodium chloride.

1. Remove the plasma from the cells and add

---

*Droplet freezer, Union Carbide Corporation, New York, N.Y.

glycerol freezing solution in a volume equal to that of the packed red cells.
2. Wait 15 to 30 minutes, then suspend the red cells in 14% v/v glycerol.
3. Freeze in 5 to 15 ml aliquots in Pyrex glass tubes or plastic tubes by immersing the container in liquid nitrogen.
4. Store in a liquid nitrogen refrigerator.
5. Thaw the samples by gently agitating the tubes in a warm-water bath (40° to 45° C) until the ice mass disappears.
6. Centrifuge and decant the supernate.
7. Wash the cells gently three times using one wash of 16% mannitol in 0.9% sodium chloride, followed by two washes in physiologic salt solution.
8. Add all washes slowly to the cells with gentle mixing. Rapid washing of the cells may result in excess trauma and hemolysis of the red cells.
9. Resuspend the washed red cells in saline, in Alsever solution, or in their original plasma.

This technic is especially useful for **preserving relatively large amounts of blood.**

PREPARATION OF ENZYME-TREATED SALINE-SUSPENDED CELLS

Proteolytic enzymes are organic substances, secreted by living cells, that catalyze the digestion of protein. In many instances the action of enzymes can be checked (quality control) by their action on the gelatin layer of x-ray films. A large drop of the enzyme solution is placed on the surface of an unexposed, unfixed gelatin (x-ray) film, and then incubated at 37° C for 1 hour or at room temperature for 2 hours. The drops must be large enough not to dry during incubation or cake during the test. The film is then washed in running water with gentle rubbing. Complete digestion appears as a clearing of the film at the area covered by the drop. Proper controls should be run. Among the enzymes used in blood grouping are trypsin, bromelin, papain, papain-activated cysteine, and ficin. These alter the membrane or surface of cells. Some blood group antibodies will not react with enzyme-treated cells. This characteristic is used as an additional means of identifying the various blood group systems.

Trypsinated saline-suspended cells

Trypsin solutions must be prepared daily. Difco Trypsin 1:250 is recommended and 0.067M phosphate buffer pH 7.4.*

1. Place about ¼ inch of trypsin in a tube 125 × 12 mm, and add enough buffer to make a supersaturated solution.
2. Centrifuge, remove the supernate, and place it in another tube.
3. Wash saline-suspended red cells four times. After the last washing, remove the supernate from the packed cells.
4. Measure 9 drops of packed washed cells in a tube and add 1 drop of the trypsin solution, shake, and incubate in a water bath at 37° C for 1 hour. Shake every 15 minutes while in the water bath.
5. Wash once with saline; add saline, centrifuge, and remove the supernate.
6. Resuspend to 5% concentration in saline (1 drop concentrated cells and 19 drops saline).

These trypsinated saline-suspended red cells will remain useable if kept in a refrigerator for 1 or 2 days. If any hemolysis occurs, wash once with saline and resuspend the cells.

Ficinated saline-suspended cells

1. Wash a saline suspension of red cells twice, and after the second washing remove the supernate.
2. Prepare 1% ficin solution in 0.067M phosphate buffer pH 7.41 or buffered saline pH 7.3, by placing 0.1 gm of ficin in a small tube and adding 9.9 ml of phosphate buffer. Stopper and mix. Do not make a supersaturated solution. Take care not to spill any solution on the hands or splash into the eyes. After the ficin has dissolved, centrifuge immediately to remove any particles or detritus and use the supernate. This solution will remain useful for 5 or 6 days if kept refrigerated. It can be stored frozen at -20° C.
3. Place 9 drops of packed washed cells in a tube and add 1 drop of 1% ficin, giving a 0.1% solution.
4. Mix thoroughly and incubate in a water bath at 37° C for 1 hour. The American Association of Blood Banks recommends 15 minutes.
5. Fill the tube with saline, mix, and centrifuge to pack the cells.
6. Remove the supernate. This is one washing.
7. Resuspend the cells in saline to a 5% concentration.

The enzyme-treated cells remain useable for several days if kept in a refrigerator.

---

*Fisher Scientific, Pittsburgh, Pa.

Alternate ficin technics

Technic 1

1. To 2 gm ficin in a tube, add 10 ml of 0.15M buffered saline and dissolve. This can be kept in the frozen state.
2. Thaw to room temperature.
3. Place 0.5 ml of stock solution in a 100 ml volumetric flask, returning the stock to the freezer.
4. Dilute to 100 ml with buffered saline.
5. Dispensed in small quantities, it lasts 2 or 3 weeks. Freeze the aliquots until needed, but do not refreeze after thawing.
6. Wash cells three times in buffered saline.
7. Add 1 vol ficin solution to 2 vol packed red cells.
8. Incubate at 37° C for 15 minutes.
9. Wash three times in buffered saline and resuspend to a 5% concentration.
10. Mix the treated cells with the serum (equal parts) and incubate at 37° C for 30 minutes.
11. Wash and if desired perform the antiglobulin test.

Technic 2

1. Place 1 drop of ficin solution in a small test tube.
2. Transfer cells, using applicator sticks, to the tube containing the enzyme.
3. Leave at room temperature 3 to 7 minutes.
4. Add the antiserum and let remain at room temperature 3 minutes.
5. Centrifuge 15 seconds and read.

As in other tests, agglutination is a positive reaction, lack of agglutination negative.

Rapid method of ficinating cells

1. Prepare a suspension of red cells in saline, wash twice with saline, and resuspend to a 3% concentration in saline.
2. Further dilute the 1% ficin solution 1:5 with saline (1 part of ficin solution to 4 parts of saline).
3. To 1 drop of the 3% suspension of twice-washed red cells in a small Kahn tube, add 1 drop of ficin solution, and mix by shaking.
4. Place in a water bath at 37° C for 15 minutes.
5. Wash once with saline and remove and discard the supernate, leaving 1 drop of ficinated red cells in the tube, to which the serum can be added directly.

If the test calls for 2 drops of cells, double the quantities. If time is an important factor, use this method when testing for unknown antibodies or autoantibodies, ex-

cept where enzyme-treated cells must not
be used (M-N-S, Lu, Fy, etc.)

Bromelin

Prepare a 0.5% bromelin solution by dissolving
0.5 gm of bromelin in 90 ml of physiologic saline
and 10 ml of 0.15M Sørensen phosphate buffer pH
5.5. Add 0.1% sodium azide and 0.05% actidione
as preservatives. Store at 4° C. Fresh solutions
should be prepared monthly.

Bromelin solutions are available ready for use
from Difco. The bromelin solution is added to the
test and not directly to the cells.

Papain

Papain and other enzyme solutions are
prepared in a manner similar to that of
trypsin. Papain solutions should be clear.
Filter through a Seitz filter with clarifying
pad or through fine-grade filter paper several times. The following method is suggested:

1. To 1 vol of 0.2M phosphate buffer pH 5.4
   add 9 vol of chilled sterile 0.9% NaCl.
2. To 495 ml buffered saline (step 1) in a 500
   ml bottle, add the following:
   Papain (BDH or Merck) 5 gm
   K₂EDTA·2H₂O (dipotassium ethylenedi-
   amine-tetra-acetate dihydrate), 5 ml of
   a 5 gm/100 ml aqueous solution

This mixture can be kept 6 months at 4° C, but
if frozen, it can be thawed, used only once, and
then must be discarded. Do not refreeze.

3. Stopper tightly, shake vigorously 10 minutes,
   then store at 4° C overnight.
4. Shake well and filter through Whatman No.
   1 filter paper at 4° C.
5. Dispense in small portions, properly labeled. Cork the tubes and store at -25° C.
   Do not use after 4 months. The final pH
   should be 4.8 to 5.0. When 2 vol of serum
   are added to 1 vol of papain-EDTA, the pH
   should be 6.3 to 6.5.

Papain-activated cysteine

1. Place 94 ml of M/15 phosphate buffer pH
   5.4 in a 100 ml flask and add 1 ml of a 5%
   aqueous solution of K₂EDTA·2H₂O and 1
   gm papain.
2. Stopper tightly, shake vigorously for 10 minutes, and centrifuge at high speed for 3
   minutes. Filter the supernate through No.
   1 Whatman paper.
3. Add freshly prepared, neutralized L-cys-
   teine hydrochloride to a final concentration
   of 0.025M by dissolving 0.4 gm of L-cys-
   teine hydrochloride in 2.5 ml of distilled
   water and add sufficient 1.0N NaOH to

bring the pH to 6.5 to 7.0, about 2 to 2.5
ml. Use either Hydrion papers or a pH meter
to measure the pH.

4. Incubate in a water bath at 37° C for 30
   minutes and check the pH. It should be
   5.2 to 5.4. When mixed with an equal volume of serum, the pH should be 6.2 to 6.4.
5. Dispense in small volumes, label and cork
   the tubes, then store at -25° C no longer
   than 4 months. Use according to the following directions.

To use enzymes in treating red cells

1. Wash the red cells twice with saline.
2. Dilute the papain, ficin, etc. tenfold with
   Bacto (Difco) Hemagglutinator Buffer pH
   7.3 immediately before use.
3. Add 4 vol of diluted extract to 1 vol of
   washed packed cells.
4. Incubate in a water bath at 37° C for 10
   minutes.
5. Wash cells three times in saline to stop the
   action of the enzyme.
6. If the cells have previously been frozen,
   treat only 10 min with the enzyme.

Sørensen M/15 phosphate buffer pH 5.4

9.07 gm KH₂PO₄, anhydrous, dissolved in a liter of distilled water	1 part
9.46 gm Na₂HPO₄ dissolved in a liter of water	24 parts

QUALITY CONTROL OF ENZYME REACTIONS

Serum and red cells must be in correct
proportions, as well as temperature and
time of reaction optimum for the enzyme
used. Centrifugation and end point determination must be standardized. If the enzyme is not active, the reaction is unreliable.

Always record the lot number and expiration date of each enzyme as received,
and do not keep any enzyme beyond the
expiration date unless used for special circumstances under rigid control, with positive and negative control cells tested at the
same time. Store powdered enzyme in the
desiccated state in a deep freeze. Let the
bottle warm to room temperature before
opening to prevent condensation of moisture inside. After the bottle has been
opened, a silica gel dryer should be added
or the enzyme put into a desiccator before
being returned to the deep freeze.

Concentrated stock solutions of most enzymes can usually be prepared and frozen for considerable periods of time, for example, bromelin, papain, and ficin. Before use the material is thawed and diluted then promptly used. Bromelin is the most stable. It can be stored at 2° to 8° C for as long as 3 weeks without losing it activity. It often turns dark as its activity decreases. Papain, ficin, and trypsin should not be stored longer than overnight. All enzyme solutions should be kept at room temperature for as little time as possible. Commercial enzyme preparations should be stored according to the manufacturer's recommendations.

There are a number of tests to determine if the enzyme is active. A simple one is that of Walker,[23] which is a modification of the test for enzymes in stool described in 1949 by Schwachman et al.[24] (See p. 242.)

PREPARATION OF 50% SUSPENSION OF RED CELLS IN THEIR OWN PLASMA (WHOLE BLOOD)

Collect blood as usual in an anticoagulant, centrifuge, remove enough supernatant plasma to leave 50% cells and 50% plasma, and then shake to mix. It is especially important when testing blood from an anemic patient that the red cells constitute 50% of the specimen. Whole blood is referred to as a **high-protein medium.**

QUALITY CONTROL OF CELL SUSPENSIONS

In preparing whole blood to be used for cell suspensions, centrifuge and remove enough plasma to bring the concentration of the cells to 50%. If the volume of red cells exceeds 50%, add 22% bovine albumin to adjust the concentration. If the blood has been allowed to clot, break up the clot by vigorous agitation with a glass rod or wooden applicator sticks. Place such a rod in each tube and then put the tubes in a mechanical shaker such as the Kahn variety, for several minutes. Decant the red cells immediately, or allow the large clots to settle and pour off the suspended red cells. Centrifuge the red cell suspension and adjust so that the ratio of

cells to supernate is 50%. Myhre[14] suggests 40% cells and 60% plasma, but we have had better results using 50% cell suspension in their own plasma or serum. The concentration is not critical outside of 40% ± 15%.

For tube tests, a difference in results can occur when the suspension is either too concentrated or too light. Most texts suggest a 2% to 5% concentration. In the methods given in this text, the optimum concentration is included in the technic. The cells must be washed in a tube in which at least twenty times the volume of cells can be prepared in saline. Wash the cells the number of times required by the specific method, then dilute them to the desired suspension. Any protein in the suspending medium of the cells should be reduced to at least 1:400 concentration or better. For accurate controls, mix the blood after dilution, remove a small portion, and count the red cells on an automatic counter. Adjust the count to yield 100,000 red cells per milliliter for a 2% suspension, 200,000 for a 4% suspension, and 250,000 for a 5% suspension. If too few cells are present, centrifuge and remove enough supernate to bring the concentration to the desired amount. If too concentrated, add more saline. This method is usually too laborious for routine work, but it should be used occasionally, and technologists should be able to learn to judge the concentration of cells visually by color or shade.

Another method is to pack the cells and then measure the volume of packed cells. For a 2% suspension, use 0.5 ml packed cells plus 24.5 ml of saline, and so on. This is not as accurate as the preceding method, but it is more practical.

Cell suspensions can be used for an entire day provided they are mixed before use and kept refrigerated. If the cells are to be kept overnight, remove the saline before placing in a refrigerator, then cover with group AB plasma or albumin. The following day, wash the cells three times with saline and again dilute them.

PREPARATION OF UNKNOWN SERUM

Remove blood from the vein in the usual manner and allow it to clot. Loosen the clot from the side of the tube with an applicator stick or glass rod, and centrifuge about 15 minutes at 1500 rpm to separate the serum from the clot. Aspirate the serum with a clean, dry capillary pipet and transfer to a clean, dry tube bearing the same label as the blood from which it was removed. Some workers prefer to pour off the serum. Small beads (Gradient Beads*) may be placed above the clotted blood, and after the blood is centrifuged, the serum may simply be poured off. No cells are present in the serum by this method. Cells carried over to the serum could constitute an interfering factor in the tests.

The serum is used fresh for most tests, but if it contains an isohemolysin that interferes with the readings, it should be inactivated at 56° C for 15 to 30 minutes and retested. Hemolyzed serum should preferably not be used. Serum should be stored in a refrigerator at 5° C until ready for use, then allowed to warm to room temperature. It is possible to maintain activity of antibodies by freezing the serum in liquid nitrogen or in a deep freeze.

OTHER REAGENTS

In addition to the blood grouping sera and standard cells, the unknown cells and unknown sera, anti-human globulin reagent is needed, as well as bovine albumin (usually 25% or 30%), Witebsky group A– and group B–specific substances, 0.85% sodium chloride in water, 0.067M phosphate buffer pH 7.41, and the various enzyme solutions.

EQUIPMENT AND GLASSWARE

Whenever possible it is best to use disposable glassware and discard it once it has been used. This prevents carry-over of any residual particles that might be present. If nondisposable glassware is used, follow the method of cleaning outlined on p. 235.

There should be a large supply of glass slides, ceramic ring or welled slides for blood grouping, droppers, straws (if capillary dropper pipets are not used), 1 ml pipets graduated in 0.1 ml, graduated 10 ml pipets for titrations, a supply of tubes containing dry anticoagulant, and test tube racks of various sizes to accommodate the variety of tubes. The tubes are 100 by 12 mm, 75 by 12 mm, 75 by 8 mm, and B-D Vacutainer tubes, either empty or containing dry anticoagulant for collecting specimens of blood if the blood is not to be taken by syringe.

There should be a microscope equipped with a scanning lens, as well as the conventional 10× and 44× objectives and a 10× eyepiece. It is best to have a thermostatically controlled water bath, or, better still, two water baths—one set at 37° C and one at 56° C. These should be kept covered.

Small angle centrifuges are preferred for the tests, but larger centrifuges for separating cells and plasma or clot and serum are also needed.

Disposable syringes and needles are recommended for collecting blood to prevent transmitting serum hepatitis when Vacutainer tubes are not used.

Various test tube racks to accommodate the different size tubes, as well as adjustable suspension test tube racks with handles (Fig. 17-4) for small tubes used in blood grouping are important. Small Kahn tube racks and Wassermann racks are also needed, as well as the standard test tube racks.

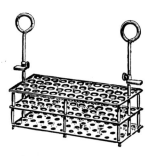

Fig. 17-4. Adjustable suspension test tube rack with handles, for small tubes used in blood grouping. (Courtesy Standard Scientific Supply Corporation, New York, N.Y.)

*Curtin Scientific, Houston, Texas.

The viewing box selected should be of the type that heats when the light is turned on. The temperature should not exceed 45° to 47° C, and a heated box should never be used when testing for the A-B-O blood group factors (Fig. 17-5).

There should be a large supply of wooden applicators and disposable droppers, 12 ply gauze pads 75 × 75 mm, a red, a blue, and a black wax pencil, 22 mm cover glasses, an electric rotating apparatus, and 250 ml glass containers of various shapes.

Absolute chemical cleanliness is a necessity, but the glassware need not be sterile except in certain instances. It must, however, be dry.

Preparation of slides

Boerner microtest slides are 88 by 58 by 2 mm, with rounded corners, and they have ten mold-pressed, raised rings, 15 mm top diameter, in two rows each, numbered consecutively from 1 to 10. Other sizes are available. The bottom of the wells should be flat. The slides are easily examined under a microscope. Ceramic ring slides can be purchased in many sizes. The rings are baked onto the slides. Both the Boerner slides and the ceramic ring slides may be used repeatedly if properly cleaned and dried. After use the slides should be soaked in large quantities of water, washed in Edisonite, rinsed many times to remove any traces of substances

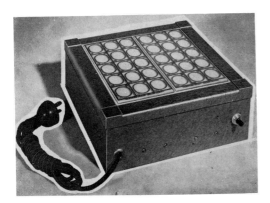

Fig. 17-5. Illuminated viewing box for blood grouping. (Courtesy Behring Diagnostics, Woodbury, N.Y.)

that could adhere to the slide, and then dried. There are also disposable slides.

Centrifuges

A number of different manufacturers have made fixed-speed centrifuges available for blood grouping purposes only. Follow the manufacturer's directions for standardization. (See p. 226.)

ABSORPTION TESTS

Absorption tests are used to identify the blood group of stains from blood, semen, vaginal fluid, saliva, gastric contents, etc. of secretors. They are also important in studying newly found antibodies and identifying them. Absorption technics can be used to remove unwanted antibodies so that the absorbed serum contains either only a single antibody or else the antibodies that the worker wishes to study without interference from species-specific antibodies, as when preparing anti-**M** and anti-**N** reagents from immune rabbit sera. These technics are also used to prepare antisera for laboratory testing purposes and to confirm the presence of weak antigens present on red cells.

The cell-serum ratio in absorption tests is higher than that in the direct agglutination tests. There must be sufficient antigen to remove the antibody from the serum, or else the serum must be diluted to a point where the antigen of the cells can remove all the antibody in the diluted material. This latter method is used in identification of blood stains. Some authorities suggest that there should be one volume of packed cells for each volume of serum that is to be absorbed.

The following steps illustrate the general method. For each test in this text in which absorption is part of the method, the appropriate technic will be presented in detail.

Cells for the absorption test must have the particular antigen with which the antibody will react. These cells are washed three to four times in saline to remove all protein that may be present. After the last washing, the red cells are centrifuged to pack them. There should be as little saline as possible remaining with the cells, and for this reason the cells are tightly packed. The saline can be removed either by vacuum aspiration, by decantation, or by rapidly turning the tube upside down perpendicularly and, with the tube still in that position, touching the lip of the tube against a thick gauze square to remove any traces of free saline.

A volume of serum equal to the volume of absorbing cells is added to the packed, washed cells and the two mixed well.

The next step is incubation in a water bath for 30 to 60 minutes, depending on the test, the antigen, and the antibody. If the antibody is a cold-reacting one, absorption should be made at refrigerator temperature. If it is a "warm" agglutinin, the absorption is carried out at 37° C in a water bath. Otherwise it may be done at room temperature.

After incubation the tube is centrifuged and the supernatant serum removed immediately. The cells may be saved for later elution tests.

The theory of this method is that the cells and antibody, being specific for one another, will combine and the antibody will be adsorbed onto the cells. The serum, after absorption, either has no antibody at all or it has residual unabsorbed antibodies, assuming that it originally had more than one kind.

If enzyme-treated cells are to be used, these may be treated with ficin, trypsin, papain, bromelin, or a special product called Spectrazyme.*

Where the antigen is in solution, as in saliva and other body secretions, the neutralization of antibody is called **inhibition,** which is similar in principle to absorption by red cells. The inhibition test is described later. Absorption tests are also useful in studies on the blood groups and specificities in nonhuman primates and in other animals.

In the Lewis system, tests are made not only on the red blood cells, using anti-**Le** serum, but also on the saliva. Two inhibition tests are needed to establish the genotypes, in addition to the tests for blood and saliva types. In this case the **Le** antiserum is inhibited by the boiled saliva for

---

*A stable enzyme solution available as a blend of ficin, papain, and bromelin from Spectra Biologicals, Oxnard, Calif.

the **Le saliva types,** and the anti-**H** lectin is inhibited by the boiled saliva to establish A-B-H **secretor status.** These tests are described later.

By use of absorption tests the presence of a specific antigen on the cells can also be determined, which forms the basis for the methods of identifying the blood groups of dried stains. The red cells or blood stains are mixed with the appropriate antiserum, and these two are allowed to remain together for a fixed period of time. The mixture is then centrifuged to remove red cells and particulate matter and the supernate tested for agglutinins. If the agglutinins that were present in the original antiserum used in the test are still there, the cells or blood stain did not have the antigen for which the antiserum is specific. If the absorbed antiserum fails to agglutinate the cells for which it is specific, the agglutinins have been removed by the cells (or stain), which therefore have the antigen for which the antiserum is specific. This is detailed later.

The absorption method is also used to determine whether an antiserum has more than one antibody and for the fractionation of antisera such as anti-**M** and anti-**Rh** by nonhuman primate red cells (Chapter 15).

ELUTION TESTS

After an antibody has become attached to its specific cells, it can be recovered by elution. The antibody thus recovered in solution is designated an **eluate.** Elution methods are useful (1) to separate and identify antibodies in sera that have more than one antibody; (2) to confirm antibody specificity; (3) to confirm the presence of weak antigens on red cells; (4) to identify antibodies that have caused hemolytic disease of the newborn, especially when the antibody seems to be of a type not previously described; (5) to identify antibodies that have caused transfusion reactions; and (6) to study antibodies in cases of acquired hemolytic anemia. Elutions can be made whether the antibodies have attached themselves to the red cells in vivo or in vitro. Variants in the A-B-O system have been identified by elution methods. In erythroblastosis fetalis the antibody on the red cells of the infant or of the umbilical cord can be eluted. This is especially useful when the mother's serum is not available for testing.

The accuracy of the methods depends on *complete* removal of unabsorbed antibody that surrounds the red cells, and therefore the cells must be washed as many as three to twelve times before attempting to elute the adsorbed antibody. Elution tests are routine in some laboratories. The serologic behavior of an eluate is not always the same as that of the antibody in the serum before absorption.

For the antibody to be eluted, the antigen-antibody complex must be broken, which often means destruction of the red cells and release of hemoglobin into the eluate. In the Landsteiner-Miller method this is accomplished by heat, in the W. Weiner method by freeze-thaw, and in the Rubin technic by ether.

When an eluate is to be stored before testing, the antibody should be eluted in 6% bovine albumin or in group AB serum; otherwise, saline is the fluid of choice.

Landsteiner-Miller heat elution method[25]

1. Prepare a heavy suspension of the cells coated with antibodies that are to be eluted, and wash with large volumes of saline until all free antibody has been removed. Test the supernate for antibody at the end of the fourth washing, and if free antibody is still present, continue the washing until there is no reaction between the supernate and the specific cells.
2. After the last centrifugation, remove the supernatant liquid thoroughly and completely and add an equal volume of saline. If the cells are to be stored, use group AB serum or 6% bovine albumin, as previously stated.
3. Mix thoroughly, place in a water bath at 56° C for approximately 10 minutes, agitating frequently during incubation, that is, every 15 seconds.
4. Immediately transfer the tube to a prewarmed centrifuge cup containing water at 56° C and centrifuge at high speed.
5. The recovered supernatant eluate will nec-

essarily be hemoglobin-tinged. Remove the eluate and test as directed in the discussion of testing the eluate (p. 250).

Heat elution at 42° to 44° C

The purpose of this method is to prepare red blood cells to be used in tests that require uncoated cells. It is *not* done to obtain a strong antibody preparation. Do not let the temperature rise above 44° C; otherwise the antigenic sites might be damaged, and the cells therefore would not be suitable for use.

1. Prepare packed washed red cells.
2. Add several volumes of saline to each volume of red cells.
3. Mix. Place in a water bath at 42° to 44° C for 30 to 60 minutes, agitating frequently.
4. Wash the cells three or four times in warm saline (42° to 44° C).
5. Test the cells by the direct antiglobulin method (p. 252).
6. If the results are positive, repeat the elution until the direct antiglobulin test is negative. This may require several elutions.

W. Weiner freeze-thaw method[26]

This is an alcohol precipitation method. It is not successful in eluting anti-**A** and anti-**B**.

1. Wash the cells as directed in the Landsteiner-Miller method, remove the last supernate from the packed cells, stopper the tube, and place the cells in a deep freeze at -6° to -35° C for 30 to 60 minutes.
2. As soon as the cells are frozen, remove and thaw at room temperature.
3. When thawing is just complete, add ten times the original red cell volume of 50% ethanol cooled to -6° C or lower. Mix rapidly, restopper, and rapidly invert to mix the alcohol thoroughly with the laked red cells.
4. Return the tube to the freezer for 30 to 60 minutes to complete precipitation of the antibody proteins.
5. Centrifuge at 3000 rpm for at least 5 minutes. There should be a dense sediment.
6. Completely remove and discard the supernate, then fill the tube with distilled water.
7. Loosen the precipitate along the side and bottom of the tube, using a clean, pointed glass rod, stopper the tube, and mix vigorously.

8. Recentrifuge at 3000 rpm for 5 minutes, and discard the supernate.
9. Add saline (or group AB serum or 25% or 30% bovine albumin), break up the sediment, and mix thoroughly with a glass rod. Determine the amount of saline to be added according to the titer of the original direct antiglobulin test. If the reaction was 3+ or 4+, add two to three times the lysed red cell volume. If the reaction was 1+ or 2+, add one fourth to one half the lysed red cell volume.
10. Place in a water bath at 37° C for 30 to 60 minutes, then centrifuge at high speed and remove the supernate for testing. See the discussion of testing the eluate (below).

Rubin ether elution method[27]

This method is particularly applicable to antibodies in the Rh-Hr system. Take care to avoid sparks or flame because of the highly volatile ether used.

1. Wash the cells, as directed previously, six times in large volumes of saline. After the last washing, pack the cells and remove as much of the saline as possible.
2. Add an equal volume of saline to the cells.
3. Add a volume of reagent grade diethyl (anesthetic) ether equal to the total volume of saline and packed red cells together, stopper the tube, and mix by inversion for 1 minute. Remove the stopper carefully so as to release the volatile ether gradually.
4. Incubate at 37° C for 30 minutes.
5. Centrifuge at 1000 g for 10 minutes or at 3000 rpm. These should be three distinct layers—the upper containing clear ether, the middle the denatured red cell stromata, and the bottom the hemoglobin-stained eluate.
6. Remove the ether and stroma layers by aspiration, with suction, or carefully insert a capillary pipet along the side of the tube to the bottom and remove the eluate to a second tube.
7. Centrifuge the eluate at high speed to remove any remaining particles.
8. Transfer the supernatant eluate to a clean tube.
9. Incubate the eluate in an unstoppered tube at 37° C for 15 minutes to evaporate any residual ether. Then test the eluate as described in the following discussion.

To test the eluate

If the antibody is of unknown specificity, test against a panel of cells, using the same method as that for an unknown blood serum. The cells that are agglutinated necessarily have the antigen for which the eluate has a specific antibody.

If this is a test for an antibody eluted from cells known to have some or any of the Rh-Hr antigens, test with at least three red cell samples having the suspected antigenic determinant and at least three cell specimens lacking the determinant, if at all possible. This will confirm the identity of the antibody.

ANTIGLOBULIN TESTS

The chapter on antibodies contains detailed information on various differences in the makeup of agglutinins, conglutinins, complete and incomplete antibodies, or, preferably, of the 7S (IgG) and the 19S (IgM) antibodies. In short, some antibodies (7S) combine with the red cells without agglutinating them, whereas others (19S) of the same specificity directly agglutinate red cells suspended in saline media. The former (7S) antibodies are of smaller molecular size and require a third substance besides antigen and antibody to cause clumping of the cells. Such antibodies coat the red cells without agglutinating them in saline media. Naturally the laboratory cannot detect antibodies that do not give visible reactions with cells. A number of tests were devised to detect such antibodies after Wiener[28] demonstrated the existence of two types of antibodies of the same specificity: one that agglutinates cells suspended in saline, the other (blocking antibody) that does not react with the cells visibly but instead coats them and blocks their agglutination by the first type of antibody. The **blocking test** of Wiener was not sensitive enough to be used clinically unless the antisera were of high titer. Later he proposed the more sensitive **conglutination test**,[29] and in the same journal Diamond and Denton[30] described the **albumin test**. Wiener et al.[31] later proposed similar tests using colloid media like dextran, acacia, etc. In 1945 Coombs et al.[32] described a test for detecting weak and incomplete Rh agglutinins, which has now become a standard laboratory procedure. It is known as the **Coombs test,** more properly the **antiglobulin test.** The test had actually been described as early as 1908 by Moreschi[33] who used it for testing bacterial antisera. Morton and Pickles,[34] in 1947, and Wiener and Katz,[35] in 1951, described the various **enzyme tests.** At the present time the enzyme tests are combined with the antiglobulin test in many instances to identify antibodies and antigens.

The purpose of the antiglobulin test therefore is to detect 7S, or IgG antibodies (also called **coating,** or **blocking antibodies**), which do not agglutinate red cells in saline media but coat them. These antibodies are globulins that are immunologically bound to red cells. If they have coated the red cells and if an anti–human globulin serum is added, the antiglobulin (itself an antibody against the human globulin that is the coating antibody) reacts with the globulin (antibody) on the red cells and the cells then clump. This can be explained as follows:

Red cells having blood group specificity (factor) + 7S antibody = coating of cells
Coated cells + antiglobulin = clumping of cells

Complement is not needed in this type of reaction. If the antibodies are complement-dependent, they require **anti–nongamma globulin.** The reaction is:

Cells with blood group specificity + antibody + complement + antiglobulin = reaction

By the use of radioiodine-labeled anti-Rh_0 serum, it has been shown that as few as 300 molecules of IgG per red cell may be sufficient to produce agglutination in the antiglobulin reaction.[36] The complement-fixing antibody consumption (CFAC) test is a research procedure (1976) that detects fewer than 35 molecules of IgG per cell. This is important in certain conditions, such as acquired immunohemolytic anemia, in which a negative antiglobulin reaction occurs when conventional methods are used, but in reality abnormally high amounts of cell-bound IgG (70 to 434 molecules per cell) are present. Red cells with fewer than 35 molecules of IgG per cell are considered to have nonimmunologically bound IgG. Thus, the conventional antiglobulin test, although inherently sensitive, fails to detect immunologically significant red cell sensitization if the red cells are coated with only 35 to 300 molecules of IgG per cell. Until the CFAC test is made feasible for routine usage, the antiglobulin test as now performed still remains a valuable procedure.

Antiglobulin reagent supplied by many serum producers is of the broad-spectrum variety that can be used in either the direct or indirect antiglobulin test.

Antiglobulin serum is prepared by injecting animals, usually rabbits or goats, with whole human serum or with purified human serum globulin. The globulin acts as an antigen and stimulates formation of antiglobulin by the injected animal. After an adequate course of injections, the animal blood containing the antiglobulin antibody (and other unwanted antibodies) is taken from the animal, the serum is separated from the clot, and the serum is then absorbed with pooled, washed (ten times) human group A, B, and O cells to remove all antibodies except the antiglobulin. The antiglobulin antibodies react with their specific antigen, human globulin; they are complete, IgM antibodies.

There are two types of antiglobulin tests: (1) the direct test, which detects red cells already coated with antibody in vivo, and (2) the indirect test, in which the red cells must first be coated with antibody in vitro and then, after suitable preparation, tested with antiglobulin serum.

The **direct test** consists of washing the already coated cells, then mixing with antiglobulin serum, centrifuging, and examining for agglutination. It is used in the diagnosis of erythroblastosis fetalis, in which the red cells of the infant or the cells of cord blood have been coated with antibody in utero; in the diagnosis of autoimmune hemolytic anemia, in which the red cells have also been coated in vivo; and in the investigation of transfusion reactions, in which a 7S, or IgG, antibody is suspected and the transfused cells would then have become coated in vivo.

In the **indirect test** the cells are suspended in saline, and 7S, or IgG (incomplete), antibody antiserum is added. After mixing and incubating to allow time for the antibody and the cells to combine, the cells are washed thoroughly to remove all free antibody and protein, the antiglobulin serum is added, and the mixture centrifuged. The reaction is read after the cells have been gently resuspended. This test is used in cross matching to detect incompatibility in which a 7S, or IgG, antibody may be involved, in detecting and identifying irregular antibodies, in detecting antigens not demonstrable by other methods, in investigative studies such as those on the blood groups of nonhuman primates, in mixed agglutination tests, and so on.

Direct antiglobulin test (Coombs test)

1. Wash the red cells four times in saline, using large quantities of saline for each washing.
2. After the last washing and centrifugation, quickly turn the tube upside down and, while still inverted, touch against a pad of gauze to remove all traces of saline.
3. Resuspend the cells to approximately 4% concentration in saline.
4. Perform the test in duplicate. Place 2 drops of washed, saline-suspended cells in a clean, dry tube 7 by 70 mm; add 2 drops of antiglobulin serum, then mix.
5. If the cells have been very strongly sensitized by coating antibodies, they clump almost immediately. Examine over a lighted viewing box.
6. If the cells have not been maximally coated in vivo, the reaction might be weak. If this is the case or if the reaction appears to be negative, allow the tube to stand at room temperature for a few minutes, then centrifuge at 500 rpm for 2 minutes, resuspend the sediment, and again read over a lighted viewing box.
7. *Readings:* Clumping is a positive reaction; absence of clumping is negative.
8. *Controls:* Use red cells coated with antibody (p. 287) and carry out the test in the same manner. This is a positive control. For a negative control, use any cells that have not been coated with antibody and proceed as above.

Drug-induced positive antiglobulin test (anti-penicillin antibodies)

A positive direct antiglobulin test may be the result of antibodies produced against certain drugs that have been administered to the patient. The most important of these drugs are penicillin, cephalothin, p-aminosalicylate, isoniazid, and alpha-methyldopa. Penicillin not only coats the red cells but also leads to the production of anti–penicillin-IgG globulin, which may act on the penicillin-sensitized red cells and produce a severe hemolytic anemia. Penicillin-sensitized red cells for testing can be produced in the laboratory. These can then be used to detect serum penicillin antibodies in the patient, or the anti-penicillin antibody may be eluted from the patient's sensitized red cells and the eluate tested against laboratory penicillin-sensitized red cells. The following procedure is modified from Bauer et al.[37]

Penicillin-coated red cells

1. Obtain 10 ml of blood, and transfer 1 ml to a tube without an anticoagulant, as a control.
2. Place 1 ml of ACD solution in a test tube and add the remaining 9 ml of blood to it and mix.
3. Reconstitute 500,000 units of buffered potassium penicillin G with 4 ml of distilled water.
4. Add 1 ml of penicillin solution to the blood in the anticoagulant.
5. Incubate the mixture at 37° C for 30 minutes and at 4° C for at least 60 minutes.
6. Wash the cells three times in saline solution to remove excess penicillin.
7. *Controls:* Known anti-penicillin serum should agglutinate penicillin-coated cells at room temperature or after conversion to the anti–human globulin test. Always run positive and negative controls.

Anti-penicillin serum is one that gives a positive direct antiglobulin test and may be obtained from a patient who has become sensitized to the drug.

Indirect antiglobulin test

1. Obtain blood in the usual manner, suspend the red cells in saline, and wash once in saline if the method requires washing of

the cells. Resuspend the washed cells to a 4% concentration in saline.

2. Make duplicate tests. Use 2 drops of saline-suspended cells with 2 drops of the serum being tested in each of the tubes.

3. Mix and let stand for the time required by the test—30 to 60 minutes at room temperature, 30 minutes in a 37° C water bath, etc.

4. If the cells have agglutinated, the indirect antiglobulin test is unnecessary. If they have not agglutinated, centrifuge at 500 rpm for 2 minutes, resuspend, and read. If they still have not clumped, proceed with the **antiglobulin test**.

5. Wash the cells four times with large quantities of saline. After the last washing, when the cells are firmly packed, remove all traces of supernatant saline.

6. Add 2 drops of antiglobulin serum to each tube, shake to mix, and centrifuge at 500 to 1000 rpm for 2 minutes.

7. Gently dislodge the sediment, tip the tube back and forth, allowing the cells to settle, and read under a scanning lens or if the clumps are large, macroscopically.

8. If the cells have agglutinated, the serum contains a 7S, or IgG, antibody specific for the antigen on the cells.

The indirect antiglobulin test may be made on cells that have been treated with enzymes. Unger used the antiglobulin test to examine all negatively reacting ficinated red cells. This is the **Unger ficinated cell antiglobulin test**. It is sensitive and useful, especially in tests with anti-**Lewis** sera.

Factors that affect the antiglobulin tests

Time and temperature of incubation. Sufficient time of incubation should be allowed to enable antibodies to coat the red cells. This refers, naturally, only to the indirect test because the antibodies are presumably already attached when a direct test is run. Most antibodies require 15 to 30 minutes, but some need a longer incubation period, as in the Fy and Jk systems. The temperature should be 37° C, and incubation should be carried out in a water bath. If a dry air incubator is used, the tests should be placed in a container of water at 37° C in the incubator. The tubes should remain at this temperature until the beginning of the washing period.

Suspending medium; enzyme treatment. The suspending medium for the red cells may vary with the blood group system under investigation. Some tests require that the cells be treated with enzymes before applying the antiglobulin test; others require only that they be suspended in saline, albumin, or fresh serum. Enzyme treatment may increase the sensitivity of the cells, but **some red cell antigens are destroyed and will not react if treated with proteolytic enzymes.**

Washing. Washing must be carried out rapidly, and once the procedure begins, it must not be interrupted. Use adequate volumes of saline. Washings may be made in regular Kahn tubes, 10 × 75 mm, in which case three to four washings generally suffice. The saline must be added with force, preferably from a measuring pump, but a dropper with a fine tip will also give sufficient force to dislodge the cells from the bottom of the tube. In any event, the finger must never be placed over the top of the tube to invert it to mix the cells. Wax paper may be used, but it must be held tightly in place when the tube is being inverted or the fluid and red cells can leak out. Protein from the skin surface, in a quantity as low as a 1:4000 dilution, can neutralize 1 drop of antiglobulin serum.

The saline must be decanted completely between each washing and the cells resuspended. If cells remain in even a small button at the bottom of the tube, enough protein may be trapped there to negate the test.

To evaluate the efficiency of washing, add an equal volume of 25% sulfosalicylic acid to the supernate removed from each washing. As long as a turbidity develops, protein is present. The supernate from the last washing must show no turbidity.

Centrifugation. In agglutination tests, it must be remembered that the antibody molecule is extremely small, and therefore any force that can bring the red cells into contact with one another facilitates their linkage by the antibody molecules. Rotating, centrifuging, and so on are therefore used to speed up agglutination. Centrifugation causes a more rapid and complete agglutination than simply allowing natural sedimentation to take place. The relative centrifugal force (expressed in numerical gravities and indicated by the letter *g*), the time of centrifugation, and the suspending medium are all important.

Inadequate centrifugation and insufficient packing of cells may lead to a false negative result. Overcentrifugation may pack the red cells so tightly together that they cannot be resuspended fully even though not coated by antibodies, resulting in a false positive report. It is best to take the advice of the manufacturer of the reagent when determining duration and speed of centrifugation.

The supernate must be clear after centrifugation; the cell button should have a sharp margin, but the cells must be easily dislodged from the bottom of the tube by gentle shaking. Cells treated with certain enzymes tend to stick together even when not coated by antibody and may be difficult to resuspend. They may have to be shaken a little harder than otherwise. **Use the least force and time of centrifugation** to produce correct reactions for the controls of known blood types.

A number of blood banks use fixed-speed centrifuges. Each centrifuge should be standardized separately.

Evaluation of results. Examine the supernate for hemolysis immediately after centrifugation. If the original serum did not contain hemoglobin but the supernate is reddish, this complete or partial hemolysis is a positive reaction, provided no water has entered the tube at any time.

To dislodge the cells from the bottom of the tube, shake gently until all cells are free, then tilt back and forth to form an even suspension of cells or clearly visible agglutinates. Examine over a light source or with a magnifying lens or a scanning lens of a microscope. Record results as on p. 227.

Controls. Check the antiglobulin serum daily, using **coated cells** * and carrying out the same method as for an unknown. Check also against noncoated cells.

Quality control of antiglobulin reactions. As in all tube tests, drop the serum, cells, and reagents into the tubes so that they go directly to the bottom and do not run along the sides. Add each in the proper quantity according to the test or directions from the manufacturer of the antiglobulin serum. Be sure to use the proper time and temperature of incubation. Always wash the cells in sufficient saline to remove any uncombined antiglobulin reagent; otherwise, the antiglobulin serum will be neutralized by the uncombined antiserum, and a false negative result will ensue. After each washing and centrifugation, completely disrupt the button of cells with a jet of saline so as not to trap any serum in the cell button. Be sure that the last drop of saline is removed.

The correct amount of antiglobulin serum must be used as soon as possible after the cells have been washed, then the button of cells dispersed by shaking the tube gently and allowing the serum and cells to remain in contact for the required period of time at the correct temperature. After this, centrifuge for the correct amount of time and *g* force.

The reagents should be stored in a refrigerator until needed and left at room temperature only as long as it takes for the temperature to become adjusted. If the reagents show any evidence of bacterial or mold growth, they should be discarded.

Some laboratories add previously sensitized red cells to any antiglobulin reaction that is negative. These cells should agglutinate. If the tests have been properly carried out and controls are used correctly, this is not necessary, but at times it is well to check the laboratory or the antiglobulin reagents. Such checking is essential when using automated equipment.

False negative results. If cells are inade-

---

*The method of coating cells with antibody is described on p. 287.

quately washed, the antiglobulin serum may be neutralized by the residual trace amounts of globulin in the supernate, leading to false negative results. Human serum will neutralize the reagent. Take special care that the dropper in the vial of antiglobulin serum does not come in contact with a mixture of cells and serum when performing the test. The entire vial of antiglobulin reagent would be rendered worthless should this occur. Be sure not to touch the top of the tube with the finger or palm of the hand when inverting the tube. Cover the top of the tube with wax paper or stopper it with a cork surrounded by wax paper.

Always complete the test immediately after it is begun. Delays may result in elution of antibody from the red cells. Maintain the correct temperature and time for maximal coating of the cells.

Do not use too heavy a cell suspension, or the cells cannot all be coated with antibody. On the other hand, a weak cell suspension yields small clumps difficult to read. Keep the suspension at 4% to 5% concentration. When washing the cells, take special care not to lose any cells during the process either by aspirating them into the capillary pipet or when inverting the tube.

If examining for complement-dependent antibodies, complement must be added. Use **fresh** neutral (group AB) serum but not plasma, since anticoagulants are anticomplementary.

If the antiglobulin serum has not been correctly standardized, there could be a prozone. Follow the manufacturer's directions precisely.

If a negative reaction is not expected but does occur, repeat the test. The antiglobulin reagent may have been omitted inadvertently. Check the speed and time of centrifugation.

False negative reactions may also be due to (1) inadequate washing of red cells, as already explained; (2) excessive packing of red cells in the washing procedure before the cells are thoroughly washed, which traps protein between the red cells and

neutralizes the reagent; (3) contamination of antiglobulin reagent with human protein that neutralizes the antiglobulin (do not use pipets that must be put into the mouth); (4) absence of complement in a serum that has a complement-dependent antibody; (5) absence of anticomplement in the antiglobulin serum; (6) insufficient incubation of cells and serum; (7) elution of antibody from red cells after prolonged contact with antiglobulin reagent; (8) elution of antibody from red cells when the washing procedure is interrupted and the cells are allowed to remain in saline for considerable amounts of time; (9) incubation at temperatures other than optimal; and (10) inadequately cleaned glassware containing either minute traces of dried blood or a detergent.

A number of diseases or immunologic abnormalities will also produce false positive results as well as false negatives in an antiglobulin reaction.

False positive results. Red cells that give a positive direct reaction must not be used for the antiglobulin test because they will agglutinate regardless of what is done. Avoid bacterial contamination, and bear in mind that cells from a septicemic patient could be agglutinated by any serum (panagglutination).

In tests on umbilical cord blood, wash the cells four times or more with saline to remove Wharton's jelly.

Extreme reticulocytosis may cause a positive result because reticulocytes react with antiglobulin serum. Saline that has been stored for a long time in glass bottles may contain colloidal silica that has been leached from the container, leading to false positive results. If the saline has been stored in containers with metal parts and metallic ions are present, the red cells may become coated with protein (see cross matching, p. 311).

Antiglobulin serum from reliable sources is generally not at fault in cases of false positive reactions. If, however, there are traces of species-specific antibodies—that is, if the antiglobulin serum has not been completely absorbed during its preparation—there can be a false positive reaction due to such antibodies.

If all the antiglobulin tests are weakly positive, look for some form of contamination in the reagents or glassware, and conduct a thorough investigation before running any more tests.

Overcentrifugation may be responsible for mistaking a negative reaction for a positive.

False positive reactions can also be due to (1) chemical contamination with copper, zinc, or iron present in saline or detergent traces on glassware; (2) poor quality of saline (hypertonic, bacterially contaminated); (3) colloidal silica from the use of glass bottles; (4) antiglobulin serum with additional antibody specificity; (5) bacterial contamination of reagents, test cells, or unknown serum; (6) serum that contains saline agglutinins; (7) cold agglutinins (cells from donor pilot tubes stored for long periods at 4° C may have naturally occurring cold agglutinins adsorbed to their surfaces); and (8) clots or fibrin particles.

REFERENCES

1. Wiener, A. S., and Cioffi, A. F.: Am. J. Clin. Pathol. 58:693, 1972.
2. Jenkins, W. J., and Marsh, W. F.: Transfusion 5:6, 1965.
3. Bird, G. W. G., Wingham, J., Chester, G. H., Hill, D. M., Kidd, P., and Payne, R. W.: Br. J. Haematol. 33:295, 1976.
4. Bird, G. W. G., Shinton, N. K., and Wingham, J.: Br. J. Haematol. 21:443, 1971.
5. Greenwalt, T. J., and Steane, E. A.: Postgrad. Med. 52:170, 1972.
6. Friedenreich, B.: The Thomsen hemagglutination phenomenon, Copenhagen, 1930, Levin & Munksgaard.
7. Bird, G. W. G., and Wingham, J.: Br. J. Haematol. 23:759, 1972.
8. Bird, G. W. G.: Rev. Fr. Transfus. Immunohématol. 19:231, 1976.
9. van Logham, J. J., Jr., van der Hart, M., and Band, M. E.: Vox Sang. 5:125, 1955.
10. Springer, G., and Desai, P.: Biochem. Biophys. Res. Comm. 61:470, 1974.
11. Crookston, J. H., Crookston, M. C., Burnie, K. L., Francombe, W. H., Dacie, J. V., Davis, J. A., and Lewis, S. H.: Br. J. Haematol. 17:11, 1969.
12. Crookston, J. H., Crookston, M. C., and Rosse, W. F.: Br. J. Haematol. 23:83, 1972.
13. Wiener, A. S.: Lab. Digest 15:11, 1952.
14. Myhre, B. A.: Quality control in blood banking, New York, 1974, John Wiley & Sons, Inc.
15. Medart, W. S.: A.S.C.P. Summ. Rep. 9(7):1, 1972.
16. Erskine, A. G. In Frankel, S., Reitman, S., and Sonnenwirth, A. C.: Gradwohl's clinical laboratory methods and diagnosis, ed. 7, St. Louis, 1970, The C. V. Mosby Co.
17. Bird, G. W. G.: Br. Med. Bull. 15:165, 1959.
18. Ottensooser, F., and Silberschmidt, K.: Nature (Lond.) 172:914, 1953.
19. Rowe, A. W., Davis, J. H., and Moor-Jankowski, J.: Primates in medicine, vol. 7, Basel, 1972, S. Karger AG.
20. Rowe, A. W., and Allen, F. H.: Transfusion 5:379, 1965.
21. Rowe, A. W., Borel, H., and Allen, F. H., Jr.: Vox Sang. 22:188, 1972.
22. Rowe, A. W., Eyster, E., and Kellner, A.: Cryobiology 5:119, 1968.
23. Walker, R. H.: A.S.C.P. Commission on Continuing Education Check Sample 1:49, 1970.
24. Schwachman, H., Patterson, P. R., and Laguna, J.: Pediatrics 4:222, 1949.
25. Landsteiner, K., and Miller, C. P.: J. Exp. Med. 42:853, 1925.
26. Weiner, W.: Br. J. Haematol. 3:276, 1957.
27. Rubin, H.: J. Clin. Pathol. 16:70, 1963.
28. Wiener, A. S.: Proc. Soc. Exp. Biol. Med. 56:173, 1944.
29. Wiener, A. S.: J. Lab. Clin. Med. 30:662, 1945.
30. Diamond, L. K., and Denton, R. L.: J. Lab. Clin. Med. 30:821, 1945.
31. Wiener, A. S., Hunt, J. G., and Sonn-Gordon, E. B.: J. Exp. Med. 86:267, 1947.
32. Coombs, R. R. A., Mourant, A. E., and Race, R. R.: Br. J. Exp. Pathol. 26:255, 1945.
33. Moreschi, C.: Zentralbl. Bakteriol. 46:49, 1908.
34. Morton, J. A., and Pickles, M. M.: Nature (Lond.) 159:779, 1947.
35. Wiener, A. S., and Katz, L.: J. Immunol. 66:51, 1951.
36. Gilliland, B. D., Leddy, J. P., and Vaughn, J. H.: J. Clin. Invest. 49:898, 1970.
37. Bauer, J. D., Ackerman, P. G., and Toro, G.: Clinical laboratory methods, ed. 8, St. Louis, 1974, The C. V. Mosby Co.
38. Prokop, O., Rackwitz, A., and Schlesinger, D.: S. Afr. J. Forensic Med. 12:108, 1965.
39. Sumida, S.: Transfusion of blood preserved by freezing, Philadelphia, 1973, J. B. Lippincott Co.

RECOMMENDED READINGS

Cohen, E., editor: Biomedical perspectives of agglutinins of invertebrate and plant origins, Ann. N.Y. Acad. Sci. **234**, 1974.

Mäkelä, O.: Studies in hemagglutinins of leguminosae seeds, Ann. Med. Exp. Fenn. **35**(supp. 11):1-133, 1957.

Sumida, S.: Transfusion of blood preserved by freezing, Philadelphia, 1973, J. B. Lippincott Co.

Technical methods and procedures of the American Association of Blood Banks, ed. 6, 1974, Washington, D.C.

Tobiška, J.: Die Phythämagglutinine, Berlin, 1964, Akademie Verlag.

18 □ Tests made in the A-B-O and Lewis blood group systems

TECHNIC OF TESTS IN THE A-B-O BLOOD GROUP SYSTEM

Certain tests are made prior to a blood transfusion to ensure that the donor blood will mix in vivo with the recipient's blood without agglutination or hemolysis. This is **compatibility testing**, or **cross matching**. Prior to this, the blood groups of the recipient and the donors are determined by testing the red cells with anti-**A** and anti-**B** typing sera, preferably also with group O serum, then confirming the results by testing the sera of the recipient and donors with groups A, B, and O cells. If the results of the two tests are inconsistent, both must be repeated, using different anti-**A** and anti-**B** reagents to test the cells and different sets of cells to test the sera. In some instances, especially when preparing large quantities of donor blood for open heart surgery in which the blood from more than one person will be used in the transfusion, it may be customary to test the bloods of the different donors against each other as well as against the blood of the recipient.

Controls are run on the antisera used to determine the blood group of cells and on the red cells used to test the sera. If the controls do not react correctly, different antisera or different control cells must be substituted and the tests and controls rerun.

To prepare for these tests, blood is taken from the recipient and the donors, the cells separated for cell suspensions, and the se-

rum removed for testing. There must be at hand anti-**A** and anti-**B** typing sera, as well as group O serum, group A cells (A_2 preferably, but A_1 will do), groups B and O red cells, ceramic ring slides for the open slide method, physiologic saline, wooden applicator sticks or toothpicks for stirring the mixtures, capillary dropper pipets, a centrifuge, and the required test tubes.

Testing unknown cells to determine A-B-O groups

Tests for the A-B-O groups may be made with cells suspended in saline, with whole blood, or with the blood cells that cling to applicator sticks dipped into a clot. For the cell suspension the red cells are suspended to a 3% concentration in saline (p. 241).

CONTROLS ON ANTI-A AND ANTI-B SERA

The controls are run simultaneously with the tests as a general rule, although there is no objection to running them separately before the tests are made.

Open slide method

1. Use two slides each with two ceramic or wax rings. If group O cells are to be included in controls, there must be three rings.
2. Label the left-hand ring "A cells," the second ring "B cells," and the third ring, if there is one, "O cells."
3. Label the first slide anti-**A** and the second slide anti-**B**, the first ring "A," the second ring "B," and the third ring "O."
4. Place 1 drop of known group A cells on the left side in the first ring, 1 drop of known group B cells in the second ring, and

258

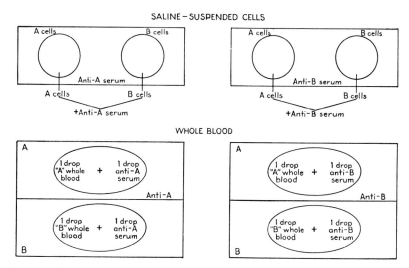

Fig. 18-1. Controls on anti-**A** and anti-**B** sera. (From Erskine, A. G. In Frankel, S., Reitman, S., and Sonnenwirth, A. C., editors: Gradwohl's clinical laboratory methods and diagnosis, ed. 7, St. Louis, 1970, The C. V. Mosby Co.)

1 drop of known group O cells in the third ring on each slide.

5. Add 1 large drop of known anti-**A** testing serum to each drop of cells on the first slide and 1 large drop of known anti-**B** typing serum to each drop of cells on the second slide.

6. Stir the contents of each ring with a separate wooden applicator or toothpick, then rotate the slides at 90 rpm or tilt them back and forth, then allow them to stand. Most commercial antisera are reactive within 10 seconds. Follow the suggested time that the manufacturer indicates in the instructions that come with the antisera. Such antisera are of high titer and avidity and so react quickly.

Read the reactions as positive (+) or negative (−). A positive reaction is indicated by large, brick-red clumps; a negative reaction is a smooth suspension of cells, without clumps, which is orange-red and pale because the red cells have been diluted.

7. Take preliminary readings, mix the drops again, add 1 drop of saline to each, mix, and reread. Be sure that the saline is added *after* and not before the reaction has had time to take place. No change in reaction should be observed after the addition of saline. The saline breaks up any rouleaux that might have formed and makes it easier to read the results.

The expected results with the controls are given in Table 18-1.

Table 18-1. Expected results in controls on anti-**A** and anti-**B** typing sera

	A cells	B cells	O cells
Anti-**A** serum	+	−	−
Anti-**B** serum	−	+	−

Table 18-2. Controls when group O serum is also used

	A cells	B cells	O cells
Group O serum	+	+	−

Group O cells should not be agglutinated by either antiserum. A positive reaction in the controls must be 4+. A clear negative (−) should be indicated when there is no agglutination.

A control on group O serum that will be used later in tests to determine the groups using unknown cells requires a third slide for testing A, B, and O cells with the group O serum, as in Table 18-2.

The use of group A_2 instead of A_1 cells is suggested because they are more weakly reactive than A_1 cells and therefore are more likely to reveal a weak anti-**A** serum in control tests. They will also detect deterioration of the anti-**A** serum sooner than will **A**$_1$ cells.

Never apply heat during this test.

If the cells for testing are obtained by dipping applicator sticks or toothpicks into a clot, the tests are performed by mixing the cells directly into the respective antisera from the sticks. Some suggest larger rings when this method is used. If whole blood is used for the tests—that is, blood taken in an anticoagulant without separating the cells and plasma—the rings should be at least 4 by 1.5 cm so that the blood may be stirred into the antiserum and then spread rather thin; otherwise, the reactions are difficult to read. If the tests are made in small tubes, the controls must also be made in tubes of the same size.

Tube method for controls

1. Use once-washed cells suspended to a 3% concentration in saline.

2. Label six small Kahn tubes, respectively, 1 to 6.

3. Label tubes 1, 2, and 3 as A, B, O, respectively, and tubes 4, 5, and 6 as A, B, O, respectively.

4. Place 1 drop of group A cells in tubes 1 and 4, 1 drop of group B cells in tubes 2 and 5, and 1 drop of group O cells in tubes 3 and 6.

5. Add 1 drop of anti-**A** serum to each of tubes 1, 2, and 3 and 1 drop of anti-**B** serum to each of tubes 4, 5, and 6.

6. Mix by shaking. Let the tubes stand at room temperature for 1 hour or centrifuge them at 1000 rpm for 2 minutes.

7. Gently dislodge the sediment and read. A hand lens or a scanning microscope may be used to read the results, but the reactions should be sufficiently strong to be read macroscopically without any enlargement.

8. The results should be as in Table 18-1.

9. If group O serum is used as a control, three more tubes should be prepared, containing, respectively, group A, B, and O cells, to each of which is added 1 large drop of group O serum. The tubes are han-

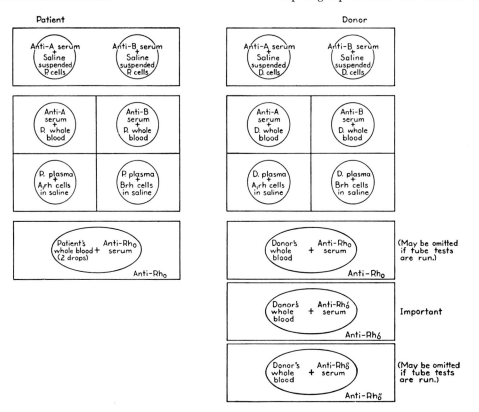

Fig. 18-2. Tests on patient and donor, open slide method. (From Erskine, A. G. In Frankel, S., Reitman, S., and Sonnenwirth, A. C., editors: Gradwohl's clinical laboratory methods and diagnosis, ed. 7, St. Louis, 1970, The C. V. Mosby Co.)

dled as above and the results read as in Table 18-2.

TESTS FOR THE A-B-O GROUPS USING CELLS AS THE UNKNOWN

This is a test for the isoagglutinogen content of the cells.

Open slide method

1. Prepare two slides with ceramic rings. If group O serum is used as a testing reagent, use three slides.
2. Label the slide with the identification of the individual whose blood is being tested and label the first ring anti-**A**, the second anti-**B**, and the third group O.
3. Place 1 drop of the unknown cell suspension in each ring.
4. Add 1 drop of anti-**A** serum to the first ring, 1 drop of anti-**B** serum to the second ring, and 1 drop of group O serum to the third ring.
5. Take care that the tips of the droppers dispensing the antisera do not touch the cell suspension. Should this occur, discard the dropper and its contents and begin the tests again using a fresh dropper.
6. Hold the antisera vials in a slanted position to help keep bacteria or particulate matter from entering them.
7. Mix the contents of each ring separately and rotate the slides. Examine macroscopically and later microscopically. Record a positive reaction when it occurs, but wait 5 minutes before recording a result as negative.
8. Add 1 drop of saline to each ring, mix, rotate, and reread, preferably under a microscope, using the low power.
9. Record agglutination as positive, even when the clumps are small (+), and absence of agglutination as negative (-). When in doubt, repeat the tests.
10. If desired, mix the contents of each ring with a separate toothpick before rotating

the slide. Do not use the toothpick for more than one ring.
11. Do not apply heat, which could interfere with the reaction.
12. Determine the blood group by consulting Table 18-3.

The importance of using group O serum, aside from its action as a control, is explained on pp. 263 and 264. Results from this test must be confirmed by testing the serum of the same individual against known A, B, and O cells, which is called reverse grouping.

Open slide method using whole blood. Whole blood is blood taken in an anticoagulant; the cells are thus already suspended in their natural plasma and not in saline. The controls in tests on whole blood must also make use of whole blood. The tests are made the same as when using cell suspensions, except for the relative quantities of blood and typing serum.

1. Prepare glass slides 75 by 50 mm by drawing oval red wax rings 30 by 20 mm with two such rings on a slide; if group O serum is to be used for testing purposes, prepare a third ring on a separate slide.
2. Label the first ring anti-**A**, the second ring anti-**B**, and the third group O serum. Identify the slides with the name or laboratory number of the individual whose blood is being tested.
3. Mix the whole blood, then transfer a small drop of the blood by just touching the slide with the end of a straw or dropper. A fraction of a drop is all that is required. Place some of the blood specimen in all three rings.
4. Add 2 drops of anti-**A** serum to the first drop, anti-**B** to the second, and group O serum to the third. There must be no delay in adding the antiserum; otherwise, drying

Table 18-3. Identification of the A-B-O blood groups using unknown cells

Unknown cells and anti-A serum	Unknown cells and anti-B serum	Unknown cells and group O serum	Blood group
−	−	−	O
+	−	+	A
−	+	+	B
+	+	+	AB
−	−	+	C (rare)

Anti-A   Anti-B
+   +
Unknown cells Unknown cells

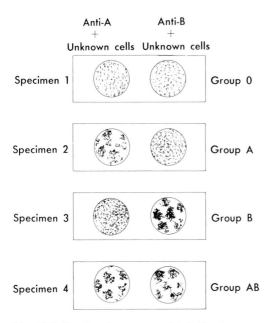

Specimen 1 — Group 0

Specimen 2 — Group A

Specimen 3 — Group B

Specimen 4 — Group AB

Fig. 18-3. Results of tests to establish blood group of an unknown cell suspension and known antisera.

may occur and the test will be worthless.
5. Mix the contents of each ring with a separate applicator stick or toothpick, spreading the mixture over the surface of the ring.
6. Place the slides on a viewing box but do not turn on the light. Allow them to remain 5 minutes, tipping the box back and forth occasionally. Then turn on the light so as to better read the results. Record agglutination as +, absence of agglutination as -.
7. Add 1 drop of saline to each ring, rock the slides gently and slowly back and forth on the viewing box, and reread. Do not read microscopically.
8. Determine the blood group by consulting Table 18-3. Adequate controls should be run simultaneously and read. The results of the controls should be as in Tables 18-1 and 18-2.
9. The controls are as follows:
   1. Group A whole blood and anti-**A** serum
   2. Group B whole blood and anti-**A** serum
   3. Group A whole blood and anti-**B** serum
   4. Group B whole blood and anti-**B** serum
   5. Group A whole blood and group O serum
   6. Group B whole blood and group O serum
Slides 1, 4, 5, and 6 must show agglutination.

The use of whole blood as a routine test is not recommended because it is difficult to regulate the ratio between whole blood and antiserum.

Open slide method using blood adhering to applicator sticks. This is the same technic as that using whole blood, except that the specimen is obtained by dipping applicator sticks into a clot and rubbing the cells that adhere to them into anti-**A** serum on the left side of the slide and rubbing a second set of cells obtained with other sticks into anti-**B** serum on the right. Do likewise with group O serum. Prepare the controls in the usual manner.

Testing unknown serum to determine A-B-O blood groups—reverse grouping

Testing the serum to determine the blood groups is called **reverse grouping.** It is a control over the results of tests previously made on the red cells. It can also be used to determine blood groups when serum (but not cells) is submitted to the laboratory, but such a procedure is not recommended for routine testing. No control is possible over the antibody content of the unknown serum, and there is no way of knowing prior to the tests whether the unknown serum has an isohemolysin along with the isoagglutinins. It is therefore well to inactivate the serum at 56° C for 15 minutes and then to let it cool to room temperature before testing. Fresh serum may be used, but if the reaction is unclear, it is advisable to inactivate the serum and rerun the tests. Isohemolysin requires complement to react. If isohemolysin and agglutinins against the same antigens are present in the same serum, the hemolysin usually reacts first. Manifestly, if the cells are dissolved, they cannot agglutinate. At times there is first a weak agglutination or no clumping at all, followed by hemolysis. Hemolysis changes the appearance of the drop, usually to reddish and transparent, although not all the cells are necessarily dissolved.

Group O cells are included in the test as a negative control.

The tests may be made either in tubes or on open slides. Since the antibody content of the serum is unknown, sufficient time must be allowed for any reaction to

Table 18-4. Identification of A-B-O groups using serum as the unknown

A₁ cells and unknown serum	B cells and unknown serum	O cells and unknown serum	Agglutinins in serum	Blood group
+	+	−	Anti-**A** and anti-**B**	O
−	+	−	Anti-**B**	A
+	−	−	Anti-**A**	B
−	−	−	Neither anti-**A** nor anti-**B**	AB

take place. The type of agglutination may vary from large, brick-red clumps to small, brownish or star-shaped clusters of cells.

Open slide method

1. Label a slide having three rings with the identification of the person whose serum is being tested. Label the first ring "A," the second "B," and the third "O."
2. Place 1 drop of known group A₁ cell suspension in the first ring, 1 drop of B cells in the second, and 1 drop of O cells in the third.
3. Add 1 large drop of the unknown serum to each ring.
4. Mix and rotate in the usual manner and record a positive reaction as soon as it occurs. Wait 7 or 8 minutes before recording a test as negative. A positive reaction may be either agglutination or hemolysis.
5. Read the reactions before surface drying can take place. After reading, add 1 drop of saline to each ring, mix, rotate, and then read again. The readings should be made under a microscope; otherwise, small clumps could be missed.
6. Determine the blood groups according to Table 18-4.

This is a test for isoagglutinin content of serum. If the serum has anti-**A** only, it will clump A but not B cells; if it has anti-**B** only, it will clump B but not A cells. If it has both anti-**A** and anti-**B**, it will clump both A and B cells. If it has neither anti-**A** nor anti-**B**, neither A nor B cells will be agglutinated. The group O cells must not be agglutinated. If they are, the unknown serum may have some antibody that has not been identified. The inclusion of group O cells is considered a negative control. A serum that agglutinates group A but not group B cells is group B. One that aggluti-

nates group B but not A cells is group A. A serum that agglutinates both A and B cells is group O, and one that does not clump either is group AB.

If the blood groups determined as a result of this test differ from those obtained by testing the cells of the same individual, there usually has been an error, and all the tests must be repeated. This test is therefore a control over the results in the direct test on the red cells. The test may also be made in tubes.

Tube method

1. Label three tubes with the name or laboratory number of the individual whose blood is being tested and also identify each with "A," "B," or "O," respectively.
2. Place 2 drops of the unknown serum in each tube.
3. Add 2 drops of known group A₁ cells to the first tube, 2 drops of group B cells to the second, and 2 drops of group O cells to the third. These are 3% saline suspensions of the cells.
4. Shake each tube to mix, and centrifuge at 1000 rpm for 2 minutes.
5. Read the reactions immediately, after gently dislodging the cells. If desired, the contents of the respective tubes may be poured onto a slide and read under a microscope, or a scanning lens may be used to read the reactions directly in the tubes.
6. If fresh (not inactivated) serum has been used, be aware that hemolysis may have occurred, which is also a positive reaction.
7. Identify the blood groups according to the results in Table 18-4.

Use of group O serum (erroneously called anti-A,B)

Group O serum may be used as a screening reagent to detect group O individuals and also as a confirmatory reagent in blood grouping tests. Its greatest value derives from the fact that the serum contains, in addition to anti-**A** and anti-**B**, a third antibody called anti-**C** (the cross-reacting antibody) that reacts with A and B cells as well as with AB but not with O. Cells of the rare group having the C antigen but no A or B could be missed if anti-**A** and anti-**B** sera alone were used, since neither of these two antisera contains anti-**C**. All cells except those of group O individuals should be agglutinated by group O serum, and only group O serum of high titer and avidity should be used for this test.

Group O serum reacts readily with group A_2 cells, which in newborn infants may be missed with ordinary anti-**A** sera. It also reacts with blood of the other subgroups of A, including group C, because of the anti-C agglutinin it contains. It is wrong to call group O serum anti-**A,B** because the serum also contains anti-**C**. Mixing anti-**A** and anti-**B** sera, which do not have anti-**C**, does not provide a serum comparable to that of group O. Before group O serum may be used as a reagent, it must be tested for reactivity against A_1, A_2, B, and O cells.

CONTROLS ON GROUP O SERUM

Controls may be made on open slides or in small tubes.

Slide test
1. Place 1 drop of 3% cell suspension in a ceramic ring on a slide.
2. Add 1 drop of group O serum.
3. Mix and rotate back and forth for 10 minutes.
4. Read microscopically and macroscopically.

Tube test
1. Place 1 drop of group O serum in a small tube and add 1 drop of 3% suspension of cells to be tested.
2. Let stand at room temperature for 1 hour or centrifuge immediately for 1 minute at 500 rpm.
3. Record clumping as a positive reaction, absence of clumping as negative.

If the cells are not agglutinated in either of these tests, the blood is group O. If clumping occurs, it is A, B, AB, or very rarely C. See Tables 18-3 and 18-5.

WEAK-REACTING A ANTIGEN

Several forms of the A antigen differ from one another, although slightly, in both qualitative and quantitative expression. The two most important subgroups of A are A_1 and A_2. A_1 is four times as frequent in occurrence as A_2. In some diseases, the A antigen may be weak. The best way to detect weak A antigens is by the use of group O serum as the antiserum, rather than by the use of anti-**A** from group B persons. The presence of the weak A antigen can be confirmed by absorption and elution methods.[1] Refer to p. 248ff for the method.

Tests for subgroups of A and AB

Subgroups of A and AB can be detected by use of absorbed anti-**A** serum, also designated anti-A_1 serum, or by anti-A_1 lectin. The red cells are tested to establish the subgroup, but it is also possible to test for anti-A_1 agglutinin, especially in the serum of subgroup A_2B, or for anti-**H** in the serum of subgroup A_1B.

The absorbed anti-**A** serum can be prepared in the laboratory; however, it is better to purchase it commercially prepared.

CONTROLS

Using absorbed anti-A serum. Time limits must be established within which it is safe to read a negative reaction whenever an absorbed serum is used. A positive reaction may be recorded as soon as it occurs, but a test should not be recorded as negative until after a specific time period. The purpose of the controls over absorbed anti-**A** serum therefore is twofold: (1) to make

Table 18-5. Reactions of cells with group O serum

Cells of group	Group O serum (see Table 18-3)
O	−
A	+
B	+
AB	+
C (rare)	+

certain that the reagent is in proper working order and will agglutinate cells that have A_1 agglutinogen but will not agglutinate cells with A_2 only and (2) to establish a time limit for reading the tests.

1. Have ready 3% suspensions in saline of known groups A_1 and A_2 cells.
2. Perform the tests on open slides with ceramic rings. Label one slide A_1, the other A_2.
3. Place 1 drop of A_1 cells on the slide labeled A_1 and 1 drop of A_2 cells on the slide labeled A_2.
4. Add 1 drop of absorbed anti-**A** serum to each, mix, and rotate periodically, watching the reactions microscopically and macroscopically.
5. Record the time required for agglutination to take place, and continue observing and periodically rotating and tilting the slide on which the absence of reaction is noted.
6. The A_1 cells should have agglutinated within 30 seconds to 1 or 2 minutes. The A_2 cells should remain unagglutinated or evenly suspended for at least 10 minutes. Since most absorbed antisera are slightly underabsorbed, eventually the A_2 cells might clump but not until after at least 10 minutes have elapsed. Allow a margin of 2 minutes for safety, and establish as the reading time a period 2 minutes shorter than that in which A_2 cells began to show some clumping. For example, if there is no clumping within 10 minutes, establish a time limit of 8 minutes for reading the results of the actual tests. Some laboratories establish an arbitrary time limit of 5 minutes for all subgrouping tests.
7. Table 18-6 gives the results expected in controls in subgrouping.

Using anti-A_1 lectin. The controls are the same as for absorbed anti-**A** serum, except that anti-A_1 lectin, prepared from the seeds

of *Dolichos biflorus*, is substituted for the antiserum and a 10% suspension of cells is used. Many laboratories prefer to carry out the tests in tubes when using the lectin.

ACTUAL SUBGROUPING TESTS

Using absorbed anti-A serum

1. Label a one-ring slide with the name of the individual being tested and the blood group, either A or AB.
2. Place a drop of cell suspension in the ring and add 1 drop of absorbed anti-**A** serum.
3. Mix and rotate the slide and read the result within the time limit set by the controls.
4. If the cells agglutinate, they are subgroup A_1 (or A_1B as the case may be). A_1B clumping is generally weaker and takes longer to appear than A_1 agglutination.
5. If the cells have not agglutinated the subgroup is A_2 (or A_2B if AB cells were tested). See Table 18-7.

Using anti-A_1 lectin. Use a 10% suspension of the red cells in saline.

Slide test

1. Place 1 drop of 10% suspension of known A (or AB) cells on a labeled slide, add 1 drop of anti-A_1 lectin, mix, and spread over an area of about 20 mm diameter.
2. Tilt the slide from side to side and observe macroscopically for agglutination, which should occur within 20 seconds to 1 minute. Read the results as in Table 18-7.

Tube test

1. Place 1 drop of anti-A_1 lectin in a 10 by 75 mm tube and add 1 drop of 3% suspension of group A (or AB) cells.
2. Mix and centrifuge at 500 to 1000 rpm for 1 minute.
3. Read immediately after twirling the tube to dislodge the sediment.
4. Cells of subgroup A_1 or A_1B remain agglutinated after the sediment has been dis-

Table 18-6. Expected results in controls on absorbed anti-**A** serum

A_1 cells + absorbed anti-**A** serum = agglutination within 1 minute
A_2 cells + absorbed anti-**A** serum = no agglutination for at least 10 minutes

Table 18-7. Possible results in testing for subgroups of groups A and AB

A cells + absorbed anti-**A** serum	Subgroup	AB cells + absorbed anti-**A** serum	Subgroup
Agglutination	A_1	Agglutination	A_1B
No agglutination	A_2	No agglutination	A_2B

lodged, but subgroup A_2 or A_2B cells will be evenly suspended. If the test is allowed to stand for a time before being read, the A_2 and A_2B cells might begin to form small clumps.

SUBGROUP $A_{1,2}$ AND ANTI-H LECTIN

Some group A bloods give weak or indefinite reactions with anti-A_1 serum, a source of error in such tests. These reactions are common in newborn infants of subgroup A_1, and it is therefore recommended that subgrouping tests not be performed on the blood of newborn infants. Among adults, blood giving such reactions is not uncommon in Negroids of group A. This blood is classified as subgroup $A_{1,2}$, or **intermediate subgroup A.**

Anti-**H** lectin, derived from *Ulex europeus* seeds, may be used to clarify some of the reactions. Subgroup A_2 cells are regularly and strongly clumped by anti-**H** lectin, whereas cells of subgroup A_1 are usually only weakly clumped or are not clumped at all, although strong reactions may also occur.

1. Prepare a 3% suspension in saline of the A or AB cells.
2. Place 1 drop of anti-**H** lectin in a small tube and add 1 drop of the cells.
3. Let stand for 2 hours at room temperature, and then examine for agglutination or its absence.

This test has its greatest value in paternity cases in which the putative father's group A blood does not agglutinate in anti-A_1 reagents and is classified as A_2, the mother is group O (or B or A_2), and the child is group A, but the child's red cells are strongly clumped by anti-A_1 serum. The man's subgroup A_2 can be confirmed by the strong clumping of his cells with the anti-**H** lectin reagent and the child's subgroup A_1 by weaker clumping or negative reaction of his cells with the same lectin.

TESTING SERUM TO DETECT IRREGULAR ANTI-A_1 AND ANTI-H ISOAGGLUTININS

As previously stated, tests may be run to detect anti-A_1 often present in the serum of blood group A_2B and anti-**H** less often present in the serum of blood group A_1B. Anti-**A** may also be found at times in group A_2 serum. Test the serum of group A_2B or A_2 against A_1 and A_2 cells in the usual manner. If the A_1 cells clump and A_2 cells do not, the serum contains anti-A_1. The American Association of Blood Banks suggests that the mixture be subjected to incubation at 4° C for a prolonged period of time. Approximately 2% of subgroup A_2 and 25% of A_2B subjects have anti-A_1 in their sera. Approximately 0.5% of A_1 and B and 3% of A_1B subjects have anti-**H** in their sera. This is often a cold antibody.

Test the serum of group A_1B against group O red cells to detect the presence of anti-**H**. Subgroup A_2 and group O cells both react with anti-**H** antibodies. For confirmation, titrate the serum against group O cells as well as against groups A_1 and B cells. The O cells should agglutinate at a higher titer if anti-**H** is present in the serum.

SUBGROUPS A_3 AND A_4

These subgroups are identified by their weaker reactions with standard antisera and not by the use of special antisera as in other subgroups. In tests with anti-**A** sera, red cells of subgroup A_3 typically show clumps on a background of unagglutinated red cells.

BLOOD GROUP C (A_0 OR A_x)

This group is identified by the fact that the cells fail to clump when mixed with anti-**A** or anti-**B** sera, but they are agglutinated by almost all group O sera (Table 18-5). The incidence is 1 in 60,000 individuals, but it is much more common in the Bantu.[2]

Other subgroups and types in the A-B-O system

The other subgroups in the A-B-O system and the Bombay type, group O_h, are discussed on p. 72ff.

Titration of anti-A and anti-B sera

All titrations, whether in the A-B-O or other blood group systems, are made by diluting the sera serially and then testing each dilution against the cells for which the antibody under investigation is reactive. The reactions are recorded according to their reactive strength from negative (−) through four plus (4+). The weakest positive reaction is rated as +w, the strongest is 4+. The **titer** is the reciprocal of the highest dilution of the serum that gives a definite reaction with its specific cells.

Sera may be titrated against more than one cell group if they have more than one antibody or if cells of different groups differ in agglutinability. For example, anti-**A** serum should be titrated against A_1, A_2, A_1B, and A_2B cells and group O serum against A_1, A_2, and B cells. The technic in all the titrations is the same; only the cells are varied. The example given here is for the titration of anti-**A** serum against A_1 cells.

1. Have at hand group A_1 cells, 5% suspension in saline.
2. Prepare serial dilutions of the inactivated serum, 1:1 (undiluted), 1:2, 1:4, 1:8, 1:16, 1:32, 1:64, 1:128, 1:256, and any further dilutions desired. Use racks that hold ten tubes per row. The dilutions and the measuring of the drops for the titration will be carried out simultaneously. The following technic will refer to tubes in which dilutions are made as **dilution tubes** and those in which the titrations are to be carried out as **titration tubes**. Similarly, the expressions **dilution rack** and **titration rack** will also be used. Dilutions are made in Kahn tubes of the wider diameter variety, titrations in 7.5 cm by 8 mm tubes.
   a. Set up nine or ten tubes per row, one row for each type of cells used.
   b. Set up a similar number of Kahn tubes for the dilutions and ten Wassermann tubes for saline that will be used to rinse the droppers between dilutions.
   c. If titrating a serum against cells of only one blood group, there will be one row of Kahn tubes in the front of the rack, then one row of small Kahn tubes in the second row of the rack. Label the dilution and titration tubes 1, 2, 4, 8, 16, 32, 64, 128, 256, 512, etc., the reciprocal of the dilutions.

3. Fill all the Wassermann tubes with 0.85% saline. As each tube is used for rinsing and the saline removed, take the tube out of the rack and lay it on the table or put it in a container of water to soak.
4. Put 1 drop of undiluted serum to be tested into the first tube of the titration row, the tube marked "1."
5. Put 10 drops of serum in the second tube in the dilution row.
6. Rinse the dropper with all the saline in tube 1 of the back row containing saline, wipe the saline off the outside of the dropper, and then place 10 drops of saline in each tube of the dilution rack, beginning with tube 2 and holding the dropper at the same angle throughout the procedure to ensure that the drops are of the same size.
7. Mix the contents of tube 1:2 of the dilutions in and out of the dropper and transfer 1 drop to the tube marked 1:2 of the titrations and 10 drops to the tube marked 1:4 of the dilutions.
8. Rinse the dropper with the saline in the next Wassermann tube, remove the excess saline from the dropper, then mix the contents of tube 1:4 of the dilutions in and out of the dropper.
9. Transfer 1 drop of the 1:4 dilution to tube 1:4 of the titration and put 10 drops of the 1:4 dilution into tube 1:8 of the dilutions.
10. Again rinse the dropper with the contents of the next large tube of saline; continue in this manner until all the dilutions have been made and there is 1 drop of each dilution of serum in its respectively labeled tube.
11. Add the opposing cells, in this case group A_1, 1 drop of a 5% saline suspension for each titration tube. Anti-**A** serum is titrated against A_1, A_2, A_1B, and A_2B cells, using group O or B cells as a negative control. Use the same dropper for dispensing cells so that each tube receives the same quantity of cells.
12. Shake the rack thoroughly and let it stand at room temperature for 2 hours.
13. Tip the rack to examine the bottoms of the tubes. Agglutinated cells tend to remain in a single round or irregular clump or button, or they may be only partially clumped. The agglutinates should be clearly visible. Negative reactions have no clumps, and the cells flow readily by gravity in more of a pear shape.
14. Flick or gently shake each tube. Pour out the contents on a properly labeled ceramic ringed slide, examine under the 10× ob-

jective of a microscope, and record the strength of the various reactions as on p. 227.

15. Reactions may also be read in the tube under a scanning lens.

16. As the dilutions progress, the antibody concentration decreases and the reactions gradually become weaker, except for prozones, in which some of the higher serum dilutions (weaker concentration) give stronger reactions than lower dilutions (stronger concentration). Some antisera do not react at all when diluted; others have titers higher than 512, and the titration then should be continued beyond the 1:512 dilution.

17. The titer is the reciprocal of the weakest (highest) dilution of serum that gives a definite positive reaction. See Table 18-8.

Titration of group O serum

When group O serum is to be titrated for anti-**A** and anti-**B** content, three titrations will be made—one using group A_1 cells, one with A_2 cells, and one with B cells. It is well also to carry out a fourth titration using group O cells as a negative control.

1. Set up a row of "dilution tubes," four rows of "titration tubes," and a row of Wassermann tubes filled with saline to rinse the dropper, as described previously. Label the dilution tubes 1:1, 1:2, 1:4, 1:8, 1:16, 1:32, 1:64, etc.

2. Label the titration tubes 1, 2, 4, 8, 16, 32, 64, etc. and also note the cells that each row will receive. The first row will be labeled A_1, the second A_2, the third B, and the fourth O.

3. Place 1 drop of undiluted group O serum under test into the first tube of the dilution rows and also into the first tube of the titration rows.

4. Carry 10 drops of the undiluted serum to tube 1:2 of the dilution tubes.

5. Rinse the dropper with all the saline in the first Wassermann tube in the back row. Wipe the outside of the dropper, then put 10 drops of saline into each of the dilution tubes, beginning with the tube marked 1:2.

6. After making sure that all the saline has been removed from the dropper, mix the contents of the 1:2 tube in and out of the dropper, transfer 1 drop of that dilution to each of the 1:2 tubes in each of the titra-rows, and add 10 drops of the 1:2 dilution to the dilution tube marked 1:4.

7. Rinse the dropper as before, wipe the outside, mix the contents of the 1:4 dilution tube, carry 1 drop to each 1:4 tube of the titration tubes, and add 10 drops to tube 1:8 of the dilution row.

8. Always hold the dropper at the same angle so that all the drops will be the same size. Take care not to admit any bubbles; continue with the dilutions and measuring of the titration drops until as many different dilutions as desired have been prepared.

9. The last dilution tube will contain 20 drops. Keep it until it becomes obvious that no further dilutions need be made, or if the titer is extremely high, use this tube to continue with the dilutions and the titrations.

10. To each tube in the first row of the titration tubes add 1 drop of 5% suspension in saline of group A_1 cells.

11. Add 1 drop of A_2 cells to each tube of the second row of titration tubes.

12. Add 1 drop of B cells to each tube of the third row of titration tubes.

13. Add 1 drop of group O cells to each tube of the fourth row of titration tubes.

14. Mix each tube and let the racks stand for 2 hours at room temperature, then record the strength of reaction for each tube after examining as on p. 227. In recording the results and the titer, record also the cells against which the titer was obtained. The reciprocal of the highest (weakest)

Table 18-8. Examples of titrations of serum in the A-B-O blood groups

1:1	1:2	1:4	1:8	1:16	1:32	1:64	1:128	1:256	1:512	Titer (units)
2+	—	—	—	—	—	—	—	—	—	1
4+	4+	2+	1+	±	—	—	—	—	—	8
4+	4+	4+	3+	3+	2+	2+	1+	1+w	—	128
4+	3+	3+	2+	1+	—	—	—	—	—	16
+w	—	—	—	—	—	—	—	—	—	½
—	—	4+	—	2+	4+	—	3+	4+	—	Error
—	—	tr	1+	2+	3+	2+	1+	—	—	128 with prozone

dilution of serum that gives a definite positive reaction is the titer.

15. The following is an example of a record of a titration of group O serum: Titer against A$_1$ cells = 256, against A$_2$ cells = 32, against B cells = 128. Results with group O cells were all negative, which is expected.

One reason for titrating the antibodies in group O serum is that when such group O is to be used as universal donor blood, the antibody titer should be below 10 units. Use of so-called universal donor blood should be discouraged.

Titration of anti-C of the A-B-O system

The following method of titration is that of Unger, modified by Wiener.[3] It is especially useful in cases of erythroblastosis fetalis due to incompatibilities in the A-B-O system. If ordinary titration methods are employed, it is not possible to differentiate between the IgM and the IgG antibodies of anti-A and anti-B specificity.

REAGENTS

Acacia

1. Dissolve 20 gm acacia (gum arabic) and 2 gm Na$_2$HPO$_4$ in 180 ml of distilled water and autoclave at 10 lb pressure for 10 minutes.
2. Use the supernatant fluid, which is slightly opalescent.

Cells

1. Use group A$_1$rh cells suspended in saline when titrating anti-A in group B or O sera, and Brh cells for titrating anti-B in group O or A sera.
2. Prepare the cells in the usual manner, wash once with saline, and resuspend to a 3% concentration in saline.

PROCEDURE

IgM antibodies

1. Prepare serial dilutions in saline of the serum to be tested: 1:1, 1:2, 1:4, 1:8, 1:16, 1:32, etc. See p. 267.
2. Add 1 drop of the opposing cells to 1 drop of each dilution of serum. If group O serum is being titrated, there will be two sets of tubes—one for titration against A cells and one for titration against B cells.
3. Incubate in a water bath at 37° C for 1 hour and then examine the sediment macro-

scopically and under a scanning lens, reporting clumping as positive and lack of agglutination as negative.

4. Record the result in each tube as the IgM, or agglutinating, antibody titer.

Acacia conglutination titer (IgM and IgG)

1. Add to each negative tube in the agglutination test 1 drop of the acacia solution, mix, and incubate in a water bath at 37° C for 1 hour.
2. Read as before and record the results as the acacia conglutination titer.

IgG antibodies

1. At the same time prepare titrations on the same serum diluted 50% with Witebsky group-specific substance 1:2.
2. Carry out the titrations exactly as directed previously and record results in the same manner.
3. Perform an antiglobulin test.
4. If there is a titer in this second set of tubes, the antibodies are due to isosensitization by A-B-O factors, since ordinarily Witebsky (group-specific) substance neutralizes IgM anti-A and anti-B antibodies, but does not neutralize the IgG antibodies. Table 18-9 is an example of a complete titration.

CONCLUSIONS

1. In Table 18-9, the titer for anti-A IgM antibodies is 32. These are the naturally occurring antibodies. When acacia was added the titer was the same.

2. The titer for anti-B IgM antibodies with the same serum is 64. When acacia was added (this is a conglutinin), the titer showed no significant change.

3. The anti-A IgG antibodies show no titer.

4. For anti-B IgG antibodies the titer is 8.

Any anti-A and anti-B agglutinins that are present at birth have been passively acquired by placental transfer from the mother. The anti-A and anti-B agglutinins that develop later are generally of heterospecific origin.

The preceding titration is used to differentiate between the IgM and IgG antibodies. Agglutinogens A and B are both characterized by a commonly shared specificity,

Table 18-9. Titration of anti-**A** and anti-**B** IgM and IgG antibodies in a group O individual

	1:1	1:2	1:4	1:8	1:16	1:32	1:64	1:128	1:256	1:512	Titer
					Dilutions						
	Group O serum, no Witebsky substance, no acacia (saline method)										IgM
A₁ cells	3+	3+	3+	2+	1+	1 + w	±	−	−	−	32
B cells	4+	4+	3+	2+	2+	1+	1+	−	−	−	64
	Same serum, acacia added										IgG and IgM
A₁ cells	3+	3+	2+	1+	1+	1 + w	−	−	−	−	32
B cells	4+	3+	2+	1+	1+	1+	1+	1 + w	−	−	128
	Same serum, Witebsky substance added, antiglobulin method										IgG
A₁ cells	−	−	−	−	−	−	−	−	−	−	0 (no titer)
B cells	2+	2+	1+	1+	−	−	−	−	−	−	8

C. Group O serum has not only anti-**A** and anti-**B** but also anti-**C** antibodies. Anti-C is usually of the IgG variety and therefore readily passes through the placental barrier, and thus it can enter the fetal circulation.

In the preceding titration, acacia is used as a conglutinin. Witebsky group-specific substance suppresses the action of the naturally occurring anti-**A** and anti-**B** antibodies, but does not suppress anti-**C**. Therefore any titer that is obtained in the third series of titrations in Table 18-9 is considered to be the anti-**C** titer. Anti-**C** can react with both A and B cells because these cells share a common specificity, **C**, as stated. Anti-**C** is also called the **cross-reacting antibody.**

Titration of group O serum for heterospecific A-B-O transfusion

The method of titration of group O serum when the blood is to be used as a "universal donor" may be varied. The technic recommended by the American Association of Blood Banks is as follows:

1. Dilute the serum 1:50 with saline by adding 0.1 ml of serum measured with a pipet to 4.9 ml of saline in a tube. Mix thoroughly.
2. Place 0.1 ml of the diluted serum in a tube labeled "A" and 0.1 ml in a tube labeled "B."
3. Add 0.1 ml of a 2% suspension in saline of group A₁ cells to tube 1 and 0.1 ml of 2% suspension in saline of group B cells to tube 2.
4. Mix each thoroughly and allow to stand at room temperature 15 minutes.
5. Centrifuge as usual.
6. Gently dislodge the cell button and observe macroscopically for agglutination. If either the A or the B cells agglutinate, the titer of agglutinins in the serum is greater than 50 units, and the blood may *not* be designated as low titer. It should not be used for any recipient other than one belonging to group O.
7. At the same time as the preceding test, prepare a test for hemolysins.
8. The serum must be fresh. Use a weak suspension, 1% or 2% in saline, of groups A₁ and B cells.
9. Place 0.1 ml of fresh, undiluted, *uninactivated* serum in a tube labeled "A" and 0.1 ml in a tube labeled "B."
10. Add 0.1 ml of A cell suspension to the first tube and 0.1 ml of B cells to the second tube.
11. Mix the contents of each tube but do not centrifuge. Incubate at 37° C for 1 hour.
12. Centrifuge and observe the supernatant fluid for evidence of hemolysis. If the supernate is reddish or tinged with red, the cells have dissolved (lysed).
13. If group O serum contains a hemolysin, it must not be used for any recipient who is not group O.

Neutralization of naturally occurring anti-A and anti-B

As detailed in the titration for anti-**C** of the A-B-O blood groups, anti-**A** and anti-**B** of the naturally occurring type of antibody can be neutralized by adding group-specific substances to group O serum, which is the only serum that contains anti-C. Group-specific substance is also designated as **Witebsky substance**. The reagent is a group-specific substance for in vitro use.

1. Place 1 ml of serum in a small tube.
2. Add 0.2 ml of reagent group-specific substance, mix, and let stand for 5 minutes.
3. Dilute the neutralized serum 1:20 with saline and mix.
4. Place 1 drop of neutralized serum in each of two tubes, labeled, respectively, "A" and "B."
5. Add 1 drop of 2% group A_1 cells in saline to the first tube and 1 drop of group B cell suspension, 2% in saline, to the second tube.
6. Mix each and incubate at 37° C in a water bath for 30 minutes.
7. Carry out an antiglobulin test: Wash the contents of each tube four times with saline and remove all traces of saline after the last centrifugation. This is accomplished by turning the tube upside down after removing the supernate and then touching the lip of the tube against a pad of gauze. Shake and add 1 drop of antiglobulin serum, incubate at 37° C for 30 minutes (some tests require only 15 minutes and some even less time). Then centrifuge at 1000 rpm for 1 minute, gently dislodge the sediment, and observe for agglutination or lack of agglutination.

If the cells have agglutinated, the serum contains anti-C of the A-B-O system (the cross-reacting, or nonneutralizable, antibody). Blood containing such an antibody should never be used to transfuse any recipient outside of group O.

It is dangerous to transfuse a recipient with blood of an individual of a different blood group. When choosing donors, choose one of the same A-B-O group and preferably subgroup. This subject is discussed in detail under cross matching (Chapter 21).

Test for A-B-H secretors

Tests for secretors of A-B-H substance are useful in classifying the Lewis genotypes and phenotypes, in identification of the group of blood stains, and in determining secretor status in certain medicolegal situations. The screening test is presented here. The more elaborate test is included in the discussion of tests in the Lewis system in this chapter.

PREPARATION OF SALIVA

1. Collect the saliva in a widemouthed tube, then place the tube immediately in a boiling water bath for 20 minutes to inactivate the enzymes that could interfere with the reactions and to destroy bacteria present in the saliva.
2. Centrifuge at high speed to separate the coagulum from the supernatant opalescent saliva. Transfer the supernate to another tube and either use immediately or store at 4° C or, better, frozen until needed.

Saliva for secretor status and for the Lewis tests is prepared in the same manner.

PREPARATION OF REAGENT

The reagent is anti-H lectin from *Ulex europeus*. The lectin should be diluted to the weakest point in which a 2+ macroscopic agglutination with appropriate cells can be seen. The titer is generally written on the pamphlet that the manufacturer supplies. If not, the lectin will need to be titrated against A, B, and O cells. The technic of the inhibition titration is given in the section on technics in the Lewis system. Dilutions should always be made in 0.85% saline. **Have available 2% suspension of group O cells in saline.**

TECHNIC OF THE TEST

1. Prepare controls as described following this technic and run simultaneously with the test. Dilute the anti-H lectin to 4 to 8 agglutinating doses.
2. Place 1 drop of diluted anti-H lectin in a tube labeled "O."
3. Add 1 drop of processed saliva to the tube, mix, and leave at room temperature for 10 minutes.
4. Add 1 drop of 2% suspension in saline of once-washed group O red cells.
5. Mix and let stand at room temperature for 30 to 60 minutes.
6. Centrifuge and look for agglutination macroscopically.

1. Add 1 drop of diluted anti-H lectin and 1 drop of saline or nonsecretor saliva to 1 drop of a 2% suspension in saline of group O cells.
2. Incubate, centrifuge, and read for agglutination. The cells should be agglutinated.

INTERPRETATION

If the cells in the test have not agglutinated, the saliva has prevented the anti-**H** lectin from acting, and therefore the individual is a secretor of the H substance. If the cells have agglutinated, there has been no inhibition, and the individual is not a secretor of H substance.

TECHNIC OF TESTS IN THE LEWIS BLOOD GROUP SYSTEM
Tests on saliva for Lewis saliva type

For the preparation of saliva, refer to p. 271. Tests on saliva are titrations of the degree of inhibition of the antibody (Table 18-10).

1. To prepare serial dilutions of the saliva, first rack up five small tubes for the dilutions and five small tubes for the titrations. Label them, respectively, with the dilutions 1:1, 1:4, 1:16, 1:64, and 1:256. Place 6 drops of saline in each tube beginning with 1:4 of the dilution tubes. Add 2 drops of saliva to the tube labeled 1:4, mix and transfer 2 drops to the next tube, mix, transfer 2 drops to the next tube, and continue until all the dilutions have been made. Then dispense 1 drop of undiluted saliva to the 1:1 titration tube, 1 drop of the 1:4 dilution to its specific tube, and so on, so that each tube of the titration rack has 1 drop of its respective dilution of saliva.
2. Add to each tube of the titration 1 drop of anti-**Le** serum, previously diluted according to its titer, that is, to the highest dilution that gives at least a 2+ macroscopic agglutination with appropriate cells.
3. Mix and allow to stand at room temperature for 15 minutes.

4. Add 1 drop of 3% suspension of ficinated type Le_1 cells to each tube, mix, and place the rack in a water bath at 37° C for 1 hour or longer.
5. Read the reactions and record. Inspect the sediment, then place the tube on a microscope stage under a scanning lens. After gently twisting the tube to dislodge the sediment, determine agglutination or lack of clumping. Handle the tubes gently; otherwise, the fragile clumps may be broken up.
6. Absence of agglutination is recorded as negative, agglutination as positive. The degree of reaction should also be recorded. A negative reaction represents inhibition of the antibody, since ordinarily anti-**Le** serum clumps Le_1 cells. If the saliva contains the Lewis substance—that is, if it has been derived from a Lewis secretor—the Le substance will inhibit agglutination when Le_1 cells are aded, thus resulting in a negative test. The last tube showing inhibition, that is, a negative reaction, is the titer. Titers are usually recorded as the reciprocal of the dilution. If all the tubes show positive results, no Lewis substance is present and the subject is saliva type nL. If there is inhibition, the individual is saliva type Les. It is customary to determine the inhibition titer.
7. At the same time that the tests are run, controls should also be made, using the same anti-**Le** serum and a saliva of known Lewis type. It is good practice to run a control using group-specific A and B substance, because this has the H substance but lacks the Lewis substance, resulting in lack of inhibition (agglutination).

Tests on saliva for simultaneous detection of both Lewis and H secretor substances

For full information regarding saliva types, the tests for Lewis and A-B-H substances should be run simultaneously.

TEST FOR H SUBSTANCE IN SALIVA

Use the same serial dilutions of saliva as those for testing for Lewis secretors.

Table 18-10. Example of inhibition tests for Lewis saliva type (Les or nL)

Dilutions of saliva	1:1	1:4	1:16	1:64	1:256	Titer	Lewis saliva type
Specimen							
1	−	−	−	−	1+	64	Les
2	−	−	−	2+	3+	16	Les
3	3+	3+	3+	3+	3+	0	nL

1. Label five Kahn tubes with the dilution of saliva, and place 1 drop of each serial dilution of saliva into its proper tube–undiluted (1:1), 1:4, 1:16, 1:64, and 1:256.
2. Add to each 1 drop of anti-H lectin made from *Ulex europeus* seeds and diluted to yield a titer of 4 units for group O cells.
3. Mix each tube separately and let the tubes stand at room temperature 15 minutes.
4. Add 1 drop of 3% saline-suspended group O cells to each tube.
5. Mix and let stand at room temperature for 1 hour or longer.
6. Read as for the Lewis test. The last tube showing a negative result (inhibition) is the titer of the H substance.

Anti-**H** lectin causes clumping of group O cells because those cells have the H substance. If the lectin did not agglutinate such cells, the saliva inhibited the action of the lectin and was thus derived from an A-B-H secretor. If the cells do agglutinate, there has been no inhibition and such a person is not a secretor of the H substance. See Tables 18-11 and 18-12.

Results

1. If the reactions in the tests for the Lewis and A-B-H substances both show inhibition, the saliva is classified as Les Sec; that is, this individual secretes both the Lewis and the H substances.
2. If the Lewis test shows inhibition and

the H test does not, the saliva is classified as Les nS; that is, this individual secretes the Lewis but not the H substance.

3. If the reactions for the Lewis test show no inhibition but the test for the H substance shows inhibition, the saliva is classified as nL Sec; that is, this individual does not secrete the Lewis substance but does secrete the H susbtance.

4. If the tests for the Lewis and the H substances both show no inhibition, the saliva is classified as nL nS, which means that this individual does not secrete either the Lewis or the H substance.

Tests for the Lewis factor of red cells

1. Prepare 3% suspensions in saline of ficinated red cells.
2. Make the tests in duplicate and include the controls simultaneously with the tests.
3. For the test, mix 1 drop of ficinated red cells with 1 drop of anti-**Le** serum in a small Kahn tube.
4. Allow to remain at 37° C in a water bath for 1 hour, then shake gently to dislodge the sediment and take a preliminary reading.
5. If the cells have agglutinated, they are classified as type Le₁. If they have not agglutinated, proceed with step 6.
6. Wash the cells four times with saline, remove the last saline completely, then add 1 drop of antiglobulin serum and mix.

Table 18-11. Examples of inhibition test for saliva types (Sec or nS)

Dilutions of saliva	1:1	1:4	1:16	1:64	1:256	Titer	Secretor type
Specimens							
1	−	−	−	−	1+	64	Sec
2	−	−	1+	2+	3+	4	Sec
3	3+	3+	3+	3+	3+	0	nS

Table 18-12. Simultaneous inhibition tests on saliva for Lewis and A-B-H secretor types

Dilutions of saliva	Inhibition titration for Lewis					Inhibition titration for H					Saliva types	Lewis red cell types
	1:1	1:4	1:16	1:64	1:256	1:1	1:4	1:16	1:64	1:256		
Specimens												
1	−	−	−	−	−	−	−	−	+	2+	Les Sec	Le₂ Le(a−b+)
2	−	−	−	+	2+	3+	3+	3+	3+	3+	Les nS	Le₁ Le(a+b−)
3	3+	3+	3+	2+	2+	−	−	−	−	±	nL Sec	le Le(a−b−)
4	3+	2+	2+	2+	2+	3+	3+	3+	3+	3+	nL nS	le Le(a−b−)

Table 18-13. Possible results in tests for the Lewis type using red blood cells

Specimen	Cells and anti-Le serum	Antiglobulin test	Lewis type
1	+	Not needed	Le₁
2	−	+	Le₂
3	−	−	le

7. Centrifuge for 1 minute at 1000 rpm.
8. Shake the tube gently and read. If the cells have agglutinated during the second stage of the test (but not the first), they are classified as type Le₂.
9. If the cells did not agglutinate in either stage of the test, they are classified as type le.
10. *Controls:* Run control tests on red cells of types Le₁, Le₂, and le. Carry out the technic in the same manner as for the tests. Determine the types according to Table 18-13.

Lewis genotypes and phenotypes

Refer to pp. 88 and 89 for tables showing possible genotypes and phenotypes in the Lewis system, as well as the frequency of the Le saliva types.

Tests for Lewis antibodies in serum

Tests for antibodies in the serum in the Lewis system are made to determine whether or not there is sensitization to the Lewis substance. Since only type nL individuals can form such antibodies, there is no need to test sera from individuals of other Lewis types for **Lewis** antibodies.

1. Have available ficinated red cells suspended in saline to a concentration of 3%. These should be of types Le₁, Le₂, and le. Type Le₁ is also designated as Le(a+) or Le(a+b−), and Le₂ is Le(a−) or Le(a−b+). Type le is also called Le(a−) or Le(a−b−). The cells must have been derived from a group O individual because the red cells of such persons have neither A nor B agglutinogen. The ficinated cells are available commercially, or they may be prepared in one's own laboratory.
2. Label the tubes according to the type of cells they will contain.
3. Place 1 drop of cell suspension of each type into its respective tube and add 1 drop of *fresh* serum to each. Only fresh serum is used because it contains complement.

4. Mix and let stand in a water bath at 37° C for 1 hour.
5. Examine for hemolysis and clumping.
6. If the patient has been sensitized to the **Le** factor, type Le₁ cells generally hemolyze, often completely. The Le₂ cells may not show hemolysis, or they may show only partial hemolysis and partial clumping. If no **Lewis** antibody is present, the cells will neither be hemolyzed nor clumped. Type le cells remain suspended and unaffected. In cases of **Le^H** sensitization (p. 87), only type Le₂ cells dissolve.
7. If there is no complement in the serum, either due to loss through age or heating, there can be no hemolysis. If, however, the **Lewis** antibody is present the cells will clump.
8. If the cells have not clumped and if there was no hemolysis, wash the cells, in the same tube in which the tests were made, four times with saline and proceed with the antiglobulin test. If the cells now clump, the serum contains anti-**Le** antibodies.

The antiglobulin serum should be of the anti–nongamma globulin type, or a broad-spectrum antiglobulin serum may be used in the Lewis test.

Tests for the blood group of seminal stains as well as those for identification of dried blood are given in Chapter 22.

REFERENCES

1. American Association of Blood Banks, Technical methods and procedures, ed. 6, Washington, D.C., 1974, The Association.
2. Wiener, A. S., and Ward, F. A.: Am. J. Clin. Pathol. 46:27, 1966.
3. Wiener, A. S., Wexler, I. B., and Hurst, J. G.: Blood 4:104, 1949.

RECOMMENDED READING

Wiener, A. S., and Socha, W. W.: A-B-O blood groups andd Lewis types, New York, 1976, Stratton Intercontinental Medical Book Corporation.

19 □ Tests made in the Rh-Hr blood group system

TESTS FOR THE Rh FACTOR IN RED CELLS

There are a number of different methods of determining whether an individual is Rh positive (**Rh testing**) and, if he is positive, the exact Rh phenotype (**Rh typing**). Screening tests for Rh typing may be made by the open slide or the rapid tube method. Routine examination in many hospitals and blood banks consists merely in determining whether the Rh_o factor is present, using a slide test with conglutinating (IgG) antiserum or a tube test using saline-agglutinating serum (IgM) followed, when necessary, by an antiglobulin test. A test for the Rh_o variant, $\mathfrak{Rh}_o$, is routine in many laboratories. Since at least 50% of the population is type Rh_1, many laboratories test for Rh_o and **rh′**, both of which are present in type Rh_1 cells.

Slide test for Rh_o in red cells (slide conglutination test)

Equipment
1. A viewing box fitted with an electric light globe that will bring the temperature on the plate to 45° to 47° C is used (Fig. 17-5). The light should be turned on at all times to keep the temperature of the glass plate steady. If tests are made infrequently, turn the light on a few minutes before use.
2. Draw large oval rings on ordinary laboratory slides, one on each slide, using a red wax pencil. Black wax seems to come loose during the tests. The oval should be about 4 by 2 cm. Slides can be purchased permanently marked in this way.
3. Applicator sticks or wooden toothpicks for spreading the mixture of blood and antiserum are also needed.

Reagents and specimen. Anti-Rh_o slide serum is used. It differs from saline-agglutinating serum (tube serum) in that it reacts with and clumps cells if whole blood is used but not if the red cells are suspended in saline. It also reacts with cells suspended in any high-protein medium, like albumin. Anti-Rh_o serum identifies all blood having the Rh_o specificity, such as types Rh_o, Rh_1, Rh_2, and Rh_Z, without differentiating among them.

Take the blood in a dry anticoagulant (p. 240) and either centrifuge it or permit it to stand to separate the cells from the plasma. The plasma should be removed but only to a point at which the volume of cells and plasma equal one another, that is, to produce a 50% suspension of cells in their own plasma. The blood and plasma are then mixed by inverting the tube several times.

Controls. Controls consist of whole blood from an Rh_o-positive person and from an Rh_o-negative person. These should be run simultaneously with the tests.

1. Label each slide with the identification of the person being tested. Label the controls Rh_o positive and Rh_o negative, respectively.
2. Place 1 large drop of anti-Rh_o slide test serum in the ring on each slide.
3. Add 2 drops of whole blood to the proper slide.
4. Mix each with a separate toothpick or appli-

Table 19-1. Results possible with **Rh$_o$** slide test

Whole blood and anti-Rh$_o$ serum	Conclusions
Agglutination	**Rh$_o$** positive
No agglutination	**Rh$_o$** negative

cator stick and spread the mixture over the surface outlined by the wax ring.

5. Place the slides on the preheated viewing box, tilt back and forth occasionally, and observe macroscopically. Record clumping as positive (+) and absence of clumping as negative (-). Record a positive result as soon as it occurs, but allow 3 to 4 minutes before recording a result as negative.

6. Tilt the box, add a drop of saline to each mixture, and let it run through the mixture on the slide. Agglutination remains unaffected. Negative reactions become easier to read after the saline has been added. Do not confuse drying around the edge of the drop with agglutination. In a positive test, the clumps of blood cells are large, brick red, and dispersed throughout the drop. There may be a single large clump of red cells that cannot be dispersed. *Do not* read under a microscope.

7. The **Rh$_o$**-positive control should exhibit clumping; the **Rh$_o$**-negative control should not.

8. Refer to Table 19-1 for reading the reactions of the unknowns.

If desired, another control may be included, consisting of the unknown cells (whole blood) and 20% to 30% bovine albumin. The cells should not clump. If they do, wash the cells three times in saline and resuspend to a 5% suspension. Then continue with the test using anti-**Rh$_o$** IgM (saline-agglutinating) serum:

1. Place 1 drop of anti-**Rh$_o$** slide serum on a labeled slide.

2. Place 1 drop of 20% to 30% albumin on a second slide.

3. Add 2 drops of 50% red cells in serum or plasma (whole blood) to each slide.

4. Spread each with a different applicator.

5. Place the slides on a heated viewing box and tilt back and forth, reading within 2 minutes.

6. Observe for agglutination.

7. Tilt the box and let a drop of saline run

through each test and control, then read again.

8. If the slide containing the antiserum shows agglutination and the slide with the albumin does not, the test is positive.

9. If the results are doubtful, wash the cells, resuspend in saline, and test with saline-agglutinating serum.

This type of control may also be performed in a test tube.

If the donor's blood is **Rh$_o$** positive, it must be used only for an **Rh$_o$**-positive recipient. If the recipient's blood is **Rh$_o$** negative, give only Rh-negative blood in a transfusion. If the donor's blood is **Rh$_o$** negative, determine the exact Rh-Hr type before using it in a transfusion.

Slide test for Rh$_o$, rh′, and rh″ specificities in red cells (screening test made on donor whole blood)

Prepare slides as in the previous method. Collect blood in a dry anticoagulant; then prepare it as in the first method. Three wax ring slides will be needed for each unknown blood and six slides for the controls. (See Fig. 19-1.) Prepare a similar set of three slides each for the positive control and the negative control (six slides in all).

1. Identify each slide with the blood being tested and the antiserum used and label the controls in a similar fashion.

2. For each blood being tested use 1 drop of whole blood with 1 drop of each antiserum, respectively, as follows:
   Unknown blood + anti-**Rh$_o$** slide serum
   Unknown blood + anti-**Rh$_o$′** slide serum
   Unknown blood + anti-**Rh$_o$″** slide serum

3. Mix and spread as in the first method, place on a preheated viewing box, and treat in the same manner as in the first method. After 3 to 4 minutes tilt the box, let a drop of saline run down through each mixture, and read. Record agglutination as a positive reaction, absence of agglutination as negative.

4. If the ring that has the anti-**Rh$_o$** serum shows agglutination, all three slides will necessarily show the same reaction because each antiserum contains anti-**Rh$_o$** (alone or with another antibody). If the drop of blood mixed with the anti-**Rh$_o$** serum does not agglutinate, either, both, or neither of the remaining drops may show agglutination. As a

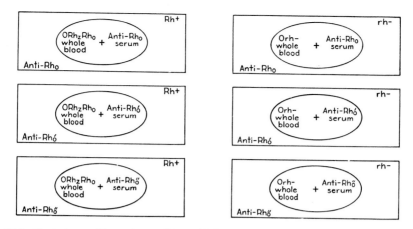

Fig. 19-1. Controls on Rh antisera. (From Erskine, A. G. In Frankel, S., Reitman, S., and Sonnenwirth, A. C., editors: Gradwohl's clinical laboratory methods and diagnosis, ed. 7, St. Louis, 1970, The C. V. Mosby Co.)

Table 19-2. Possible results in open slide screening test for donor blood in the Rh-Hr system

Whole blood plus			
Anti-Rh$_0$ serum	**Anti-Rh$_0'$ serum**	**Anti-Rh$_0''$ serum**	**Conclusions**
−	−	−	Type rh (Rh negative); test for $\Re$h$_0$
+	+	+	**Rh$_0$** specificity present
−	+	−	**rh′** specificity present; test for $\Re$h$_0$
−	−	+	**rh″** specificity present; test for $\Re$h$_0$
−	+	+	**rh′** and **rh″** specificities present; test for $\Re$h$_0$
+	−	−	Error*
+	−	+	Error*
+	+	−	Error*

*If the red cells are agglutinated by anti-Rh$_0$ serum, they have the **Rh$_0$** specificity and will therefore be agglutinated by the other two antisera, both having anti-Rh$_0$.

rule, this test is made only on the blood of prospective doners. See Table 19-2 for possible results and interpretation.

Anti-**Rh$_0'$** serum causes agglutination of red cells having either **Rh$_0$** or **rh′**, or both, such as types Rh$_0$, Rh$_1$, Rh$_2$, Rh$_z$, rh′, and rh$_y$. Anti-**Rh$_0''$** serum agglutinates red cells with either **Rh$_0$** or **rh″**, or both, as in types Rh$_0$, Rh$_1$, Rh$_2$, Rh$_z$, rh″, and rh$_y$.

Interpretation

1. If a prospective **donor** lacks **Rh$_0$** but has either **rh′** or **rh″**, or both, for transfusion purposes he is considered Rh positive and his blood is given only to Rh-positive recipients. It has antigens that could isosensitize a type rh person.

2. If a prospective **recipient** lacks **Rh$_0$** but has either **rh′** or **rh″**, or both, consider the recipient Rh negative and give only Rh-negative blood in a transfusion unless blood of the identical Rh type as the recipient is available.

3. When tests show that **Rh$_0$** is not present in the cells, always test for the Rh$_0$ variant, $\Re$h$_0$.

This is a screening test only and is not

recommended except in cases of extreme emergency. It is best to test all donor blood by the tube method, as well as by the antiglobulin technic.

This test can also be made using clotted blood. Simply dip a number of applicator sticks into the clot and carry over the amount of blood cells needed for the test, mixing with the appropriate antisera. Take care not to admit any clots, since these might be mistaken for agglutinates and thus interfere with accurate reading.

Tube test to determine Rh types

All Rh-negative donors should be tested by the tube technic to ascertain the exact Rh type. To determine the "complete" Rh-Hr phenotype, the test must be combined with tube tests for the Hr factors.

Reagents. Have at hand anti-Rh_o, anti-rh′, anti-rh″ saline agglutinating (tube test) sera, and anti-Rh_o slide test (conglutinating) serum.

Prepare a suspension in saline of the unknown blood cells, wash once in saline, and resuspend to a 3% concentration.

Antiglobulin serum is needed to test for the Rh_o variant.

Use 7.5 cm by 8 mm tubes for each test.

Procedure

1. Label each tube with the identifying mark and the antiserum used. Four tubes are required for each blood tested. Prepare a duplicate set, as in Fig. 19-2.
2. Place 1 drop of cell suspension in each of the four tubes, using the same size drop in each. Hold the dropper (or straw) at the same angle when dispensing the drops (Fig. 19-3).
3. Place 1 drop of respective antisera into the tube for each test as follows:
   1—anti-rh′ saline agglutinating serum
   2—anti-rh″ saline agglutinating serum
   3—anti-Rh_o saline agglutinating serum
   4—anti-Rh_o slide test serum. Tube 4 will be completed only if the result in tube 3 is negative. It is a test for the Rh_o variant.
4. Mix the contents of each tube and place the rack in a water bath at 37° C for 1 hour.
5. Take a preliminary reading from the bottoms of the tubes at the end of the hour by tipping the rack and observing the pat-

tern of the sediments. Positive reactions tend to remain round; negative reactions run down and then tend to look pear-shaped.

6. Spread the mixture thin in the tube and read over a lighted viewing box. Read also under a scanning lens of the microscope. Record clumping as positive (+) and lack of clumping as negative (−).
7. To make it easier to read, centrifuge the tubes at low speed for 1 minute, then gent-

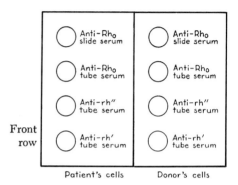

Fig. 19-2. Tube test for Rh factors. (From Erskine, A. G. In Frankel, S., Reitman, S., and Sonnenwirth, A. C., editors: Gradwohl's clinical laboratory methods and diagnosis, ed. 7, St. Louis, 1970, The C. V. Mosby Co.)

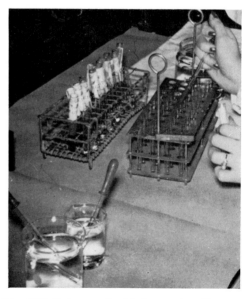

Fig. 19-3. Tube test for Rh factors in cell suspensions. (From Erskine, A. G. In Frankel, S., Reitman, S., and Sonnenwirth, A. C., editors: Gradwohl's clinical laboratory methods and diagnosis, ed. 7, St. Louis, 1970, The C. V. Mosby Co.)

ly dislodge the sediment and read again, or allow the tubes to remain at room temperature for 1 hour before reading after removal from the water bath.

8. If the result in tube 3, containing anti-**Rh₀** saline agglutinating serum, is negative, wash the cells in tube 4 four times with saline, remove all traces of saline after the last washing, and proceed with the **antiglobulin test** as follows:

9. Add 1 drop of antiglobulin serum and mix thoroughly.

10. Centrifuge at 500 to 1000 rmp for 2 minutes, then rotate gently to dislodge the sediment.

11. Read over a lighted viewing box and under a scanning lens. Do not use tube 4 if the result in tube 3 is positive.

12. Consult Table 19-3 for results. If anti-**rh'** serum causes the cells to clump, they have **rh'** specificity. If the cells are agglutinated by anti-**rh"** serum, they have **rh"**. If they are agglutinated by anti-**Rh₀**, they have **Rh₀**. If anti-**Rh₀** tube serum fails to clump the cells, but they are agglutinated at the end of the antiglobulin test, they have ℜh₀.

Type Rh₀ has only specificity **Rh₀**; type rh' has only **rh'**; type rh" has only **rh"**; type rhᵧ has both specificities **rh'** and **rh"**; type Rh₁ has both **Rh₀** and **rh'**; type Rh₂

Table 19-3. Possible results in the tube test for the Rh factors*

Unknown cells plus				
Anti-rh' serum	Anti-rh" serum	Anti-Rh₀ tube serum	Anti-Rh₀ slide serum and antiglobulin test	Conclusions: Rh type†
−	−	−	[−]	rh (Rh negative)
+	−	−	[−]	rh'
−	+	−	[−]	rh"
+	+	−	[−]	rhᵧ
−	−	+		Rh₀
+	−	+		Rh₁
−	+	+		Rh₂
+	+	+		Rhᵤ
−	−	−	[+ / −]	ℜh₀
+	−	−	[+ / −]	ℜh₁
−	+	−	[+ / −]	ℜh₂
+	+	−	[+ / −]	ℜhᵤ

*Box, ⌐ , represents the results of the antiglobulin test.
†The arrangement of the types in this table was suggested by Wiener as the "natural" one, for reasons given by him in J.A.M.A. 99:988. 1967.

Table 19-4. Reactions of the eight standard Rh blood types

| | Blood having Rh$_o$ specificity (Rh$_o$ positive) | | | | Blood without Rh$_o$ specificity (Rh$_o$ negative) | | |
| | Reactions with antisera | | | | Reactions with antisera | | |
Types	Anti-Rh$_o$	Anti-rh'	Anti-rh"	Types	Anti-Rh$_o$	Anti-rh'	Anti-rh"
Rh$_o$	+	−	−	rh	−	−	−
Rh$_1$	+	+	−	rh'	−	+	−
Rh$_2$	+	−	+	rh"	−	−	+
Rh$_z$	+	+	+	rh$_y$	−	+	+

Note: The symbol Rh$_1$ is short for Rh$_o'$; Rh$_2$ is short for Rh$_o''$; Rh$_z$ is short for Rh$_o'''$; rh$_y$ is short for rh'rh", or rh' ". Type Rh$_1$ has both specificities Rh$_o$ and rh'; type Rh$_2$ has Rh$_o$ and rh"; Rh$_z$ has Rh$_o$, rh', and rh"; and rh$_y$ has rh' and rh". Type rh has none of the standard Rh factors (specificities).

has both **Rh$_o$** and **rh"**; and type Rh$_Z$ has **Rh$_o$**, **rh'**, and **rh"**.

The eight principal, or standard, Rh blood types and their reactions with three anti-Rh antisera are shown in Table 19-4.

Rapid tube test for Rh specificities in cells (tube conglutination test)

1. Place a large drop of anti-Rh$_o$ slide test serum in a small tube 7 to 8 mm inside diameter.
2. Dip a wooden applicator stick into the sample of blood that is to be tested (whole oxalated blood or clotted blood) to pick up some of the red cells.
3. Transfer enough unknown cells on the applicator stick(s) to the tube containing the antiserum so that a 3% suspension of the cells results.
4. Place the tubes in a water bath at 37° C for a few minutes to warm and then centrifuge at 500 rpm for 1 minute.
5. Twist the tube gently to dislodge the sediment. If the reaction is positive, the sediment will come away in a single clump or in several large clumps. In negative reactions the cells disperse to form a homogeneous suspension.
6. Check the readings microscopically, using a scanning lens.
7. The tubes may be kept in the water bath for as long as 1 hour in lieu of centrifuging them. Read the reactions under a scanning lens after twisting gently to dislodge the sediments.
8. Run positive and negative controls along with all tests.

The glassware must be clean and dry, and the specimens must be fresh or properly stored in a refrigerator. The blood must not be permitted to freeze; higher temperatures are also to be avoided. Do not store specimens that have been diluted with aqueous solutions like saline.

Precautions to be observed for tube tests

If the temperature of the water bath rises above 40° C, the red cells may be damaged, leading to weak reactions. Temperature, as well as speed and duration of centrifugation, is important. Avoid excessively strong centrifugation.

Sources of error in tube tests

In performing tube tests for the Rh specificities, care must be taken to avoid certain sources of error.

1. Poor blood samples should be avoided. Whole blood can be used for typing tests for as long as 5 to 7 days if it is kept refrigerated, either as a blood clot or in a dry oxalate. Blood cell suspensions should be prepared only on the day of use. In warm weather, these suspensions may deteriorate in a few hours. Never use hemolyzed blood. Avoid the use of wet syringes, and take care that there is no alcohol in the syringes. Use apparatus at room temperature. If blood is taken by finger puncture, the specimen may contain an admixture of cells, plasma, and tissue juices, with resulting poor reactions. Avoid the use of specimens contaminated by bacteria. When in doubt, obtain a fresh specimen, preferably by venipuncture.

2. Too weak a cell suspension gives poor results; the same is true of too strong a suspension.

3. Use small tubes, preferably 7 to 8 mm in diameter. Evaporation takes place more rapidly in the wider tubes, with resulting indistinct reactions. If the tubes are too narrow, they are difficult to manage.

4. Maintain the temperature of the water bath at 37° C for consistent results.

5. Rough handling of the tubes can break up weak agglutination. It is best to roll or twist the tubes to dislodge the sediment, but do not shake them. Whenever possible, read the reactions in the tube in which the test was made.

6. Do not mistake swirls of cells and small clots for agglutinates. In a true positive reaction the cells will be strongly clumped, with few if any free cells among the clumps.

7. Citrate solutions should not be used to prepare blood cell suspensions. Use 0.85% sodium chloride.

8. Discard soapy, dirty, or old, etched tubes. Use only scrupulously clean tubes or, preferably, disposable tubes.

9. Round bottom tubes are preferred, but conical tubes may also be used.

10. Avoid the use of contaminated or deteriorated antisera.

11. Controls must be run simultaneously with all tests. Include at least one known positive specimen and one known clear negative.

Testing red cells for rhʷ specificity

The test for the **rh**ʷ factor is not made routinely. It can be run if specific active antisera are available. Anti-**rh**ʷ serum reacts with cells having the **rh**ʷ specificity, present only in Rh types that have the **rh′** factor such as Rh₁, rh′, rh$_y$, Rh$_z$, ℜh₁, and ℜh$_z$. Blood having **rh**ʷ reacts more weakly with anti-**rh′** serum than does blood without the **rh**ʷ specificity.

The tests are made to determine sensitization to the **rh**ʷ factor in hemolytic transfusion reactions and in erythroblastosis fetalis when the mother lacks the specificity that is present in the fetal blood cells. Anti-**rh**ʷ serum will subdivide type Rh₁ into two subtypes, as shown in Table 19-5.

Table 19-5. Subdivision of type Rh₁ by use of anti-**rh**ʷ serum

Rh types	Reactions with anti-rhʷ serum	Rh subtypes
Rh₁Rh₁	+	Rh₁ʷRh₁
	−	Rh₁Rh₁ (proper)
Rh₁rh	+	Rh₁ʷrh
	−	Rh₁rh (proper)

1. Wash the cells once in saline and resuspend to a 3% concentration in saline.
2. Place 1 drop of saline-suspended cells in a small tube, 7 mm diameter.
3. Add 1 drop of anti-rhʷ serum and mix.
4. Incubate in a water bath at 37° C for 1 hour.
5. Centrifuge at 500 rpm for 1 minute.
6. Gently dislodge the sediment, then read macroscopically and under a scanning lens of a microscope. Record clumping as positive (+) and absence of clumping as negative (−).
7. Run controls using rhʷ-positive and rhʷ-negative blood at the same time as the tests.
8. Cells that are agglutinated by the anti-rhʷ serum have the rhʷ specificity.
9. The distinction between a positive and a negative reaction is usually clear-cut, but it might be necessary to centrifuge the tube for 1 minute at 500 rpm before reading the results.

Testing red cells for rh$_i$ specificity

Anti-**rh**$_i$ is sometimes mistaken for anti-**rh′**, resulting in incorrect typing of Rh$_z$ blood as type Rh₂. Anti-**rh**$_i$ serum reacts with blood having agglutinogens produced by genes $r′$ and R^1 but not with any of the other six standard Rh-Hr agglutinogens. Genes r^y and R^z are very rare. Anti-**rh**$_i$ reactions therefore closely parallel anti-**rh′** in specificity, and the two reagents are easily confused. There is evidence that a number of the commercially available anti-**rh′** sera are in reality anti-**rh**$_i$.

The tests are made in a tube, using anti-**rh**$_i$ serum against the cells and following the same method as outlined previously in the test for anti-**rh**ʷ. Table 19-6 shows the usefulness of anti-**rh**$_i$ serum in a case of exclusion of paternity.

Table 19-6. False exclusion of paternity (after Wiener)

| Blood of | Original report | Correct report | | Anti-rh′ | Anti-rh$_i$ | Anti-hr |
		Phenotype	Genotype			
Putative father	Rh$_z$Rh$_1$	Rh$_z$Rh$_1$	R^zR^1, R^1r', or R^1r^y	+	+	−
Mother	Rh$_1$rh	Rh$_1$rh	R^1r, R^1R^o, or R^or'	+	+	+
Child	Rh$_2$rh	Rh$_z$rh	R^zr, R^zR^o, or R^or^y	+	−	+

Table 19-7. Reactions of red cells with anti-rh′ and anti-rh$_i$ antisera

| Gene | Corresponding agglutinogen | Reaction with | |
		Anti-rh′	Anti-rh$_i$
r	rh	−	−
r'	rh′	+	+
r''	rh″	−	−
r^y	rh$_y$	+	−
R^o	Rh$_o$	−	−
R^1	Rh$_1$	+	+
R^2	Rh$_2$	−	−
R^z	Rh$_z$	+	−

The child was originally incorrectly typed as phenotype Rh$_2$rh before it was found that the anti-rh′ serum used in the test was in reality anti-rh$_i$, with which the cells of the child did not react. When the typing was repeated and the red cells reacted with anti-rh′ but not with anti-rh$_i$, the correct Rh type and phenotype were discovered, and paternity was therefore not excluded.

Table 19-7 compares the reactions with the two antisera, anti-rh′ and anti-rh$_i$, which are so often confused with one another because of faulty preparation or labeling by the suppliers of the antisera.

Testing cells for rh^G, rh^{w2}, and rh$_{ii}$ specificities

The tests for these specificities, defined by their specific antisera, are conducted as for the other Rh-Hr factors. Refer to pp. 119 to 122 for a discussion of these specificities.

Testing red cells for cognates of Rh$_o$

The cognates of **Rh$_o$** are **Rh^A**, **Rh^B**, **Rh^C**, and **Rh^D** and their variants. The method described here is that of Wiener and Unger. It is made when an Rh-positive woman has delivered an erythroblastotic infant and her serum has an antibody resembling anti-**Rh$_o$** in specificity.

1. Prepare the red cells by the rapid ficination technic (p. 309). Carry out the ficination in four tubes labeled, respectively, anti-**Rh^A**, anti-**Rh^B**, anti-**Rh^C**, and anti-**Rh^D**. Place 1 drop of the ficinated red cells in each of the tubes.
2. Add 1 drop of the antiserum to its respectively labeled tube, anti-**Rh^A** in the tube labeled anti-**Rh^A**, etc.
3. Mix the contents of each tube and place in a water bath at 37° C for 1 hour.
4. Examine the bottoms of the tubes in the usual manner and record agglutination as positive (+) and absence of agglutination as negative (−). Confirm the readings by gently dislodging the sediment and reading under a scanning lens of a microscope. In negative reactions, centrifuge and take a second reading.
5. If the cells have clumped, they have the cognate identified by the antiserum; that is, if anti-**Rh^B** causes agglutination of the cells, they have **Rh^B**, etc.
6. If the cells do not agglutinate, the missing factor is designated by the appropriate small letter, for example, Rh^a, Rh^b, Rh^c, Rh^d, Rh^{ac}, etc.

TESTS MADE ON RED CELLS FOR Hr SPECIFICITIES

Tests for Hr factors of red cells are made (1) to determine the phenotypes in the Rh-Hr system and (2) in cases of isosensitization, primarily to the **hr′** factor (or to **hr^s** or others), to identify the antigenic stimulus. In the **symbols for the phenotypes** in the Rh-Hr system, the left half represents the results of tests for Rh factors, the right half the results of tests for the Hr speci-

Table 19-8. Phenotype determination by Hr testing of red cells

Rh type	Results of Hr testing	Rh-Hr phenotype
rh′	**hr′** negative	rh′rh′
	hr′ positive	rh′rh
rh″	**hr″** negative	rh″rh″
	hr″ positive	rh″rh
rh$_y$	**hr′** and **hr″** positive	rh$_y$rh
	hr′ negative; **hr″** positive	rh$_y$rh′
	hr′ positive; **hr″** negative	rh$_y$rh″
	hr′ and **hr″** negative	rh$_y$rh$_y$
Rh$_1$	**hr′** negative	Rh$_1$Rh$_1$
	hr′ positive	Rh$_1$rh
Rh$_2$	**hr″** negative	Rh$_2$Rh$_2$
	hr″ positive	Rh$_2$rh
Rh$_z$	**hr′** and **hr″** positive	Rh$_z$Rh$_o$
	hr′ negative; **hr″** positive	Rh$_z$Rh$_1$
	hr′ positive; **hr″** negative	Rh$_z$Rh$_2$
	hr′ and **hr″** both negative	Rh$_z$Rh$_z$

ficities. Because Hr antisera are not easily obtainable and wasting the antisera or performing unnecessary laboratory work should be avoided, when bloods of types Rh$_1$ and rh′ are examined, test only with anti-**hr′** serum, since anti-**hr″** serum will invariably give positive results, except in a few rare instances in which the blood lacks both the **rh″-hr″** pair of factors. Likewise, in testing types Rh$_2$ and rh″ bloods, test only with anti-**hr″**, since tests with anti-**rh′** serum will almost invariably be positive. Rh-negative bloods need not be tested as a rule because they react positively with anti-**hr′** and anti-**hr″** sera except in extremely rare instances (Rh$_{null}$).

The phenotypes are determined as in Table 19-8. The genotype corresponding to phenotype rh is always *rr*. The second half of the symbol rhrh is redundant and is therefore omitted (type rh). To determine the exact phenotypes of Rh$_z$ or rh$_y$ types, an additional antiserum, anti-**hr**, is of value. If the tests of the cells against anti-**Rh$_o$**, anti-**rh′**, anti-**rh″**, anti-**hr′**, and anti-**hr″** are all positive, the cells would be classified as

type Rh$_z$Rh$_o$. For further information see Chapter 8 and Tables 8-3, 8-9, and 8-11.

The exact technic to be used with anti-Hr reagents depends on whether they are IgM or IgG. (Follow the manufacturer's directions when using commercial reagents.) When tests by the conglutination method give weak reactions, centrifuge the blood sample, remove the plasma, and replace it with an equal volume of compatible normal adult plasma; then resuspend the red cells and proceed with the test. This method may also be used when a patient's blood shows marked pseudo-agglutination, as in certain hyperproteinemic states like myeloma or in diseases or conditions associated with a high fibrinogen content of the blood such as pneumonia and pregnancy.

The open slide method is used more or less as a screening test. When the reactions are negative, retest the blood by the tube method.

Slide test for Hr specificities in red cells

Anti-**hr′** and anti-**hr″** sera for slide tests (conglutinating, IgG) and whole, oxalated blood are needed for the slide test. Rh-negative blood may be used as a positive Hr control because it has both **hr′** and **hr″** factors.

1. Prepare slides with large ovals made with a red wax pencil as directed for the slide test for Rh specificities. Label with identifying number or name and the antiserum used. Two slides are needed for each blood.
2. Place 1 drop of anti-**hr′** slide serum on one slide and 1 drop of anti-**hr″** slide serum on the other.
3. Add 2 drops of oxalated whole blood to each slide.
4. Mix each with a separate toothpick or wooden applicator stick, and spread the mixture over the surface outlined by the wax ring.
5. Place the slides on a preheated viewing box and tilt the box back and forth slowly. Wait 2 minutes before recording a result as negative. Do not alow the test to dry. Record a positive reaction as soon as it is evident.
6. Tilt the box and let a drop of saline solution run down through each test. If rouleaux formation of the red cells is present, the saline

Table 19-9. Possible results in Hr slide testing

Anti-hr' serum and whole blood	Anti-hr" serum and whole blood	Conclusions	Second half of phenotype symbol
−	−	**hr'** and **hr"** negative	rh_y or Rh_z
+	−	**hr'** positive and **hr"** negative	rh" or Rh_2
−	+	**hr'** negative and **hr"** positive	rh' or Rh_1
+	+	**hr'** and **hr"** positive	rh or Rh_o

will break up the rolls of cells. Read again after adding the saline. Report clumping as positive (+) and absence of clumping as negative (−).

7. Run positive controls using type rh whole blood at the same time as the tests. If **hr'**-negative and **hr"**-negative bloods are available, run controls using these. Table 19-9 gives the possible results in this test.

Tube method for Hr specificities in blood cells

Using ficinated red cells

1. Wash the red cells twice in saline and then suspend to a 3% to 5% concentration in saline.
2. Place 2 drops of the suspension in each of two labeled Kahn tubes, one tube for anti-**hr'** and one for anti-**hr"** serum.
3. Add 1 drop of 1% ficin diluted 1:5 (p. 243) to each tube.
4. Mix thoroughly and incubate in a water bath at 37° C for 15 minutes.
5. Mix again, wash once in saline, centrifuge, then remove and discard the supernate.
6. Add 1 drop of anti-**hr'** tube serum to the first tube and 1 drop of anti-**hr"** tube serum to the second tube, and mix each thoroughly. These antisera are IgM (saline agglutinating) reagents.
7. Incubate again in a water bath at 37° C for 1 hour.
8. Tilt the tubes and observe for clumping or absence of it. If the results are negative, the sediment usually flows down the tilted tube bottom in a pear-shaped form. Gently dislodge the sediment and examine under a scanning lens of a microscope. Agglutination is a positive result.
9. Record the results of the tests just as those in the slide method and refer to Tables 19-8 and 19-9 for conclusions. See also Tables 8-3 and 8-9.

Using untreated red cells (saline agglutinating method)

1. Use a tube for each antiserum and label with identifying number or name and the name of the serum, anti-**hr'** or anti-**hr"**.

2. Place 1 drop of 3% suspension of once-washed red cells in saline in each tube.
3. Add 1 drop of anti-**hr'** agglutinating (tube, or IgM) serum to the first tube and 1 drop of anti-**hr"** agglutinating (tube, or IgM) serum to the second.
4. Mix the contents of each tube separately and place in a water bath at 37° C for 1 hour.
5. Read the sediment by slanting the racks, then read each tube over a lighted viewing box and under a scanning lens of a microscope.
6. Record results and draw conclusions by referring to Tables 19-8 and 19-9. See also Tables 8-3 and 8-9.

TESTS MADE ON BLOOD SERUM FOR ANTI-Rh ANTIBODIES (SENSITIVITY TESTING)

Tests of serum for anti-Rh or other irregular antibodies are called **sensitivity testing.** As previously shown, there are two distinct kinds of antibodies of Rh and Hr specificity, agglutinating, IgM, or 19S antibodies, which react with cells suspended both in saline and in high-protein media; and conglutinating, IgG, or 7S antibodies, which coat the cells in saline media without clumping them. The latter have also been called **blocking,** or **incomplete, antibodies** because in vitro there is no clumping, even though the cells have been coated by the antibody. For these cells to clump, a third substance, preferably antiglobulin serum, must be added, although in some cases a high-protein medium will suffice. If the cells are suspended in their own plasma or in a fortified protein medium, any conglutinating antibody present will then react and agglutination will ensue.

Fig. 19-4 is a diagrammatic representation of the difference between an agglutination reaction and a blocking reaction.

Some human sera containing anti-Rh an-

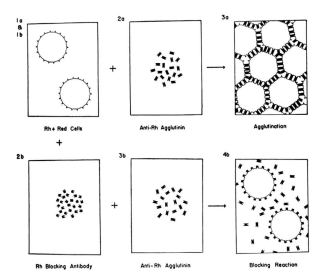

Fig. 19-4. Comparison of Rh agglutination and blocking reaction (test in saline media). (From Wiener, A. S.: Lab. Digest 14(6), 1950.)

tibodies exhibit a marked **prozone effect,** that is, they react when diluted, but in the undiluted state or when only slightly diluted they fail to bring about agglutination of the cells for which they are specific. Some workers have attributed such prozones to lack of "optimal proportions," that is, an excessive amount of antibody by comparison with antigen, or an excessive amount of antigen in proportion to antibody. This may appear satisfactory in the case of the precipitin test, but it is not so in agglutination tests. Wiener[1] presented evidence that the occurrence of prozones in titrations of anti-Rh sera by the saline agglutination method is due to the presence in the reagent of a mixture of anti-Rh_0 IgM and IgG antibodies. Significantly, when the same reagent is titrated by the high-protein (conglutination) method or when the antiglobulin technic is employed, the prozone does not occur. He also observed[*] that when certain freshly obtained antisera of specificities other than anti-Rh are titrated by the saline agglutinating method, prozones may occur due to the action of complement. When such sera are inactivated to destroy complement, prozones are no longer observed.

[*]Wiener, A. S.: Personal communication, Dec., 1971.

Test for Rh-Hr antibodies in serum

The test for Rh-Hr antibodies in serum consists of two parts:

Part I
1. Use group O type Rh_zRh_0 red cells. Group O is used because such cells do not have A or B agglutinogens and therefore are not agglutinable by anti-**A** or anti-**B** agglutinins that may be present in the unknown serum Type Rh_zRh_0 red cells are employed because they have all five standard Rh-Hr specificities, **Rh_0, rh′, rh″, hr′,** and **hr″,** which can detect any of the five opposing antibodies in an unknown serum. Two different cell suspensions are necessary, one untreated and suspended in saline to a 3% concentration, the other treated with proteolytic enzymes and suspended to a 5% concentration in saline.
2. Label two tubes, 7.5 cm × 8 mm, to indicate the contents.
3. Place 1 drop of untreated saline-suspended cells in the first tube and 1 drop of enzyme-treated cell suspension in the second tube.
4. Add 1 large drop of serum being tested to each of the tubes.
5. Mix the contents of each tube separately and incubate both in a 37° C water bath for 1 hour.
6. Tilt the tubes back and forth gently over a lighted viewing box and examine for agglutination or absence of agglutination, then confirm the reading under a scanning lens of a microscope.
7. If agglutinates are seen in either tube, the

serum presumably contains an anti-Rh antibody, the specificity of which has not yet been determined.

8. If there is no agglutination, proceed with Part II.

Part II (antiglobulin test)

9. Add saline to each tube to its full capacity and mix by covering tightly with a piece of wax paper and inverting the tube. Take care not to lose the cells.

10. Centrifuge to pack the cells, pour off the supernate, shake, and add saline again, then continue with the washing process four times.

11. After the last washing and centrifugation, invert the tube and press it against a gauze pad to remove remaining traces of saline, then shake to suspend the cells.

12. Place in a water bath at 37° C for 5 minutes.

13. Add 1 drop of antiglobulin serum to each tube and mix.

14. Centrifuge at 500 to 1000 rpm for 1 minute.

15. Gently dislodge the sediment, tip the tube back and forth gently, and read under a scanning lens of a microscope.

16. If the cells have agglutinated, the serum presumably contains an Rh-Hr IgG antibody, the specificity of which has not yet been determined.

When Part II as well as Part I of this test is performed, the entire test is called the **indirect antiglobulin test.** When ficinated cells are used and an antiglobulin test subsequently performed, it is the **Unger test,** or the **ficinated cell antiglobulin test.** This is an important laboratory procedure.

When agglutination occurs in Part I, using saline-suspended, untreated red cells and without antiglobulin serum, the antibody is of the IgM, or agglutinating, type. If agglutination occurs with enzyme-treated cells as well as with the untreated cells, there could be both agglutinating and coating antibodies. If agglutination occurs only with the enzyme-treated cells in Part I, there are no agglutinating IgM antibodies, but the IgG variety is present. If antiglobulin serum is needed to complete the agglutination reaction, that is, if the results in the first part are both negative but are positive in the second part, the antibodies are definitely of the IgG variety.

If the serum is from a prospective donor, that donor's blood should not be used in a transfusion because it has antibodies that could be harmful to a recipient. If the serum is from a prospective recipient, the presence of antibodies must be reported to the attending physician, and donor blood must be found that lacks the antigen with which the antibody reacts.

In the preceding technic, if group O type Rh_zRh_o blood cells are not available, use as many different Rh types of blood as are needed to identify all the five standard Rh-Hr antibodies. Group O Rh_1 has **Rh$_o$** and **rh′** as well as **hr″** specificities; group O Rh_2 has **Rh$_o$**, **rh″**, and **hr′**; and group O rh has **hr′** and **hr″**. These three cell suspensions may be used to identify anti-**Rh$_o$**, anti-**rh′**, anti-**rh″**, anti-**hr′**, and anti-**hr″** in an unknown serum. Prepare the red cell suspensions from these bloods, one set untreated and saline suspended, the other enzyme treated and saline suspended. Then make tests on each blood type in both sets. Panel cells that contain all the antigens are available commercially.

Conglutination test for anti-Rh and anti-Hr antibodies in blood serum (Wiener)

The test is performed as in the preceding method, except that the red cells for testing purposes are suspended in their own plasma or in a plasma-albumin mixture.

Indirect test for Rh$_o$ IgG antibodies (Wiener)

1. Use untreated, saline-suspended cells of group O, preferably type Rh_zRh_o. If only anti-**Rh$_o$** is to be tested for, cells may be from type Rh_o, Rh_1, Rh_2, or Rh_z.

2. Place 1 drop of the unknown serum in a small Kahn tube. Add 1 drop of the saline suspension of group O Rh-positive cells.

3. Mix and place in a water bath at 37° C for 1 hour.

4. Centrifuge at 1000 rpm for 1 minute, then read the reactions under a scanning lens of a microscope. If agglutination has occurred, **Rh$_o$** agglutinating antibodies (IgM) are pres-

ent and the test is ended. If the cells have not agglutinated, proceed with step 5.

5. Resuspend the sedimented cells and add to the tube 1 drop of anti-Rh$_o$ IgM (tube) serum.
6. Mix and place in a 37° C water bath for 1 hour and then read.
7. Centrifuge for 1 minute at 1000 rpm, shake gently to dislodge the sediment, and take a second reading.
8. If there now is agglutination, the serum has neither IgM (from result of the first part of the test) nor IgG (from result of the second part of the test) antibodies; otherwise, the result would be negative. If IgG antibodies are present, they coat the Rh-positive red cells and prevent the anti-Rh agglutinating serum from acting. When agglutination has occurred, the anti-Rh serum has reacted, which demonstrates that there was nothing in the serum under test to "block" the reaction and no IgG antibodies are present. On the other hand, if the red cells do not agglutinate, the antibodies in the serum under test have coated the red cells that were added, which blocked the reaction when the anti-Rh serum was added, so that the added anti-Rh serum could not react with its specific Rh-positive cells.

Theoretically, this test could be used to detect specificities other than Rh$_o$, provided the agglutinating serum is specific for the antigen present in the test cells. In practice, however, the test does not work for antibodies of other specificities such as anti-hr′ with the reagents available at present.

Direct antiglobulin test (direct Coombs test)

This test is used routinely to detect antibodies that react to antiglobulin, that is, antibodies that have coated red cells. These are the 7S, IgG antibodies that can also be detected by the blocking, conglutination, or enzyme technics. The test does not identify the antibodies as to specificity; it merely tells whether or not they are present. (In a newborn infant the antibodies that coat the red cells have been derived from the isosensitized mother.)

1. Wash the red cells four times with saline. After the last washing and centrifugation, invert the tube and touch the lip on a gauze pad to remove any traces of saline.

2. Resuspend the cells to a 5% concentration in saline.
3. Label small tubes, 7 by 70 mm, that have been thoroughly cleaned and dried.
4. Place 2 drops of the washed, saline-suspended red cells in the tube.
5. Add 2 drops of antiglobulin serum and mix.
6. If the cells have been strongly coated (sensitized), they should clump almost immediately. Read the reactions over a lighted viewing box.
7. If the reaction appears to be negative or only weakly positive, let the tube stand at room temperature for 15 to 30 minutes, then centrifuge at 500 rpm for 2 minutes or at 1000 rpm for 1 minute and read again.
8. It may be necessary to read under a scanning lens, although the reaction is usually plainly visible without the use of a lens.
9. If the cells have agglutinated, they have been coated with antibodies of the 7S, IgG type that readily pass through the placenta. In the infant this means that the mother has been isosensitized.

Controls

1. Carry out controls in the same size tubes used in the test and simultaneously with the test.
2. In tube 1 of the controls mix 2 drops of infant's (or other patient's) washed cells with 2 drops of saline.
3. In tube 2 of the controls, mix 2 drops of saline-suspended Rh-positive cells with 2 drops of antiglobulin serum.
4. In tube 3 of the controls, mix 2 drops of Rh-positive sensitized cells (cells previously coated with anti-Rh IgG antibodies) in 5% suspension in saline with 2 drops of antiglobulin serum.
5. Handle the controls in the same manner as the tests.
6. Tubes 1 and 2 should show no agglutination (−); tube 3 should show agglutination (+).

Table 19-10 gives the results that may occur in the direct antiglobulin test, including the controls.

False negative reaction. If the unknown cells have been coated with a minimal amount of antibody, there could be a false negative direct or indirect reaction.

Coating red cells with antibody

1. Suspend the Rh-positive red cells in saline to a 3% concentration.
2. Add 2 drops of the suspension to 2 drops of known anti-Rh slide IgG serum, mix, and incubate in a 37° C water bath for 30 minutes. *The cells should not agglutinate.*

Table 19-10. Possible results of the direct antiglobulin test

Unknown cells and antiglobulin serum	Unknown cells and saline	Rh-positive cells and antiglobulin serum	Coated Rh-positive cells and antiglobulin serum	Conclusions
+	−	−	+	Cells have been coated with antibody
−	−	−	+	Cells have not been coated with antibody

3. Centrifuge and remove the supernatant fluid.
4. Wash three times with saline. The cells remaining in the tube should now be coated with antibody.
5. To test these cells, mix in equal parts with antiglobulin serum. They should then agglutinate.

Quantitative direct antiglobulin test (Wiener)

This test measures the degree of coating of red cells by antibody.

1. Wash the red cells four times with an excess of saline, then resuspend to a 5% concentration.
2. Dilute the antiglobulin serum serially, 1:1 (undiluted), 1:2, 1:4, etc.
3. Perform the direct antiglobulin test on the unknown cells with each dilution of the antiglobulin serum (titration).
4. Titrate the same antiglobulin serum against maximally coated Rh-positive cells.
5. Calculate the percentage of coating of the unknown cells by dividing the titer of the antiglobulin serum for these cells by its titer for maximally coated Rh-positive cells, then multiply by 100.

Comment. This method can be used to determine the relative number of antigenic sites in the discoplasm for agglutinogens of different blood group systems and can be applied to the blood of babies with erythroblastosis fetalis as an additional criterion of severity of the disease. It is also useful in patients with acquired hemolytic anemia, in which case the degree of coating correlates well with the severity of the clinical manifestations. A rise in the degree of coating may be associated with a hemolytic crisis, a decrease with a remission. In disseminated lupus erythematosus there is a milder manifestation of autosensitization.

The titer is expressed as the reciprocal of the weakest dilution of the antiglobulin serum that gives a positive reaction.

For false results possible in the antiglobulin test, see p. 209.

Antiglobulin test control

Negative antiglobulin reactions should be checked by the use of group O Rh-positive sensitized (coated) red cells, prepared in the laboratory or purchased. In this test, coated red cells are added to each tube showing a negative reaction. The coated cells should agglutinate. If they do not, it is possible that the antiglobulin serum was inadvertently omitted from the tube, that the serum protein was not completely removed from the cells during the washing process, that the antiglobulin serum is unreactive and incapable of clumping sensitized red cells, or that the technic used was incorrect.

1. Resuspend the coated red cells by inverting the vial several times.
2. Add 1 drop of coated cell suspension to each *negative* antiglobulin test.
3. Mix, centrifuge the tube for 1 minute at 2000 rpm, and examine.
4. Record agglutination as positive (+), absence of clumping as negative (−).

Interpretation. If the antiglobulin test system used can detect sensitized cells, the reaction should now be positive. If negative, the antiglobulin test was inaccurate. Repeat the tests using a different antiglobulin serum.

IDENTIFICATION OF ANTIBODIES IN SERUM
Use of multiple antigens to identify antibodies

Multiple-antigen and panel cells are used to detect irregular antibodies in serum. These are suspensions of red blood cells having as many as possible of the blood group antigens but not necessarily all such antigens in each vial. As an example, one vial may have Rh_o, rh′, rh″, hr′, hr″, Fy^a, Le^a, P, M, N, and Xg^a. Another may have none of the Rh antigens but may contain hr′ and hr″, as well as some of the other blood group specificities.

It is the practice in many laboratories and blood banks to screen the sera of all donors and recipients for isoantibodies that could give rise to hemolysis. For this purpose a number of manufacturers have made available a panel of cells especially prepared and preserved, each vial containing particular antigens.*

The principle of using these cells is as follows: Each vial contains red cells having some but not all of the various blood group antigens. In the example presented here, there are ten vials. Tests are run using the unknown serum (the serum under test) against each cell suspension, ten suspensions or ten tests in all, using both the saline agglutinating and the antiglobulin tests. Other technics may also be used.

If the cells are agglutinated, those antigens in the cells of that vial identify one or more of the antibodies in the unknown serum. The next vial has different antigens, and also some of the same antigens as in vial No. 1. If these cells are also agglutinated, the antibody in the serum reacts with one or more of their antigens. If the antigens in vial No. 2 differ from those in vial No. 1, in that some of those in the first vial are absent from the cells in the second vial and some in the second vial are absent from the cells in the first vial, some of the antigens so determined may be eliminated.

---
*Manufacturers are listed on p. 305, footnote.

Accompanying the vials of cells is a sheet supplied by the manufacturer giving the contents of each vial. All the antigens are listed at the top of the sheet, and the antigens in each vial are designated either by a "+" ("x") or by an "O," the "+" designating presence of the antigen, the "O" its absence. As an example, in vial 10 in Table 19-11, the following antigens are present: hr′, hr″, hr, K, k, Kp^b, Js^b, Fy^a, Fy^b, Jk^a, Le^b, M, N, S, s, Lu^b, and Xg^a. If the tests made on the unknown serum with the red cells in each vial are positive, all antigens in that vial that are designated by an "O" are eliminated from the results. If the results are negative, any antigen designated by a "+" is eliminated from the results.

Stated in another manner, if the results of testing with vial 1 are negative (see the last five columns in Table 19-11), cross out all the "+" symbols in the first vial. If the reaction is positive, as in vial 2, cross out all the "O" marks on the line for vial 2. Continue in the same manner with each vial (one tube is run for each cell suspension per vial). If a line has been drawn in any (perpendicular) column, eliminate the antigen heading that column. The antigen or antigens remaining determine the antibody in the serum.

By using multiple-antigen cell panels, the antibody in a serum can be identified as to specificity, except when none of the vials has the antigen that is specific for this antibody.

Procedure
1. Resuspend the cells in their vials by gentle inversion.
2. Set up and label a series of ten small Kahn tubes. Set up an eleventh tube as a control.
3. Add to each tube 1 drop of its respective cell suspension, that is, 1 drop of cell suspension from vial 1 to tube 1, 1 drop from vial 2 to tube 2, and so on.
4. Add to each tube 2 drops of the unknown serum.
5. In the control tube place 1 drop of 5% to 8% cell suspension of the patient's own cells and add 2 drops of his own serum. This is a test for autoantibodies.
6. Centrifuge the eleven tubes immediately for 1 minute at 1500 rpm, read, and record

Table 19-11. Use of cell panels for antibody identification (example, antibody is identified

Vial		rh'	Rho	rh"	hr'	hr"	rhw	hr	hrV	K	k	Kpa	Kpb	Jsa	Jsb	Fya	Fyb	J
1	Rh₁Rh₂	∤	∤	∤	∤	∤	O	O	O	O	∤	O	O	O	O	∤	∤	
2	Rh₁Rh₁	+	+	Ø	Ø	+	Ø	Ø	Ø	+	Ø	Ø	+	Ø	+	Ø	+	
3	Rh₂Rh₂	O	∤	∤	∤	O	O	O	O	O	∤	O	∤	O	∤	O	∤	
4	rh'rh	+	Ø	Ø	+	+	Ø	+	Ø	+	+	Ø	+	Ø	+	Ø	+	
5	rh"rh	O	O	∤	∤	∤	O	∤	O	O	∤	O	∤	O	∤	∤	∤	
6	rh K+	Ø	Ø	Ø	+	+	Ø	+	Ø	+	+	+	+	Ø	+	Ø	+	
7	rh Fyᵃ	O	O	O	∤	∤	O	∤	O	O	∤	O	∤	O	∤	∤	O	
8	Rho	O	∤	O	∤	∤	O	∤	∤	O	∤	O	∤	∤	∤	O	∤	
9	rh	O	O	O	∤	∤	O	∤	O	O	∤	O	∤	O	∤	∤	∤	
10	rh	Ø	Ø	Ø	+	+	Ø	+	Ø	+	+	Ø	+	Ø	+	+	+	

*Provided by Dr. John D. Bauer, DePaul Hospital Division, St. Louis, Mo.

the results of each tube. The manufacturers call this "immediate spin." Use the master list supplied by the manufacturer.* If the test is positive, draw a line through all antigens that show an "O" in the master list. If it is negative, draw a line through all that have the "+" mark in the master list. Proceed in a like manner for each tube.

7. If cold antibodies are suspected, place the mixture of serum and cells in a refrigerator at 4° C, but use tubes having only antigens that are likely to react in the cold, for example, Lewis or P.

8. Incubate all the tubes at 37° C for 30 to 60 minutes, centrifuge at 1500 rpm, and examine, again noting the reaction. This is the 37° C reading.

9. Wash, four times with saline, the contents of each tube that shows a *negative* reaction, and after the last centrifugation remove all traces of saline, shake, then add 2 drops of antiglobulin serum to each.

10. Mix and centrifuge at 1500 rpm for 1 minute, then examine for agglutination.

11. Record on the chart as previously and determine the antibody or antibodies present.

12. If more than one antibody is present, perform an absorption and elution test (pp. 247 to 250) for identification of each.

---

*The O and + marks are printed on the list supplied by the manufacturer. The laboratory worker simply draws a line through the symbol at the top of the chart representing the antigen present in the cells.

Test for only Rh-Hr antibodies in serum

This is a test to determine whether the individual has antibodies that react against any of the Rh-Hr specificities, but it does not identify the specificities. It is an excellent method of screening the bloods of donors and recipients.

The cells used must have all the standard Rh-Hr specificities, **Rho, rh', rh", hr',** and **hr",** and must be derived from a group O person, since group O cells have neither A nor B agglutinogen. Type RhzRho blood has all the standard Rh-Hr factors and is therefore used in this test. This type blood is available commercially, or it may be prepared in one's own laboratory.

1. Prepare two cell suspensions of group O RhzRho blood, one untreated, the other treated with proteolytic enzymes, and resuspend them to 3% concentration for the untreated cells and 5% for the treated cells.

2. Label two tubes for each serum, identifying each with the name or laboratory number assigned to the serum and whether the cells are untreated or enzyme treated. The tubes should be 7.5 cm by 8 mm.

3. Place 2 drops of the untreated, saline-suspended group O type RhzRho cells in tube 1 and 2 drops of the enzyme-treated cells in tube 2.

ti-K) *

	Leᵃ	Leᵇ	P₁	M	N	S	s	Luᵃ	Luᵇ	Xgᵃ	Immediate spin	Room temp.	Albumin	37° C	Coombs enzyme
	O	≠	≠	≠	≠	≠	≠	O	≠	≠	O	O	O	O	O
	Ø	+	+	+	Ø	+	Ø	Ø	+	Ø	O	O	O	O	3+
	≠	O	≠	≠	O	O	≠	O	≠	+	O	O	O	O	O
	Ø	+	+	+	+	Ø	+	Ø	+	+	O	O	O	O	3+
	O	O	≠	≠	≠	O	≠	≠	≠	O	O	O	O	O	O
	+	Ø	+	+	+	Ø	+	Ø	+	+	O	O	O	O	3+
	O	≠	≠	O	≠	≠	O	O	≠	O	O	O	O	O	O
	O	≠	≠	≠	O	O	O	O	+	+	O	O	O	O	O
	O	≠	≠	≠	≠	≠	≠	≠	O	+	O	O	O	O	O
	Ø	+	Ø	+	+	+	+	Ø	+	+	O	O	O	O	3+

4. Add 1 large drop of the serum being tested to each tube. Shake each tube.

5. Incubate in a 37° C water bath for 30 minutes.

6. Tilt the tubes back and forth gently and observe for agglutination. Also read over a lighted viewing box and under a scanning lens of a microscope.

7. If there are any agglutinates, the individual from whom the serum was derived has been sensitized to one of the Rh-Hr factors.

8. If the results are negative, proceed with the antiglobulin test, p. 286.

9. If there is no clumping after the antiglobulin test has been made, there are no Rh-Hr antibodies in the serum. If, however, the cells have agglutinated, the serum contains Rh-Hr antibodies, but the specificity has not been determined.

10. If the saline-suspended cells have agglutinated, the antibody is of the IgM variety. If only the enzyme-treated cells have agglutinated, or if the saline-suspended cells were agglutinated only after antiglobulin serum was added, the antibody is of the IgG variety.

11. If the donor's serum contains antibodies, the donor's blood is rejected for all time. If the patients' serum contains antibodies, a compatible donor must be found, that is, one lacking the antigen(s) for which the patient's antibodies are specific.

Some laboratories routinely titrate the antibodies found in a patient's serum.

Conglutination test for Rh-Hr antibodies (Wiener)

The conglutination test for Rh-Hr antibodies uses red cells suspended to a 5% concentration in their own plasma or in **plasma-albumin mixture (4:1)**. The test is the same, then, as the preceding test.

Indirect test for Rh₀ IgG antibodies (Wiener)

The indirect test for Rh₀ IgG antibodies is described on p. 286.

TITRATION OF Rh-Hr ANTIBODIES[2]

The purpose of titrating serum for anti-Rh antibody concentration is to determine the concentration of such antibodies in the serum of isosensitized pregnant or postpartum women and thus the probabilities of delivering an erythroblastotic infant. The first titration should be made before the third month of pregnancy to determine if the antibody is being carried over from previous pregnancies or previous transfusions. Titrations are then usually made again at monthly intervals until the seventh month, then at biweekly intervals until the last month, when they should be made weekly. However, if the titration results at the third month show little or no titer, no further studies need be made until the seventh month. A rising titer after the third month shows that immunity is stimulated and in the case of an Rh-negative mother that the fetus is Rh positive. If the titer does not change, the fetus may be either Rh positive or Rh negative.

Titrations should be made on the bloods of all Rh-negative sensitized individuals and on all other bloods as requested. The red cells against which the serum is titrated should be group O (having neither A nor B agglutinogen) type $Rh_z Rh_o$, which has all five standard Rh-Hr specificities, **Rh_o**, **rh'**, **rh''**, **hr'**, and **hr''**. If no such blood is available, use types Rh_1, Rh_2, and rh blood. In this case three separate titrations will have to be made. Type Rh_1 has **Rh_o** and **rh'**, type Rh_2 has **Rh_o** and **rh''**, and type rh has **hr'** and **hr''**.

Titrations are made against the red cells untreated and saline suspended and against enzyme-treated cells. The antiglobulin test is run on negatively reacting tests.

Titrations may also be carried out against a specific antigen once the antibody has been identified.

1. Prepare serial dilutions of the unknown serum, using the method detailed on p. 267. Dilutions should be 1:1, 1:2, 1:4, 1:8, 1:16, 1:32, 1:64, and as many further dilutions as deemed necessary. Manifestly, if a former

Table 19-12. Examples of Rh-Hr titration results on an unknown serum

Specimen	Cells	Dilutions of serum							Conclusions
		1:1	1:2	1:4	1:8	1:16	1:32	1:64	
1	Untreated	4+	3+	3+	− [+]	− [−]	− [−]	− [−]	Agglutinating antibody titer = 4 units. Antiglobulin titer = 8 units
	Enzyme treated	4+	4+	4+	3+	3+	− [+]	− [−]	Enzyme-treated cell antibody titer = 16 units. Enzyme-treated cell antiglobulin titer = 32 units

In this example, both agglutinating and small-molecule antibodies are present; when both are in the serum in the same concentration, they cannot be separated by titration.

Specimen	Cells	1:1	1:2	1:4	1:8	1:16	1:32	1:64	Conclusions
2	Untreated	− [+]	− [+]	− [+]	− [−]	− [−]	− [−]	− [−]	No agglutinating antibody
	Enzyme treated	3+	2+	+w	− [+]	− [+]	− [−]	− [−]	Univalent antibody titer = 16

In this example there is only one type of antibody, the univalent, 7S, or IgG, variety. The titer is 4 units by the saline-antiglobulin technic and 16 units by the enzyme-treated antiglobulin method.

Specimen	Cells	1:1	1:2	1:4	1:8	1:16	1:32	1:64	Conclusions
3	Untreated	4+	4+	2+	2+	1+	+w	± [−]	Agglutinating antibody titer = 32
	Enzyme treated	4+	4+	4+	3+	1+	+w	− [−]	

In this example there appears to be only one type of antibody, the saline-agglutinating type. This antibody is detected when cells are untreated and saline-suspended and, likewise, in most cases when the cells are also enzyme-treated, although there are some cases in which the antigen is not reactive when the cells are treated with enzymes such as in the M-N-S system.

Specimen	Cells	1:1	1:2	1:4	1:8	1:16	1:32	1:64	Conclusions
4	Untreated	− [−]	− [−]	− [−]	− [−]	− [−]	− [−]	− [−]	No antibodies against test cells have been demonstrated.
	Enzyme treated	− [−]	− [−]	− [−]	− [−]	− [−]	− [−]	− [−]	

Note: The box, ⌐|, represents the results of the antiglobulin test.

titration of this individual's antibodies yielded a titer of 32, then dilutions at this time would begin at 1:16, 1:32, 1:64, 1:128, 1:256, etc. Prepare the dilutions of serum in 0.85% saline solution.

2. Place 1 drop of each dilution of serum in its respective tube. There will be two tubes for each dilution—one for the untreated red cells, the other for those treated with enzyme.

3. To each tube in the first rack, containing the different serum dilutions, add 1 drop of untreated saline-suspended group O Rh_ZRh_0 red cells.

4. To each tube of the duplication titration rack, add 1 drop of group O type Rh_ZRh_0 enzyme-treated cells.

5. Mix the contents of each tube and incubate the rack in a 37° C water bath for 1 hour.

6. Read the reactions in each tube under a scanning lens of a microscope and record the degree of reaction.

7. Perform antiglobulin tests on all negatively reacting tubes, first washing the cell and serum mixture four times with saline and removing the saline after the last washing.

8. Add 1 drop of antiglobulin serum, shake the tubes, and centrifuge at 1000 rpm for 1 minute, then gently dislodge the sediment and read.

9. The reciprocal of the highest dilution of serum giving a positive reaction is the titer. An example of a titration is given in Table 19-12.

In erythroblastosis fetalis due to isosensitization of the mother, the important antibody is the small molecule that readily traverses the placenta, that is, the 7S, IgG variety, which is not detected when the cells are suspended in saline without enzyme treatment, unless an antiglobulin test is also performed.

TEST OF SERUM FOR ANTI-Hr ANTIBODIES

The test for Hr antibodies is made in the same manner as that for anti-Rh antibodies in serum, except that ficinated hr' and hr″ cells are used. The two specificities, hr' and hr″, are present in type rh (Rh-negative) blood. The unknown serum must first be tested against Rh-positive blood cells to make sure that it does not contain anti-Rh₀, anti-rh', or anti-rh″ antibodies. If it is important that the specificity of the Hr antibodies be known, two tests are run. Otherwise, the following simplified test will suffice.

1. Use group O type rh cells. Wash the red cells twice with saline and discard the supernatant fluid after the last washing. Resuspend to a 5% concentration. Some prefer to use a third or a fourth washing.

2. Place 2 drops of the cell suspension in a small Kahn tube, add 1 drop of 1:5 ficin (p. 243) and mix.

3. Incubate in a 37° C water bath for 15 minutes, shaking the tube frequently.

4. Wash once with saline. After the last centrifugation remove and discard the supernatant fluid.

5. Add 1 large drop of the unknown serum and mix.

6. Incubate in a 37° C water bath for 60 minutes.

7. Gently dislodge the sediment and read, then examine under a scanning lens of a microscope.

8. If the cells did not agglutinate, wash four times with saline, remove the saline after the last centrifugation, and leave only a trace of the liquid.

9. Shake, add 1 drop of antiglobulin serum, mix, and centrifuge at 1000 rpm for 1 minute, then read.

10. If there still is no agglutination (whether in the first or the second part of the test), there are no anti-Hr antibodies in the serum.

11. If the cells agglutinated in the first half of the test or after the antiglobulin serum was added, the unknown serum contains an anti-Hr antibody, the specificity of which has not been identified.

Test to determine the specificity of anti-Hr antibody

Blood cells of type Rh_1Rh_1 react with anti-Rh₀, anti-rh', and anti-hr″ but not with anti-hr' or anti-rh″. Such cells have the specificity hr″ and can therefore be used to test for anti-hr″ antibodies, provided the serum being tested does not react with any of the Rh factors. Similarly, type Rh_2Rh_2 cells react with anti-Rh₀, anti-rh″, and anti-hr', and therefore these have the hr' specificity but not hr″ or rh'. These cells can thus be used to test for anti-hr' antibodies in an unknown serum.

The tests are conducted in the same

Table 19-13. Possible results in testing for specificity of Hr antibodies

Tube	Cells used	Reaction	Conclusion
1	O Rh₁Rh₁	+	Serum contains anti-**hr″**
2	O Rh₁Rh₁	−	No anti-**hr″** in serum
3	O Rh₂Rh₂	+	Serum contains anti-**hr′**
4	O Rh₂Rh₂	−	No anti-**hr′** in serum

manner as in the previous technic, but instead of using type rh cells against the unknown serum, types Rh_1Rh_1 and Rh_2Rh_2 red cells are used. The cells must all be group O.

When using group O Rh_1Rh_1 cells, the tubes may be labeled hr″; when using group O Rh_2Rh_2 cells, label the tubes hr′.

If the unknown serum reacts positively with the Rh_1Rh_1 cells and it has previously been shown that this same serum does not have any Rh antibodies, it has now been proved that the anti-**hr″** antibody is present.

If it reacts with the Rh_2Rh_2 cells and has been shown not to have any anti-**Rh₀** antibodies, it can be stated that the serum has anti-**hr′** antibodies.

Table 19-13 gives the possible results in tests for specificity of anti-Hr antibodies.

DETECTION OF FETAL RED CELLS IN THE PRESENCE OF ADULT ERYTHROCYTES
Kleihauer technic,[3] modified by Clayton et al.[4]

The Kleihauer technic is a method of eluting hemoglobins A, S, and C, leaving only fetal hemoglobin F in the erythrocytes. Erythrocytes that appear granular with a blue background are reticulocytes. Pink-staining, clear cells that have a heavy rim of cell membrane are erythrocytes having a high percentage of fetal hemoglobin. Adult erythrocytes appear simply as a cell wall or "ghost cells."

Reagents
1. Ethyl or isopropyl alcohol, 80%
   a. Dilute 80 ml of 95% alcohol with distilled water to a total of 95 ml.
2. Citric acid-phosphate buffer pH 3.2
   a. Solution A—0.2 M sodium phosphate, dibasic: Dissolve 14.2 gm Na_2HPO_4, mol wt 141.98, in distilled water and dilute to 500 ml with distilled water. Refrigerate at 4° to 6° C to prevent growth of molds.
   b. Solution B—0.1 M citric acid: Dissolve 9.6 gm $C_6H_8O_7$, mol wt 192.12, in distilled water and dilute to 500 ml with distilled water. Refrigerate at 4° to 6° C.
   c. Mix 14.25 ml solution A with 35.75 ml solution B. Check the pH on a pH meter. The pH must be exactly 3.2. Vary the amounts of the two solutions as necessary to obtain the proper pH, then add 0.25 gm new methylene blue to 50 ml of the buffer.
3. Giemsa counterstain: Immediately before use, add 20 drops of Giemsa stain to 50 ml Sørensen phosphate buffer, 0.067M pH 6.5.
4. Sørensen buffer pH 6.7
   a. Solution A—Place exactly 9.47 gm Na_2HPO_4, anhydrous, in a liter volumetric flask, dissolve in water, and dilute to 1 L with distilled water.
   b. Solution B—Place exactly 9.08 gm KH_2PO_4 in a liter volumetric flask, dissolve in water, and dilute to 1 L with distilled water.
   c. Sørensen buffer, 0.067M, pH 6.7—Mix 43.5 ml solution A with 56.5 ml solution B.
   d. Sørensen buffer, 0.0067M, pH 6.7—Dilute 100 ml 0.067M buffer to 1 L with distilled water. This solution is used for washing the slides after fixation, laking, and staining.
   e. Sørensen buffer, 0.067M, pH 6.5—Mix 31.7 ml solution A with 68.3 ml solution B. Use this to dilute the Giemsa stain.

Procedure
1. Place 5 ml venous blood in a tube containing a mixture of 6 mg ammonium oxalate and 4 mg potassium oxalate. This is the same dry oxalate used in taking blood for the Rh-Hr tests.
2. Mix the contents of the tube thoroughly but gently and refrigerate until the films are to be made, but do not freeze. Blood films should be made within 24 hr.
3. Prepare very thin blood films and allow to dry in the air.
4. Fix immediately for 5 min. in a Coplin jar containing 80% alcohol.
5. Wash thoroughly but gently, 5 to 6 dips, in 0.0067M Sørensen buffer pH 6.7.
6. Preheat, in a Coplin jar, citric acid-phosphate buffer pH 3.2, containing new meth-

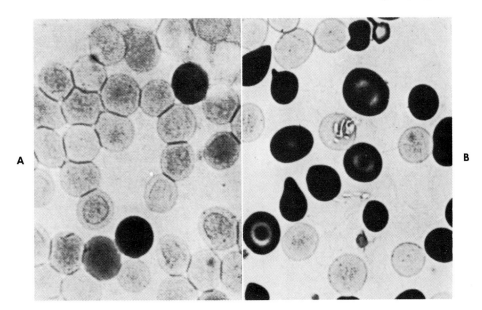

Fig. 19-5. Kleihauer test to demonstrate fetal hemoglobin. **A,** Thalassemia minor–Hb F 1.8%; Hb A₂ 3.8%. **B,** Thalassemia major–Hb F 45%; Hb A₂ 3.5% transfused. (From Kleihauer, E., and Betke, K. In Merher, H., editor: Zyto- und Histochemie in der Hämatologie, Berlin, 1963, Springer-Verlag.)

ylene blue, and leave the jar and its contents in a 50° C water bath. As soon as the solution warms, bubbles will form. Let the solution cool to 37° C in a water bath.

7. Immerse the blood films completely in the Coplin jar and leave uncovered for 15 min. Gently agitate the slides occasionally during this time.
8. Wash the blood films carefully, 5 to 6 dips, in 0.0067M buffer pH 6.7.
9. Place the slides in diluted Giemsa stain in a Coplin jar for 45 min.
10. Wash carefully, 5 to 6 dips, in 0.0067M phosphate buffer pH 6.7.
11. Allow to dry in the air and examine under low or high power. Oil immersion is not necessary.
12. Count 1000 cells under the microscope, keeping enumeration of the cells with fetal hemoglobin in a separate column, and then determine the percentage of such cells by dividing by 10. (See Fig. 19-5.)

Errors. If too little oxalate has been used, the blood will clot; if too much is present, the red cells will be crenated. EDTA or other sequestering agents produce cell distortion and artifacts that make the slides unreadable and should not be used. Blood specimens must not stand at room temperature for any appreciable time. The slides must not be shaken too vigorously during the staining or washing processes. The slides must never be placed in the laking buffer before the temperature reaches 37° C.

REFERENCES

1. Wiener, A. S.: Proc. Soc. Exp. Biol. Med. **56:** 173, 1944.
2. Erskine, A. G. In Frankel, S., Reitman, S., and Sonnenwirth, A. C., editors: Gradwohl's clinical laboratory methods and diagnosis, ed. 7, St. Louis, 1970, The C. V. Mosby Co.
3. Kleihauer, E., Braun, H., and Betke, K.: Klin. Wochenschr. **35:**637, 1957.
4. Clayton, E. M., Feldhaus, W. D., and Phythyon, J. M.: Am. J. Clin. Pathol. **40:**487, 1953.

20 □ Tests made in the M-N-S, P-p, K-k, Fy, and I-i blood group systems

TESTS MADE IN THE M-N-S BLOOD GROUP SYSTEM

Tests for the M and N specificities in red cells

Blood for the M-N tests should be collected in dry oxalate, as previously described. Either venous or capillary blood from skin puncture may be used. In paternity cases, blood from infants may be collected in small tubes, 7 to 8 mm in diameter, containing a few drops of ACD solution in the proportion of 5 to 10 drops of blood to 1 drop of ACD. Blood from skin puncture of adults or children can be collected in small tubes without an anticoagulant, allowed to clot, and the clot shaken in sufficient saline solution to make a 3% suspension of red cells. The method is not recommended as a routine procedure. It is best to obtain venous blood. **The red cells must not be treated with proteolytic enzymes.**

It should be noted that influenza viruses destroy the principal antigens of the M-N-S-s system. *Vibrio cholerae* and *Clostridium perfringens* have receptor-destroying enzymes (RDE).

REAGENTS

Two antisera made in rabbits are needed —anti-**M** and anti-**N**. Anti-**N** lectin made from *Vicia graminea* seeds is recommended for checking the results of the tests for the N specificity.

Anti-N lectins. Lectins of anti-N specificity are uncommon. Such anti-N lectins were first obtained from seeds of *Vicia graminea* by Ottensooser and Silberschmidt[2] in 1953. Other anti-N lectins have been prepared from *Bauhinea variegata* by Mäkelä[3] and by Bird and Wingham[4] from seeds of *Moluccella laevis* (also known as Belles of Ireland, shell flower, Molucca balm). Wiener[5] used anti-N lectin from *V. graminea* for studies on homologues of the human M-N types in nonhuman primates. See Chapters 15 and 24.

Moon and Wiener[1] prepared an extract of the leaves of the Korean *Vicia unijuga, Al. Braun* var. *Ouensanensis leveile*, which proved to be a powerful anti-N reagent. Comparative tests of the anti-N lectin by the tube method at body and refrigerator temperatures showed no significant differences in titer. The tests gave satisfactory results both by the well slide and the tube methods at room temperature.

Crude extracts of *V. unijuga* may agglutinate type M red cells as well as those of types N and MN. Absorption must be carried out with type M cells.

Refer to p. 237ff for a discussion of other lectins.

The antisera are available commercially. In the preparation of rabbit anti-**M** and anti-N sera, the species-specific antibodies are absorbed. A negative reaction therefore must be read within a specified time limit; otherwise, the red cells might eventually agglutinate, since the antisera are often slightly underabsorbed during the manufacturing process. When such delayed agglutination occurs, it could be

Table 20-1. Possible results in M-N tests

Reactions of red cells with		Type
anti-M serum	anti-N serum	
+	−	M
−	+	N
+	+	MN
−	−	Error

Table 20-2. Expected results with controls in M-N tests

	M cells	N cells	MN cells
Anti-**M** serum	+	−	+
Anti-**N** serum	−	+	+

mistaken for a positive reaction. True positive reactions are prompt and clear-cut, with large clumps of cells, except for some subgroups of N for which the reactions may be difficult to read.

As previously noted (p. 97), there is a specificity, M^e, shared by the M and He antigens, which can be a source of error in laboratory tests for the M-N types. It is essential that the antiserum used be standard anti-**M** and not anti-M^e.

TECHNIC

1. Use a freshly prepared 3% suspension of red cells in saline.
2. Place 1 drop of cell suspension in each of two rings on a ceramic ring slide labeled with the name of the individual from whom the blood has been derived and anti-**M** at the left side and anti-**N** at the right. Welled slides may also be used. (See Fig. 17-3.)
3. Add 1 drop of anti-**M** serum to the left ring and 1 drop of anti-**N** serum to the right ring. The mixture should fill the wells or rings.
4. Mix and rotate either by hand or on a rotating machine for 10 minutes.
5. Read macroscopically and confirm microscopically.
6. After the first reading, add 1 drop of saline to each ring, twirl, and read again. Record agglutination as positive (+) and absence of agglutination as negative (−).
7. Determine the M-N types according to Table 20-1.
8. **Controls** must be run at the same time as the tests, using all three cell types—M, N, and MN—against each antiserum:
   a. Prepare three slides, each with three rings. Label the first ring M, the second ring N, and the third ring MN on each slide. Then label the first slide anti-**M** and the second anti-**N**.
   b. Place 1 drop of type M cells in the rings so labeled, 1 drop of type N cells in the N rings, and 1 drop of MN cells in the MN rings on each slide.
   c. Add 1 drop of anti-**M** serum to each of the three rings on the first slide and 1 drop of anti-**N** serum to each of the three rings on the second slide.
   d. Mix and rotate as for the tests and record the results.
   e. Table 20-2 gives the expected results with the controls.
   f. If the controls give incorrect reactions, obtain different antisera and repeat.

Tests for other specificities in the M-N-S system

Tests for other specificities in the M-N-S system are carried out in a similar manner, using proper specific antisera: anti-**S** for detection of S, anti-**s** for detection of s, anti-**U** to detect U, and so on. These antisera are in short supply and therefore such tests are made only under special circumstances. As with all the blood grouping tests, these may also be made in small tubes. **The red cells must *not* be treated with proteolytic enzymes.**

Tests of serum for antibodies in the M-N-S system

Detection of antibodies in the M-N-S system is best done by use of panels of cells that may be purchased from certain manufacturers of blood grouping reagents (p. 239). The tests are then conducted on those cells having the various antigens. If such cells are available in the blood bank, there is no reason why they could not be used to test the unknown serum. **The cells should *not* be enzyme treated.** Anti-**M** and anti-**N** antibodies occur only rarely in human serum.

Production of anti-M and anti-N testing sera

Since anti-**M** and anti-**N** testing sera are available commercially, the method of preparing them is omitted. (For detailed information consult references 6 to 8.)

TESTS MADE IN THE P-p BLOOD GROUP SYSTEM
Test for P specificity in red cells and the P types

The following method is that of Wiener and Unger, modified:

1. Prepare a suspension of the red cells in saline, wash once in saline, and resuspend to a 5% concentration without enzyme treatment.
2. Place 1 drop of the cell suspension in each of two small, properly labeled Kahn tubes, 7 mm inside diameter.
3. Add 1 drop of anti-**P** serum to the first tube and 1 drop of anti-**p'** serum to the second.
4. Mix each tube thoroughly and refrigerate at 4° C for 2 hours.
5. Gently dislodge the cells by tilting the tube and read the reactions macroscopically and under a scanning lens of a microscope. Do not let the tube warm during the reading. Keep the rack containing the tubes in ice water or on a tray of ice until the readings have been completed.
6. Do *not* perform an antiglobulin test.
7. Record the results as positive (+) or negative (−) and determine the phenotype according to Table 20-3.
8. Always include positive and negative controls with the tests, made like those for identifying the unknown cells.

For other designations of phenotypes in the P-p system, refer to Chapter 10.

Since the anti-**P** and anti-**p'** antibodies are cold agglutinins, the reactions must be carried out in the cold and the tubes must not be permitted to warm to room temperature. On humid days, moisture may condense on the tubes. This must be wiped off before reading the reactions.

The tests for antibody in the serum must also be made in the cold. In using panel cells that have the P antigen, tests must be carried out not only at room temperature and at 37° C. for the other antibodies but also at refrigerator temperature (pp. 289 and 290).

Anti-**P** has been prepared by immunizing rabbits with P-like antigens from mucilaginous plants (p. 158).

TESTS FOR K-k AND Js SPECIFICITIES IN RED CELLS

Enzyme-treated cells must *not* be used when testing for the K-k blood group specificities. Red cells that have been treated with an enzyme often fail to react with anti-**K** and anti-k sera. Anti-**K** gives best reactions when the indirect antiglobulin method is used, as does anti-k, although anti-**K** also reacts well by the plasma conglutination method.

Tests for the K specificity (Wiener)
Plasma conglutination method

1. Have at hand fresh oxalated blood plasma derived from a group AB individual (no anti-**A** or anti-**B** agglutinins are present in group AB plasma). Plasma from the blood of a person compatible with that of the individual whose blood is being tested may also be used. The plasma must be prepared from blood taken in dry oxalate and not in a liquid anticoagulant.
2. Prepare a suspension in saline of the cells to be tested, wash once with saline, then resuspend to a 3% concentration.
3. Place 1 drop of washed, saline-suspended

Table 20-3. Identification of the P-p types*

Reactions of red cells plus antiserum		Phenotypes	Isoantibodies that can be in the serum
Anti-**P**	Anti-**p'**		
−	−	p (rare)	Anti-**P** and anti-**p'**
−	+	p' (rare)	Anti-**P**
+	−	P (formerly P negative)	Anti-**p'**
+	+	P₁ (formerly P positive)	None

*Modified from Wiener, A. S.: Lab. Digest **31**(4):6, 1968.

red cells in a small tube, 7 to 8 mm inside diameter, properly labeled.

4. Add 1 drop of anti-**K** serum and mix.
5. Incubate in a 37° C water bath for 1 hour, at which time the cells will have settled to the bottom of the tube.
6. Remove the supernate as completely as possible, using a fine capillary dropper.
7. Add 2 large drops of oxalated group AB plasma and resuspend the sediment in it.
8. Incubate in a 37° C water bath for 1 hour.
9. Shake gently to dislodge the sedimented cells, then read macroscopically and under a scanning lens of a microscope. Agglutination is a positive reaction (+).
10. If the cells have agglutinated, they have the **K** specificity. If they have not agglutinated, the **K** specificity is not present.

Antiglobulin technic

1. Prepare a saline suspension of red cells to be tested, wash once in saline and resuspend to a 3% concentration.
2. Place 1 drop of the cell suspension in a small tube, 7 mm inside diameter, labeled with the name or identifying number.
3. Add 1 drop of anti-**K** serum and mix.
4. Incubate in a 37° C water bath for 30 to 60 minutes.
5. Wash rapidly with saline four times and remove all the supernate after the last washing and centrifugation.
6. Add 1 drop of antiglobulin serum and shake to mix.

Table 20-4. Possible results with anti-**K** and anti-k sera

Reactions with			Corresponding genotype
Anti-**K**	Anti-**k**	Phenotype	
+	−	K	*KK*
−	+	k	*kk*
+	+	Kk	*Kk*
−	−	Error or rare atypical blood	

Table 20-5. Possible results using anti-Js^a and anti-Js^b sera

Reactions with		Phenotype
Anti-Js^a	**Anti-Js^b**	
+	+	Js(a+b+)
+	−	Js(a+b−)
−	+	Js(a−b+)
−	−	Js(a−b−) (rare)

7. Centrifuge at 500 rpm for 1 minute.
8. Gently dislodge the sediment and read macroscopically and under the scanning lens of a microscope.
9. If the cells have agglutinated, they have the **K** specificity. If they have not agglutinated, the **K** factor is not present.

Test for the k specificity in red cells

The antiglobulin method is recommended because the anti-k serum antibody in most available reagents is 7S, IgG.

1. Prepare a fresh specimen of the cells to be tested, wash once with saline, and resuspend to a 3% concentration in saline.
2. Place 1 drop of cell suspension in a small tube, properly labeled.
3. Add 1 drop of anti-**k** serum and mix.
4. Incubate in a 37° C water bath for 60 minutes.
5. Wash rapidly four times with saline and remove all but 1 drop of supernatant saline after the last washing and centrifugation.
6. Add 1 drop of antiglobulin serum and mix.
7. Centrifuge at 500 rpm for 1 minute.
8. Gently dislodge the sediment and read the reaction. Read macroscopically and under the scanning lens of a microscope.
9. Record agglutination as positive (+), absence of agglutination as negative (−). If the cells have agglutinated, the **k** specificity is present. If they have not clumped, the **k** factor is not present.

Determining the phenotypes in the K-k system

The phenotypes are determined according to the results in Table 20-4.

Test for Js^a and Js^b specificity in red cells

Carry out the tests as for the **K-k** factors, using anti-**Js^a** and anti-**Js^b** testing sera and determine the type by consulting Table 20-5.

TEST FOR Fy SPECIFICITIES IN RED CELLS

The anti-**Fy^a** antibody is usually of the 7S, IgG type, for which reason these tests are made by the indirect antiglobulin method. The red cells do not react when trypsin and especially papain are used to treat the cells, but enzyme-treated Fy(a+)

Table 20-6. Possible results in testing red cells with anti-**Fy**^{a} and anti-**Fy**^{b} sera

Reactions with			
Anti-Fy^a	Anti-Fy^b	Phenotype	Genotype
+	+	Fy(a+b+)	*Fy^{a}Fy^b*
+	−	Fy(a+b−)	*Fy^{a}Fy^a* or *Fy^{a}fy*
−	+	Fy(a−b+)	*Fy^{b}Fy^b* or *Fy^{b}fy*
−	−	Fy(a−b−)	*fyfy*

Table 20-7. Possible results using anti-**Jk**^{a} and anti-**Jk**^{b} serum against unknown cells

Reactions with			
Anti-Jk^a	Anti-Jk^b	Phenotype	Genotype
+	+	Jk(a+b+)	*Jk^{a}Jk^b*
+	−	Jk(a+b−)	*Jk^{a}Jk^a* or *Jk^{a}jk*
−	+	Jk(a−b+)	*Jk^{b}Jk^b* or *Jk^{b}jk*
−	−	Jk(a−b−)	*jkjk*

cells do react in the trypsinated cell antiglobulin test.[9-13] The papain-antiglobulin test is always negative.

1. Prepare a saline suspension of red cells to be tested, wash once, and resuspend in saline to a 3% concentration.
2. Place 1 drop of the cell suspension in each of two small tubes, 7 mm diameter, properly labeled.
3. Add 1 drop of anti-**Fy**^{a} serum to the first tube and 1 drop of anti-**Fy**^{b} serum to the second tube.
4. Mix the contents of each tube separately and incubate in a 37° C water bath for 30 to 60 minutes.
5. Wash rapidly with saline four times, leaving 1 drop of saline in the tubes after the last washing, centrifugation, and decantation.
6. Resuspend the cells in the drop of saline and add 1 drop of antiglobulin serum to each tube. Mix.
7. Centrifuge for 1 minute at 500 to 1000 rpm.
8. Gently dislodge the sediment and read the reactions.
9. Record agglutination as positive (+) and absence of clumping as negative (−).
10. Refer to Table 20-6 for possible results.

To avoid false negative reactions, washing with saline must be done rapidly. The red cells are fragile and may undergo spontaneous clumping or hemolysis if kept in saline suspension too long.

TEST FOR THE Jk SPECIFICITIES IN RED CELLS

Identification of the Jk antigens must be made by the antiglobulin method, since other tests usually fail to detect them. The antisera tend to lose their reactivity on storage because the reactions are complement-dependent and the complement that is naturally present in the serum deteriorates with time. Controls must always be included, and the blind test should also be made. Cells must *not* be enzyme treated unless the trypsin-antiglobulin test of Unger is used. If complement is included in the tests in the form of fresh group AB serum, the results are usually good, but better results may be obtained by suspending the red cells in fresh group AB serum instead of in saline. If enzyme-treated cells are used, weak to moderate hemolysis is often observed. Antiglobulin serum with anti–nongamma components are required for best results.

1. Prepare a 3% cell suspension in saline or, preferably, in fresh group AB serum.
2. Label two tubes, 7 mm in diameter, with identification of the specimen and of the antisera.
3. Place 1 drop of cell suspension in each of the two tubes.
4. Add 1 drop of anti-**Jk**^{a} serum to the first tube and 1 drop of anti-**Jk**^{b} serum to the second.
5. Mix the contents of each tube separately and incubate in a 37° C water bath for 1 hour.
6. Read the reactions macroscopically and under a scanning lens of a microscope.
7. If there is no agglutination, wash four times with saline and, after the last washing and centrifugation, remove all traces of saline. Invert the tubes over a gauze square to absorb remaining traces of saline.
8. Add 1 drop of antiglobulin serum (anti–nongamma globulin) to each tube and mix.
9. Centrifuge immediately at 500 to 1000 rpm for 1 minute.
10. Gently dislodge the sediment, then read

macroscopically and under a scanning lens of a microscope.

11. Run positive and negative controls at the same time as the tests.
12. If the controls give correct readings, agglutination in the test means that the specificity delineated by the antiserum is present in the unknown red cells. Read results as in Table 20-7.

TESTS FOR ANTI-P, ANTI-K, ANTI-k, ANTI-Fyᵃ, ANTI-Fyᵇ, ANTI-Jkᵃ, AND ANTI-Jkᵇ IN SERUM

Unless there is suspicion that a certain one of these antibodies is present in the serum to be tested, the tests for such antibodies are usually made employing a panel of cells, as described on p. 289ff. However, the identity of each antibody can be established separately by testing the unknown serum against cells containing the antigen for which the antibody under question is specific. The methods of performing tests for antibodies include the use of untreated, saline-suspended red cells, cells treated with enzymes, the antiglobulin test, or a combination of the enzyme and antiglobulin tests, as described previously (p. 250ff). The temperatures at which the antibodies react optimally are discussed in the chapters dealing with the individual antigens and in the technics for detecting such antigens.

TESTS MADE IN THE I-i BLOOD GROUP SYSTEM
Tests for I and i specificities in red cells

Essentially all newborn babies are I negative and i positive. All cord blood is I negative and not agglutinated by anti-I serum. Adult red cells, with hardly any exceptions, are I positive. Anti-I serum therefore agglutinates almost all adult red cells but not cord cells, although in some instances cord cells are weakly agglutinated. On the other hand, anti-i serum agglutinates cord cells and essentially no adult cells except for the few adults who are i positive, about one in 5000 persons. Wiener found four Negroids and one Caucasian adult subject who were I negative

and therefore i positive among 22,000 people tested.[14] For these reasons, tests in the I-i blood group system are limited to detection and identification of anti-I and anti-i in the serum.

Test for anti-I and anti-i in blood serum

The unknown serum must be tested against a battery of adult cells and also against cord cells. Cord cells are regularly I negative. If the serum fails to agglutinate adult red cells (group O) but does agglutinate cord cells, it contains anti-i, since the cord cells have the i antigen. If the serum clumps the adult cells but not the cord cells, it has anti-I. If neither the adult nor the cord blood cells are agglutinated by the serum, there are no anti-I or anti-i antibodies present.

Anti-I and anti-i are cold agglutinins. The test gives strongest reactions at refrigerator temperature.

1. Prepare at least ten red cell suspensions derived from ten different group O adults. Wash and resuspend to 5% concentration in saline.
2. Prepare a 5% suspension of group O cord red cells in saline.*
3. Label ten small tubes with the identifying label. Mark the first eight tubes "A" for adult cells, the ninth tube "C" for cord cells, and the tenth tube "P" for patient's cells.
4. Place 1 drop of washed group O adult cells from eight different individuals in each of the first eight tubes, respectively.
5. Place 1 drop of 5% suspension of group O cord cells in tube 9.
6. Place 1 drop of patient's own cells in tube 10. This is to test for autoantibodies in the patient's serum and to serve as a negative control for cases in which there are no autoantibodies present.
7. Add to each tube 2 drops of the serum to be tested. Mix the contents of each tube separately.
8. Centrifuge all tubes at 1000 rpm for 30 seconds, read, and record the results. Then place the tubes in a refrigerator at 4° C in a glass of cracked ice for 30 minutes.
9. Centrifuge the tubes in ice for 30 seconds

---

*Cord cells, ready for use, are available from Behring Diagnostics, Woodbury, N.Y.

Table 20-8. Results of tests for anti-**I** and anti-**i** antibodies in serum

	Tubes									
	1	**2**	**3**	**4**	**5**	**6**	**7**	**8**	**9**	**10**
Specimen 1										
Reactions with										
Adult cells	4+	4+	4+	4+	4+	4+	4+	4+		
Cord cells									−	
Patient's cells										−
Specimen 2										
Reactions with										
Adult cells	−	−	−	−	−	−	−	−		
Cord cells									4+	
Patient's cells										−

Interpretation:

Serum specimen 1 contains anti-**I** antibody.

Serum specimen 2 contains anti-**i** antibody.

If none of the cell suspensions exhibit agglutination, there is no antibody.

at 1000 rpm and again place them in the 4° C ice bath.

10. Wait 5 minutes, then read again and record the results.

11. Table 20-8 gives examples of results using unknown serum in a test for anti-**I** and anti-**i** antibodies.

REFERENCES

1. Moon, G. J., and Wiener, A. S.: Vox Sang. **26**:167, 1974.
2. Ottensooser, F., and Silberschmidt, K.: Nature (Lond.) **172**:914, 1953.
3. Mäkelä, O.: Ann. Med. Exp. Fenn. **35** (supp. 11): 1957.
4. Bird, G. W. G., and Wingham, J.: Vox Sang. **18**:235, 1970.
5. Wiener, A. S., Gordon, E. B., Moor-Jankowski, J., and Socha, W. W.: Haematologia (Budap.) **6**:86, 1972.
6. Wiener, A. S.: Blood groups and transfusion, ed. 3, Springfield, Ill., 1943, Charles C Thomas, Publisher; reprinted New York, 1962, Hafner Publishing Co.
7. Wiener, A. S., Zinsher, R., and Selkowe J.: J. Immunol. **27**:431, 1934.
8. Erskine, A. G. In Frankel, S., Reitman, S., and Sonnenwirth, A. C., editors: Gradwohl's clinical laboratory methods and diagnosis, ed. 7, St. Louis, 1970, The C. V. Mosby Co.
9. Race, R. R., and Sanger, R.: Blood groups in man, ed. 5, Philadelphia, 1968, F. A. Davis Co.
10. Morton, J. A.: Thesis, University of London, 1972.
11. Unger, L. J., and Katz, L.: J. Lab. Clin. Med. **38**:188, 1951.
12. Haber, G., and Rosenfield, R. E.: Andresen, P. H., papers in dedication of his 60th birthday, Copenhagen, 1957, Munksgaard, International Booksellers & Publishers, Ltd.
13. Issitt, P. D., and Jerez, G. C.: Transfusion **6**:155, 1966.
14. Wiener, A. S., and Wexler, I. B.: Heredity of the blood groups, New York, 1958, Grune & Stratton, Inc.

21 □ Tests made before a transfusion; coding of blood group reactions; automation

TESTS MADE BEFORE A TRANSFUSION

The numerous tests of patient's and donors' blood before a transfusion are for the purpose of selecting the donor(s) whose blood will be beneficial to the recipient. Such blood supplies the cellular and chemical elements needed to restore the recipient to health. The incoming cells of the donor(s) must therefore not agglutinate or hemolyze in vivo, and the plasma in which the cells are naturally suspended must not react unfavorably with the recipient's own cells. In other words, the donor's and recipient's bloods must be compatible with one another in all respects.

A medical history of prospective donors is taken prior to the laboratory tests. Whether to accept or reject a donor on the basis of this history is the prerogative and responsibility of the attending physician. This will not be discussed in this text nor will the methods of carrying out transfusions. Only those laboratory tests immediately related to the subject of blood grouping will be presented.

The following tests are made on donor(s) and recipient before a transfusion. When numerous donors' bloods are to be used for the same recipient, as in open heart surgery and organ transplantation, the respective donors' bloods should be compatible with one another and with that of the recipient although compatibility tests among donors are not usually performed.

1. Test for the A-B-O blood group, using cell suspensions against known anti-**A** and anti-**B** sera and preferably also against group O serum (**major**).

2. Run controls on the anti-**A** and anti-**B** sera to make certain that they are in correct working order and also for comparative purposes in reading reactions.

3. Test the serum against groups A, B, and O cells (**reverse grouping, minor**). (If hemolysis occurs, which is a positive reaction, inactivate the serum and repeat the test.) If the result in this test differs from that in step 1, repeat the entire procedure, using different anti-**A** and anti-**B** sera for testing the cells and different group A and B cells for checking the serum.

4. If further confirmation is needed, test whole blood of the recipient as well as whole blood from the donor against anti-**A** and anti-**B** sera. The resulting blood groups should be the same as in step 1.

5. Although not essential for transfusion, some blood banks subgroup all group A and AB bloods, using either absorbed anti-A serum or anti-A_1 lectin against the cells.

6. Test the patient's blood for Rh_0 by the open slide or rapid centrifugation method with whole blood, taken in a dry oxalate, against anti-Rh_0 slide serum (IgG).

7. At the same time, test the donor blood against anti-Rh_0, anti-Rh_0', and anti-Rh_0'' slide sera, using whole blood.

8. If the recipient is Rh positive by the open slide technic, transfuse with blood from an Rh-positive donor.

9. If the recipient is Rh negative by the open slide method, transfuse with blood from an Rh-negative donor.

10. If tube tests instead of slide tests are made and if the recipient is Rh_0 positive, select Rh_0-positive donors for the transfusion.

11. If the tube tests show the **recipient** to be type rh, rh', rh'' or rh_y, use only Rh-negative blood for the transfusion unless a donor of the identical type as the recipient can be found.

12. If the **donor** is type rh', rh'', or rh_y, do *not* give this blood to an Rh-negative recipient. It may be used, however, for an Rh-positive recipient.

13. Cross match (1) the donor's cells against the recipient's serum and (2) the recipient's cells against the donor's serum. The first half of the test is called the "major" half because it detects antibodies reactive for the donor's red cells. The second half is called the "minor" half because it detects antibodies for the recipient's cells. Such antibodies would be diluted in the recipient's circulation during the transfusion and therefore ordinarily would not be harmful.

14. If any agglutinates are observed in the cross-matching tests, do not use that donor's blood for this particular recipient.

15. At the same time perform tests for antibodies in the recipient's and donors' sera against Rh-Hr and other blood specificities. If the donor's serum contains such antibodies, reject that donor for all time.

16. If the recipient's serum contains such antibodies, select a donor(s) whose red cells do not have an antigen(s) specific for these antibodies.

17. Test for autoantibodies in both the recipient's and the donor's sera using their ficinated cells against their own sera.

18. In all cases of unexplained erythroblastosis fetalis in which the mother is in need of a transfusion, test her serum for all irregular antibodies using a panel of cells, as outlined on p. 239.

Under no circumstances should one depend on cross-matching tests alone without preliminary tests to determine the blood groups of the recipient and donors when preparing for a transfusion. It is also dangerous simply to obtain donor blood of the same group and type as that of the recipient and to transfuse it without preliminary cross-matching tests because of the possibility of intragroup incompatibility and subsequent transfusion reactions.

Cross-matching tests should be made on bloods of recipient and donor who are of the same A-B-O and Rh-Hr blood types. Bloods of incompatible A-B-O groups will give positive agglutination reactions in the cross-matching tests, under which circumstances the donors would be rejected.

Universal donor

It was believed at one time that group O blood could be safely used to transfuse individuals of any blood group because group O red cells do not have A or B iso-agglutinogens and therefore are not agglutinable by anti-**A** (in group B serum) or by anti-**B** (in group A serum). (Group AB serum has neither anti-**A** nor anti-**B**.) Group O blood has both anti-**A** and anti-**B** agglutinins, however, in addition to anti-**C**; if these are present in high concentration, the dilution that the incoming donor blood undergoes in the recipient's circulation may not be sufficient to reduce its agglutinin concentration below the point where it cannot react with the recipient's cells. This could lead to an unfavorable transfusion reaction. In addition, group O blood might also contain certain natural or immune antibodies antagonistic to the cells of the recipient. Group O blood should therefore never be transfused to anyone outside of group O unless its anti-**A** and anti-**B** agglutinin titers are low and it does not contain any irregular antibodies. Even so, the universal donor idea has fallen into disrepute because of the number of cases of sensitization resulting from transfusion of antigens outside the A-B-O system into individuals who lack them. On the other hand, group O packed cells may be used for transfusions of individuals outside group O if the cells do not have antigenic specificities lacking from the recipient's blood.

If it is ever necessary, however, to transfuse group O blood into individuals not of group O, the anti-**A** and anti-**B** agglutinins may be neutralized by adding **group-specific substances** A and B, also called **Witebsky blood group substances,** to the group O blood. Group-specific substances, however, usually do not neutralize the natural anti-**C** present in group O sera because these are IgG antibodies, and group-specific substances do not neutralize such antibodies.

Universal recipient

Group AB serum does not have anti-**A** or anti-**B** agglutinins, and therefore there is no isoantibody to react with cells of group A, B, or AB should such blood be used to transfuse group AB recipients. For this reason, at one time group AB was designated universal recipient. It is not safe, however, to transfuse group AB people with blood outside their own group. There are subgroups of group AB such as A_1B and A_2B. Individuals having such subgroups may have isoantibodies in their sera. One example is subgroup A_2B, which often has anti-A_1 that could react with blood cells from groups A_1 and A_1B. The blood plasma of group AB is not necessarily compatible with other blood groups nor even with other group AB blood. It can be dangerous to use the universal recipient idea in selecting donors for a group AB patient.

Technics of cross matching

After the A-B-O blood groups, Rh types, etc. of the recipient have been determined, donors are selected of the same A-B-O blood group and Rh type. If the recipient is **Rh**$_o$ positive, a donor belonging to the same A-B-O blood group who is **Rh**$_o$ positive is selected. If the recipient is type rh, or even rh′, rh″, or rh$_y$, donors must be Rh negative unless a donor of the identical type is available. Cross matching is the last

opportunity before the transfusion to detect an error in blood grouping and correct it.

The test consists of two parts, major and minor (p. 304). Some institutions omit the minor half. This should always be omitted if group O blood is to be used to transfuse a person not of group O because it will invariably be positive.

A routine cross-matching test includes the following:

1. Donor's cells + recipient's serum
2. Recipient's cells + donor's serum
3. Recipient's cells + recipient's serum (for autoantibodies)
4. Sensitivity testing of the patient and donors should also be made at the same time, consisting of the following:
   a. Patient's serum + group O mixed antigen cells,* untreated and saline-suspended
   b. Patient's serum + group O mixed antigen cells, enzyme treated
   c. Donor's serum + group O mixed antigen cells, untreated, saline-suspended
   d. Donor's serum + group O mixed antigen cells, enzyme treated

Tube method of cross matching (recommended)

1. Use 7.5 cm by 8 mm tubes and set up the tests in duplicate.
2. Have at hand 5% suspensions in saline of once-washed red cells from the recipient and from each prospective donor.
3. Prepare blood serum from the recipient and from each prospective donor.
4. Four tubes will be needed for simple cross matching (not counting the tests for autoantibodies). The four tubes are needed because the tests are made in duplicate. If cells are lost during the various washings, the duplicate tubes can be used.
5. Place the tubes in a rack in two rows. Label the front tubes "PS" for patient's serum and the back tubes "DS" for donor's

---

*Mixed antigen cells, that is, cells containing a number of different blood group antigens, are available from Pfizer & Co., New York, N.Y.; Spectra Biologicals, Oxnard, Calif.; Ortho Diagnostic Division, Raritan, N.J.; Hyland Laboratories, Costa Mesa, Calif.; and others. See footnote on p. 239.

serum. Identify each set of tubes with the proper laboratory number or name.

6. Place 2 drops of patient's serum in each front tube.
7. Place 2 drops of donor's serum in each back tube.
8. Add 1 drop of donor's cells, 5% in saline, to the two front tubes.
9. Add 1 drop of recipient's cells, 5% in saline, to the two back tubes.
10. Mix the contents of the four tubes separately and incubate in a 37° C water bath for 30 to 60 minutes. In urgent cases, reduce the incubation period to 15 minutes.
11. Centrifuge at 500 rpm for 2 minutes or at 1000 rpm for 1 minute and examine for hemolysis. If there is hemolysis, the bloods are incompatible and another donor must be selected. In such cases, the supernatant fluid will be clear but tinged with red.
12. Twist to dislodge the sediment and look for a button of clumped red cells. If there is such a button, the red cells have agglutinated and the bloods are incompatible. Reject the donor.
13. If neither hemolysis nor agglutination has occurred, proceed with the antiglobulin test.
14. Wash the contents of all four tubes four times with saline and remove and discard the supernatant fluid after the final washing. All traces of saline and all protein must be removed before adding the antiglobulin serum.
15. Shake the tubes to loosen the cells.
16. Add 1 drop of antiglobulin serum to each tube and mix by shaking.
17. Centrifuge at 1000 rpm for 1 minute, gently dislodge the sediment, and read macroscopically, under a scanning lens of a microscope, and, if desired, under the low power of the microscope.
18. If there is any agglutination, reject the donor. If clumping does not occur, the bloods are compatible. When A-B-O compatibility is evident in this test but there is clumping in the antiglobulin test, the serum apparently contains antibodies other than anti-A and anti-B, which can be identified by use of a panel of cells, as outlined on p. 239.

Open slide method of cross matching using high-protein media (Unger). This is a screening test only. If the test shows incompatibility between the blood of the donor and that of the recipient, it is not necessary to perform the longer tube tests, since this donor will necessarily be rejected for this recipient. If the test shows compatibility, however, the longer tube tests must also be run.

1. Obtain blood serum from both recipient and donor, as well as whole blood taken in a dry anticoagulant (double oxalate). Remove enough plasma to produce a proportion of 50% blood cells, and 50% plasma. In the case of anemic patients, centrifuge the blood and remove enough plasma to give a 50% suspension of red cells. Then shake thoroughly but gently to mix.
2. Draw a large wax ring approximately the length of the slide and at least half the width, using a red wax pencil. Prepare three such slides.
3. Label the first slide "PS" for patient's serum, the second "DS" for donor's serum, and the third "PS + PC" for patient's serum + patient's cells (test for autoantibodies).
4. Place 2 drops of donor's whole blood on slide 1, 2 drops of recipient's whole blood on slide 2, and 2 drops of recipient's whole blood on slide 3.
5. Add 1 drop of recipient's serum to slide 1, 1 drop of donor's serum to slide 2, and 1 drop of recipient's serum to slide 3.
6. Add to each slide 1 drop of 30% bovine albumin.*
7. Mix the contents of each ring with a separate toothpick or wooden applicator and spread the mixture throughout the full surface of the ring.
8. Wait 5 minutes, then examine over a viewing box.
9. Tilt the box, then add 1 drop of saline to the top of each ring and let the saline run down through the mixture to break up any rouleaux present.
10. If there is any agglutination, reject the donor for this patient.
11. If slide 3, with patient's serum + patient's cells, shows agglutination, the recipient's serum has an autoantibody.
12. If the slides show no incompatibility, proceed with the tube test.

Tube conglutination method of cross matching. Some laboratories prefer to carry out the tests in tubes rather than perform-

---

*Bovine albumin solution may vary in strength from 15% to 22% to 30%, depending on the manufacturer. This albumin solution is available from most manufacturers who prepare blood grouping antisera and other reagents, including Armour Laboratories, Chicago, Ill.; Pentex, Kankakee, Ill.; and Hyland Laboratories, Costa Mesa, Calif.

ing either of the previous two methods. When the conglutination test is made, it is still desirable to perform an antiglobulin test. The conglutination method does not detect anti-**Fy** antibodies; if anti-**Fy** is under consideration, the antiglobulin method must be used.

1. Use small Kahn tubes, 7.5 cm by 8 mm, and label.
2. Place 2 drops of recipient's serum in the tube marked PS and 2 drops of donor's serum in the tube marked DS.
3. Add 1 drop of 30% bovine albumin to each tube and mix.
4. Using applicator sticks, transfer enough red cells from a clot of the donor's blood to the tube marked PS (tube 1) to make a 3% suspension of red cells in serum. This is the direct (major) match.
5. In tube 2 (DS) transfer enough of the recipient's red cells, using applicator sticks, to the mixture of serum and albumin, making a 3% suspension of these cells in the mixture (minor match).
6. Mix the contents of each tube separately and incubate in a 37° C water bath for 3 to 5 minutes.
7. Centrifuge at 1000 rpm for 2 minutes.
8. Gently dislodge the sediment. Avoid excessive shaking, which might break up agglutination. Examine. If there are any agglutinates, reject this donor for this recipient.
9. If A-B-O compatibility has been proved, agglutination in the tube labeled PS means that the recipient has been sensitized to an antigen outside the A-B-O system, which is present in the donor's red cells; other donors must be sought and matched.
10. When Rh-positive recipients have been sensitized to Rh-positive blood of another Rh type (Rh₁rh recipient, Rh₂rh donor), or when Rh-negative recipients have erroneously been designated Rh positive and are isosensitized, incompatibility with the donor blood can usually be detected by this method.

Routine cross-matching tests including simultaneous tests for autoantibodies and other antibodies in serum. Tests for autoantibodies and other antibodies (sensitivity tests) may be made simultaneously with the cross-matching tests, in which case seven tubes will be needed for the recipient and each donor. Also needed will be 5% red cell suspensions in saline from

the recipient and donor, and saline suspensions of group O mixed antigen cells* and group O enzyme-treated mixed antigen cells.* Group O is used because such cells have neither A nor B isoagglutinogen.

1. Set up seven tubes for each donor being tested with a specific recipient. If only one donor is tested there will be seven tubes, if two donors, there will be fourteen tubes, etc. See Fig. 21-1.
2. Label the tubes as follows: Tube 1, PS; tube 2, DS; tube 3, PS + PC; tube 4, PS + UC (untreated cells); tube 5, PS + Ez (enzyme-treated cells); tube 6, DS + UC; tube 7, DS + Ez. Tubes 4 through 7 represent sensitivity testing of the respective sera.
3. Place 2 drops of recipient's serum in tube 1 and add 2 drops of donor's cells, 5% suspension in saline.
4. Place 2 drops of donor's serum in tube 2 and add 2 drops of recipient's red cell suspension, 5% in saline.
5. Place 2 drops of recipient's serum in tube 3 and add 2 drops of recipient's saline-suspended red cells for the autoantibody test.
6. Place 1 drop of recipient's serum in tube 4 and add 1 drop of group O mixed antigen cells, untreated and saline-suspended.
7. Place 1 drop of recipient's serum in tube 5 and add 1 drop of group O mixed antigen cells, enzyme treated then saline-suspended.
8. Place 1 drop of donor's serum in tube 6 and add 1 drop of group O mixed antigen cells, untreated and saline-suspended.
9. Place 1 drop of donor's serum in tube 7 and add 1 drop of group O mixed antigen cells, enzyme treated then saline-suspended.
10. Mix the contents of each tube separately and place the rack in a 37° C water bath for 30 minutes.
11. Examine the bottoms of the tubes. Positive reactions tend to remain in a button of cells, but negative results will not form the button; instead the cells will run down the tube when it is tilted. Small clumps may be present. If there is any agglutination, do not use this donor for this patient. If the results are negative, proceed to step 12.
12. If there are no agglutinates, wash the contents of each tube four times with saline

---

*Mixed antigen cells, that is, cells containing a number of different blood group antigens, may be prepared in one's own laboratory or they may be purchased. See footnote on p. 239 for sources of such cells.

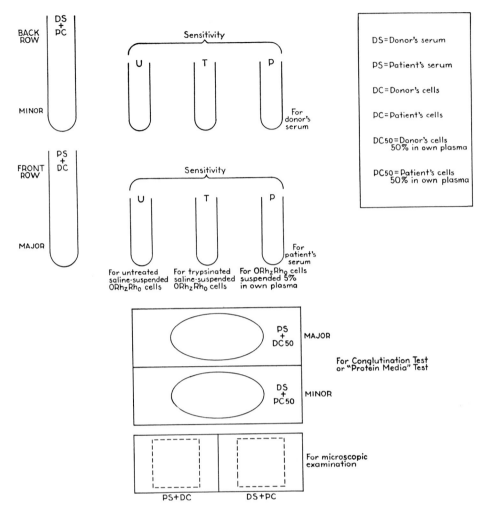

Fig. 21-1. Cross matching and Rh-Hr sensitivity testing for antibodies in serum. (After Unger; from Erskine, A. G. In Frankel, S., Reitman, S., and Sonnenwirth, A. C., editors: Gradwohl's clinical laboratory methods and diagnosis, ed. 7, St. Louis, 1970, The C. V. Mosby Co.)

and after the last washing and centrifugation, remove all traces of saline in the usual manner.

13. Add 1 drop of antiglobulin serum to each tube, mix thoroughly, then centrifuge at 1000 rpm for 1 minute. Dislodge the sediment gently and read.

14. If agglutination appears in tube 1 or 2, the bloods of the recipient and donor are incompatible and another donor must be sought.

15. If there is no agglutination, the bloods are compatible and the donor's blood may be used.

16. If there is agglutination in tube 3, the recipient's serum has autoantibodies.

17. If the donor's serum has irregular antibodies, as shown by a positive reaction with

mixed antigen cells, do not use that donor's blood.

18. If the patient's blood has an irregular antibody, as shown by the use of mixed antigen cells, the antibody may be identified, using the method on p. 289.

19. Table 21-1 gives the possible results with this method.

If no group O mixed antigen cells are available, use group O type Rh_zRh_0 cells, which will detect any of the standard anti-Rh antibodies because it has the five standard specificities, Rh_0, rh′, rh″, hr′, and hr″.

Anti-Fy^a does not react with enzyme-treated cells.

When testing for **Le** and **P** specificities

Table 21-1. Possible results in complete cross-matching test

Tubes	Contents	Reaction	Conclusions
1 (PS + DC)	Patient's serum + donor's cells	+	Incompatible*
		−	Compatible
2 (DS + PC)	Donor's serum + patient's cells	+	Incompatible*
		−	Compatible
3 (PS + PC)	Patient's serum + patient's cells	+	Autoantibodies present
		−	No autoantibodies
4 (PS + UC)	Patient's serum + group O mixed antigen, untreated cells	+	Irregular antibody
		−	No irregular antibody
5 (PS + Ez)	Patient's serum + group O mixed antigen, enzyme-treated cells	+	Irregular antibody
		−	No irregular antibody
6 (DS + UC)	Donor's serum + group O mixed antigen, untreated cells	+	Irregular antibody*
		−	No irregular antibody
7 (DS + Ez)	Donor's serum + group O mixed antigen, enzyme-treated cells	+	Irregular antibody*
		−	No irregular antibody

*Reject the donor.

the tubes are placed in cracked ice in a refrigerator at 4° C and duplicate tests are also made at room temperature. If the cells have not been enzyme treated, the refrigerator temperature is mandatory for testing for the **Le** factor.

If mixed antigen cells in saline suspension are refrigerated overnight, they should be washed with saline before use.

Rapid ficinated or bromelin-treated cell method for the autoantibody test in cross matching

1. Place 1 drop of washed red cells of the patient in a small Kahn tube.
2. Add 1 drop of 1:5 ficin or bromelin (1% solution diluted 1:5 with saline).
3. Mix thoroughly and place in a 37° C water bath for 15 minutes.
4. Wash once in saline and resuspend the cells to a 4% concentration. This will require about 1 or 2 drops of saline, added to the sediment.
5. Mix and add 2 drops of the patient's serum.
6. Mix and place in a 37° C water bath for 30 minutes.
7. Read the sediment under a scanning lens, after gently dislodging the cells.
8. Agglutination indicates presence of autoantibodies. (An antiglobulin test at this point may give false positive results and is not recommended.)

Results in a simple cross-matching test

Table 21-2 shows the various results that may occur in a simple cross-matching test in which an antiglobulin test has also been made.

RhoGAM* cross match

RhoGAM is the name of a product* that is administered intramuscularly to Rh_o-negative or $\mathfrak{R}h_o$-negative women immediately after delivery of an Rh_o-positive or $\mathfrak{R}h_o$-positive infant. The purpose of the injection is to suppress the antibody response of the mother to the Rh_o- or $\mathfrak{R}h_o$-positive fetal cells. It is also administered to Rh_o-negative women after abortion, miscarriage, or ectopic pregnancy.

Each package of RhoGAM also contains a serum vial with a 1:1000 dilution of the same lot number of RhoGAM as that contained in the package. This vial is used to cross match the mother's cells with the RhoGAM.

Method

1. Label one tube "S" for saline agglutination, and one "A" for albumin cross match.

*Ortho Diagnostics, Raritan, N.J.

Table 21-2. Results that may occur in cross matching*

Donor's cells and recipient's serum	Recipient's cells and donor's serum	Conclusions
−] / −	−] / −	Compatible
−] / −	+] / −	Incompatible
+] / −	−] / −	Incompatible
+] / −	+] / −	Incompatible
−] / −	+	Incompatible
+	−] / −	Incompatible
+	+	Incompatible
+	+] / −	Incompatible

*Box,], represents the antiglobulin test results. No antiglobulin test need be made when the original reaction is positive.

2. Wash the mother's cells once with saline, drain the saline solution after centrifugation, and prepare a 4% suspension of the cells in saline.
3. Add 1 drop of maternal cell suspension to each tube.
4. Add 2 drops of saline to tube S and 2 drops of 22% bovine albumin to tube A.
5. Add 2 drops of 1:1000 dilution of RhoGAM to each tube.
6. Centrifuge at 1000 rpm for 1 minute, then examine microscopically and macroscopically for agglutination or hemolysis, or both.
7. Perform an indirect antiglobulin test on tube A (if negative) and again examine microscopically and macroscopically for agglutination.

Results

If there is no agglutination, RhoGAM may be administered to the Rh-negative postpartum mother.

If the cells are weakly agglutinated, RhoGAM should not be administered because there is a possibility that the mother is $\mathfrak{Rh}_o$.

If there is mixed-field agglutination, there has been fetomaternal hemorrhage and the mother's blood contains a mixture of her Rh_o-negative blood and her fetus' Rh_o-positive cells. This is not a contraindication to the administration of RhoGAM, but the mother's cells should be tested again for the presence of $\mathfrak{Rh}_o$, using an incubation period of 30 minutes and washing the cells four times instead of the usual three. If there has been fetomaternal hemorrhage, the Rh-positive cells of the fetus will agglutinate, but the cells of the Rh-negative mother will remain free, giving a mixed-field pattern. (Confirm the presence of fetal cells by the Kleihauer method, pp. 294 and 295.) In such a case the dose of RhoGAM should be *increased!*

Problems in cross matching

Introduction of incompatible donor cells into a recipient's circulation can be dangerous, but infusion of plasma containing antibodies that may react with the recipient's cells is usually not hazardous. For this reason, some hospitals limit their matching tests to the major match, that is, donor's cells plus patient's serum.

Except for those of the A-B-O, Rh-Hr, K-k, and a few other specificities, most of the more than a hundred known blood group factors of human red cells are only weakly antigenic. When, however, the patient's or donor's serum contains an antibody, this should be identified by use of a panel of cells. If the preliminary grouping tests of recipient's and donor's blood have been correctly conducted, almost all crossmatching tests show compatibility. The few incompatible results can be costly in time consumed trying to trace either the cause of the incompatibility or the presence of an error. There are a few problems in cross matching, however, that can be avoided, as follows:

1. If the cross-matching test shows incompatibility between the donor and recipient bloods, one problem is to determine the **specificity of the antibody** involved. In some instances no compatible blood can be found, as in sensitization to the high-frequency blood factors or in multiple sensitizations, but in many instances

the antibody in the patient's serum can be identified by using cell panels, and compatible blood can then be obtained from one of the blood bank centers.

If the search for a compatible donor requires more time than the referring physician believes is safe because of need for an immediate transfusion, and if he insists on the use of blood that the laboratory finds incompatible, he should sign a release from responsibility or liability of the blood bank for each unit of blood he obtains. In such cases the technologist and hospital would be exonerated should the recipient experience any untoward effect from the transfusion.

2. One source of problems in cross matching is **centrifugation.** The speed and length of centrifugation are both critical. The centrifuge should be checked for accuracy in speed, and the tests should be repeated at the proper centrifugal force and time. If reactions still occur, they were not due to improper centrifugation.

Constant speed centrifuges are available for blood grouping use exclusively. These are usually of the small size variety. Centrifuges should be standardized from time to time, following the manufacturers' directions. The tendency is to use many small centrifuges instead of the larger ones in vogue for so long a time.

3. The **temperature of the water bath** is critical. It should be set at 37° C ± 0.5°. Only thermostatically controlled apparatus should be used, and the temperature should be checked at frequent intervals throughout the day.

4. Certain **cations** in distilled water can cause improper cross-matching results. Heavy metal cations at times occur in saline because the water from which the saline was prepared flowed through the wrong grade of metal tubing or some tin was present in the still. High-valence cations effectively reduce the surface charge of erythrocytes and thus give rise to false positive results. The best water is that from a still, but water prepared by use of ion exchange resins is also recommended.

5. If the recipient's serum clumps all the cells in a panel, there is a possibility of **autosensitization.** Autosensitization tests of the patient's serum should be routine in cross matching. Autoantibodies usually cause agglutination not only of the individual's own cells but also of those of all other humans. Whenever possible, transfusions should be avoided under such circumstances. See polyagglutinability, p. 230.

6. **Pseudoagglutination** due to rouleaux formation of the red cells, a cause of some errors, is common in multiple myeloma and in some cases of Hodgkin's disease, as well as in other states characterized by an accelerated sedimentation rate. If the cells are in rouleaux formation due to the protein in the serum in such conditions, dilution with saline is not always effective in suspending them. Some instances of rouleaux formation may be prevented by washing the cells in saline several times before performing the cross-matching tests, but when agglomerates of the cells cannot be broken, the **biologic test** must be relied on by the person performing the transfusion. Transfuse the first 50 ml of blood slowly, over a period of 1 hour; if no untoward reaction occurs and there is no rise in serum bilirubin content, proceed with the rest of the transfusion, first removing a tube of blood and examining the serum for hemolysis or icterus index. If hemolysis is evident or if there is a rise in the icterus index, discontinue the transfusion.

See p. 229 for method when rouleaux formation is present.

7. If the patient's serum agglutinates all cells in the panel except the patient's own cells, his serum most likely has an antibody that is active against some **high-frequency factor** like **Vel, U,** etc. If the antibody proves to be anti-**Vel,** the patient's *fresh* serum will usually hemolyze the red cells of all random individuals, especially if such cells have been enzyme treated, but his own cells and cells of Vel-negative people will remain unaffected. Anti-U antibodies react well with saline-suspended, untreated cells plus the antiglobulin test, but they do not react with enzyme-treated cells. All antibodies in the M-N-S system are similarly

characterized so that when testing for M-N-S specificities and other factors in this system, the cells must not be enzyme treated.

8. If all the cells of the panel have been agglutinated by the serum of the patient and none of the high-frequency antibodies are present, there can be a **mixture of antibodies,** which should be identified. The blood of siblings is usually tested to obtain donors in these cases.

9. When possible, all patients scheduled for surgery should be tested before there is any need for a transfusion. In this way the serum can be screened for antibodies and all the numerous tests made. If the physician waits until the patient is going into surgery before requesting blood grouping tests, there may not be enough time to carry out all the required methods.

10. **Nonspecific agglutination** in cross matching may be due to autoagglutination, rouleaux formation, high sedimentation rate, or the presence of cold agglutinins. Over-centrifuging can give false positive results. Shaking a tube too hard, on the other hand, could break up weak agglutinates. In the antiglobulin test the methods vary with the different antiglobulin serum manufacturers; their directions must be closely followed.

11. If the serum contains anti-**I** antibody, continue with the transfusion, but use warmed blood because anti-**I** antibody does not react at body temperature.

12. When one puts pipets into the mouth, **saliva** may enter the pipet. Saliva has group-specific substances that can interfere in blood grouping. Straws or droppers are useful in blood grouping tests.

13. If cells are washed and improperly resuspended, the antiglobulin test may be negative, which is a **false negative** cross-matching reaction. Saline should be pure. Mouth pipets must not be used. Any saliva reaching the antiglobulin serum can inhibit its reacting ability.

14. **Cell suspensions** should be 5% concentration. During the washing process some cells are lost and the concentration becomes less than 5%. After numerous washings the eventual concentration may become so weak that reactions, if they do occur, are difficult to read or there could be a false negative result. All cross-matching tests should be performed in duplicate.

15. **Fresh serum** is used as a rule in cross matching. If the serum has hemolyzing antibodies, the opposing cells dissolve and there is no visible agglutination. Such a hemolytic reaction is considered positive, but at times it is difficult to read. **Hemolysis** occurs only if complement is present, and in fresh serum it is invariably present. Blood from the blood bank is not necessarily freshly drawn on the day of the cross-matching test so that hemolysis is usually no problem in using such blood. If there is any doubt about whether hemolysis has occurred, inactivate the serum and repeat the test. The **Lewis** antibody is often hemolytic but does not produce lysis except in the presence of complement.

16. When cells have been treated with a proteolytic enzyme and tests are conducted in a cold room, **nonspecific agglutination** can occur. Although negative enzyme tests are of great value in screening for antibodies, the use of enzyme-treated cells for cross matching is nevertheless not recommended as a routine procedure.

17. Whenever the patient is to have a transfusion, always insist on obtaining a freshly drawn sample of blood and test the serum for **irregular antibodies,** even though this might not be the first transfusion of that patient in that hospital.

18. Always **double check** to make sure that the sample of blood on which the tests are being made has indeed been drawn from the individual for whom the tests should be made. There have been serious errors due to interchange of specimens.

19. **In case of doubt,** repeat the blood grouping tests and then cross match the bloods again.

Cross matching when strong rouleaux formation is present

If rouleaux formation is present in the saline-antiglobulin cross match test, recentrifuge the serum-cell mixture, remove the supernatant serum, and replace it with an equal volume of saline. Mix and centrifuge. Resuspend and read. The saline should disperse the rouleaux. If the cells now appear clumped, this is true agglutination.

Posttransfusion reaction "work-up"

If, despite all precautions, a transfusion reaction does occur, it is necessary to perform certain tests in an attempt to discover its cause. All tests on both recipient and donor, especially the A-B-O and Rh-Hr tests, should be repeated. In such a case the blind test would serve well (p. 233).

1. Test for all the Rh factors and types, and perform sensitivity tests on the recipient's serum against a panel of cells, each having a known blood group antigen. Do not use pooled or mixed antigen cells.
2. Make similar tests of the donors' sera.
3. Use both untreated and enzyme-treated red cells, except when testing for Fy and M-N-S antigens.
4. Retest all sera of all donors used for this recipient in previous transfusions, as well as that of the present donor.
5. Repeat the autoantibody test—that is, the recipient's serum against the recipient's own cells—using the blood taken before the transfusion.
6. Repeat the cross-matching test on the pretransfusion specimens and perform cross-matching tests on blood taken after the transfusion. Include enzyme-treated cells in the test even when these are not routinely used in cross matching.
7. Test all glassware and the saline used, as well as the centrifuge, to determine if these are in standard condition.
8. A **cell survival test** often gives clues. If the transfused cells have survived and the recipient has no demonstrable antibody, the reaction was due to a cause other than incompatible transfusion. As an example, if the recipient lacked the **M** specificity in his red cells and the transfused blood was **M** positive, and if M cells are present in the recipient's blood, the transfused cells have survived. If the recipient is type Rh_1, as an example, and has received blood from a donor whose blood cells have Rh_0 and rh'' (type Rh_2 or Rh_z), and if the rh'' specificity is still present in the recipient's blood, the reaction was not due to hemolysis of the transfused blood.

Prevention of Rh sensitization after a mismatched transfusion

In 1970 Schellong and Grimm[2] reported a case of a 29-year-old Rh-negative woman erroneously transfused with 400 ml of group O Rh-positive blood. To neutralize in vivo the incompatible Rh-positive red cells circulating in the patient's blood and thus to prevent sensitization, she was given anti-Rh_0 immunoglobulin (anti-Rh_0 IgG) to a total of 6500 μg administered in sixteen doses on 9 consecutive days, most of it intravenously. By the tenth day there were no donor cells present in the patient's blood and there were no side effects from the injections. The injected Rh_0 antibodies were still demonstrable up to eleven months after the transfusion and then disappeared. The patient has since been successfully delivered of an Rh-positive child without forming Rh antibodies.

There are other cases similar to this one. It now is apparently possible to prevent Rh sensitization after Rh-positive transfusion into an Rh-negative individual if treatment with anti-Rh_0 IgG is undertaken promptly and in sufficiently high dosage, probably in excess of 1000 μg/100 ml of Rh-positive blood, in divided doses over a period of 3 or 4 days.

COUNTERELECTROPHORESIS (IMMUNOELECTRO-OSMOPHORESIS) METHOD
(Fig. 21-2)

Counterelectrophoresis is a method of immunodiffusion that is modified by electrophoretically driving antigen and antibody toward one another. It is used primarily in the detection of the **Australian antigen** (hepatitis-associated antigen, or **HAA**). HAA appears to be a hepatitis virus related to serum hepatitis and can be transmitted from one individual to another through blood transfusion. Whereas antibodies against HAA have been found in multitransfused patients, they are also found in patients who have never been transfused, but who may have acquired the antigen by the oral route.

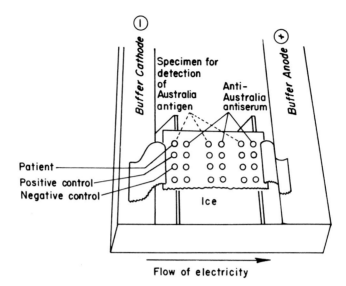

Fig. 21-2. Counterelectrophoresis. Diagram of electrophoresis chamber. (From Bauer, J. D., Ackermann, P. G., and Toro, G.: Clinical laboratory methods, ed. 8, 1974, The C. V. Mosby Co.)

A counterelectrophoresis method utilizes three basic principles in the detection of HAA:

1. Diffusion: molecules of a dissolved substance tend to migrate from a region of greater concentration to a region of lesser concentration.

2. Electrophoresis: when charged particles are placed in an electric field, a force is exerted on them that is proportional to the amount of charge on the particles and the intensity of the electrical field.

3. Electro-osmosis (counterflow of buffer): the aqueous component, in the presence of buffer ions and a stabilized colloid (agarose gel), tends to flow toward the negative electrode (cathode).*

HAA is dispensed into one well (precut in agarose) located on the positive side of the agarose plate. Control HAA or a test sample is dispensed into the other well of the pair, located on the negative side of the plate. As the specific antigen and specific antibody migrate, molecules of each meet between their respective wells and react, and an insoluble antigen-antibody

complex is formed. This complex forms a visible precipitin line between the two wells. The visibility of the line improves with the time as more of the antigen and antibody combine to form the precipitate. Improvement in visibility will stop when no more antigen or antibody is available for combination.

In the method given here,[1] a large number of specimens can be tested simultaneously, making the test useful for the blood bank. It is relatively sensitive, and only a short time is required to complete the test.

Counterelectrophoresis is also useful for testing blood stains. The tests take 90 minutes and are four to eight times as sensitive as the ring test. When stains are partly denatured, contaminated, and minute in quantity, the test is valuable. It eliminates centrifugation and filtration of cloudy contaminated stains because the agar does the filtering and lets only the protein through.

Reagents

1. Barbital buffer, 0.06M, pH 8.2

Sodium barbital	24.7 gm
Barbituric acid	11.1 gm
Sodium azide	2.0 gm

Place in a 2 L volumetric flask and add approximately 1500 ml distilled water. Heat on

---

*HepaScreen, by Spectra Biologicals, Oxnard, Calif., is an HAA detection system.

a hot plate until dissolved. Cool and dilute to volume with distilled water.

2. HAA antibody, or in the case of blood stains, precipitin serum
3. Controls, both positive and negative
4. Agarose slides, which are available commercially°

Each slide can hold a maximum of eleven sets of wells, two wells to a set, each measuring 2 mm in diameter and being 5 mm apart.

Electrophoresis

1. Place identifying marks on the anode of the electrophoresis chamber and the anode end of the agar slide. At the same time, prepare an identification guide of the slide with the arrangement of the patients' sera and the control sera.
2. Fill one vertical row of cathode (-) wells with unknown sera and known positive and negative control sera, respectively, using capillary pipets. Fill each well exactly to the top.
3. Fill the other vertical row of anode (+) wells with HAA antibody or anti–human precipitin serum.
4. Submit the plates to electrophoresis for 90 minutes at 30 ma (for each plate).
5. Remove the slide immediately after electrophoresis and examine at once.

Results

1. Examine the agar for precipitation lines between the anode and cathode wells of each set of tests, using a hand lens and oblique illumination against a dark background.

2. Examine the controls for precipitation lines of identity. If the lines between antiserum and unknown sera are similar to those of the positive control, this indicates a positive reaction.

3. Absence of precipitation lines should be reported as "not detected," or in the case of the precipitin test for human blood, as negative.

CODING OF BLOOD GROUP REACTIONS†

The introduction of computers into medicine and the medical laboratory has created a need for codes to store, analyze, and

retrieve results of the blood grouping tests. Wiener suggested such a code based on the binary system. With the use or adoption of such a code, blood grouping test results would be presented in two distinct manners: (1) the scientific symbols used in textbooks and journals and (2) the codes used for electronic transmission of information and the storing and retrieving of data in computers.

Unfortunately in blood grouping the scientific symbols are not as yet universally standard (pp. 16 and 17) except for the blood groups in the A-B-O system, in which O means zero, or absence of the A and B agglutinogens; A means presence of A agglutinogen; and B means presence of the B agglutinogen. The designation group AB shows at once that both A and B agglutinogens are present on the red cells, group A says that A is present but B is not, B says that B is present but A is not, etc. These symbols have not always been accepted; the Moss and Jansky Roman numerals were used for many years. Now they have been dropped, but the same type of confusion remains in the Rh-Hr blood type nomenclature. This has been discussed elsewhere in this text and will not be repeated here. See p. 16.

In coding results of tests in the Rh-Hr system, one should follow the order Rh_o, rh', rh'', hr', hr'', and so on. In this way a binary code can be established that may be universally accepted. This is the coding system of Wiener. It spells out the information in detail and shows the exact reaction of the blood cells with various antisera. Throughout the text the binary code is included in the different tables.

The A-B-O system

The antisera should be arranged in the order anti-**A**, anti-**B**, anti-**A**₁. If this order is changed, so is the code, and therefore a **standard system of arrangement** of reactions should also be devised and followed for coding the blood group reactions in all the other systems. With the antisera in the preceding order, the codes in the binary

---

°Cordis Corporation, Miami, Fla.
†Much of the material for this section is derived from publications of A. S. Wiener.[3]

system for the A-B-O groups would be as follows:

Group O	000
Group A₁	101
Group A₂	100
Group B	010
Group A₁B	111
Group A₂B	110

Codes must not be used when scientific symbols are required, as in preparing a dissertation, a textbook, or a journal article. They are for use only in computers.

The Rh-Hr system

In the Rh-Hr system the binary code[3] number follows the order of blood specificities such as **Rh₀, rh′, rh″, hr′, hr″,** and **hr.** The antisera are therefore in the order anti-**Rh₀,** anti-**rh′,** anti-**rh″,** anti-**hr′,** anti-**hr″,** and anti-**hr.** If the cells react with anti-**Rh₀,** for example, this is coded as 1 in the Rh₀ column. If they fail to react with anti-**rh′,** for example, that is coded as 0 in the rh′ column. The binary code, as adapted to the Rh-Hr system, would be as in Table 21-3.

Since there are variants of the Rh factor and instances in which the blood lacks all the specificities (Rh₍null₎), as well as other factors like the "w" in rhʷ, the Wiener system[4] provides for these also. These codes can be added to the table or a separate table of codes for such specificities may be compiled as in Table 21-4.

Codes can be worked out in the other blood group systems by preparing a protocol of reactions after arranging the blood types in logical sequence, as in this text. The codes then would follow the scheme as demonstrated in Tables 21-3 and 21-4. Refer to the chapters on the various blood group systems for their codes.

Other coding methods have been suggested. The binary code scheme seems to hold most promise for use in computers.

AUTOMATION IN BLOOD GROUPING

The use of automated equipment in chemical investigation is now standard, routine laboratory practice. Automation has also been introduced into the field of blood grouping, and this poses some interesting problems that are much different from those in biochemistry or syphilis serology, where it is also used. Although biochemical tests may be repeated on the same patient a number of times, blood grouping tests are made as a rule just once, or at least once before each transfusion of that patient. Once the blood group of a patient is established by the laboratory, it becomes a matter of record for that laboratory or that physician, and the tests need not be repeated unless there is some doubt about their accuracy or unless the patient transfers to another physician or hospital. Blood sugars, for example, may be made hourly, daily, weekly, or only when the patient first reports to his physician for an examination. If there has been a gross error in the biochemical tests, this is rather easily detected and corrected by repeating the test. The same is not always true with the blood groups, unfortunately. In general, an error in a chemical test as a rule will not affect the patient's life or well being, which a mismatched transfusion will most assuredly do. Once a blood group has been determined in the laboratory and cross-matching tests have been performed, that is usually final unless there is an untoward transfusion reaction.

Automated tests for biochemical examinations have enabled the laboratory to give more rapid service and to devote more time to difficult manual tests, as well as to repeat tests when results are in doubt, and such repetitions do not unduly increase the workload. On the other hand, in blood grouping there are so many blood group specificities and so many unforeseen reactions that can occur, which automation cannot at present resolve, that the value of the present types of equipment seems to be limited. However, newer automation methods are constantly being devised and researched so that the future may hold many surprising developments in the automation field.

Table 21-3. Wiener binary code in the Rh-Hr system, with six standard antisera*

Reaction of cells with antisera						Binary code number	Rh phenotypes
Anti-Rh$_o$	Anti-rh'	Anti-rh"	Anti-hr'	Anti-hr"	Anti-hr		
−	−	−	+	+	+	000111	rh
−	+	−	−	+	−	010010	rh'rh'
−	+	−	+	+	+	010111	rh'rh
−	−	+	+	−	−	001100	rh"rh"
−	−	+	+	+	+	001111	rh"rh
−	+	+	+	+	−	011110	rh'rh"
−	+	+	+	+	+	011111	rh$_y$rh
−	+	+	−	+	−	011010	rh$_y$rh'
−	+	+	+	−	−	011100	rh$_y$rh"
−	+	+	−	−	−	011000	rh$_y$rh$_y$
+	−	−	+	+	+	100111	Rh$_o$
+	+	−	−	+	−	110010	Rh$_1$Rh$_1$
+	+	−	+	+	+	110111	Rh$_1$rh
+	−	+	+	−	−	101100	Rh$_2$Rh$_2$
+	−	+	+	+	+	101111	Rh$_2$rh
+	+	+	+	+	−	111110	Rh$_1$Rh$_2$
+	+	+	+	+	+	111111	Rh$_z$rh
+	+	+	−	+	−	111010	Rh$_z$Rh$_1$
+	+	+	+	−	−	111100	Rh$_z$Rh$_2$
+	+	+	−	−	−	111000	Rh$_z$Rh$_z$

*Modified from Erskine, A. G. In Frankel, S., Reitman, S., and Sonnewirth, A. C., editors: Gradwohl's clinical laboratory methods and diagnosis, ed. 7, St. Louis, 1970, The C. V. Mosby Co.

Table 21-4. Wiener system of code numbers for Rh specificities and agglutinogens (not phenotypes)

Reactions of red cells with antisera				Code number	Rh agglutinogens
Anti-Rh$_o$	Anti-rh'	Anti-rh"	Anti-rh^{w1}		
−	−	−	−	0000	rh
−	+	−	−	0100	rh'
−	+	−	+	0101	rh'^{w}
−	−	+	−	0010	rh"
−	+	+	−	0110	rh$_y$
−	+	+	+	0111	rh$_y^w$
+	−	−	−	1000	Rh$_o$
+	+	−	−	1100	Rh$_1$
+	+	−	+	1101	Rh$_1^w$
+	−	+	−	1010	Rh$_2$
+	+	+	−	1110	Rh$_z$
+	+	+	+	1111	Rh$_z^w$
+	−	−	−	10x0	$\bar{R}h_o$*
+	−	−	−	1xx0	$\bar{R}h_o$*
+	−	−	+	1xx1	$\bar{R}h^w$*
±	−	−	−	w000	$\mathfrak{R}h_o$

*The single and double bar Rh$_o$ types cannot be determined without the use of Hr antisera. The single bar Rh$_o$ lacks the **rh'-hr"** contrasting factors, whereas the double bar Rh$_o$ lacks both **rh'-hr'** and **rh"-hr"**. Double bar Rh$_o$ agglutinogen ($\bar{\bar{R}}h_o$) is the type designated as —D— by the British workers.

The automated equipment available from Technicon Corporation, Ardsley, New York,[5] has a small round platform with a number of small bottles containing the blood specimens, arranged around the periphery. A sampling device removes portions of the red cells and plasma from each bottle of blood in turn as the platform rotates. The plasma sample is divided among three channels to be tested against standard red blood cells of group O, A_1, and B.

The red blood cells of the subject are diluted and then divided among five channels to be tested against anti-**A**, anti-**B**, anti-**Rh**$_o$, and anti-**Rh**$'_o$'' sera, and a saline control containing 1.3% sodium chloride with bromelin.

As the red cells are mixed with appropriate antisera or the plasma is mixed with appropriate standard red cells, they move along in parallel channels, with small airspaces separating the individual sets of eight mixtures each (three for the plasma and five for the cells), and lose their identity in the confines of the machine. When they emerge at the other end, they are deposited on a moving strip of fine-grade filter paper, and the sets then are identified with the individual whose blood is being tested. This is accomplished by means of an automatic counter and printer.

The reactions are read with the naked eye and the A-B-O groups and Rh reactions recorded.

As the test progresses, all the mixtures are subjected to the identical short incubation at room temperature in the machine. Polyvinyl-pyrrolidone (PVP), bovine albumin, bromelin, and other substances are added to increase the speed and sensitivity of the reactions.

The antisera are used in tenfold and twentyfold dilutions over that utilized in manual tests. Additives are not used in manual tests because they tend to produce nonspecific clumping of red cells.

The antisera and standard red cell suspensions used for the tests are aspirated through tubes that dip into open Erlenmeyer flasks exposed to the air of the room.

The automated method is said to recognize blood samples of the subgroup A_2B, which has at times been mistakenly identified as group B; but dangerous reactions do not as a rule occur in transfusing group A_2B recipients. Transfusion reactions are sometimes due to gross errors in technic, weak or nonspecific typing sera, and clerical errors such as giving group A blood to a group O or group B patient, giving Rh-positive blood to an Rh-negative recipient, etc. There are enough checks and balances, controls, and so on in blood grouping so

that no incompatible blood should ever be administered to a patient. A patient's life is involved whenever a transfusion is given; only highly trained personnel with a thorough understanding of the principles and pitfalls of blood grouping should be permitted to supervise or use the automated equipment. Since blood grouping is a most complex subject, the use of automated equipment demands much foresight and knowledge. Individuals must be trained to recognize when a machine is out of order and must be prepared either to repair it or to call in an expert, meanwhile carrying out the tests by manual methods. These people should always be prepared to conduct manual tests either on randomly selected specimens or on control specimens to check their efficiency.

Wiener pointed out that to his knowledge, no hospital or pathologist has ever been sued for an incorrect serum cholesterol test, but there have been numerous costly lawsuits when errors in "simple" blood grouping tests have caused serious or fatal transfusion reactions or when young Rh-negative women have been isosensitized by injection of Rh-positive blood. He also noted that a single such lawsuit will cost far more than can possibly be saved by reducing the staff of laboratory personnel when automation is introduced.

Brittin and Brecher[6] have evaluated automation in blood grouping and believe that the results in A-B-O and Rh-Hr typing are more accurate as a rule than those of the manual methods, provided the laboratory personnel has higher standards of knowledge and skill than the usual personnel engaged in performing manual tests. Nevertheless, detection of irregular antibodies in the serum by the automated method is more difficult than ordinary blood grouping. The conditions required for agglutination of red cells in the various antigen-antibody systems differ from one another. It is difficult, if not impossible, to choose reagent red cells in which the antigens always react with the corresponding antibodies. For example, although treatment of red cells with protease is effective for detecting Rh antibodies, it alters some antigens and fails to detect from 5% to 13% of irregular antibodies, especially those in the Fy and Jk systems. Even the automated Coombs reaction gives only 90% correct results.

This is not intended to imply that automation in blood grouping is not to be used; objections can be overcome if the procedures are properly conducted to prevent errors. All the tests should be run independently by two different technicians on duplicate sets of specimens and on different machines, and the results should be read and interpreted independently of both workers. If the results are identical, the transfusion may proceed. If they differ, the work must be repeated, preferably manually while the apparatus is being repaired or checked.

Cross-matching tests must be conducted manually after the proper donor(s) has been selected.

Weakly reacting antigens and weak antibodies are more easily detected by manual methods, although at present elution technics are being devised and tested for identification of such antigens and antibodies by automation.

Some of the objections to the use of automation in blood grouping are (1) the danger of carry-over from specimen to specimen; (2) the absence of microscopic reading that seriously limits the reading; (3) the absence of control over antibodies in unknown serum; (4) the danger of misidentification of bloods when the automatic counter is used, because if the apparatus is "off one," disaster could result; and (5) the danger of reducing specificity of the clumping reactions because of the additive substances used to increase sensitivity of

reaction. The use of automation in blood banking is not safe at present, and is impractical and therefore remains primarily a research tool. If the objections can be overcome, automation will be of great service to the blood bank.

Other automated equipment includes automated cell washers,[7] with automatic addition of anti–human globulin, microtiter hemagglutination technics,[8-12] and automated data handling.

REFERENCES

1. Bauer, J. D., Ackermann, P. G., and Toro, G.: Clinical laboratory methods, St. Louis, Mo., 1974, The C. V. Mosby Co.
2. Schellong, G., and Grimm, W.: Dtsch. Med. Wochenschr. **95**:2555, 1970.
3. Wiener, A. S.: Haematologia (Budap.) **2**:205, 1968.
4. Wiener, A. S.: J. Forensic Med. **15**(3):106, 1968.
5. Sturgeon, P.: Technicon Symposium: Automation in Analytical Chemistry, Ardsley, N.Y., 1965, Technicon Corporation.
6. Brittin, G. M., and Brecher, G.: Progress in hematology, vol. 7, New York, 1971, Grune & Stratton, Inc.
7. Dale, I.: Vox Sang. **23**:232, 1972.
8. Conrath, I. B.: Handbook of Microtiter procedures, Cambridge, Mass., 1972, Dynatech Corporation.
9. Crawford, M. N., Gottman, F. E., and Gottman, C. A.: Transfusion **10**:258, 1970.
10. Howell, E., and Parkins, H. A.: Transfusion **8**:33, 1968.
11. Wegmann, T. G., and Smithies, O.: Transfusion **8**:47, 1968.
12. Wegmann, T. G., and Smithies, O.: Transfusion **6**:67, 1966.

RECOMMENDED READINGS

American Association of Blood Banks: Technical methods and procedures, ed. 6, Washington, D.C., 1974.
Myhre, B. A.: Quality control in blood banking, New York, 1974, John Wiley & Sons, Inc.

22 □ Tests used in the medicolegal applications of blood grouping

Several principal considerations are involved in a discussion of the medicolegal aspects of blood grouping:

1. Conclusions based on tests that depend on a knowledge of heredity
   a. Disputed paternity and maternity
   b. Mixed baby cases in nurseries
   c. Stolen babies and kidnapping
   d. Immigration and citizenship claims
   e. Estate problems when kinship with the deceased must be established
   f. Personal identification
2. Identification of stains from blood or body secretions such as semen, saliva, and gastric juice
   a. Suspected sexual assault
   b. Hit-and-run driving
   c. Identification after death from drowning
   d. Murder when the similarity or difference between blood stains on the victim and blood groups of the suspect must be established
3. Lawsuits growing out of the following
   a. Mismatched transfusions
   b. Transfusion reactions
   c. Isosensitization due to the use of blood belonging to the wrong blood group

TESTS BASED ON GENETICS OF BLOOD GROUPS

Genetics in general is discussed in Chapter 4, and the genetics of blood groups in Chapters 12 and 13. The basic principle on which forensic examinations of blood are made is that once the blood group of an individual is established, it remains unchanged for life. Even after receiving a transfusion of blood with specificities other than those of the recipient's blood cells, such factors disappear shortly, since red cells survive only for a few months at most after a transfusion, and the recipient's own bone marrow has been busy during and after the transfusion producing cells with the same serologic specificities as before the transfusion. If, therefore, the recipient is type N, for example, and has received either type M or MN cells, all the transfused red cells having M antigens disappear shortly after the transfusion and the recipient's type remains as N.

For changes in red cell antigens due to disease, see pp. 78 and 79.

Evidence based on blood tests is accepted in many courts, and there are also many states with statutes that empower their courts to order such tests. Although in a number of European countries, results of blood grouping tests were admitted as evidence in paternity cases as early as the 1920s, in the United States the first state to adopt such a law was New York in 1935. From the institution of this law until November 17, 1949, no man had ever been adjudged the father of a child if the blood tests excluded him. However, in 1949 this record was broken when the accused man was declared the father of a child although two independently performed blood examinations clearly excluded him as a possible parent.[1,2] Despite this incident, the reliability of blood grouping tests is so great that no other evidence can approach it.

Tests in disputed parentage

Disputed parentage cases include instances in which a child is born to an unmarried woman or to a married woman whose husband is not the father of the child. If the child was conceived before the marriage of the mother to a man who is not the father, or during a period of separation from her husband, the child may be regarded as illegitimate. **Illegitimacy** is determined by the legal status of the mother with reference to her paramour, the child's actual father, to whom she is not married. The purpose of the law in cases of disputed parentage is to protect the child.

It must be kept in mind that each parent contributes one gene for each blood group characteristic. The two genes thus inherited by the fetus constitute the genotype of that fetus and thus determine the blood group. If the genes from each parent are alike, the offspring is **homozygous** for that characteristic; if they are unlike, the offspring is **heterozygous.** A homozygous individual can contribute genes for only one characteristic; for example, a homozygous group A_1 (genotype A^1A^1) can transmit only A^1 genes. A heterozygous group A_1 (A^1A^2 or A^1O) can transmit A^1 or A^2 or A^1 or O. Expressed differently, if an individual is homozygous for a blood group gene, the product of such a gene must appear in all the children. Unfortunately, no laboratory tests have yet been devised that will establish the genotypes directly. It may be possible, however, by means of blood group studies, to exclude a certain man as the father of a certain child. Table 22-1 shows which of the A-B-O groups cannot occur in the father of a certain child, in the cases in which the mother's and child's blood groups have been determined by laboratory tests.

Problems in disputed parentage cases can be resolved only in a negative way, as a rule. This means that a man accused of fathering a child can be excluded as a parent if tests show that genetically he could not have sired the child. If, however, the mother and putative father are, for example, both blood group O and the child is also group O and the mother, putative father, and child are all type N and Rh negative, and if there are no discrepancies in any of the other blood group systems, the most that can be said is that this man could be the father of the child; this does not prove, however, that he is in fact the father. On the other hand, in the case of certain rare blood groups, in which a specific factor appears in only 1 in 1000 to 1 in 100 of the population and this factor is present in both the putative father and the child but is absent from the mother, this is circumstantial evidence that the man is probably the father. Even in such a case, however, there is no absolute proof.

Cases of disputed parentage occur (1) when a man is accused of being the father of a child born out of wedlock and denies the charge; (2) when a man denies implication in rape and therefore claims that he is not the father of a child conceived as a result; (3) when a husband denies that the child born in wedlock is his; (4) when two newborn infants have been interchanged in a hospital; (5) when a woman simulates pregnancy and childbirth, then claims that a child is hers, either to induce a man to marry her or to claim an estate; (6) when an immigrant claims kinship with a citi-

Table 22-1. A-B-O blood groups that cannot occur in the father*

Mother's blood group	Child's blood group			
	O	**A**	**B**	**AB**
O	AB	O, B	O, A	Not possible
A	AB	None	O, A	O, A
B	AB	O, B	None	O, B
AB	Not possible	None	None	O

*Modified from Wiener, A. S., and Socha, W. W.: A-B-O blood groups and Lewis types, New York, 1976, with permission of Stratton Intercontinental Medical Book Corporation.

zen of a country to gain entrance to that country or to remain there once he arrives; or (7) when a man claims to be the father of a child but the mother denies the claim.

In disputed parentage cases, blood specimens must be obtained from the mother, the child or children in question, and the putative father or fathers. All specimens must be carefully identified by the individual taking the blood; the person from whom the blood is withdrawn should present identification such as a driver's license, automobile registration, social security card, draft board registration, or be identified by the other party involved. The signatures of the individuals whose blood is being tested should be obtained, whenever possible, not only for comparison purposes but also for consent to the tests, and fingerprints should be taken for absolute identification.

All individuals involved in a particular case should be tested in the same laboratory, whenever possible, and all specimens from these subjects should be taken in the same laboratory if at all possible. All reagents used for the tests on various individuals must be the same in each instance. Adequate controls are mandatory.

In the laboratory the specimens must be carefully identified by number and name, and all tubes and slides used in the examination must bear similar identification.

All tests should be made in duplicate by separate laboratory personnel working independently of one another, and the results should be read blind so that the individual reading the results has no knowledge of the person from whom the specimen was derived. As with all blood grouping tests, proper and complete controls must be included along with the tests. When the two sets of results have been completed, they must agree in all respects; otherwise, all the tests must be repeated, preferably by another person. A qualified expert must be responsible for the final recording of results and drawing of conclusions. The interpretation must be decisive and in language that is simple enough to be understood by any-

one—even a person who is not well versed in the terminology and significance of tests in immunohematology and immunogenetics.

Only fully qualified experts should engage in these tests. Technical personnel who are well qualified to test blood prior to a transfusion but whose medicolegal experience is either nonexistent or too limited to qualify them as experts should not perform these tests or draw conclusions. Serious errors have been made by unqualified laboratory personnel. Some tests are so extremely delicate that they require specific precautions in running them and in reading the reactions.

The specimens of blood taken from the mother, child or children, and putative father or fathers are each given a separate identification label. Two tubes of blood from each person are needed, one taken in a dry tube and allowed to clot, the other collected in dry double oxalate and mixed to prevent clotting.

Assuming that the test to be used in disputed parentage cases gives clear, reproducible results and that the hereditary mechanism of the types defined is clearcut, the usefulness of the test will depend primarily on the distribution of the types in the population from which the persons involved derive. Thus, if the trait in question has a very high or very low frequency, the test will have hardly any value because of the limited degree of polymorphism; the individuals tested will usually be all positive or all negative. Therefore the formulas for the chances of excluding paternity are usually given in terms of the gene frequencies.

In cases of a blood group system that has only two types, D+ and D−,* paternity will be excluded only when both the mother and the accused man are D− and the child is D+. Obviously, the frequency with which both mother and the falsely accused man

---

*The letter "D" is used as an example of a hypothetical blood type and is not to be confused with the British type D of the Rh-Hr system.

will be D– is $r^2 \times r^2 = r^4$, where r^2 expresses the frequency of type D– in terms of gene frequencies. The chances that the child will be D+ depend on the frequency p of the gene D derived from the actual father. Therefore the chance of exclusion of a falsely accused man is pr^4.

Since $p = 1 - r$, the chance of exclusion is $P = pr^4 = (1 - r)r^4 = r^4 - r^5$. It is easy to show, by applying differential calculus, that when frequencies of two genes, r and p, are 80% and 20%, respectively, the maximum chances of exclusion are 8.2%. In other words, 8 out of 100 falsely accused men could be excluded on the basis of tests for blood type D.

In practice, these maximum chances are often not achieved. For example, in the case of Kell types, the chance of exclusion for whites is only 3.5 percent. For Negroids, who have a very low percentage of Kell-positive individuals, the exclusion rate is only 0.5%; for Chinese, in whom there are hardly any Kell-positive individuals, the exclusion rate is virtually zero.

A frequent situation is one involving a system with two contrasting, codominant alleles, having three phenotypes and three corresponding genotypes, for example, the M-N types. If m and n represent the frequencies of two respective alleles, the chance P of excluding paternity is given by the following formula:

$$P = mn(1 - mn)$$

In this case, the maximum chance of excluding paternity is 18.75%, as when $m = n = 0.5$.

In the case of the four A-B-O groups, the formula for the chances of excluding paternity can be derived similarly. For simplicity and to conserve space, the reader is referred to the literature for details.[3] The maximum chances of excluding paternity by A-B-O tests alone are about 20%; tests for the subgroup of A increase the chances by only 2% or 3%. If the Rh-Hr system is used alone, the exclusion rate is 25%. If the M-N-S system is used in place of the M-N specificities alone, that is, if S

and s are included, the chances of excluding paternity are 23.9%.

Usually, in cases of disputed paternity, blood tests include more than one system. It is easy to see that the chances of excluding paternity are not obtained by simply adding the chances for each individual system because there are cases of overlap in which the same man is excluded by more than one of the tests. The correct procedure is to determine the chances of nonexclusion for each system. The product of these individual chances then gives the chance that none of the tests will exclude an innocent man. Therefore, by subtracting this product from unity (or from 100%), one obtains the chance that at least one test will exclude a falsely accused man, as in the formula

$$P = 1 - (1 - P_1)(1 - P_2) \ldots (1 - P_n)$$

where P is the probability of exclusion, n is the number of independent systems tested for, and P_1, P_2 ... P_n are the individual chances of exclusion for each system.

Most cases of disputed parentage can be resolved by testing for red cell specificities in the A-B-O, M-N, and Rh-Hr systems. If these three systems are utilized, the combined chances of exclusion are 56.4%. Utilizing other blood group systems and including some of the more recently discovered factors in the Rh-Hr system, a few percentage points may be added. It is not difficult to see that as more and more independent tests are included, the chances of excluding paternity become closer and closer to 100%, without actually achieving that goal (the ideal situation in which every falsely accused man would be excluded so that if not excluded, he must necessarily be the actual father). Unfortunately, attempts to raise the exclusion rate become less and less rewarding.

Wiener and Socha[4] pointed out the fallacy of adding more and more tests in parentage exclusion to reach an efficiency of 100%. The cost in terms of time, effort, and materials increases exponentially as the chances of exclusion increase. As an example, when tests have reached the 50% rate of exclusion, any new test can operate at only 50% efficiency because half of the exclusion demonstrated by the new test has already been detected by the previous tests. Again, when 90% exclusion rate is reached, it becomes ten times as expensive as initially to raise the exclusion rate. At the 95% level, it is twenty times as expensive. Where should the line be drawn?

Despite the clear-cut nature of the heredity of the secretor types as a simple mendelian dominant, and the high reproducibility of the tests, these tests are used only rarely in paternity disputes. Collection of the saliva samples is troublesome and time consuming, especially from infants and younger children. The tests themselves are also time consuming and must be carried out by the titration method if the results are to be considered reliable. Moreover, in Caucasians and Negroids the frequency of nonsecretors is about 25%, so that the chances of exclusion are $pr^4 = (0.5)(0.5)^4 = 0.03125$, or only slightly over 3%. In Asiatic populations, in which there are no nonsecretors, the test is of course entirely useless. Therefore, considering the low rate of exclusion by secretor types, they are not sufficiently rewarding in proportion to the cost in time and effort.

Other factors in not increasing the number of tests are that certain reagents are in very short supply (anti-**hr** serum, anti-**s**, anti-**Kidd**, anti-**P**, and anti-**Xg**^{a}). Some of these reagents also are very weak. In addition, the more tests that are added, the more there is chance for error and thus miscarriage of justice.

If the Court accepts the qualifications of the expert and that expert has utilized tests in the other blood group systems, these may be additionally used in exclusion tests; otherwise, only the A-B-O, M-N, and Rh-Hr systems are accepted. It must be reemphasized that blood grouping tests in paternity suits are interpreted only in a negative way, that is, to exclude parentage and not to identify the parents specifically.

Application of blood grouping tests for solving problems of disputed parentage is based on the assumption that the hereditary transmission of blood groups follows established genetic patterns, and that the phenotypic expression of the blood group does not change during the life of the individual. Although this has been proved to be true in most of the cases in everyday practice, one must not forget that there are very rare phenomena that may invalidate that assumption. There are **mutations,** in which there is an accidental modification of a gene, the frequency of which has been estimated to be 1 in 50,000 gene-generations. When a new mutant gene occurs in homozygous form it is often lethal; therefore mutations are seldom, if ever, important in these studies. No convincing example of a blood group gene mutating between two generations has been found.[5] Temporary, acquired changes have been reported in **leukemia** and in **radiation** or **chemical exposure,** but the examining expert is aware of these and knows if the client falls into any of the categories and so can act accordingly.

Even in exchange transfusions, in which the entire blood content is exchanged for another (Rh negative for Rh positive), the **life of the transfused red cells** is only 60 to 100 days, and in the meantime the individual is rapidly replacing worn-out or effete red cells from the donor with his own type cells. Such a temporary alteration in blood type therefore does not present any serious problems.

There are **racial differences** in the distribution of the various blood group specificities. Such specificities can be useful in paternity testing. As an example, **K** for Caucasians, and **Js**^{a} for Negroids are the most useful antigens. Unequivocal exclusion occurs if the child is Kell-positive and the mother and putative father are both Kell negative, or if the child is Js^a positive and the mother and putative father are both Js^a negative.

The following are some of the genotype (or phenotype) frequencies:

1. In the Kell system the frequency of *KK* is 0.12%; *Kk*, 6.75%; and *kk*, 93.12%.

2. In the P system 98% of Negroids are

P positive, 78% of Caucasians, and 30% of Asiatics.

3. In the Lu system Lu^aLu^a comprises 1% of the population; Lu^aLu^b, 7%; and Lu^bLu^b, 92%.

4. In the Fy system 20% of Caucasians are Fy(a+b−), 34% are Fy(a−b+), 46% are Fy(a+b+), and 0.1% are Fy(a−b−), whereas 70% of Negroids are Fy(a−b−).

5. In the Jk system 24.5% are Jk^aJk^a; 52.7%, Jk^aJk^b; and 22.5%, Jk^bJk^b.

6. The **Di** specificity has been found only in Chinese, Japanese, and Amerindians.

These figures are important at times in determining whether or not to test for specificities in systems outside the A-B-O, M-N, and Rh-Hr.

Procedure

1. All tests must be made in duplicate, using two different sets of antisera. Take care to use antisera of adequate potency and specificity.

2. Take venous blood from the mother, the child, and the putative father—one portion collected in a dry tube without anticoagulant, the remainder in a tube with dry double oxalate anticoagulant.

3. Loosen the clots in the clotted specimens with a wooden applicator stick and centrifuge. Remove the supernatant serum, placing in tubes previously labeled.

4. If only clotted blood specimens have been submitted, use applicator sticks to dip into the clot to obtain the red cells. The concentration of serum-suspended cells should be 50%.

5. Prepare suspensions of the various red cell specimens in saline, then wash once and resuspend to a 5% concentration.

6. Have at hand the following antisera: anti-**A**, anti-**B**, and anti-**A₁** lectin or absorbed anti-**A** serum for the A-B-O tests; anti-**M** and anti-**N** for the M-N tests; and anti-**Rh₀**, anti-**rh′**, anti-**rh″**, anti-**hr′**, and anti-**hr″** tube agglutinating sera (IgM) for use with saline-suspended cells, as well as anti-**Rh₀** conglutinating serum (IgG) to detect a possible **Rh₀** variant and to determine the Rh-Hr phenotypes. Test to be certain that anti-**rh′** is in reality anti-**rh′** and not anti-**rh₁** (p. 121) and that anti-**M** is not anti-**Mᶜ**. Have available anti-**rhʷ** and anti-**hr** sera to use as needed.

7. Test the red cells of the mother, child, and putative father using anti-**A** and anti-**B** sera, and if the blood group is A or AB,

proceed to test with anti-**A₁** to determine the subgroup. Although the tests may be made by the open slide method, many workers prefer the tube tests. Use proper controls. The technic is on p. 258ff.

8. Confirm the results in step 7 by testing the respective sera against known group A and group B cells suspended in saline, If there is a problem of hemolysis, inactivate the sera at 56° C for 15 minutes, let them cool to room temperature, and continue with the tests. If there are no discrepancies between the results in steps 7 and 8, conclusions may be drawn as to the A-B-O groups and subgroups. The tests for A-B-O blood groups must be carried out at room temperature. It is best to include a control using group O serum against the unknown cells, as described on pp. 263 and 264.

9. Test the cells with anti-**M** and anti-**N** reagents, either by the open slide or tube method, or both, using proper controls. Follow the method on p. 296ff.

10. Prepare three sets of four small tubes, 7 to 8 mm diameter. Label each set with the identifying mark and antiserum used—one set for the mother, one set for the child, and one set for the putative father. Follow the setup as given in Table 22-2. This is to determine the Rh type.

11. Mix the contents of each tube separately and incubate the rack in a 37° C water bath for 1 hour.

12. While the tubes are incubating, prepare ficinated red cells of the mother, child, and putative father, using the rapid method outlined on p. 243. This will be used to test for the **hr′** and **hr″** specificities of the red cells. It is not necessary, as a rule, to test for **hr′** if tests for **rh′** are negative, since the reaction will almost invariably be **hr′** positive. There are very rare exceptions. Likewise, if tests for **rh″** are negative, it is not usually necessary to test for **hr″** because these tests will almost invariably be positive. Exceptions occur in type $\bar{\bar{\text{Rh}}}_0$, which lacks both pairs of contrasting specificities, **rh′-hr′** and **rh″-hr″**, and in some extremely rare Rh$_{null}$ bloods (pp. 119 and 283).

13. Test for **hr′** and **hr″** in the red cells of all three individuals. Tests for **hr** are made only in certain cases that may indicate a probable exclusion of paternity, for example, putative father type Rh$_z$Rh$_0$, mother Rh₁Rh₁, child Rh₁rh (p. 125). For the Hr specificities, use ficinated red cells. Mix 1 drop of unknown ficinated cells with 1 drop of anti-**hr′** and 1 drop of the unknown cells with 1 drop of anti-**hr″** serum. Incubate in a 37° C water bath for 40 to 60 minutes

Table 22-2. Setup for each blood in disputed paternity to determine Rh type[*]

Back row for $\mathfrak{R}h_o$	1 drop of unknown cells + 1 drop anti-**Rh_o** conglutinating (slide) serum
Third row for **Rh_o**	1 drop of unknown cells + 1 drop anti-**Rh_o** agglutinating (tube) serum
Second row for **rh″**	1 drop of unknown cells + 1 drop of anti-**rh″** serum
Front row for **rh′**	1 drop of unknown cells + 1 drop of anti-**rh′** serum

[*]From Erskine, A. G. In Frankel, S., Reitman, S., and Sonnenwirth, A. C., editors: Gradwohl's clinical laboratory methods and diagnosis, ed. 7, St. Louis, 1970, The C. V. Mosby Co.

Table 22-3. Identification of the eighteen Rh-Hr phenotypes using five standard antisera[*]

Antisera used					
Anti-Rh_o	**Anti-rh′**	**Anti-rh″**	**Anti-hr′**	**Anti-hr″**	**Designation of types**
−	−	−	+	+	rh
−	+	−	−	+	rh′rh′
			+	+	rh′rh
−	−	+	+	−	rh″rh″
			+	+	rh″rh
−	+	+	+	+	rh_yrh
			−	+	rh_yrh′
			+	−	rh_yrh″
			−	−	rh_yrh_y
+	−	−	+	+	Rh_o
+	+	−	−	+	Rh_1Rh_1
			+	+	Rh_1rh
+	−	+	+	−	Rh_2Rh_2
			+	+	Rh_2rh
+	+	+	+	+	Rh_zRh_o
			−	+	Rh_zRh_1
			+	−	Rh_zRh_2
			−	−	Rh_zRh_z

[*]From Erskine, A. G. In Frankel, S., Reitman, S., and Sonnenwirth, A. C., editors: Gradwohl's clinical laboratory methods and diagnosis, ed. 7, St. Louis, 1970, The C. V. Mosby Co.

and read as usual. The test may also be made on open slides, using the appropriate anti-Hr slide sera.

14. After the tests for Rh-Hr specificities have incubated sufficiently (steps 10 and 11), read in the usual manner after gently dislodging the sediment. If tests for **Rh_o** are negative, proceed with the examination for the **Rh_o** variant by washing the contents of the back tubes (tube 4) four times with saline, and after the last washing and centrifugation, remove all the saline. Then perform an antiglobulin test and proceed as usual.

15. If the blood proves to be type Rh_1, Rh_z, rh′, or rh_y, and if it is necessary to test for **rh^w**, carry out the test for this specificity as outlined on p. 281. If the results are negative, proceed with the antiglobulin test and reread.

16. Record the results of the tests. Consult Table 22-3 to establish the correct Rh-Hr phenotypes when the five standard anti-Rh and anti-Hr sera are used. For phenotypes

Table 22-4. Example of method of drawing conclusions in disputed paternity cases

	Blood group	Possible genotypes	Remarks
A-B-O system			
Putative father	B	BB or BO	
Mother	A_1	A^1A^1 or A^1A^2 or A^1O	Only A^1O is possible
			if child is group O
Child	O	OO	
M-N system			
Putative father	MN	MN	
Mother	M	MM	
Child	MN	MN	
Rh-Hr system			
Putative father	Rh_1Rh_2*	R^1R^2 or R^1r'' or R^2r'	
Mother	Rh_1rh	R^1r or R^1R^o or R^or'	
Child	Rh_2rh	R^2r or R^2R^o or R^or''	

*Assuming that the blood is hr negative.

and genotypes in the various blood group systems, see Chapter 13.

Table 13-20 summarizes conclusions drawn to exclude paternity or maternity by use of the Rh-Hr blood types. The table is applied only when at least one of the parents is Rh_o positive. If both parents lack the Rh_o specificity—that is, if they are type rh, rh', rh'', or rh_y—there can be no Rh_o-positive children. See also Table 13-19.

The laws of heredity of blood groups are on pp. 52ff, 198, and 199. These should be consulted when drawing conclusions in exclusion cases. The genotypes possible in all the blood group systems are given in Chapter 13, together with a method of determining the possible children in the various matings. That chapter should be consulted in disputed parentage cases.

To summarize the test results, prepare a chart showing the phenotypes and possible genotypes of the putative father(s), the mother, and the child or children in all three blood group systems, as in Table 22-4.

Next, determine what children are possible in each system by consulting Chapter 13. In the example in Table 22-4 the children that could result from this mating would be group O, A_1, A_2, B, A_1B, or A_2B in the A-B-O system but not all in the same

family. Thus there has been *no* exclusion on the basis of the A-B-O tests. (As an example, an individual of type A_1 is genotype A^1A^1 *or* A^1A^2 *or* A^1O, but *not* all three. Blood groups of siblings help in establishing genotypes.)

In the M-N system the children possible to this mating are M or MN but *not* N, and therefore there is no exclusion here.

In the Rh-Hr system the children possible to this mating would be determined as follows. Record all possible combinations of genotypes in this mating, which would be $R^1r \times R^1R^2$; $R^1r \times R^1r''$; $R^1r \times R^2r'$; $R^1R^o \times R^1R^2$; $R^1R^o \times R^1r''$; $R^1R^o \times R^2r'$; $R^or' \times R^1R^2$; $R^or' \times R^1r''$; and $R^or' \times R^2r'$. After drawing the nine diagrams, then converting the genotypes to phenotypes and eliminating duplications, the following children would be found possible to this mating: rh'rh, rh'rh', rh''rh, rh'rh'', Rh_1rh, Rh_1Rh_1, Rh_2rh, and Rh_1Rh_2, but not all in the same family. The following children would not be possible to this mating: rh, rh''rh'', rh_y, Rh_o, Rh_2Rh_2, and Rh_z. It can be seen that there is no exclusion in the Rh-Hr system by these tests in this example.

The final conclusion from the above tests is that the putative father is not excluded.

In all paternity or parentage cases, con-

Table 22-5. Results of a test for exclusion of paternity (case cited in Table 22-4)

	Anti-A serum / cells	Anti-B serum / cells	Absorbed anti-A serum (anti-A$_1$) / cells	Anti-M serum / cells	Anti-N serum / cells	Anti-rh' serum (tube) / cells	Anti-rh" serum (tube) / cells	Anti-Rh$_0$ serum (tube) / cells	Anti-Rh$_0$ serum (slide) (conglutinating) / cells	Anti-hr' serum / cells	Anti-hr" serum / cells	Anti-hr* serum / cells	Blood groups
Putative father	−	+	Not needed	+	+	+	+	+	Not needed	+	+	−	B MN Rh$_1$Rh$_2$
Mother	+	−	+	+	−	+	−	+	Not needed	+	+	Not needed	A$_1$ M Rh$_1$rh
Child	−	−	Not needed	+	+	−	+	+	Not needed	+	+	Not needed	O MN Rh$_2$rh

*Anti-hr serum is used only when needed. It is not necessary for determination of phenotypes of the mother and child in this example. The A-B-O groups are confirmed by testing the serum against group A, B, and O cells. See text for conclusions in this case.
Note: Anti-A$_1$ lectin may be used in place of absorbed anti-A serum.

firmation of A-B-O grouping is made by testing the serum against known A, B, and O cells. The test for the **Rh$_0$** variant is not necessary when the individual reacts positively with anti-**Rh$_0$** saline-agglutinating serum.

Table 22-5 is a suggested form to be used in recording the results of the blood tests of the putative father, the mother, and the child, filled in as for the example given here.

In 1957 the Committee on Medicolegal Problems of the American Medical Association[6] made certain suggestions contained in a report, from which the following is quoted. "Because the use of two systems of nomenclature for the Rh-Hr system leads to confusion and misunderstanding, the Committee on Medicolegal Problems of the American Medical Association recommends adoption of a single uniform system for medicolegal reports. It is recommended that, unless and until some other convention can be agreed upon, the original Rh-Hr notations be kept as the standard and sole nomenclature for preparing approved medicolegal reports on Rh types.

"It is recommended that routine medicolegal applications of blood grouping be restricted at present to tests for the four blood groups, O, A, B, and AB of the A-B-O system; the three types M, N, and MN of the M-N-S system; and factors **Rh$_0$**, **rh'**, **rh"**, and **hr'** of the Rh-Hr system. Tests for additional factors and systems are considered insufficiently established for routine use at present, although they may provide evidence in particular selected cases. Such evidence should be submitted in a separate letter not part of the standard report and should be presented with proper caution. Similarly, the value of rare combinations of groups providing indication of paternity, in contrast to the conventional use of tests to establish only nonpaternity, should be recognized in unusual cases, but should be treated with caution in a separate communication not part of the definitive report."

Tests made in baby mixing, stolen baby, and kidnapping cases

The tests in these cases are the same as in disputed parentage. Tests should be made for all the standard blood group factors in the three systems, A-B-O, M-N, and Rh-Hr, and conclusions drawn as for disputed paternity cases described previously. It may be necessary to test for other blood group specificities such as rh^w, rh_i, **hr**, and some of the rare factors if the conclusions from the standard tests are in dispute.

Establishing kinship

Tests to establish kinship are not easily made, especially if the one to whom the individual claims relationship has died. However, this is not an impossible undertaking if siblings, descendants, and forebears are still available for examination. Many such problems have been presented, along with their solutions, in a series entitled "Problems in Immunohematology and Immunogenetics" by A. S. Wiener.[7]

Every person has a pair of allelic genes for each of the blood group agglutinogens. One of the two genes in his genotype is derived from the mother and one from the father. In kinship cases, if the presumed father is dead but his parents are alive, tests should be made to establish the blood groups and types in both parents (grandparents of the subject in question). The paternal genotype was derived from the grandparents, one gene from the maternal and one from the paternal grandparent. The child who wishes to establish kinship should therefore have one, and only one, of the four genes that the paternal grandparents have. If tests are made for the A-B-O, M-N, Rh-Hr, and Kell types of both the mother and the child, as well as of the two parents of the dead putative father, the chance of excluding paternity if the charge has been falsely made is about 27%, which is just about half the chance of excluding paternity if the man were alive. For example, if the two paternal grandparents were either O or A and the mother of the child is also O or A, paternity is excluded if the child is group B or AB. If both paternal grandparents are type M and the child is type N, paternity is excluded irrespective of the M-N type of the mother.[8]

For other examples of exclusion of parentage, consult Sussman.[9]

Personal identification

So many different blood group specificities exist that it is not unreasonable to predict, as Landsteiner did, that at some time in the future identifying each person by a study of his blood group specificities could be possible. This time has not as yet arrived. Except for monozygotic twins, it is probably true that each person is distinctive with respect to his blood groups. Certain blood types or specificities seem to be virtually limited to certain separate racial groups, which is another factor in individual identification. For example, hr^V, Js^a specificities, and the blood type Fy(a–b–) are found almost exclusively in Negroids, whereas Di(a+) is seen mostly in South American Indians, Japanese, and Chinese.

IDENTIFICATION OF SUSPECTED BLOOD STAINS

Specimens suspected of containing blood are received in the laboratory on a variety of objects, in various states of decomposition or preservation, and in different quantities. Some of these have been obtained by the police, but a private citizen or a person outside the profession might have asked for an examination. In all cases the specimens must be carefully labeled in indelible ink or crayon, and they must be kept for possible later introduction as evidence in court.

Gradwohl[10] stressed the importance of maintaining the **integrity of the chain of evidence** in all criminal proceedings. All evidence should be received by members of the laboratory staff and by no other person, and the laboratory staff must work in close harmony with the homicide squad. Material for examination should be brought to the office of the laboratory director, entered in the laboratory specimen record books as to time of collection, time of delivery, names or other identification, name and identification of the person submitting the specimen, and date. A receipt should be given to the person bringing the specimen, and that person should also make a written statement that he has delivered the material to the laboratory. All these records must be available if necessary for evidence during the trial of the case.

The stains may be on paper, wood, metal, plastic, cloth, glass, cotton, wool, hair, and clothing, even shoes. Since the tests are delicate and readily subject to error, only specially qualified and trained personnel should be permitted to examine the specimens. When there is sufficient material, all tests should be made in duplicate, preferably by two different workers, each examining the specimens separately.

At times there is ample stain with which to perform all the tests. At other times there is little with which the laboratory can work. This should be noted in the reports. Great care must be exercised to avoid contamination of the specimen from any source whatsoever. It is best to use disposable glassware or plastic tubes and slides that can be thrown away after a single use. The bare hands must never be used in examining evidence.

The identification of stains suspected as being blood presents three problems:
1. Is the stain blood?
2. Is it human blood?
3. What is the blood group?

Before any test is made, the area of the material on which the stain has been found must be clearly marked with the initials of the individual who cuts it from the cloth or removes it from other material. A similar area from an unstained portion must also be identified and used as a control.

Caution. Clothing that has been subjected to cleaning fluids cannot be satisfactorily tested for human blood stains; this is also true of the "permanent-press" fabrics. Heat and the cleaning fluid apparently denature the proteins, and they no longer

precipitate with anti–human precipitin serum. Even the benzidine test for blood, if positive, is not reliable because it is a nonspecific test for peroxidase present in other stains of animal and vegetable origin as well as of blood.

Is the stain blood?
CHEMICAL TESTS

The benzidine and the reduced phenolphthalein (phenolphthalin) tests have been the methods of choice, but benzidine is now believed to be carcinogenic and is therefore not much used. It is difficult to obtain.

Benzidine test. The benzidine test may be made directly on the stained area or on an extract of or scrapings from the stain. A control is made at the same time on an unstained area. Do not use the entire stain for this test; otherwise, there may not be enough left for other tests that determine its species specificity or blood group. If the stain is on cloth, tease out a fiber and use the stained area of the fiber for the test.

1. Prepare an extract of the stained area in saline, using a minimal amount of saline.
2. Prepare a saturated solution of benzidine, special for blood, in glacial acetic acid. (Benzidine dihydrochloride may be used, but the technic is different.) Place a small amount of benzidine in a clean small tube, free from blood, and add about 0.5 to 1 ml of glacial acetic acid. Shake vigorously. If all the crystals dissolve, add more until a supersaturated solution is obtained. Allow the undissolved crystals to settle and use the supernatant fluid. This solution must be freshly prepared for each test. It is very unstable.
3. Add an equal volume of 3% hydrogen peroxide and mix thoroughly. If a green or blue color develops, discard the solution and prepare a fresh reagent using different glassware or different chemicals.
4. Place a drop of the extract or a fiber containing the stain on a clean (new) slide, and add a drop of benzidine reagent. This may be applied with a wooden applicator stick or a toothpick, or a small-diameter glass rod. The reagent may be added directly to the stained area if desired.
5. Perform a similar test on an unstained portion. It should be negative.

6. A dark green or blue color indicates the presence of blood. If the test remains colorless, the stain is not blood and no further examinations are indicated. If the test is positive, proceed with the precipitin test to determine whether or not it is human blood. If the tests made on the unstained portions of the specimen are positive, no further tests should be made because the controls show that the material itself, on which the stain is present, reacts with the reagent and thus the test is unreliable.

Reduced phenolphthalein (phenolphthalin) test (Gettler-Kaye[11])

1. Prepare the reduced phenolphthalein reagents by dissolving 20 gm of sodium hydroxide in 200 ml of distilled water in a 500 ml Erlenmeyer flask and adding 1 gm of phenolphthalein. When completely dissolved, add 20 gm of granulated zinc, 20 to 30 mesh. Using a reflux condenser to prevent loss by evaporation, slowly boil the mixture until the red color of the alkaline phenolphthalein disappears, leaving a colorless or faintly yellow solution. This may require 2 or 3 hours. When cool, place it in a brown bottle and stopper with a rubber stopper. Add some of the zinc to keep the phenolphthalein in the reduced phenolphthalein form (phenolphthalin). The reagent is stable many months in a cool, dark place.
2. Add a few drops of the reduced reagent to the extract of stain, then add about half as much 3% hydrogen peroxide. A pink or red color indicates blood.
3. Make similar tests on the unstained portion of the evidence.

SPECTROSCOPIC EXAMINATION

When a solution of blood is examined in a spectroscope, certain absorption bands will be formed in the solar spectrum (Fig. 22-1).

1. Prepare a solution of the blood stain in distilled water.
2. Place the solution in a small glass chamber with parallel sides so arranged that the rays of light will pass directly through it. After placing the chamber with the solution into the spectroscope, adjust the instrument so that the spectrum is clearly visible. If the solution contains blood, it will absorb some of the light rays from the spectrum, resulting in characteristic absorption bands that vary with the type of blood pigment present, as follows:

Oxyhemoglobin—two bands in the yellow between the Fraunhöfer lines D and E.

Hemoglobin—a broad band between D and E, with a small rim over the D on the red side of the spectrum.

Carboxyhemoglobin—similar to oxyhemoglobin. Addition of ammonium hydroxide reduces oxyhemoglobin to hemoglobin but leaves carboxyhemoglobin unchanged.

Methemoglobin—dark band in the red between C and D but nearer C. If the solution has been properly diluted, it splits into bands resembling the bands of acid hematin.

Acid hematin—sharp band between C and D, nearer to C, also a broad band not clearly defined between D and F.

Alkaline hematin—band between C and D; it also absorbs the violet end of the spectrum.

Hemochromogen—sharp, dark band between D and E and a pale, broader band over E.

Hematoporphyrin in alkaline solutions—faint line between C and D, a broader band at D extending toward E, a band between D and E but nearly at E, and a broad band between E and F.

Diluted old blood stains give hemoglobin and oxyhemoglobin bands. If a weak alkali is added, they form alkaline hematin; with a weak acid they form acid hematin. Old and decomposed blood stains yield positive tests for hematoporphyrin after addition of strong alkali to a portion of the suspected blood solution.

Is this human blood?

Once the stain has been identified as blood, it must be established as human blood. The standard test is the precipitin test. The standard precipitin test is the ring test. Other methods are the agar double diffusion technic and counterelectrophoresis.

Precipitin tests are based on the fact that when rabbits are injected with human blood serum, they form a precipitating antibody that reacts with human serum to form a precipitate. The original experiments were performed in 1901 by Uhlenhuth,[12] who at first believed that the anti–human precipitin serum produced by the rabbit was absolutely specific for human

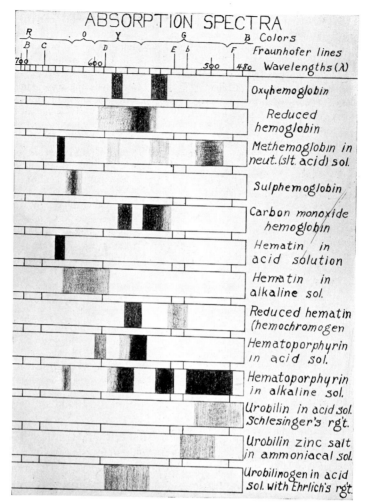

Fig. 22-1. Absorption spectra. (From Bauer, J. D., Ackermann, P. G., and Toro, G.: Bray's clinical laboratory methods, ed. 7, St. Louis, 1968, The C. V. Mosby Co.)

blood. In 1901 Nuttall,[13] pursuing the original experiments of Uhlenhuth, gave a classic account of blood relationships of various animals by means of the precipitin test and showed that a common property exists in the blood of certain groups of animals and that this property has persisted throughout the ages elapsed during our possible evolution from a common ancestor. In 1952 and 1953 Gradwohl[14-16] found that chimpanzee blood gives a ring reaction indistinguishable from that of human blood with anti–human precipitin serum and that human blood gives an identical ring reaction with anti–chimpanzee precipitin serum. He found the same results using blood from the gorilla and the olive baboon (*Papio anubis*).

The precipitins formed in animals as a result of injection of blood are reactive not only for serum proteins but also for other body proteins as well, and this test can therefore be used to identify seminal stains as of human origin, bone fragments, meat adulteration like addition of chopped horse meat to chopped beef, and so on.

The precipitin sera react with **groups** of mammalian bloods. **Specific** anti-rabbit, anti-dog, anti-beef, anti-cat, etc. precipitins are available commercially. The sera must

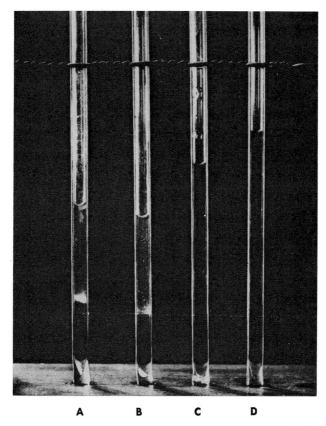

Fig. 22-2. Precipitin ring test. **A,** Anti-chimpanzee serum vs chimpanzee blood. **B,** Anti-chimpanzee serum vs human blood. **C,** Anti-chimpanzee serum vs guinea pig blood. **D,** Anti-chimpanzee blood vs rabbit blood. (From Gradwohl, R. B. H.: Lab. Digest **15**[5]:4, 1952.)

be potent, and the material under investigation must be dilute when the test is made. Anti–human precipitin sera should react with the blood of primates but not with that of other lower animals. Shupe* (1968) pointed out that some anti–human precipitin sera also give positive reactions even with raccoon blood, and we have confirmed this in our own laboratories. Since the precipitin ring test does not differentiate between human and nonhuman primate blood, it is of no value in regions of the world where nonhuman primates may have been in the vicinity of a crime. In other areas, for example, the United States, this fact may be ignored in criminal cases, and a positive precipitin ring test may be interpreted as designating the blood as having been derived from a human source.

*Shupe, L. M.: Personal communication, 1968.

The method of preparing anti–human precipitin serum is available in many texts and will not be repeated here.[19]

PRECIPITIN RING TEST

1. Use 5 mm tubing with a 2 mm bore that has a heavy-walled, narrow opening. Cut it into 8 cm lengths and seal one end in the flame. The tubes must be clean and dry and should be used only once, then discarded (Fig. 22-2).
2. Prepare an extract of the stained area and one from a nonstained portion of the evidence. If the stains have been exposed to high temperatures, it may be necessary to soak them in saline for as long as 72 hours to extract the stain and in a refrigerator to prevent bacterial growth. If the extract contains debris or is cloudy, centrifuge and use the clear supernate for the test. Always use a minimum amount of saline in making the extract. The extract should foam on shaking. Prepare several different

Table 22-6. Possible results in the ring precipitin test

Anti-human precipitin serum plus						
Stain extract	**Human serum**	**Bovine serum**	**Canine serum**	**Saline**	**Unstained area extract**	**Conclusions**
+	+	–	–	–	–	Stain derived from human source
–	+	–	–	–	–	Stain not derived from human source
?	+	+	–	–	–	Error
+	+	–	–	–	+	Results unreliable; unstained area should not react
?	+	–	+	–	–	Error
?	+	–	–	+	–	Error
–	–	–	–	–	–	Results unreliable; precipitin serum does not react with human blood

Tube 2 should show a positive result; tubes 3, 4, 5, and 6 should be negative.

dilutions of the extract: 1:100, 1:1000, and so on. The 1:1000 dilution should show only scanty foam on shaking.

3. Dilute known serum from a human source, about 1 drop of the serum to 50 ml of saline, as a positive control.
4. Prepare similar dilutions of sera from a bovine and a canine source. If preferred, use two control sera, one bovine and the other canine. This is the negative control.
5. Label the small-bore tubes with the respective sources of the specimen. Using capillary droppers with long, thin capillary ends, place anti–human precipitin serum in each of the six tubes, at the bottom of the tube.
6. The precipitin serum should be at a depth of several millimeters.
7. Stratify an equal volume of extract (or saline as in tube 5) of the various stains or unstained portions and the various diluted sera. In tube 1, use the unknown stain extract; in tube 2, the diluted human serum; in tube 3, the diluted bovine serum; in tube 4, the diluted canine serum; and in tube 5, saline. If extracts have been prepared from more than one portion of the evidence, use a separate tube for each extract. Tubes 3, 4, and 5 are the negative controls. Tube 2 is the positive control. Use a different capillary for each extract, diluted serum, and saline.
8. Let the tubes stand at room temperature for 5 minutes, and observe. A white line at the point of contact between the precipitin serum and the extract or diluted serum is a positive reaction. A negatively reacting serum will show only the point of contact between the two layers.
9. Tube 2, with the diluted human serum, should show a positive reaction. All the other controls should be negative.
10. If the extract of the unknown stain shows a white line at the interface between the precipitin serum and the extract, the stain was made by human blood. If it does not, it is not human blood.
11. If the results are negative and if this is not human blood, it may be necessary to identify the source of the blood. In this case, the extract must be tested with a battery of different precipitin sera that react with many different species of animal blood—duck, dog, chicken, cattle, and so on.
12. Some laboratories allow the tubes to stand overnight at room temperature after taking the first reading, to confirm the reactions. The precipitate will drop to the bottom of the tube. Unfortunately, any turbidity that may be present, especially when due to particulate matter, may also precipitate, and this method is therefore not in general use.

Human blood stains dried for as long as 10 to 15 years or longer may still give a positive reaction. Even extracts of tissue from mummies 4000 to 5000 years old have given positive reactions with this test. In cases in which bloods from several different species of animals are mixed together in the stain or extract, there can still be a positive reaction if any of the blood was derived from a human subject. Human blood stains that have been washed in water and have left only a faint color of the blood on a garment still may show the reaction.

With fresh stains, the unfixed portion of the blood serum is readily extracted by aqueous solutions, but in older stains the degree of fixation does not readily permit the serum to pass into solution with water. Prolonged steeping in saline, however, may successfully extract a sufficient quantity to yield a positive reaction. Stains that have been soaked in soap powder solutions will not react properly, and the precipitin test cannot be relied on in such cases. Blood stains on various woods, leather, and so on will yield a positive reaction.

Consult Table 22-6 for possible results in the ring precipitin test.

AGAR DOUBLE DIFFUSION PRECIPITIN TEST

Agar-covered slides, ready for use, are available commercially. The slides may, of course, be prepared in one's own laboratory. The principle of the test is that as the precipitin serum and the extracted stain for the test or controls diffuse through the agar gel toward one another, a precipitate will form where they meet if human serum is present.

The controls are prepared as in the ring test; that is, the various animal sera are diluted, but not as much as for the capillary tube method, and an extract is also made of the unstained portion of the evidence (Fig. 22-3).

1. To prepare the slides, flood each with 4 ml of 1% melted agar. The slides should be twice the width of the ordinary laboratory slides, 5 by 7.5 cm. Keep them in moist chambers after the agar has solidified and maintain them at 4° C.
2. The recommended pattern for wells to be cut into the agar on the slides is a center well for the precipitin serum, with the other wells surrounding this in a circular fashion. The wells should be equidistant from one another and from the center well. Devices for cutting standard wells may be purchased.
3. Place 0.01 ml of anti–human precipitin serum in the center well.
4. Place 0.01 ml of the extract of the stain in one of the surrounding wells, 0.01 ml of saline in one, 0.01 ml of diluted human serum in another, 0.01 ml of diluted nonhuman serum in another, and 0.01 ml of ex-

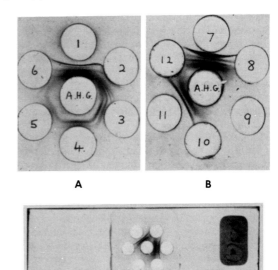

C

Fig. 22-3. Results of the precipitin test of dilutions of human serum from 1 in 1 to 1:1000 against an anti–human globulin rabbit serum (undiluted) placed in the central well. **A,** *1,* Undiluted human serum; *2* to *6,* serial dilutions of human serum, 1:10, 1:100, 1:200, 1:500, 1:1000. **B,** *7,* Human serum; *8,* cat serum; *9,* mouse serum. **C,** Ouchterlony-type gel diffusion test for species identification. Arrangement of gel diffusion test on a microscope slide. (From Camps, F.: Gradwohl's legal medicine, Bristol, England, John Wright & Sons, Ltd. By permission of the author and publisher.)

tract of an unstained portion of the evidence in another. The wells should be identified.

The controls are prepared as for the ring test. Any animal serum may be used as a negative control except that from a nonhuman primate. The positive control consists of 0.01 ml of diluted human serum.

5. Keep the slide in a moist chamber for 24 hours, then read. Let stand an additional 24 hours and read again.
6. Bands of precipitation of the positive control, continuous with precipitating components produced by the contents of other wells containing the stain extract, identify the stain as of human origin, provided that the negative controls show no precipitation bands.

ANTIGLOBULIN INHIBITION TEST

The precipitin test does *not* differentiate the bloods of the anthropoid apes and man;

in fact, there is no simple, practicable method available at this time to distinguish among the bloods of man, apes, and Old World monkeys. Wiener et al.[17] reported the results of an **inhibition test for immuno-globulins** to be used to differentiate human from nonhuman sera. This is a test of the relative ability of sera from various origins to inhibit agglutination reactions of anti–human immune rabbit serum with human Rh_o-positive red cells coated with anti-Rh_o IgG antibodies, which cells are used as indicator.

Chimpanzee[17] serum strongly inhibits the reaction but to a slightly lower titer than human serum. Gorilla blood serum also inhibits the reaction but to a much lower titer. With orangutans and gibbons as well as with monkeys, there is little or no inhibition. Later, rabbits were immunized with rhesus monkey globulin and inhibition tests were performed. Four different inhibition tests were used by these authors:

1. Anti–human globulin prepared in rabbits, titrated against Rh_o-coated red cells to determine the titer, then diluted to a titer of 10 units; used for the inhibition test
2. Anti–rhesus globulin prepared in rabbits, titrated against C^{rh}-positive* rhesus monkey cells and coated with anti-C^{rh} antibody, then diluted to a titer of 10 units; also used in the inhibition test
3. Anti–human globulin prepared as described previously and titrated against rhesus monkey cells having been coated with anti-C^{rh} and diluted to a titer of 10 units
4. Anti–rhesus monkey globulin diluted to a titer of 10 units against human group O Rh_o-positive coated cells

Before the test the unknown sera were absorbed with packed, washed, pooled human and rhesus monkey red cells to remove heteroagglutinins.

Serial dilutions of the absorbed sera were made in the usual manner, doubling each

---

*See Chapter 16 for nomenclature of blood groups of nonhuman primates.

dilution. Next, 1 drop of each dilution (undiluted, 1:2, 1:4, 1:8, etc.) of the absorbed serum was placed in each of a series of small tubes, and 1 drop of the diluted antiglobulin serum (titer 10 units) was added to each tube. The mixtures were allowed to stand for 30 minutes, then 1 drop of the appropriate coated red cells was added as indicator to each tube and the tubes shaken. After 30 minutes the tubes were centrifuged at low speed for 1 minute and the reactions read.

1. With anti–human globulin serum, using coated human red cells as indicator, human serum gave the highest inhibition titers, followed closely by chimpanzee; gorillas gave lower titers, and no inhibition occurred with sera of other apes or of monkeys.

2. With anti–rhesus globulin serum, using coated rhesus monkey cells as indicator, high inhibition titers were obtained with sera of rhesus monkeys and other Old World monkeys but none with sera of humans, apes, and New World monkeys.

3. With anti–human globulin serum, using coated rhesus monkey cells as indicator, high inhibition titers were obtained with sera of Old World monkeys and with sera of humans and apes (except gibbons), but none with sera of New World monkeys.

4. With anti–rhesus globulin serum, using coated human red cells as indicator, high inhibition titers were obtained with sera of humans and apes (except gibbons) and with sera of Old World monkeys but none with sera of New World monkeys.

Duncan-Taylor and Gordon[18] introduced an alum absorption method for identification of human blood, but the absorbed serum was of poor potency. The technic is available elsewhere.[18]

What is the blood group?

The methods used in determining the blood group of a blood stain differ from ordinary blood grouping tests. When blood dries, the red cells disintegrate. The antigens in the dried cells remain and are capable of absorbing their corresponding antibodies. The A-B-O antigens withstand heat, the passage of time, and so on, but those of the M-N and Rh-Hr systems do not, except for the M antigen. The agglutinins in the blood (serum) disappear shortly after the stain has dried.

There are a number of tests used in identifying the group to which a stain belongs: the blood "crust" test, the agglutinin-absorption test (Wiener, 1943[22]), the elution-absorption test (Kind, 1960,[23] Nickolls and Pereira, 1962,[24] Lincoln and Dodd, 1973[25]), and automated equipment like AutoAnalyzers.

The crust test requires a minimum of up to 1 mg of dried blood. The minimum requirement for the agglutinin-absorption test is that the blood group antigen be capable of absorbing and thus inhibiting the action of more than half the antibody in the reagent serum with which it is being tested. The elution method requires only small amounts of stained material. Automated equipment makes use of eluates from stains.

In the elution process the antibody is absorbed by or adsorbed onto the red cells. When the blood is in the form of dried stains, the antibody should be absorbed at the optimum temperature for the specific absorption—4° C for the A-B-O antigens and 37° C for Rh-Hr. The specifically bound antibody can be recovered by causing it to dissociate from the antigen. The best method for blood stains is by heat at 56° to 60° C (p. 249). The eluate containing the antibody is mixed with the appropriate red cells (A for anti-**A**, B for anti-**B**, etc.). The cells should be at a very dilute concentration,[23] about 0.1%. Even in some cases when the agglutinin inhibition test is negative or doubtful, the elution method may often give positive results.[24] Smaller amounts of material are required in the elution technic. Dodd uses enzyme-treated red cells for eluted Rh antibodies.

When stains are on hard surfaces and the elution method is to be used, cotton threads dampened with distilled water are placed in the dried blood to pick up the stain. According to Dodd,[5] not only can **A, B,** and **M** be detected in dry stains, but the elution method also detects **H, N, S, s,** the principal Rh-Hr factors, **K, Fy**[a], **Fy**[b], and **Jk**[a].

For practical purposes, investigation into the blood group of a stain is limited to a search for the blood specificities **A** and **B** of the A-B-O system and **M** of the M-N-S system. Although there have been reports of identification of Rh specificities in dried blood, as yet there is no confirmation of these, nor is there any proof of the accuracy of the tests. Such tests are based primarily on elution technics. The **N** specificity rapidly disappears from dried blood, but the **M** factor remains. Tests for M-N types, in general, are disappointing. They may show (1) that a blood specificity, **M,** for example, is present or (2) that it could be present, but there may be failure of the reaction.

The reason for identifying the blood group of a stain is to prove that a certain stain could have come from a certain individual. For the most part the test is valuable in determining that a stain could *not* have come from a certain individual; that is, it is a good exclusion test. If the suspect and victim of a crime are of the same blood group, no conclusion can be drawn from this test except that the stain could have been derived from the victim or the suspect. If the blood groups are different, however, the accused is not exonerated, on the basis of this test, if the stain found on the suspect is of the same blood group as that of the victim but different from that of the suspect.

There may be blood group receptors from the individual on whom the stain was found. Underclothing that has been worn for several days almost always has the A-B-H receptors of the wearer when such receptors are present in his blood and sweat, that is, if he is a secretor of A-B-H substances.

At times, unhemolyzed liquid blood is submitted to the laboratory. The tests on such blood are made just as they would be before a transfusion—the red cells are tested against various antisera, and the serum is tested against the different blood group antigens.

If the dried blood stain submitted for testing is on a nonabsorbent surface such as glass or metal, in the form of a crust, and if the crust is fairly fresh and of sufficient size, the crust test may be useful.

CRUST TEST FOR IDENTIFICATION
OF BLOOD GROUP OF A BLOOD STAIN
(COVERSLIP METHOD OF LATTES)

When blood dries, the red cells disintegrate and a suspension of the crust will show no red cells, but the isoagglutinins remain for a short time. This forms a basis for the following test. A minimum of a few square millimeters of a thin crust of blood, weighing 0.1 to 1 mg, is often sufficient for the crust test.

1. Remove the crust from such nonabsorbent surfaces as glass, stone, or shoe leather with a scalpel or razor blade.
2. Have ready 2% suspensions in saline of group A₁, B, and O cells. The test cells should be highly sensitive. The group O cells serve as a control against aggregation due to nonspecific causes.
3. Label a glass slide with "A" at the left side and "B" at the right and the identifying number or name. Label another slide "O."
4. Place 2 or more small, thin crusts of blood on the opposite ends of the first slide, and the same quantity on the slide labeled "O."
5. Add 1 drop of A₁ cell suspension adjacent to the crust on the left side of the first slide, the same quantity of B cells on the right side, and the same amount of group O cells on the slide labeled "O."
6. Place a cover glass over each preparation so that the liquid comes into contact with the edge of the crust. If the crust is too thick, the coverglass will be raised too high and development of the reaction will be difficult if not impossible. Avoid the introduction of air bubbles that might separate the crust from the liquid. Place the cover glass on the mixtures immediately after they have been prepared but avoid pressure.
7. Wait a few minutes, then examine all the preparations microscopically for agglutination. The cover glasses may be momentarily subjected to light pressure at this point to break up any rouleaux that may have formed.
8. If there is no agglutination, wait 30 minutes, examining the slides from time to time. Weak reactions require more time to develop than do strong ones.
9. Record agglutination as positive (+), absence of agglutination as negative (−). The reactions occur at the border of the cell suspension adjacent to the blood crust. The high sensitivity of the test depends on the diffusion of the agglutinins into this interface so that the bulk of the red cells do not take part in the reaction.
10. The slide with the group O cells must show no agglutination. If these cells agglutinate, the test is unreliable.
11. If the group A cells agglutinate, the stain contains anti-A.
12. If the group B cells agglutinate, the stain contains anti-B.
13. Consult Table 22-7 for possible results with the crust test.
14. The results of the blood crust test should always be confirmed or denied by the agglutinin absorption method results, provided there is enough material for those tests. Refer to sources of error in these tests discussed on pp. 342 to 344.
15. Instead of scraping some of the dried blood and using it as a crust, it is possible to extract the entire quantity from the material with minimal amounts of distilled water, then evaporate the resulting solution to dryness on glass at room temperature. Then scrape the powder off the glass, mix with very small quantities of distilled water to make a paste, and allow to dry in the proper place on glass slides. The test cells in suspension can be added directly to this dried extract and the tests conducted as above.
16. The slides with the crusts and their respective cells can be kept in a moist chamber while waiting the 30 minutes. At first only the cells immediately adjacent to the crust will clump because that is where the concentration of agglutinins is strongest. Eventually the clumps may be seen throughout the specimen. The artificial blood crusts do not give as satisfactory reactions as do the natural ones.
17. In the test of blood crusts, only positive reactions are significant.

AGGLUTININ ABSORPTION TEST FOR
IDENTIFICATION OF BLOOD GROUP

Blood cells lose their agglutinability when they dry because the cells disinte-

Table 22-7. Possible results with the blood crust test

Blood crust plus			Agglutinins in stain	Conclusions
A$_1$ cells	B cells	O cells		
+	+	−	Anti-**A** and anti-**B**	Blood derived from group O person
−	+	−	Anti-**B**	Blood derived from group A person or else there is failure of reaction with group A cells
+	−	−	Anti-**A**	Blood derived from group B person or else there is failure of reaction with group B cells
−	−	−	None	Blood derived from group AB person or else there is failure of reaction due to disappearance of the isoagglutinins
+	+	+	—	Test is unreliable; agglutination is due to nonspecific causes

Note: In the case of groups A and B it is possible that identification can be correct, but it is also possible that the blood could have come from a group O person who had both anti-A and anti-B in the serum, but one or the other of the isoagglutinins disappeared during the drying process.

grate, and without free erythrocytes there can be no agglutination. A direct test for agglutinogen content of the cells therefore cannot be done. The group-specific substances of the red cells remain in the dried blood, however, and retain their ability to remove, by absorption, any agglutinin in serum for which the substances are specific. For example, the A-specific substance neutralizes anti-A in anti-A serum, B substance neutralizes anti-B, M neutralizes anti-M, and O and other groups neutralize anti-H.

If a serum of known titer is added to an unknown blood stain and is later retested, and if the serum has lost its ability to cause agglutination of its specific cells or if the titer has been lowered, it may be concluded that the stain contained the agglutinogen corresponding in specificity to the agglutinin in the antiserum, always assuming that proper controls have been made and the observations were correct.

The agglutinin absorption test is unreliable in detecting the **N** specificity because of the tendency for nonspecific absorption of anti-N reagents. Similarly, no test has as yet been devised that will accurately identify any of the specificities of the Rh-Hr system in dried blood stains.

Sweat, bacteria, dirt, and other particulate substances on soiled garments may render the agglutinin absorption test unreliable. Even under ideal conditions, the tests may be difficult to interpret. They require the experience and patience of experts in carrying out the technics and in drawing conclusions from the results.

With the agglutinin absorption test, it is difficult to differentiate between blood groups A$_2$ and O. One of the most difficult blood groups to identify is group A$_2$B.

Negative results are not significant. They may indicate failure of the tests. Only positive reactions may be relied on. For example, if the blood stain fails to neutralize anti-A and anti-B reagents, the stain must not be identified as group O because failure of absorption may occur when the stain has been denatured or when it is insufficient in amount, and the failure to absorb is not therefore necessarily due to lack of agglutinogens in the stain. Insufficient stain will give negative results.

If a stain neutralizes anti-**B** but not anti-**A**, it presumably contains group B blood. The tests for stains of groups A and B thus have an **internal control** so that these two groups can usually be readily identified. Group A$_1$B stains neutralize both anti-**A** and anti-**B** reagents, but if both reagents are neutralized, it does not necessarily follow that the stain was derived from a group A₁B person. There is always the possibility of **nonspecific absorption** of the agglutinins in the reagents due to dirt or bacteria in the stain. This is one of the reasons why adjacent unstained material must always be included as a control.

The use of anti-**H** lectin reagents provides the internal control over groups O and AB that they lack in themselves, unlike the internal control in groups A and B. Group O stains neutralize anti-**H,** but group A₁B stains do not. This is a means of differentiation that can be relied on. Anti-**H** lectins react with almost equal intensity with red cells of groups O and A₂, less strongly with most cells of group B, and negatively or weakly with most cells of groups A₁ and A₁B. The anti-**H** reagent is prepared from extracts of seeds of *Ulex europeus* and is available commercially.* The method of preparation has been published elsewhere.[19]

---

*Hyland Laboratories, Costa Mesa, Calif.

Procedure. Dilute anti-**A** and anti-**B** sera and anti-**H** lectin with saline to yield a titer of 4 to 8 units, and use the diluted reagents in the tests and controls.

1. If the specimen is in the form of a crust or powder, grind it into a very fine powder and put 10 mg in each of three small tubes, labeled, respectively, anti-**A**, anti-**B**, and anti-**H**. This can be done only *if there is sufficient specimen.*
2. Add 0.1 ml of anti-**A** testing serum to the first tube, 0.1 ml of anti-**B** to the second tube, and 0.1 ml of anti-**H** *Ulex europeus* lectin to the third tube, using the diluted reagents.
3. Mix each tube thoroughly, using a separate tiny-bore stirring rod for each tube, then allow the mixture to remain in a refrigerator overnight to complete the absorption.
4. Centrifuge and transfer the supernatant dark red fluid to fresh tubes to test for agglutinin content. Add the correct cell suspensions to their respective tubes: group A₂ cells for the tubes containing anti-**A** serum; group B cells for the tubes with anti-**B**; and group O cells for the tubes with anti-**H**. Read microscopically for agglutination or its absence. Refer to Tables 22-8 and 22-9 for setup of controls and test and to Tables

Table 22-8. Setup for controls using cloth containing known stains

Tubes	A₁-stained cloth	A₂-stained cloth	B-stained cloth	O-stained cloth
		Serum added		
1	Anti-**A**	Anti-**A**	Anti-**A**	Anti-**A**
2	Anti-**B**	Anti-**B**	Anti-**B**	Anti-**B**
3	Anti-**H**	Anti-**H**	Anti-**H**	Anti-**H**
		Refrigerate overnight		
		Cells added		
1	A₂	A₂	A₂	A₂
2	B	B	B	B
3	O	O	O	O

Table 22-9. Setup for agglutinin absorption test*

Anti-**A** serum + stained area	Anti-**B** serum + stained area	Anti-**H** Ulex + stained area	Anti-**M** reagent + stained area
	All absorbed in a refrigerator overnight		
		Cells added	
A₂ cells	B cells	O cells	M cells

*Similar tests must also be set up for the unstained material adjacent to the stain.

22-10 and 22-11 for interpretation of results.

5. *If the stain has been absorbed,* as it will be when on clothing, paper, or other absorbent materials, cut out portions of the stained as well as the unstained areas, of approximately equal size. Identify each area from which the stain has been cut, using an indelible pencil, marking with the initials of the person who cut out the specimen and the date. This may be needed if the case is presented in court.

6. Use 7 mm diameter tubes. Cut portions of both the stained and the unstained material of approximately equal size to use in the test, taking care not to touch with the fingers. Use disposable glassware.

7. Prepare duplicate sets of tubes for the tests and one set for each of the controls. Eight tubes will be needed for the tests, four in each duplicate set, as well as twelve for the controls. Label each of the test sets as tubes 1, 2, 3, and 4. Label the tubes for the controls A_1 tube 1, A_1 tube 2, A_1 tube 3; A_2 tube 1, A_2 tube 2, A_2 tube 3; B tube 1, B tube 2, B tube 3; and O tube 1, O tube 2, O tube 3, as follows:

Tests	Controls			
1–2–3–4	A_1 A_1 A_1	A_2 A_2 A_2	B B B	O O O
1–2–3–4	1 2 3	1 2 3	1 2 3	1 2 3

8. Dilute anti-**A**, anti-**B**, and anti-**M** antisera and anti-**H** lectin to a titer of 4 to 8 units with saline.

9. Put a small piece of the stained specimen into each of the four duplicate tubes for the test (Table 22-9).

10. Put a small piece of A_1-stained cloth (below) into each of its three tubes, a piece of A_2-stained cloth into each of its three tubes, a small piece of B-stained cloth into each of its three tubes, and a small piece of O-stained cloth into each of its three tubes.

11. Add enough anti-**A** serum to each tube 1 of the test and to each tube 1 of the controls, anti-**B** to each tube 2 of the tests and of the controls, anti-**H** lectin to each tube 3

of the tests and controls, and anti-**M** to each tube 4 of the test, to just saturate the cloth.

12. Prod the contents of each tube with a separate tiny-caliber glass rod to cause the cloth to absorb the serum. There should be no runoff of serum when the tube is tilted. Use a different rod for each tube.

13. Refrigerate all the tubes, both test and controls, overnight.

14. On the following day, aspirate the serum from each tube using a thin capillary dropper with a rubber bulb, pressing against the cloth while exerting suction. Use a different capillary pipet for each tube. Transfer the aspirated serum to small tubes bearing the same label as the tube from which the serum was withdrawn.

15. Add 1 drop of 2% suspension of group A_2 cells to each tube 1 of the tests and controls.

16. Add 1 drop of 2% suspension of group B red cells to each tube 2 of the tests and the controls.

17. Add 1 drop of 2% suspension of group O cells to each tube 3 of the tests and of the controls.

18. Add 1 drop of 2% suspension of type M cells to each tube 4 of the tests.

19. Mix each tube separately.

20. Put the tubes with anti-**H** plus group O cells in a refrigerator for 2 hours, but leave the other tubes at room temperature during that time. If desired, the A, B, and M tests may be made in welled slides.

21. Read and record the reactions in each tube, agglutination as a positive (+) reaction, absence of agglutination as a negative (–).

22. If the controls show incorrect results, the tests results are unreliable and the entire procedure will have to be repeated or discarded.

23. The expected results in the controls are given in Table 22-10.

24. If the control tubes show the correct reactions, proceed to read the results in the tests according to Table 22-11.

Table 22-10. Results expected in controls using known dried blood stains

	Tube 1 A_2 cells	Tube 2 B cells	Tube 3 O cells
A_1-stained cloth	–	+	+ or –
A_2 stained cloth	–	+	–
B-stained cloth	+	–	+ or –
O-stained cloth	+	+	–

If desired, controls may be made using M-stained cloth and A_1B- and A_2B- stained cloth and the procedure carried out as described previously.

Tube 1 contains the anti-**A** serum, tube 2 the anti-**B**, and tube 3 the anti-**H**.

Table 22-11. Results in agglutinin absorption test for blood stains

Specimen	Tubes				Conclusions
	1	2	3	4	
1	+	+	−		Group O
2	−	+	+ or −		Group A; A_2 cells react regularly with anti-**H**
3	+	−	+		Group B
4	−	−	+		Group AB
				+	**M** specificity not present in stain
				−	**M** specificity present in stain

+ = agglutination = no inhibition.
− = no agglutination = inhibition.

Controls may be prepared and kept in a refrigerator. A sample of each known A_1, A_2, B, O, M, A_1B, and A_2B blood is poured on its own piece of cloth or cotton, allowed to dry, labeled with the group or type letter, and kept in a refrigerator until needed.

ACACIA METHOD FOR ISOAGGLUTININS IN DRIED BLOOD STAINS (WIENER)[25]

Acacia enhances the sensitivity of the test for agglutinins when the titer of isoagglutinins in a dried blood stain is low.

Acacia solution
1. Dissolve 10 gm of gum acacia and 1 gm of dibasic sodium phosphate (Na_2HPO_4) in 90 ml of distilled water.
2. Sterilize at once at 10-pound pressure for 10 minutes in an autoclave. The resulting opalescent solution is stable indefinitely if sterility is maintained in a refrigerator.

Procedure
1. Cut out a portion of the blood-stained cloth and place in a wide tube.
2. Add just enough saline to saturate the material thoroughly.
3. Prod with a heavy glass rod to express the saline, then allow the cloth to reabsorb the saline. Repeat many times until the expressed fluid is dark. The stain should be sopping wet, and there should be little or no run-off liquid when the tube is tilted.
4. Let stand 30 to 60 minutes, then squeeze the material with the rod or other device to express as much extract as possible.
5. Transfer the extract to a clean, small tube and centrifuge at high speed for 15 to 30 minutes or longer to remove all suspended particles.
6. Transfer 5 to 10 drops of the extract to each of three properly labeled tubes, A_1, B, and O.

7. Add 1 drop of 1% suspension of group A_1 cells to the first tube, 1 drop of group B cells to the second, and 1 drop of group O cells to the third. The cells must be freshly prepared.
8. Prepare controls in the same manner using the unstained portion of the cloth.
9. Place all the mixtures in a cup of ice water in a refrigerator for 30 minutes.
10. Centrifuge in cups containing cracked ice.
11. Completely decant the dark supernatant fluid.
12. Add to each tube 1 drop of saline and shake, then read the reactions.
13. Add 2 drops of acacia solution to each tube and shake.
14. Let stand at room temperature for 2 hours, then read again, after gently dislodging the sediment.
15. Centrifuge at 500 rpm for 1 minute and read again, after first gently dislodging the sediment.
16. Interpret the results according to Table 22-12.

SOURCES OF ERROR IN TESTING DRIED STAINS FOR BLOOD GROUP

1. In the preliminary titration of the antisera, if the results are satisfactory, if a 3+ or 2+ reaction is obtained against the known cells that are to be used in retesting the serum after absorption, and if in the actual test the control from an unstained area gives even only a 1+ or ± reaction, some group substance is present, derived from sweat, saliva, urine, etc., which inhibited the activity of the antiserum. No conclusions may then be drawn concerning the blood group of the stain unless a different test is made. When possible, a second test

Table 22-12. Results possible with extracts of large stains, acacia method

Stain extract + A₁ cells	Stain extract + B cells	Stain extract + O cells	Blood group of stain
+	+	−	Group O
−	+	−	Group A, or O with anti-**A** deteriorated
+	−	−	Group B, or O with anti-**B** deteriorated
−	−	−	Inconclusive

+ = agglutination = no inhibition.
− = no agglutination = inhibition.

should be performed on unstained material removed from an area closer to the stain. This will help in telling whether the interfering substance is localized or general.

2. In the preliminary titration of the antisera to be used later in the test, the known cells against which such antisera are titrated or tested must be the same as those to be used in the actual test. If these cells give a 3+ or 2+ reaction with the serum, and if, in the test after the serum has been subjected to absorption by the stain, known or unknown, a ± result is obtained, group-specific substance has reduced the reactivity of the serum. In such a case either (1) the stain is old and has been incompletely absorbed, or it has been exposed to conditions unfavorable for preservation of the group substance, (2) there is not enough blood in the stain for an accurate test, or (3) the antiserum used is of too high a titer. In the controls the first two reasons may be eliminated by using only freshly prepared, adequate samples. The last possibility may be eliminated by performing another test on another portion of the stain, using serum of lower titer (accomplished by diluting the original serum with an equal volume of saline) and testing this serum to make sure it is still reactive. Clear-cut negative reactions must be obtained in the controls when blood stains of known type are used. For preparation of the control stains (known blood groups), see p. 342.

3. When tests of unstained material, known group O blood, and the corresponding known stain in the controls give 3+ or

2+ results, a negative or ± result with the unknown indicates inhibition of the reactivity of the antiserum, attributable to group-specific substances in the unknown stain.

4. In an unknown stain, a positive result (agglutination) may occur not because the antigen is lacking in the original blood from which the stain was derived but because the group factor in the dried stain has disappeared as a result of age, exposure to unfavorable physical conditions, or other causes or because there is an insufficient quantity of stained material. Identification of an unknown stain as group O is provisional, except when anti-**H** is used. Group O stains may be identified absolutely by testing for and finding both iso-agglutinins present in the stain, as in the crust technic or the agglutinin extract method.

5. The A_2 specificity is much weaker than A_1. A ± reaction or a marked reduction in titer of the anti-A serum, as from a 3+ to a 1+ reaction, indicates only partial removal of anti-A agglutinin. The stain should be retested using a lower titered serum as confirmation of the probable presence of A_2.

6. Absence of group-specific factors in the stain does not necessarily signify that the blood is group O, since it could have been derived from a group A_2 person. Likewise, if a stain contains agglutinogen B, there is a possibility that it could have been derived from an A_2B blood.

When testing for the blood group of dried stains, technic, experience, and knowledge on the part of the investigator are of paramount importance. The condition of the stain—exposure to elements, age, amount of stain, and where it was found—contributes to the delicacy of the test. The use of anti-**H** lectin (*Ulex europeus*) is of great help in resolving some of the problems of this work.

IDENTIFICATION OF BODY SECRETIONS AND BODY FLUIDS
Medicolegal examination of seminal stains

The identification of seminal stains consists in determining (1) whether or not the stain is indeed semen, (2) if it is derived from a human source, and (3) what is the blood group of the individual from whom the specimen was derived. These tests are made in cases of alleged rape, sexual homicide, or adultery. The specimen may be dried on clothing, at times it is admixed with blood or vaginal secretions, and sometimes the material is present in dry masses adherent to hair.

IS THIS SEMEN?

If the specimen is examined by ultraviolet light, seminal stains will give a greenish white fluorescence that helps locate the stained areas, but this fluorescence is by no means specific for semen. Further tests must be made, such as the acid phosphatase stain and the search for spermatozoa. If spermatozoa can be demonstrated under the microscope, the stain can be definitely identified as having been derived from semen. The spermatozoa are destroyed when the stain has been subjected to much washing or to exposure to air; otherwise they remain. When they dry they are brittle, and the tail is easily separated from the head. Unless both head and tail are found so that the spermatozoon is intact, microscopic examination may not be dependable. When the specimen is liquid and fresh, motility can be demonstrated, but such motility is absent from dried stains. Because of the delicacy of the spermatozoa, the technician who handles the specimen must proceed with gentle precautions.

Spermatozoa are slender, elongated, flagellated structures, 50 to 70 μm long, with a head, a neck, a body or connecting piece, and a tail. In a fresh specimen they are actively motile. The head is pear shaped, 3 to 6 μm in width, and takes a characteristic two-tone stain. The neck has an anterior centrosome. The body is rodlike and connects the head and neck with the tail. The tail has two portions, the chief piece and the end piece.

Seminal fluid is a mixture of secretions of the epididymis, the ductus deferens, the seminal vesicles, the prostate, the bulbourethral (Cowper's) glands, and the urethral (Littre's) gland. The average amount of ejaculate is 2.5 to 6 ml. Each milliliter should contain 100 million or more spermatozoa.

There are a number of methods of staining spermatozoa: Cary-Hotchkiss,[26] Gelarie,[27] Holbert,[28] Williams-McGugan-Carpenter,[29,30] Pollák-Joël,[31] and others. Giemsa stain is often used.

Spermatozoa may also be stained in cloth by the method of Baecchi[34] and of Hektoen and Rukstinat,[35] and there are still other methods of microchemical testing such as the Florence test and the Peltzer test.[32] The Florence test, which was used in many laboratories for years, is not reliable because other body fluids give a positive reaction. A negative reaction, however, usually indicates that the suspected substance is *not* semen.

The specimen may be tested for pH and for fluorescence or ultraviolet light reaction. The best way to identify a stain as of seminal origin is to perform the acid phosphatase test, using either the Walker acid phosphatase test or the Phosphatabs-acid reagent.* We have had considerable success with the Phosphatabs-acid reagent in place of the Walker test. The details of the Walker test are available in *Gradwohl's Clinical Laboratory Methods and Diagnosis.*[32]

---

*Warner-Lambert Pharmaceutical Co., Morris Plains, N.J.

Phosphatabs-acid test (acid phosphatase)

1. Cut a 1 cm by 1 cm portion of the cloth and put the section in a 50 ml beaker.
2. Add 10 ml of distilled water.
3. After 30 minutes remove the cloth, stir the liquid in the beaker, and let the particles settle.
4. Place 4 drops of the clear supernate in one of the wells in the kit.
5. Add a silver foil tablet, crushed with a glass rod, and allow the mixture to remain at 20° C for 22 minutes. The time varies with the temperature.
6. Add a gold foil tablet and crush it.
7. A high acid phosphatase content is indicated by an immediate dark purple color.

This test is especially valuable when spermatozoa cannot be found. Kaye[33] found that male ejaculate produces a high acid phosphatase activity as compared with the low acid phosphatase activity of other body fluids like saliva, perspiration, urine, etc. and the common vegetable and fruit juice stains. The differences are so marked and definite that there can be little doubt of the interpretation of the results. **Average seminal fluid** contains approximately 2500 King-Armstrong units of acid phosphatase per ml, the upper limit being 3500 units and the lower 500 units. Ejaculates in **aspermia** give comparable high results. **Other body fluids** generally give values of less than 5 King-Armstrong units per ml. The enzyme is resistant to all known body fluids, including vaginal secretions. It might be inhibited by vaginal disinfectants and contraceptives. Semen does not readily

lose its acid phosphatase activity even after as long as 6 months.

WAS IT DERIVED FROM A HUMAN SOURCE?

The precipitin test is used to determine if the semen was derived from a human source, although this test is not considered necessary by many forensic experts.

Precipitin test for human origin of semen. The method of preparing anti–semen precipitin is described by Reitman.[32]

1. Extract the suspected stain in saline for 4 to 8 hours, using the smallest quantity of saline possible.
2. Centrifuge and transfer the supernatant fluid to a clean, dry tube.
3. Dilute with saline until the amount of foam on shaking indicates a 1:1000 dilution. The extract should have a neutral reaction.
4. Prepare an extract of an unstained portion of the cloth in a similar manner to be used as a control.
5. Prepare another control (positive control) from an extract of known human semen diluted in the same manner as that of the test.
6. Use thick-walled tubes with a very small bore, prepared by sealing one end of heavy-walled capillary tubing. Label the first "T" for test, the second "+" for positive control, the third "C" for control on the unstained portion of the specimen.
7. Using a thin capillary dropper, place 0.1 ml of anti–semen precipitin serum in the bottom of each tube.
8. Stratify the extract of **stain** over the precipitin serum in **tube 1**, the extract of known **semen** in **tube 2**, and the extract of the **unstained area** in **tube 3**. There should be a distinct line at the point of contact between the two liquids. Do *not* mix.
9. Let the tubes stand at room temperature for 1 hour, examining every 10 to 15 minutes. Look for a white coagulum, or precipitate, at the point of contact. Consult Table 22-13 for interpretation of results.

WHAT IS THE BLOOD GROUP?

The agglutinin inhibition test to determine the blood group of the individual from whom the semen was derived is made with extracts of the seminal stain and is adaptable to saliva and other body fluids (pp. 272 and 273). It should be made quantitatively similar to the inhibition test

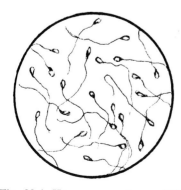

Fig. 22-4. Human spermatozoa. (×400.)

Table 22-13. Results possible in precipitin test for human semen

Unknown stain	Positive control	Negative control (unstained area)	Conclusions
+	+	−	Stain from human semen
−	+	−	Stain not from human semen
−	−	−	Result unreliable because positive control reacts negatively
+	+	+	Result unreliable because unstained portion reacts positively
+	−	−	Error; positive control reacts negatively
+	−	+	Result unreliable because unstained portion reacts positively and positive control reacts negatively

on saliva. The following is a qualitative test.

Dilute the anti-**A** and anti-**B** sera and the anti-**H** lectin to a titer of 4 to 8 units.

1. Prepare concentrated extracts of the stain and of the unstained portion. Do not dilute.
2. Label eight small Kahn tubes for identification of the antisera used.
3. Place 1 drop of the extracted stain in tubes 1, 3, 5, and 7.
4. Place 1 drop of the extracted unstained portion in tubes 2, 4, 6, and 8.
5. Add 1 drop of diluted anti-**A** serum to each of tubes 1, 2, 3, and 4.
6. Add 1 drop of diluted anti-**B** serum to tubes 5 and 6.
7. Add 1 drop of diluted anti-**H** lectin to tubes 7 and 8.
8. Mix and let stand at room temperature 1 hour, shaking occasionally.
9. Add 1 drop of A_1 cells to tubes 1 and 2, 1 drop of A_2 cells to tubes 3 and 4, 1 drop of B cells to tubes 5 and 6, and 1 drop of group O cells to tubes 7 and 8. These are 3% suspensions of red cells in saline.
10. Mix each tube and let the tubes stand at room temperature 60 minutes.
11. Observe macroscopically for agglutination and confirm by placing a small amount of the mixture from each tube on a labeled glass slide. Examine microscopically.
12. Cork the tubes and refrigerate 24 hours then read again.
13. Tubes 2, 4, 6, and 8 are controls and should all show agglutination.
14. If the reactions in tubes 1 and 3 are negative, the stain contains group-specific substance A, which neutralizes anti-A_1 and anti-A of the anti-**A** serum.

15. If the result in tube 5 is negative, the stain contains B.
16. If the first 6 tubes show positive reactions (agglutination), there are no group-specific substances in the stain, and it is therefore presumed either to have been derived from group O, or there was failure of inhibition. If it is group O, tube 7 should be negative, if the person from whom the stain was derived is a secretor.
17. If group-specific substance A is present without B, the blood group is A; if B is present without A, it is group B; if both A and B are present, it is group AB.
18. If the stain came from a nonsecretor of blood group–specific substances, there will be no inhibition of agglutinins anti-**A**, anti-**B**, or anti-**H**.

Table 22-14 shows the setup for the inhibition test on semen. Table 22-15 shows what results are possible in such a test.

The test depends on the power of group-specific substances to neutralize their corresponding agglutinin in a serum, so that when the proper cells are added (cells with which the agglutinin should react), there is no reaction. If there is agglutination, the agglutinin has not been neutralized. Group-specific substance A neutralizes anti-A and anti-**H**, substance B neutralizes anti-**B** and anti-**H**, and O neutralizes anti-**H** lectin alone. The antisera should be diluted to a titer of 5 to 10 units, at which point they should still be strongly reactive with their specific cells. See p. 271ff for **identification of secretor substances in saliva.**

Table 22-14. Setup for inhibition test to determine blood group of seminal stain

Tubes	1	2	3	4	5	6	7	8
1 drop of extract of +	Stain	Unstained portion	Stain	Unstained portion	Stain	Unstained portion	Stain	Unstained portion
1 drop of	Anti-**A** serum	Anti-**A** serum	Anti-**A** serum	Anti-**A** serum	Anti-**B** serum	Anti-**B** serum	Anti-**H** lectin	Anti-**H** lectin
			Mix and let stand at room temperature for 1 hour					
Add 1 drop of	A₁ cells	A₁ cells	A₂ cells	A₂ cells	B cells	B cells	O cells	O cells

Leave at room temperature 30 minutes, shaking each 5 minutes.

Record agglutination as positive (+), absence of agglutination as negative (−).

Table 22-15. Results of inhibition tests to determine blood group of seminal stains

			Tubes					
1	2	3	4	5	6	7	8	Conclusions
	+		+		+		+	Controls are correct
+	+	+	+	+	+	−	+	Stain derived from group O person
−	+	−	+	+	+	−	+	A₁ group-specific substance present
+	+	+	+	−	+	−	+	B group-specific substance present
−	+	−	+	−	+	−	+	Both A₁ and B group-specific substances present

Note: In the case of a nonsecretor of group-specific substance, there will be failure of inhibition, resulting in agglutination in all tubes.
+ = agglutination = no inhibition.
− = no agglutination = inhibition.

Table 22-16. Result of quantitative inhibition test for semen identification

Reagent	Test cells group	Undiluted	1:2	1:4	1:8	1:16	1:32	1:64	1:128	Conclusions
Anti-**A**	A	—	−	−	−	−	±	+ +	+ +	Group A
Anti-**B**	B	+ +	+ +	+ +	+ +	+ +	+ + ±	+ + +	+ + +	
Anti-**H**	O	−	±	+	+ +	+ +	+ +	+ + +	+ + +	
				Controls on unstained portion						
Anti-**A**	A	+ + +	+ + +	+ + +	+ + +	+ + +	+ + +	+ + +	+ + +	
Anti-**B**	B	+ + +	+ + +	+ + +	+ + +	+ + +	+ + +	+ + +	+ + +	
Anti-**H**	O	+ + +	+ + +	+ + +	+ + +	+ + +	+ + +	+ + +	+ + +	

Control tests are carried out just as the tests on the stained area. If the extract of the unstained portion inhibits the antisera, the results of the tests are unreliable.

Quantitative inhibition test for identification of seminal stains

1. Prepare the extract of the stain as described previously and identify it as human semen.
2. Prepare serial dilutions of the extract in saline: 1:2, 1:4, 1:8, 1:16, 1:32, 1:64, and 1:128 in the usual manner.
3. Test the undiluted extract and each of the dilutions as in the preceding test; mix 1 drop of the respective dilution of seminal stain with 1 drop of anti-**A** serum previously diluted to a titer of no more than 10 units (preferably 5 units), 1 drop with 1 drop of anti-**B** serum previously diluted to proper titer, and 1 drop with 1 drop of anti-**H** lectin.

4. Mix and let stand at room temperature for 1 hour.

5. Then add 1 drop of A_2 cells to the mixture of diluted extract and anti-**A** serum, 1 drop of B cells to the mixture of diluted extract and anti-**B** serum, and 1 drop of group O cells to the mixture of diluted extract and anti-**H** lectin.

6. Leave at room temperature 30 minutes, shaking each 5 minutes, then read.

7. Record agglutination as positive and the degree of agglutination from − to +++; absence of agglutination is recorded as negative (−).

Table 22-16 shows the results of one such test.

REFERENCES

1. Schatkin, S. B. In Gradwohl, R. B. H.: Legal medicine, St. Louis, 1954, The C. V. Mosby Co.
2. Schatkin, S. B.: Disputed paternity proceedings, ed. 4, New York, 1967, Matthew Bender & Co., Inc.
3. Wiener, A. S., and Socha, W. W.: A-B-O blood groups and Lewis types, New York, 1976, Stratton Intercontinental Medical Book Corporation.
4. Wiener, A. S., and Socha, W. W.: J. Forensic Sci. 21:42, 1976.
5. Dodd, B. E. In Camps, F. E.: Gradwohl's legal medicine, ed. 3, Bristol, England, 1976, John Wright & Sons, Ltd.; also Chicago, Year Book Medical Publishers, Inc.
6. Committee on Medicolegal Problems of the American Medical Association; J.A.M.A. 164:2036, 1957.
7. Wiener, A. S.: Lab. Digest 32(3-6), 1968; 33(1-6), 1969; 34(1-6), 1970; 35(1-6), 1971; 36(1-6), 1973.
8. Wiener, A. S.: Acta Genet. Med. Gemellol. (Rome) 18:285, 1969.
9. Sussman, L. N.: Paternity testing by blood grouping, ed. 2, Springfield, Ill., 1976, Charles C Thomas, Publisher.
10. Gradwohl, R. B. H.: Lab. Digest 18(10):10, 1955.
11. Gettler, A., and Kaye, S.: Milit. Surg. 93:2, 1943.
12. Uhlenhuth, P.: Deutsch. Med. Wochenschr. 27:1901.
13. Nuttall, G.: Blood immunity and blood relationship—the precipitin test for blood, Cambridge, England, 1904, Cambridge University Press.
14. Gradwohl, R. B. H.: Legal medicine, St. Louis, 1954, The C. V. Mosby Co.
15. Gradwohl, R. B. H.: Lab. Digest 15(9):4, 1952.
16. Gradwohl, R. B. H.: Lab. Digest 17(4):8, 1953.
17. Wiener, A. S., Gordon, E. B., Socha, W. W., and Moor-Jankowski, J.: Int. Arch. Allergy 39:368, 1970.
18. Duncan-Taylor, J. E., and Gordon, I.: Cited in Gradwohl, R. B. H.: Legal medicine, St. Louis, 1954, The C. V. Mosby Co.
19. Erskine, A. G. In Frankel, S., Reitman, S., and Sonnenwirth, A. C., editors: Gradwohl's clinical laboratory methods and diagnosis, ed. 7, St. Louis, 1970, The C. V. Mosby Co.
20. Wiener, A. S.: Blood groups and transfusion, ed. 3, Springfield, Ill., 1943, Charles C Thomas; reprinted New York, 1962, Hafner Publishing Co.
21. Kind, S. S.: Nature(Lond.) 185:397, 1960; 187:789, 1960.
22. Nickolls, L. C., and Pereira, M.: Med. Sci. Law 2:172, 1962.
23. Lincoln, P. J., and Dodd, B. E.: J. Forensic Sci. 13:37, 1973.
24. Lincoln, P. J., and Dodd, B. E.: Med. Sci. Law 15:94, 1975.
25. Wiener, A. S.: J. Forensic Med. 10:39, 1963.
26. Meaker, S. R.: Human sterility, Baltimore, 1934, The Williams & Wilkins Co.
27. Gelarie, A. J.: Am. J. Obstet. Gynecol. 21:1065, 1936.
28. Holbert, P. E.: J. Lab. Clin. Med. 22:320, 1936.
29. Williams, W. W., McGugan, A., and Carpenter, H. D.: J. Urol. 32:201, 1934.
30. Williams, W. W.: N. Engl. J. Med. 217:946, 1937.
31. Pollák, O. J., and Joël, C. A.: J.A.M.A. 113:395, 1939.
32. Reitman, S. In Frankel, S., Reitman, S., and Sonnenwirth, A. C., editors: Gradwohl's clinical laboratory methods and diagnosis, ed. 7, St. Louis, 1970, The C. V. Mosby Co.
33. Kaye, S. In Frankel, S., Feitman, S., and Sonnenwirth, A. C., editors: Gradwohl's clinical laboratory methods and diagnosis, ed. 7, St. Louis, 1970, The C. V. Mosby Co.
34. Baecchi: Vjschr. Gerichtl. Med. 34:1, 1912.
35. Hektoen, L., and Rukstinat, G. J.: Arch. Pathol. 6:96, 1928.

RECOMMENDED READING

Camps, F. E.: Gradwohl's legal medicine, ed. 2, Bristol, England, 1972; ed. 3, Bristol, England, 1976, John Wright & Sons, Ltd.

Prokop, O.: Lehrbuch der gerichtlichen Medizin, Berlin (GDR) 1960, VEB Verlag Volk und Gesundheit.

23 □ Mathematics and blood groups

In blood grouping a little mathematics can go a long way. The purpose of this chapter is to demonstrate how greater insight can be acquired into the blood groups and their heredity by applying elementary knowledge of algebra and probability theory.

THE M-N SYSTEM

The M-N system is used as the first example because of its simplicity. Even though the works of Wiener (1971) and of Springer (1971) indicate that the genetics is somewhat more complicated than commonly believed (pp. 103 and 104), the original simple two-gene theory of Landsteiner and Levine is still useful and suffices for the present, since for practical purposes the conclusions are the same.

According to the theory of Landsteiner and Levine, there are two allelic genes, M and N, that determine the corresponding agglutinogens M and N, respectively. In this case therefore tests with a single reagent suffice to identify each agglutinogen so that here there seems to be a 1:1:1 correspondence among gene M, agglutinogen M, and specificity **M**, as well as among gene N, agglutinogen N, and specificity **N**. Actually, the situation is more complex because each agglutinogen has multiple corresponding specificities. In the present context, however, the concept of a 1:1:1 correspondence will not interfere with the accuracy of the results or give rise to any errors. In this simple case there is also a 1:1 correspondence between phenotype and genotypes as follows: type M, genotype MM; type N, genotype NN; type MN, genotype MN.

Six different kinds of matings are possible, one being the mating M × M, in which case each parent is genotype MM and therefore can produce germ cells carrying gene M only. When fertilization occurs, the resulting zygotes are of genotypes MM only. In the mating M × M therefore all the children will be type M.

The most complex mating is MN × MN, which is analyzed by the checkerboard method as follows:

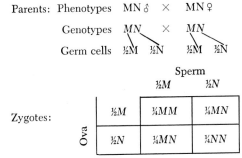

Parents: Phenotypes MN ♂ × MN ♀
Genotypes MN × MN
Germ cells ½M ½N ½M ½N

	Sperm ½M	½N
½M	¼MM	¼MN
½N	¼MN	¼NN

Zygotes: (Ova)

Children: Genotypes ¼MM; ½MN; ¼NN
Phenotypes 25% M; 50% MN; 25% N

In this analysis, use has been made of the **law of probability** that if an event has a **frequency**, or **probability**, p, and another independent event has a frequency, or probability, q, the chance that both events will occur simultaneously is the product of the two probabilities, or pq. For example, since in this case half of the sperm carry gene M and half of the ova also carry gene M, then one fourth of the zygotes will be genotype MM ($\frac{1}{2} \times \frac{1}{2} = \frac{1}{4}$). In the same

349

way the other matings are worked out with the results for all six matings as shown in Table 23-1.

The most extensive studies on the heredity of the M-N types were those of Wiener et al.[1] A summary of their findings for the years 1929 to 1962 is shown in Table 23-2. A study of the table shows that the **arithmetical fit** between the observations and expectations under the theory is close, even though there are seven children that do not seem to belong, but these seven exceptions were evidently all due to illegitimacy.

The genetic theory can also be tested by studies on the distribution of the M-N types in the general population, applying the methods of **population genetics**. In this case, instead of analyzing each kind of mating separately, the population as a whole is considered as undergoing **random mat-

ing (panmixia)**. Instead of considering the frequency of germ cells carrying genes M and N in the two parents of a single family, the frequencies of these germ cells in the population are considered as a whole. Since the distribution of the M-N blood types is the same in the two sexes, so must the frequencies of germ cells carrying M and N be the same in the two sexes. To germ cells carrying gene M, the frequency m may thus be assigned and to germ cells carrying gene N, the frequency n; thus $m + n = 1$ or 100%. Assuming panmixia, the following checkerboard results:

		Sperm cells	
Gene frequency		M (m)	N (n)
Ova $\{$ M	(m)	MM; m^2	MN; mn
N	(n)	MN; mn	NN; n^2

Frequencies of zygotes:
Genotype $MM = m^2$; genotype $MN = 2mn$
genotype $NN = n^2$

If the values m and n, respectively, are assigned to the frequencies of genes M and N among the germ cells, and $m + n = 1$, the three M-N types and corresponding three genotypes will be distributed in a population undergoing panmixia according to the three terms of the following expanded binomial:

$$(m + n)^2 = m^2 + 2mn + n^2$$

This is known as the **Hardy-Weinberg law**[2,3] because it was first stated in 1908 by Hardy, a British mathematician and by

Table 23-1. Heredity of the M-N types in families

Matings (parents)	Percent of children of types		
	M	**N**	**MN**
M × M	100	0	0
N × N	0	100	0
M × N	0	0	100
M × MN	50	0	50
N × MN	0	50	50
MN × MN	25	25	50

Table 23-2. Studies on heredity of the M-N types from 1929 to 1962[*]

Parents	Number of families		Children of types			
			M	**N**	**MN**	**Totals**
M × M	195	Number	397	0	(2)[†]	399
M × N	215	Number	(1)[†]	0	443	444
N × N	77	Number	0	135	0	135
M × MN	585	Number	626	(1)[†]	574	1,201
		Percent	52.1 ± 1.0	0.8	47.8 ± 1.0	
N × MN	425	Number	(3)[†]	453	482	938
		Percent	0.3	48.3 ± 1.1	51.4 ± 1.1	
MN × MN	499	Number	260	249	523	1,032
		Percent	25.2 ± 0.9	24.1 ± 0.9	50.7 ± 1.0	
Totals	1,996		1,287	838	2,024	4,149

[*]Modified from Wiener et al.: Exp. Med. Surg. **21**:89, 1963.
[†]These apparent contradictions to the laws of heredity are believed to be due to illegitimacy.

Weinberg, a German physician, independently of one another.

It is possible to estimate the frequency of the genes *M* and *N* from the distribution of the three M-N types in a population. One method is the so-called **square root method,** as follows:

Since

$$\overline{M} = m^2 \qquad (1)$$

$$\overline{MN} = 2mn \qquad (2)$$

$$\overline{N} = n^2 \qquad (3)$$

then:

$$m = \sqrt{\overline{M}} \qquad (4)$$

$$\text{and } n = \sqrt{\overline{N}} \qquad (5)$$

(The bar above the symbol for the type is used to indicate that the *frequency* of the type in the population is intended.)

The fact that when *m* and *n* are calculated in this way it is found that $m + n = \sqrt{\overline{M}} + \sqrt{\overline{N}}$ closely approximates unity, or 100%, is support for the genetic theory.

The second method of estimating the gene frequency is by **direct count,** which is possible in this case because each phenotype has only a single corresponding genotype. Thus all the germ cells of type M persons carry gene *M*, all the germ cells of type N persons carry gene *N*, and half the germ cells of type MN persons carry gene *M* and half carry gene *N*. Therefore:

$$m = \overline{M} + \tfrac{1}{2}\overline{MN} \qquad (6)$$

$$n = \overline{N} + \tfrac{1}{2}\overline{MN} \qquad (7)$$

The preceding estimates of the frequency of genes *M* and *N* are more precise than those given by the square root formulas and correspond to the so-called "maximum likelihood" estimates of Fisher; there is the additional advantage that they necessarily add up to 100%.

Having now derived the frequency of genes *M* and *N* with the aid of **direct count** formulas 6 and 7, the **expected frequency** of the three M-N types can be calculated with the aid of formulas 1 to 3. Then the χ^2 test is applied to compare the expected phenotype frequencies with those actually observed, as a test of the genetic theory.[4]

The purpose of the χ^2 test is to determine what is the probability of obtaining merely *by chance* a deviation from the expected ratio greater than that shown by observed data. In other words, the purpose of this test is to find out whether the calculated value of χ^2 is sufficiently great to refute a **null hypothesis** that the discrepancy between theoretically expected frequencies of the three M-N types and those actually observed could have arisen by chance. Example: if for the three phenotypes the following frequencies (or numbers of individuals) are observed, $\overline{M} = a$, $\overline{MN} = b$, and $\overline{N} = c$, then

$$\chi^2 = \frac{(b^2 - 4ac)^2 \, V}{(2a + b)^2 (b + 2c)^2}$$

where V is the total number of individuals tested.

Table 23-3 shows the application of the χ^2 test to a few population studies, as a test of the two-allele theory.

In Table 23-3, values of χ^2 were calculated separately for each set of observations. The values ranged from as little as 0.0089 to as much as 12.17. To find the **probability** (P) that the χ^2 of a given magnitude will be obtained if chance alone is responsible for the deviation, a **table of the distribution of** χ^2 must be consulted. Since, in general, χ^2 is bound to be larger as the number of items of data increases, this must be taken into consideration by ascertaining the number of **degrees of freedom** with which the table for χ^2 should be entered. The number of degrees of freedom is obtained as the number of classes whose frequency may be assigned arbitrarily without changing the total number of items. In our example, for instance, there is one degree of freedom; by consulting the table of distribution of χ^2 for one degree of freedom, corresponding values of P are found. Most of the sets of observations cited in Table 23-3 show a **good fit** with expectation, the values of P being well above 0.05 (5%), which is considered to be the borderline of **statistical significance.**

With the exception of the report of Lattes and Garrasi, the observations support the genetic theory. The findings of Lattes and Garrasi are so strikingly out of line that they point up another application of mathematics in blood grouping, that is, as a method of detecting errors in blood typing. As previously shown, the frequency of type MN $= 2\ mn$. Since $m + n = 1$, type MN has its maximum frequency when $m = n = \frac{1}{2}$, that is, the **maximum possible** frequency for type MN is $2(\frac{1}{2})(\frac{1}{2})$ or

50%. However, in the series of 430 persons tested by Lattes and Garrasi, the frequency 57.4% was obtained, so that at least thirty persons must have been incorrectly typed in this relatively short series.

The occurrence of gross technical errors in M-N typing is also evident when the reports on family studies are analyzed. In the mating MN × MN, there should be 25% type M children, 25% type N, and 50% type MN. However, in many of the pub-

Table 23-3. Chi-square (χ^2) test of the theory of Landsteiner and Levine on heredity of the M-N types[*]

Investigator	Frequency of type			Number of individuals examined	χ^2	P
	MN	M	N			
Landsteiner-Levine						
Whites (N.Y.)	53.6	26.1	20.3	532	3.04	0.09
Negroids	47.5	27.6	24.9	181	0.35	0.55
American Indians	35.12	60.00	4.88	205	0.021	0.89
Wiener-Vaisberg						
Families (Brooklyn)	48.23	30.53	21.24	904	0.66	0.42
Schiff						
Berlin	49.44	30.94	19.62	3,333	0.0089	0.92
Thomsen-Clausen						
Copenhagen	44.57	29.86	25.57	442	1.36	0.24
Lattes-Garrasi						
Italians	57.4	27.2	15.4	430	12.17	<0.001

[*]Modified from Wiener, A. S.: Blood groups and transfusion, ed. 3, Springfield, Ill., 1943, Charles C Thomas, Publisher; reprinted New York, 1962, Hafner Publishing Co.

Table 23-4. Analysis of mating MN × MN from reported studies on heredity of the M-N types[*]

Investigators	Number of families	Types of children				Percent of type MN children[†]
		M	N	MN	Totals	
Dahr	57	29	24	165	218	75.7 ± 1.9
Matta	20	9	10	45	64	70.3 ± 4.4
Taylor and Prior	23	10	8	38	56	67.5 ± 4.2
Lattes and Garrasi	54	16	17	65	98	66.3 ± 3.2
Dahr, Offe, and Weber	33	25	17	62	104	59.6 ± 3.2
Landsteiner and Levine	11	17	7	31	55	56.4 ± 4.5
Schiff	33	18	22	48	88	54.5 ± 3.7
Wiener et al.	499	260	249	523	1,032	50.7 ± 1.0
Harford	34	24	14	37	75	49.3 ± 3.9
Hauge	26	26	22	44	92	46.0 ± 3.3
Blaurock	23	25	25	40	90	44.4 ± 3.8
Totals (a)[‡]	1,068	630	565	1,510	2,705	55.8 ± 0.7
Totals (b)[§]	569	370	316	987	1,673	59.0 ± 0.8

[*]Modified from Wiener et al.: Exp. Med. Surg. 21:89, 1963. [‡]Totals of all investigators, some of whom are not listed here.
[†]Figure after the ± sign represents the probable error. [§]Totals not including the data of Wiener et al.

lished findings a great excess of children of type MN has been reported, as shown in Table 23-4. This was interpreted by Race and Sanger in the first edition of their book *Blood Groups in Man* as an example of "the phenomenon of the heterozygote being favoured by selection." However, it takes but a glance at the table to show that the reported findings are grossly heterogeneous, and it is inconceivable that the frequency of type MN children reported by Dahr, 75.7 ± 1.9, which deviates from that reported by Wiener et al., 50.7 ± 1.0, is merely due to statistical chance. It is also inconceivable that the theory could hold in New York City where Wiener did his studies and fail in Germany where Dahr worked. The tests of Dahr must have included a high percentage of technical errors, presumably due to using underabsorbed reagents, which would give rise to false positive reactions.

A-B-O GROUPS

The statistical analysis for the A-B-O groups is similar in principle to the M-N types, although it is somewhat more complicated because of the larger number of allelic genes involved. According to the original theory of von Dungern and Hirszfeld, the four A-B-O groups were assumed to be inherited by two independent pairs of allelic genes, *A-a* and *B-b*, respectively, with genes *A* and *B* determining the corresponding agglutinogens A and B, and genes *a* and *b* determining their absence. According to this theory, the possible genotypes corresponding to the four blood groups are as shown in Table 23-5.

Table 23-5. Theory of von Dungern and Hirszfeld

Blood groups (phenotypes)	Genotypes
O	*aabb*
A	*AAbb* and *Aabb*
B	*aaBB* and *aaBb*
AB	*AABB, AaBB, AABb,* and *AaBb*

Since the gene pairs *A-a* and *B-b* are independent, then, as Bernstein[5] pointed out, as a result of random mating over thousands of generations, the agglutinogens A and B should be distributed in the population independently of one another; that is, the frequency of agglutinogen A in persons having agglutinogen B should be the same as among persons lacking agglutinogen B. This would give rise to the following equation:

$$\frac{\overline{AB}}{\overline{B} + \overline{AB}} = \frac{\overline{A}}{\overline{O} + \overline{A}}$$

Clearing fractions and canceling like terms:

$$\overline{O} \times \overline{AB} = \overline{A} \times \overline{B} \qquad (8)$$

However, when Bernstein[6] applied this formula to the data published by the Hirszfelds, who typed population groups in the Macedonian front during World War I, he found that in general $\overline{A} \times \overline{B}$ was considerably larger than $\overline{O} \times \overline{AB}$ so that the theory did not hold.

Bernstein then proposed his own **theory of triple allelic genes,** which has already been described in this text, in which allele *A* determines agglutinogen A, allele *B* determines agglutinogen B, and allele *O* is an amorph. If the method of population genetics as described for the three M-N types is applied to this theory, then to the frequency of gene *A* could be assigned the value of *p*, to the frequency of gene *B* the value of *q*, and to gene *O* the value or *r*. The following **checkerboard** then results:

		Sperm cells		
		A(p)	*B(q)*	*O(r)*
Ova	*A(p)*	*AA(p²)*	*AB(pq)*	*AO(pr)*
	B(q)	*AB(pq)*	*BB(q²)*	*BO(qr)*
	O(r)	*AO(pr)*	*BO(qr)*	*OO(r²)*

Thus the frequencies of the six genotypes corresponding to the six terms of the expanded trinomial $(p + q + r)^2$ and the frequencies of the four phenotypes in terms of the frequencies of the genes are as follows:

$$\overline{O} \ (OO) = r^2 \qquad (9)$$

$$\overline{A} \ (AA \text{ and } AO) = p^2 + 2pr \qquad (10)$$

$$\overline{B} \ (BB \text{ and } BO) = q^2 + 2qr \qquad (11)$$

$$\overline{AB} \ (AB) = 2pq \qquad (12)$$

In this case the gene frequencies cannot be estimated by direct count because groups A and B have more than one corresponding genotype, and **square root formulas** must be used as follows:

$$r = \sqrt{\overline{O}} \qquad (13)$$

$$\overline{O} + \overline{B} = r^2 + 2\ qr + q^2 = (q + r)^2$$

Thus:

$$q + r = \sqrt{\overline{O} + \overline{B}}$$

and

$$p = 1 - (q + r) = 1 - \sqrt{\overline{O} + \overline{B}} \qquad (14)$$

Similarly:

$$q = 1 - \sqrt{\overline{O} + \overline{A}} \qquad (15)$$

but

$$p + q + r = 1$$

Therefore:

$$(1 - \sqrt{\overline{O} + \overline{B}}) + (1 - \sqrt{\overline{O} + \overline{A}}) + \sqrt{\overline{O}} = 1 \ (16)$$

or

$$\sqrt{\overline{O} + \overline{A}} + \sqrt{\overline{O} + \overline{B}} - \sqrt{\overline{O}} = 1$$

The equation $p + q + r = 1$ represents an ideal situation that, in practice, rarely materializes. In most studies, the sum of three gene frequencies, p, q, and r, does not equal 1.00 exactly. To obtain better estimates of gene frequencies, a simple method devised by Bernstein can be used: The raw values of p and q (obtained by formulas 14 and 15) are multiplied by a correction factor

$$1 + \frac{D}{2}$$

where

$$D = \sqrt{\overline{O} + \overline{A}} + \sqrt{\overline{O} + \overline{B}} - \sqrt{\overline{O}} - 1$$

The corrected value of r (r') is then found from

$$r' = 1 - p' - q'$$

where p' and q' represent the corrected values of p and q.

For most practical purposes, however, the simplest way of adjusting the estimated gene frequencies is merely by dividing each one of the raw values, p, q, and r, by the sum of $p + q + r$.

The fact that the population statistics of the Hirszfelds cited previously satisfied the formula 16 was evidence in support of Bernstein's triple allele theory in contrast to the theory of two independent pairs of alleles. Points of controversy, however, were the published reports of family studies. According to the triple allele theory, parents of group AB (genotype *AB*) could not have group O (genotype *OO*) children and parents of group O could not have group AB children. However, these combinations could occur according to the theory of von Dungern and Hirszfeld, provided that the group AB person was doubly heterozygous, genotype *AaBb*. The contradictions to the Bernstein theory could not all be ascribed to illegitimacy because included in the reports were mothers of group AB with group O children and vice versa. Bernstein asserted that the numerous published contradictions to his genetic theory were due to technical errors in blood grouping. This argument was supported by the fact that family studies carried out *after* Bernstein announced his theory suddenly included hardly any contradictions to the theory.

Wiener called attention to another way of checking for the occurrence of errors in blood grouping by analyzing the mating A × B. This particular mating gives the same results according to both theories, as shown in Table 23-6, and since children of all four groups—O, A, B, and AB—can occur in these families, apparently no attention was paid to them when the results of family studies were analyzed.

If the first kind of mating includes *a* children, the second kind of mating 2*b* children, the third 2*c* children, and the fourth 4*d* children, then in the combined results of all four kinds of A × B matings there will be *d* group O children, (*b* + *d*) group A, (*c* + *d*) group B, and (*a* + *b* + *c* + *d*) group AB children. Therefore

Table 23-6. Analysis of mating A × B, according to the two theories of heredity of the A-B-O blood groups

Genotypes of parents according to		Percent of children of group			
Triple allele theory	Theory of independent pairs of alleles	O	A	B	AB
$AA \times BB$	$AAbb \times aaBB$	0	0	0	100
$AA \times BO$	$AAbb \times aaBb$	0	50	0	50
$AO \times BB$	$Aabb \times aaBB$	0	0	50	50
$AO \times BO$	$Aabb \times aaBb$	25	25	25	25

$$\overline{AB} - \overline{O} = (a + b + c + d) - d = a + b + c$$
$$\overline{A} - \overline{O} = b$$
$$\overline{B} - \overline{O} = c$$

so that

$$(\overline{AB} - \overline{O}) \geqq (\overline{A} - \overline{O}) + (\overline{B} - \overline{O})$$

However, as Wiener showed in the combined published reports between the years 1910 and 1927, not including the work of Snyder, Schiff, or Thomsen, there were 483 A × B families that produced 1123 children, of which there were 188 group O, 367 group A, 298 group B, 270 group AB. Thus

$$\overline{AB} - \overline{O} = 82$$

whereas

$$(\overline{A} - \overline{O}) + (\overline{B} - \overline{O}) = 179 + 110 = 289$$

This indicates that there must have been at least 200 mistakes in blood grouping in this series of 1123 children from A × B families. Buining, on the other hand, in 1932, reported family studies including 336 A × B matings in which there were 225 group O children, 285 group A, 274 group B, and 338 group AB. In these families therefore

$$\overline{AB} - \overline{O} = 113$$

whereas

$$(\overline{A} - \overline{O}) + (\overline{B} - \overline{O}) = 60 + 49 = 109$$

In Buining's families therefore there was an excellent fit with the expectations independent of the theory of heredity.

This analysis shows how a little elemen-tary algebra or arithmetic can expose errors in technic. It also points up the vast numbers of mistakes made in the early days of blood grouping, which may seem inconceivable to those accustomed to modern methods using commercially prepared high-titered reagents. It may be salutary to point to the high frequency of mistakes in blood grouping that occurred as recently as the 1940s when mass blood grouping of the armed forces resulted in errors as high as 11% in simple A-B-O grouping. This high incidence of error, however, was due in part to confusion in nomenclature, which was terminated when the Division of Biological Standards instituted labeling of the antisera simply as anti-**A** and anti-**B** and not as group III and group II, respectively. This analysis also vindicates Bernstein's decision that the seeming contradictions to the triple allele theory in family studies were actually due to errors in blood grouping. His genetic theory is presently accepted. The theory of von Dungern and Hirszfeld is seldom even mentioned in modern textbooks. It is discussed here only because of its historic and instructive value.

The analysis according to the method of population genetics can readily be extended to include the subgroups of A, bearing in mind that it is now necessary to postulate the four allelic genes O, A^1, A^2, and B instead of three alleles.

If one indicates the frequencies of the four alleles by the symbols p_1, p_2, q, and r, respectively, the derivation of the formulas for the gene frequencies in terms of the observed phenotype frequencies follows, in general, the same rules as when dealing with three allelic genes, with the exception that p is split into two new values, p_1 and p_2.

First, the gene frequencies p, q, and r are calculated as already described. Then the two relationships are considered:

$$\overline{O} = r^2$$
$$\overline{A}_2 = p_2^2 + 2p_2 r \qquad (17)$$

Thus

$$\overline{O} + \overline{A}_2 = (p_2 + r)^2 \qquad (18)$$

or

$$p_2 + r = \sqrt{\overline{O} + \overline{A}_2} \qquad (19)$$

so that

$$p_2 = (p_2 + r) - r \qquad (20)$$

or

$$p_2 = \sqrt{\overline{O} + \overline{A}_2} - \sqrt{\overline{O}} \qquad (21)$$

The value of p_1 is then easily calculated, since it equals $p - p_2$.

Rh-Hr TYPES

In the first studies on the heredity of the Rh-Hr blood types, only a reagent with a single specificity, anti–rhesus monkey guinea pig serum, and its counterpart, human anti-Rh serum, were available for testing. These reagents define only two types, Rh positive and Rh negative. In the first family studies by Landsteiner and Wiener in 1941 (Table 23-7), it was necessary to postulate only a pair of allelic genes, Rh, determining the Rh agglutinogen, and rh, determining its absence, so that there were three genotypes, corresponding to the two phenotypes as follows:

Rh positive ⟨ Genotype *RhRh* / Genotype *Rhrh*

Rh negative   Genotype *rhrh*

Rh-positive individuals could be either homozygous or heterozygous, whereas Rh-negative persons were always necessarily homozygous. In their early studies, Landsteiner and Wiener found 15.4% Rh-negative persons among 448 tested. From this, the frequencies of the two allelic genes could be estimated from the square root formulas as follows:

$$rh = \sqrt{\text{Rh negative}} = \sqrt{0.154} = 39.2\%$$

$$Rh = 1 - rh = 1 - 39.2\% = 60.8\%$$

Using these gene frequencies, the proportion of homozygous and heterozygous Rh-positive persons could readily be calculated as follows:

Genotype *RhRh* $= (0.608)^2 = 36.96\%$

Genotype *Rhrh* $= 2 \times 0.608 \times 0.392 = 47.67\%$

Slightly more than half of the Rh-positive individuals are therefore heterozygous.

It may be mentioned in passing that in families having babies with Rh hemolytic disease, the great majority of the Rh-positive fathers are homozygous for the Rh factor, the reason for which should be apparent.

The application of population genetics to the Rh-Hr system becomes more complex as more and more reagents are included in the tests, but the principles are unchanged. One must bear in mind, however, that there is not a 1:1 correspondence between

Table 23-7. Hereditary transmission of the Rh factor[*]

Mating	Number of families	Number of children		
		Rh positive	Rh negative	Totals
Rh+ × Rh−	42	151	7	158
Rh+ × Rh−	12	37	11	48
Rh− × Rh−	6	0	31	31
Totals	60	188	49	237

[*]From Landsteiner, K., and Wiener, A. S.: J. Exp. Med. 74:309, 1941.

the agglutinogens and blood factors (serologic specificities). Table 23-8 shows the situation when only the six standard anti–Rh-Hr sera are taken into account, in which case a minimum of eight allelic genes must be postulated.

The assumption of eight allelic genes implies thirty-six possible genotypes (for n allelic genes there are $\frac{1}{2}n[n + 1]$ genotypes). Using the six antisera, anti-**Rh$_o$**, anti-**rh'**, anti-**rh''**, anti-**hr'**, anti-**hr''**, and anti-**hr**, twenty different phenotypes can be distinguished so that there are obviously, in this case, many more genotypes than phenotypes.

The phenotypes corresponding to any given genotype are determined by simply adding reactions that the two genes comprising the genotypes produce, as in Table 23-9.

Since the same results are produced by adding the reactions of genes R^1 and R^o and of genes R^o and r', there are altogether three genotypes corresponding to the

Table 23-8. The eight "standard" Rh-Hr allelic genes and their corresponding agglutinogens (after Wiener)

Gene	Agglutinogen	Blood factors (specificities)
r	rh	**hr'**, **hr''**, and **hr**
r'	rh'	**rh'** and **hr''**
r''	rh''	**rh''** and **hr'**
r^y	rh$_y$	**rh'** and **rh''**
R^o	Rh$_o$	**Rh$_o$**, **hr'**, **hr''**, and **hr**
R^1	Rh$_1$	**Rh$_o$**, **rh'**, and **hr''**
R^2	Rh$_2$	**Rh$_o$**, **rh''**, and **hr'**
R^z	Rh$_z$	**Rh$_o$**, **rh'**, and **rh''**

Table 23-9. Reactions of phenotype corresponding to genotype R^1r

	Reaction for					
Genotype R^1r	Rh$_o$	rh'	rh''	hr'	hr''	hr
Gene R^1	+	+	−	−	+	−
Gene r	−	−	−	+	+	+
Sum of reactions	+	+	−	+	+	+

phenotype Rh$_1$rh, which are genotypes R^1r, R^1R^o, and R^or'. This is the way that Table 8-3 was constructed, although that table is slightly more complex because it includes the reactions of a seventh antiserum, anti-**rh^w**.

Gene frequency analysis is the same in principle as for the A-B-O and M-N types. The formulas derived by Wiener for the six more common genes are as follows:

$$r = \sqrt{rh} \tag{22}$$
$$r' = \sqrt{rh' + rh} - \sqrt{rh} \tag{23}$$
$$r'' = \sqrt{rh'' + rh} - \sqrt{rh} \tag{24}$$
$$R^o = \sqrt{Rh_o + rh} - \sqrt{rh} \tag{25}$$
$$R^1 = \sqrt{Rh_1 + rh' + Rh_o + rh} - \sqrt{rh' + rh} - \frac{}{\sqrt{Rh_o + rh} + \sqrt{rh}} \tag{26}$$
$$R^2 = \sqrt{Rh_2 + rh'' + Rh_o + rh} - \sqrt{rh'' + rh} - \frac{}{\sqrt{Rh_o + rh} + \sqrt{rh}} \tag{27}$$

Some authors have suggested estimating the frequencies of the rare genes r^y and R^z by subtraction from 100%, but this method is fallacious, since, because of the statistical error, the sum of the estimated gene frequencies listed in the six formulas 22 through 27 could by chance exceed 100%, which would give the genes r^y and R^z an impossible negative frequency. Instead therefore Wiener suggested estimating the frequencies of the rare genes r^y and R^z directly from the frequencies of rare phenotypes having these genes. For example, phenotype Rh$_z$Rh$_1$ comprises the three genotypes R^zR^1, R^zr', and R^1r^y, but the last two are much rarer than the first and may therefore be disregarded when estimating the frequency of the gene R^z. Therefore to the phenotype Rh$_z$Rh$_1$ one may assign the frequency $2 \times R^z \times R^1$, where here the symbols R^z and R^1 represent the frequencies of the corresponding genes; but the frequency R^1 can be estimated by formula 26. Therefore

$$R^z = \frac{\overline{Rh_zRh_1}}{2\overline{R}^1}$$

in which $\overline{Rh_zRh_1}$ represents the observed frequency of the rare type Rh$_z$Rh$_1$ and $\overline{R}^1$ the estimated frequency of gene R^1.

Once the frequencies of six allelic genes have been calculated, the frequencies of the thirty-six different genotypes can be calculated, and even the frequencies of extremely rare phenotypes such as $rh_y rh_y$ can be estimated, as shown in Table 8-3.

THE Xg TYPES

The population genetics for the Xg system is different in that a sex-linked gene is involved. If the symbol Xg^a is used for the gene determining the agglutinogen Xg^a and the allelic gene xg is an amorph, then there are three genotypes among females and two genotypes among males as follows:

Xg(a+) females Genotype $Xg^a Xg^a$ (homozygous)
                Genotype $Xg^a xg$ (heterozygous)
Xg(a–) females Genotype $xg\, xg$
Xg(a+) males   Genotype $Xg^a Y$
Xg(a–) males   Genotype $xg\, Y$

Note that Xg(a+) females can be either **homozygous** or **heterozygous**, whereas Xg(a–) females are necessarily all homozygous. On the other hand, all males carry but a single Xg gene, whether Xg(a+) or Xg(a–), and are therefore said to be **hemizygous**. As noted on p. 185, tests on 342 Caucasoids showed the distribution to be females, 88.83% positive; males, 61.69% positive. The gene frequencies in the males is obvious by direct count, as in the following:

$$Xg^a = 0.6169 \text{ and } xg = 1 - 0.6169, \text{ or } 0.3831$$

In females the gene frequency must be estimated by square root formulas as follows:

and
$$xg = \sqrt{Xg(a-)} = \sqrt{0.1117} = 0.3344$$
$$Xg^a = 1 - xg = 0.6656$$

Theoretically the gene distribution should be the same in males and in females. As can be seen, the estimated gene frequencies for the two sexes do not differ more than one would expect, allowing for the size of the series.

CONTINGENCY TABLE

Whenever a new antibody is discovered and sufficient amount of data has been amassed, statistical methods are applied to determine whether the newly discovered specificity is or is not related to blood groups already known. In this way it is often possible to connect the new blood factor with one or another of the blood group systems. The simplest and most frequently used method of testing **association** (or **independence**) between two factors is by the so-called **2 x 2 contingency table.**

Assume that specificities X and Y are identified by the sera anti-X and anti-Y, respectively. When many blood samples are tested side by side with the two sera, four types of reactions may occur: ++, +–, –+, and ––. The results observed can be organized in the form of a 2×2 table, as shown in Table 23-10.

If the symbols a, b, c, and d represent the absolute numbers of blood samples that give reactions of four types, and if a + b = e, c + d = f, a + c = g, b + d = h, and e + f + g + h = N, the χ^2 test can be applied using the following formula:

$$\chi^2 = \frac{(ad - bc)^2\, N}{efgh}$$

As for the number of degrees of freedom in this case, one must bear in mind that in a 2×2 table the frequency of only one class can vary arbitrarily, whereas the frequencies of the three remaining classes are fixed by the totals; thus, there is only one degree of freedom. By consulting tables of the distribution of χ^2 for one degree of freedom, one can obtain the probability (P) of a value of χ^2 of the observed mag-

Table 23-10. 2×2 contingency table

	Reactions with anti-Y serum		
	+	–	Totals
Reactions with anti-X serum +	a	b	e
Reactions with anti-X serum –	c	d	f
Totals	g	h	N

nitude resulting from chance alone. If χ^2 is very large so that P is inordinately small, the findings are considered to have refuted the hypothesis of independence of the two blood factors X and Y. In other words, the χ^2 test indicates that there is a possibility of an association between factors X and Y. Obviously, the statistical test cannot solve the problem of the nature of that association; it suggests only that the two blood factors may prove to be inherited by corresponding allelic genes.

When the test is applied to two blood factors such as **A** and **M** of human blood, which belong to two different blood group systems, it will be found that the obtained value of χ^2 is small, in conformity with the requirements for independence.

The reader should be warned against indiscriminate use of the χ^2 test, particularly in cases when numbers of items are very small. When individual compartments in a 2×2 table contain five or less items, the obtained value of χ^2 may be greatly exaggerated, falsely indicating association between two actually unrelated factors. In such cases, a correction "for continuity" devised by Yates should be employed to artificially lower the value of χ^2. It is achieved by decreasing by one half those classes in a 2×2 table that exceed expectation and increasing by one half classes that are less than expected value.

The application of mathematical methods has proved not only useful but even irreplaceable in solving problems dealing with serology and heredity of blood groups. It has prevented some errors in the interpretation of data and has helped to avoid the drawing of sweeping conclusions from too short series of cases, by indicating the frequency with which similar observations could have resulted from chance alone. Unfortunately, it has also led, now and then, to some abuses of mathematics and to somewhat uncritical application of statistics by serologists who lack mathematical training and knowledge or by biometricians who, in turn, have no knowledge or understanding of serology to interpret their findings.

For example, as Wiener pointed out, there is a tendency among workers in the field of blood grouping to resort to the so-called maximum likelihood method to obtain highly accurate estimates of gene frequencies. Maximum likelihood calculations are complex and laborious and require a mastery of mathematics that few workers possess. Even in the hands of experts, gross errors have resulted when carrying out the laborious computations so that such calculations are not only expensive but also impractical and dangerous. As shown by Wiener, the results obtained by this highly sophisticated method differed only in the third decimal place from the values obtained by him with the aid of simple square root formulas. It is far more important to concentrate one's efforts on avoiding technical errors when performing blood grouping tests that can affect the accuracy of the first and second significant figures, than to waste valuable time in carrying out complex mathematical computations to achieve a dubious increase in "accuracy" that would affect the third or fourth significant figure.

The use of readily accessible calculators prompts many workers in the field to present the results of their computations with an exorbitant number of significant figures. In fact, no more significant figures should be used than are justified by the size of the series. For example, when frequencies of blood groups (or genes) are given for a population of a thousand individuals, introduction of more than three significant figures would be hardly justified.

REFERENCES

1. Wiener, A. S., Gordon, E. B., and Wexler, J. P.: Exp. Med. Surg. **21**:89, 1963; cited in Wiener, A. S.: Advances in blood grouping, vol. 2, New York, 1965, Grune & Stratton, Inc.
2. Hardy, G. H.: Science **28**:49, 1908.
3. Weinberg, W.: Jh. Ver. vaterl. Naturk, Wüttenb. **64**:368, 1908.
4. Wiener, A. S.: Med. Proc. **10**:559, 1964; reprinted in Wiener, A. S.: Advances in blood grouping, vol. 2, New York, 1965, Grune & Stratton, Inc.
5. Bernstein, F.: Klin. Wochenschr. **33**:1495; 1924; Z. Ind. Abst. Vererbgsl. **37**:237, 1925;

also reprinted in Selected contributions to the literature of blood groups and immunology, vol. 2, part 2, Ft. Knox, Ky., 1971, U.S. Army Medical Research Laboratory.
6. Bernstein, F.: Selected contributions to the literature of blood groups and immunology, vol. 4, part 1, Ft. Knox, Ky., 1971, U.S. Army Medical Research Laboratory.

RECOMMENDED READINGS

Carter, C. O.: Human heredity, Baltimore, 1951, Penguin Books, Inc.

Colin, E. C.: Elements of genetics, New York, 1956, McGraw-Hill Book Co., Inc.

Garlington, W. K., and Shimota, H. E.: Statistically speaking, Springfield, Ill., 1964, Charles C Thomas, Publisher.

Hoffmann, R. G.: Statistics for medical students, Springfield, Ill., 1963, Charles C Thomas, Publisher.

Levitan, M., and Montagu, M.: Textbook of human genetics, ed. 2, New York, 1977, Oxford University Press.

Li, C. C.: First course in population genetics, Pacific Grove, Calif., 1976, The Boxwood Press.

Moody, P. M.: Genetics of man, New York, 1967, W. W. Norton & Co., Inc.

Moroney, M. J.: Facts from figures, Baltimore, 1962, Penguin Books, Inc.

Rieger, R., Michaelis, A., and Green, M. M.: A glossary of genetics and cytogenetics, New York, 1968, Springer-Verlag.

Stern, C.: Principles of human genetics, ed. 2, San Francisco, 1973, W. H. Freeman Co.

Strickberger, M. W.: Genetics, New York, 1968, The Macmillan Co.

Wiener, A. S., and Wexler, I. B.: Heredity of the blood groups, New York, 1958, Grune & Stratton, Inc.

24 □ Methodology of blood grouping of apes and monkeys

The principles involved in human blood grouping can also be applied to determining the types in nonhuman primates so that only those aspects peculiar to blood grouping of simians need be discussed.

Tests on nonhuman primates fall into two main categories: tests for human-type blood factors and tests for simian-type blood factor.[1] Tests for human-type blood factors, as the term implies, are made with reagents originally prepared for typing human blood, and therefore detect homologues of the human blood groups. On the other hand, tests for simian-type blood factors are prepared by heteroimmunization and isoimmunization of animals using red cells of apes and monkeys for injection. Some of the simian-type blood factors detected by these reagents have been shown to be analogues of human blood groups.

DETERMINATION OF HUMAN-TYPE BLOOD GROUPS
A-B-O typing of apes

With the exception of gorillas, A-B-O typing of apes is done with the same technics as those used for testing human blood. However, prior to their use, the anti-**A** and anti-**B** sera of human origin have to be absorbed with group O red cells of chimpanzees to remove the nonspecific heteroagglutinins reactive for ape red cells. In tests for agglutinogen A, lectins from lima beans (*Phaseolus vulgaris*) as well as anti-**A** snail agglutinins (*Helix pomatia*) may be used without prior absorption, since they

do not contain heteroagglutinins. The snail agglutinins are very potent and can be highly diluted for testing.

All group A bloods from apes are further tested with anti-**A**$_1$ reagents. Anti-**A**$_1$ lectin (*Dolichos biflorus*) has the advantage that it can be used without prior absorption.

The A-B-O blood grouping results must be confirmed by reverse blood grouping tests on animal serum against human red cells of groups A$_1$, A$_2$, B, and O (used as a control) after the serum has been absorbed with human group O cells to remove nonspecific heteroagglutinins.

A-B-O typing of gorillas and Old World monkeys

Red cells of neither gorillas nor Old World monkeys can be used for A-B-O grouping because they do not react with anti-**A**, anti-**B**, or anti-**H** reagents. However, all gorillas and monkeys have proved to be secretors of the A-B-H substances in their saliva. The saliva is tested by inhibition technics, as in man, and reverse blood grouping tests for anti-**A** and anti-**B** are made on the sera of these animals. For the inhibition tests, the anti-**A**, anti-**B**, and anti-**H** reagents are diluted, depending on their titers, to yield reagents with 4 to 8 agglutinating units. The indicator cells for anti-**A** are human group A$_2$ red cells; human group B red cells are used for anti-**B**, and human group O cells for anti-**H**. The reagents do not have to be absorbed with

Table 24-1. Example of a protocol of the A-B-O blood grouping tests (quantitative saliva inhibition tests and reverse serum tests) in Old World monkeys

	Saliva inhibition test*															Serum test				Human-type A-B-O group
	Anti-A serum diluted 1:40 and group A_2 red cells					Anti-B serum diluted 1:5 and group B red cells					Anti-H lectin (Ulex) diluted 1:10 and group O red cells					Against human red cells of group				
	Dilutions of saliva																			
Saliva and serum of	1/1	1/4	1/16	1/64	1/256	1/1	1/4	1/16	1/64	1/256	1/1	1/4	1/16	1/64	1/256	O	A_1	A_2	B	
Baboons																				
1	-	-	-	-	+	++	++	++	++	++	-	-	-	-	-	-	-	-	+++	A
2	-	-	-	-	+	-	-	-	-	+	-	-	-	-	-	-	-	-	-	AB
3	++	++	++	++	++	-	-	-	-	+	-	-	-	-	+	-	+++	++	-	B
4	++	++	++	++	++	-	-	+w	-	+w	-	-	-	-	-	-	++	++	-	B
5	-	-	++	++	++	++	++	++	++	++	-	-	-	-	+	-	-	-	-	AB
Gelada	++	++	++	++	++	-	-	-	-	-	-	-	-	-	-	-	-	-	-	O(?)
Rhesus																				
1	++	++	++	++	++	++	++	++	++	++	-	-	-	-	+	-	++	++	-	B
2	++	++	++	++	++	-	-	+	++	++	-	-	-	-	-	-	+++	++	-	B
Human controls																				
A, Sec	-	-	-	-	+	++	++	++	++	++	-	-	-	+w	+					
B, Sec	++	++	++	++	++	-	-	-	+	++	-	-	-	+w	+					
O, Sec	++	++	++	++	++	++	++	++	++	++	-	-	-	-	+w					
nS	++	++	++	++	++	++	++	++	++	++	++	++	++	++	++					

*+w, one plus weak (or a weak one plus).

chimpanzee group O red cells before use because the indicator cells are of human origin, so that nonspecific heteroagglutinins are not involved. When carrying out the inhibition tests, it is better not to depend on a one-tube test. Instead, test the saliva in five fourfold dilutions to determine the inhibition titer. Table 24-1 shows a typical protocol of A-B-O blood grouping tests on saliva and serum samples from Old World monkeys.

M-N typing

For M-N typing, anti-**M** and anti-**N** reagents prepared from rabbit antisera are used as in routine human blood typing. Interference from heteroagglutinins is largely avoided by diluting these reagents so that, with some exceptions, they can be used directly and with the same technics as for man. Anti-**N**^{V} lectin (*Vicia graminea*), which detects an N-like specificity on human and ape red cells, can also be used with excellent results. In cases of weak reactions, when there may be some uncertainty as to whether the factor in question, for example **M**, is really present on the ape red cells, the reagent is absorbed with human M cells. This should eliminate the reactivity also for ape red cells if the weak reactions with the unabsorbed anti-**M** reagents were actually due to an **M** specificity of ape red cells.

Rh-Hr typing

Rh-Hr antisera of human origin are used for Rh-Hr typing, and the same methods are applied as for testing human red cells. In our hands, the ficinated red cell technic gives dependable results with the least effort. Further tests are necessary to determine whether the reagents contain nonspecific heteroagglutinins for ape blood; no simple method has been devised to remove these without weakening the type-specific antibodies. However, when the reagents give negative reactions in direct tests on ape blood, the specificity being tested for is obviously absent from the tested cells. If, on the other hand, positive

reactions are observed, further tests are required to determine whether these are type specific or due to other antibodies in the reagent. One of the methods used is to titrate with the positively reacting simian red cells in parallel with Rh-positive human red cells. Since the reagents used are of high titer, similarity of titers may be considered evidence that the reactions are indeed type specific.

Other human-type blood factors

The reagents for testing most other human blood groups are generally of low titer; therefore the results are poorly reproducible even in man, and the reagents are unsuitable for testing simian red cells because of the interference of nonspecific heteroagglutinins.

DETERMINATION OF SIMIAN-TYPE BLOOD GROUPS
Production of reagents

The simian-type reagents have been produced mostly by isoimmunization, thus avoiding the interference of heteroagglutinins. In most instances, the immunizations are carried out by intramuscular injections, at monthly intervals, of a mixture of 1 ml of packed, washed red cells and an equal volume of complete (or incomplete) Freund's adjuvant. Usually, after three or four courses of immunization, the recipient animals respond with a sufficient titer and are subjected to plasmapheresis while the titers are at their peak. Titers of 1:16 and over are considered to be adequate for routine blood grouping work in apes and monkeys.

The tests

The methods of testing and titrating the antisera obtained are the same as in human blood typing: the saline agglutination, the antiglobulin, the ficinated red cell methods, and, at times, the ficinated red cell antiglobulin technic. In most cases, the antiglobulin sera used for the tests are prepared by immunizing rabbits with the serum of the species being studied, but anti–human rabbit globulin can also be used with almost as good results. However, the anti–human as well as anti–monkey globulin sera must first be absorbed with pooled, washed simian red cells.

The reason that all three methods— saline agglutination, antiglobulin, and ficin —should be used is that different antibodies react by different technics, and not so infrequently several fractions can be separated from one and the same serum merely by the use of different methods.[2] Moreover, the specificities on the simian red cells can at times be classified according to their reactivity by different methods. For example, specificities reactive by the antiglobulin method but not by the ficin technic are supposed to belong to blood group systems analogous to the human M-N-S and the chimpanzee V-A-B systems. Specificities reactive by the ficin as well as the antiglobulin technic presumably belong to blood group systems analogous to the human Rh-Hr system and the chimpanzee C-E-F system.

One pitfall is the occurrence of a prozone in titrations of freshly obtained simian sera using the ficin method. Obviously, if only one-tube tests were done with such antisera, false negative reactions could result. If the serum is inactivated, however, by heating for half an hour at 56° C, the prozone disappears, showing that it was due to interference from complement present in the fresh serum. The presence of complement is sometimes apparent when hemolysis occurs in the first few tubes of the titration. Instead of inactivating the serum, the titration can be converted to the antiglobulin method by washing the red cells in each tube and then adding antiglobulin serum, whereupon the prozones disappear.

Isoimmune sera can be used not only for blood typing within the same species but also in closely related species; for example, isoimmune rhesus sera can be used for typing crab-eating macaques, chimpanzee isoimmune sera can be used for typing gorillas, and, as shown recently, also for typing human red cells.[3]

A different kind of reagent is produced by immunization with blood from closely related species. Example, baboons cross immunized with gelada red cells produced antibodies not only reactive for gelada red cells but also defined individual differences in baboons.[4]

REFERENCES

1. Wiener, A. S., Moor-Jankowski, J., and Socha, W. W.: Transplant. Proc. **4**:101, 1972.
2. Socha, W. W., Wiener, A. S., Gordon, E. B., and Moor-Jankowski, J.: Transplant. Proc. **4**:107, 1972.
3. Socha, W. W., and Moor-Jankowski, J.: Int. Arch. Allergy Appl. Immunol. Int. Arch. Allergy **56**:30, 1978.
4. Moor-Jankowski, J., Wiener, A. S., Socha, W. W., Gordon, E. B., and Davis, J. H.: J. Med. Primatol. **2**:71, 1973.

Glossary

The meanings of the following terms are restricted to their use in blood grouping serology, immunohematology, and immunogenetics.

absorption Removal of antibodies from a serum by mixing cells having the appropriate antigen with the serum for a time long enough to permit the antibodies to attach themselves to the red cells. The antibody-antigen complexes thus formed are removed from the serum, usually by centrifugation; the remaining serum is then virtually free of the absorbed antibody (as well as the added antigen).

adsorption The process by which antibodies are attached to the surface of the red cells having the specific antigen. The antibodies can then be eluted from the red cells.

agglutination Clumping of cells. In blood grouping, it is clumping of red cells by action of an antibody in serum (**agglutinin**) on the antigen (**agglutinogen**) in or on the cells. The reaction between an antibody and an antigen is an **antigen-antibody reaction** and is the means by which the antigen is identified if the antibody is known or the antibody is identified if the antigen is known. The reaction is a **specific reaction** and is the usual basis for identification of the blood groups.

agglutinin Immune substance, or antibody, present in serum and so named because it causes agglutination. It is formed as a result of an antigen stimulus and reacts with the antigen that called it into being. Agglutinins are present in plasma and removable also in serum. They may be either **naturally occurring** or **induced**. Cross-reactions can occur, such as selected anti-A sera that react with sheep red cells having an A-like agglutinogen, as well as with human red cells of groups A and AB. Antibodies are proteins.

agglutinogen Substance present on the surface of the red cells that combine with a specific anti-body with a resulting reaction, usually clumping (**agglutination**), but in some cases **hemolysis**. Each agglutinogen (**intrinsic attribute**) has multiple **serologic specificities** (**extrinsic attributes**), that is, an agglutinogen can react with more than one antibody; the specificities are also called **blood group factors** in the case of red cells. Each factor, or specificity, of an agglutinogen may stimulate production of or combine with a different specific antibody. Thus agglutinogen Rh_1, for example, has the factors Rh_o, rh', Rh^A, Rh^B, Rh^C, Rh^D, hr'', among others.

alleles; allelic genes; allelomorphic genes Different genes located at the same point, or **locus**, of a particular pair of **chromosomes**. Each kind of allele affects a particular characteristic somewhat differently from the others. All the alternate genes that can be situated at a given locus are allelic, or allelomorphic. Frequently, the ultimate gene products, in this case the antigen or agglutinogen, are antithetical to one another, like $r'-h'$ genes of antigens rh'-hr', $r''-h''$ genes for agglutinogens rh''-hr'', Fy^a-Fy^b genes for agglutinogens Fy^a-Fy^b. The **set** of all the different possible alleles that can be present in a given locus constitutes a system of **multiple alleles**. The locus for genes of the A-B-O groups is on a different pair of chromosomes from the locus for the allelic genes of the M-N-S system, and the locus for the Rh-Hr system is on still another pair of chromosomes. The three blood group systems are therefore inherited independently of each other. When genes for two distinct characteristics are at different loci on the same pair of chromosomes, they are said to be **linked;** when they are on different chromosomes, they are said to be **independent**.

alloantibody See isoantibody.

alloimmunization See isoimmunization.

amorph Gene that is present but fails to cause a specific antigenic determinant to develop, in this case agglutinogen. Examples are genes O and $\bar{r}$. In the case of the so-called amorphs in the blood grouping category, it might be that

365

they do produce an agglutinogen, but the agglutinogen is not detectable as yet by laboratory methods, or it could be that they cannot be identified by serologic technics. An amorph is an inactive allele that acts as a genetic block to normal biosynthesis. As used in this text, it is an inoperative allele, one that fails to produce a measurable effect; it may even represent the absence (**deletion**) of a gene.

anamnestic response Sharp increase in titer after introduction of an antigen into an animal previously immunized to the same antigen.

antibody; red cell antibody Specifically reacting serum globulin, usually IgG (7S) or IgM (19S), formed by an animal body in response to the introduction of an antigen stimulus. The antibody reacts with the antigen that called it into being. It is present in the plasma and recoverable in either the serum or plasma. **Cross-reactions** are not uncommon. In laboratory tests, as well as in vivo, the antibody combines with the antigen and causes **visible reactions** such as agglutination and hemolysis, Antigen-antibody tests are the basis of all blood grouping.

antigen; red cell antigen Any substance (usually a protein, but possibly a polysaccharide, polypeptide, or polynucleotide) that when introduced into the animal body, often but not necessarily by a parenteral route, stimulates formation of an antibody capable of reacting with or destroying the antigen. Red cell antigens are found on the surface of the red cell and are determined by corresponding genes. In the A-B-H system the blood group antigens are also present in solution in certain body fluids and secretions in individuals designated **secretors.**

antigenic determinant; combining site Site on the antigen molecule that combines with a specific antibody. The number of antigenic sites on the agglutinogen molecule varies according to the antigen. Antigenic determinants are estimated by many methods, including quantitative antiglobulin tests, ^{131}I-labeled anti-Rh_o serum, antiglobulin fixation, and anti-Rh_o-^{125}I-labeled anti–gamma globulin. The more combining sites a molecule has, the easier the tests are to read. Antigenic determinants, or combining sites, are **intrinsic attributes** of the antigen molecule and must not be confused with serologic specificities (blood factors), since each combining group generally has multiple specificities, or **extrinsic attributes.**

antigenicity Capacity of an antigen to stimulate production of an antibody.

antiglobulin Antibody produced by an animal that has been injected with serum globulin. In human blood grouping, this would necessarily be human globulin; in nonhuman primate blood grouping, this would be primate globulin. Antiglobulin is also known as **Coombs serum.** When red cells are coated in saline media with an IgG, 7S, gamma globulin antibody, the cells usually do not clump; however, when antiglobulin serum is added, the antiglobulin unites with the globulin attached to the surface of the red cells, and the cells then clump. There are a number of varieties of antiglobulin.

antiglobulin test; "developing" test; indirect Coombs test Method of testing for "univalent," 7S, IgG antibodies that coat blood cells without clumping them. The IgG antibodies coating the red cells are human serum globulin, so that when anti–human globulin is added it combines with the antibody gamma globulin on the cell surface and clumps the cells. In the **indirect test** the undiluted or diluted serum is mixed with a saline suspension of red cells, and the cells become sensitized, or coated, with the antibody in the serum. After the cells have been washed to remove human serum proteins from the supernate, antiglobulin serum is added. If the cells then clump, they have been coated by IgG, 7S antibodies present in the serum. If they do not clump, they were not sensitized, or coated, by the antibody in the serum.

antiglobulin test (direct) Method of testing for IgG (7S) antibodies in which the cells to be tested have been coated with antibodies in vivo and not by artificial means. The cells are washed four or more times with saline to remove supernatant human or animal protein, then they are mixed with antiglobulin serum. They will clump if they have been coated with an IgG antibody.

anti-Hr sera Antisera specific for the Hr factors, hr′, hr″, hr, hr^s, hr^V, etc. The antisera are used primarily to determine the exact phenotype or probable genotype in the Rh-Hr system. The symbols for the Rh-Hr phenotypes consist of two parts; the reactions with the sera of various Rh specificities are indicated by the left half of the symbol, and the reactions with anti-Hr sera are indicated by the right half. For example, Rh_1rh means the red cells were agglutinated by anti-**Rh_o** and anti-rh′ sera, as well as by anti-hr′, anti-hr″, and anti-hr sera.

anti–nongamma globulin Antibodies that clump cells only in the presence of complement, that is, anti–human globulin that requires complement to complete the reaction.

anti-Rh sera Any of the antisera used in testing blood cells for the various Rh factors, for example, anti-Rh_o, anti-rh′, anti-rh″, anti-Rh_o', and anti-Rh_o'' and the antisera for the cognates of Rh_o'' (Rh^A, Rh^B, Rh^C, Rh^D, etc.). Anti-Rh sera may be IgG or IgM; that is, they may cause agglutination of cells only in a protein medium or by the antiglobulin test, or they may clump cells in a saline medium. Although most anti-Rh testing sera for laboratory reagent purposes are produced by deliberately immunizing normal Rh-negative males, some are obtained from naturally isosensitized patients.

anti-Rh$_o$ serum; standard anti-Rh serum (pl., sera) Antiserum specific for the Rh$_o$ factor, present in types Rh$_o$, Rh$_1$, Rh$_2$, and Rh$_z$. Anti-Rh$_o$ serum of human origin is preferable for diagnostic purposes because anti–rhesus immune animal serum clumps all blood specimens from newborn infants.

anti-rhesus serum Original antiserum produced in guinea pigs and rabbits by Landsteiner and Wiener, which identified the "new" blood factor rhesus, or Rh. It has no relation to the so-called anti-**LW** serum of Levine (pp. 177 to 179).

antiserum (pl., **antisera**) Serum containing specific antibody or antibodies, used for testing purposes in the laboratory. The term is used by some authors to signify any serum that contains an antibody. Antisera are designated by the prefix anti-, followed by the designation of the specificity they detect. Anti-**A,** for example, clumps cells having **A** specificity, anti-**M** agglutinates cells with **M** specificity, anti-**S** clumps cells with **S,** anti-rh" with rh", etc.

Australia antigen See **HAA; HB ag.**

autoagglutination Clumping of an individual's blood cells by his own blood serum because of the presence in the serum of autoagglutinins that act against his red cells. Although an in vitro reaction, it can also occur in vivo.

autoagglutinin An antibody in the serum that causes agglutination of one's own cells. Autoagglutination may take place at low temperatures, in which case the antibody is called a **cold autoagglutinin.** In some cases of hemolytic anemia of the cold autoagglutinin type, tests must be made at 37° C to avoid autoagglutinin reactions. Most autoagglutinins act on all other human cells, as well as on the subject's own, and are then also designated as **panagglutinins.** Frequently, however, cold agglutinins have a specificity for the blood factor **I** and occasionally for **i.**

autoantibody An antibody, not necessarily an agglutinin, that reacts with an individual's own cells.

autograft See under **homograft.**

autologous; autologous transfusion Transfusion of an individual with his own blood. This implies previous withdrawal, processing, and storage of the blood. The word "autologous" means belonging to or coming from an individual's own tissue. Transfusion of blood from another individual of the same species is referred to as **homologous.**

autosomes See **chromosomes.**

avidity of reaction Strength, or potency, of an antiserum in acting against a specific antigen, along with the rate of reaction.

bilirubin One of the bile pigments, which is derived from hemoglobin released from destroyed red cells inside and outside the liver. Bilirubin is constantly circulating in the blood. It is formed in excessive amounts under conditions of massive destruction of red cells, such as in any hemolytic anemia, especially in hemolytic disease of the newborn, or erythroblastosis fetalis. The bile pigments may accumulate in the brain of an infant, resulting in **kernicterus,** or **nuclear jaundice,** and eventual damage to the brain. Bilirubin is identified by specific laboratory tests.

bivalent (complete, IgM, 19S, saline agglutinating) antibodies Large molecule variety antibodies usually formed early in immunization. They are relatively thermolabile, and since they are IgM antibodies, are held back by an intact placenta. They cause clumping of red cells suspended either in saline or in protein media. The term is seldom used any more.

blocking (coating, IgG, incomplete, 7S, univalent) antibody; blocking serum Antibody of the smaller molecule variety, which usually appears late in the course of immunization. It is relatively thermostable and readily passes through the intact placenta. In saline media the red cells are coated with the antibody and do not clump unless a third substance such as antiglobulin is present. The cells will be clumped by the antibody when they are suspended in high-protein media. This term is seldom used today.

blood group factor; blood factor Serologic specificity of an agglutinogen that renders it capable of reacting with specific antibody so that the red cells having the agglutinogen, thus the factor, will clump. The agglutinogen is recognized by its specificities, and it can and does have multiple factors. Each agglutinogen has more than one factor, demonstrated by the fact that it can react with more than one antibody. As an example, human agglutinogen M reacts with anti-**M** and also with anti-**M$_1$,** anti-**M$_{11}$,** anti-**M$_{111}$,** and so on. Agglutinogen Rh$_1$ reacts with anti-**Rh$_o$,** anti-**rh',** anti-**rh$_1$,** and the antibodies that detect the specificities **Rh^A, Rh^B, Rh^C, Rh^D, rh^G, hr", hr^S,** etc. Blood factors (specificities) and agglutinogens must not be confused with one another. The factor is an **extrinsic attribute** of the agglutinogen, and each agglutinogen can have multiple factors. New blood factors are generally identified when an antibody has been found in a serum after a transfusion or a series of transfusions or after or during pregnancy. The **number of blood factors** is theoretically unlimited; according to some authors at least 240 have been identified to date. In the case of the Rh-Hr specificities in particular, the agglutinogens are inherited by means of allelic genes, and the agglutinogens have all their factors in a **set** or a **block** so that the gene for Rh$_1$ (R^1) causes formation of agglutinogen Rh$_1$ with its multiplicity of factors. The specificity, or factor, an extrinsic attribute of an agglutinogen, differs from an **antigenic determinant,** which is an **intrinsic attribute** of the agglutinogen molecule. Thus it can be seen that there is not necessarily a 1:1 correspondence between agglutinogen and antibody but rather between a specific factor, or specificity, and its own antibody. The term **specificity** is used today to denote blood group factor.

blood group systems Collection of the various blood types and groups into categories, depending on their hereditary transmission by genes at the same locus or chromosomal segment. Knowledge of such transmission most often results from family or population genetic studies, as well as from serologic investigations. When, for example, it is found that certain "new" factors tend to be associated with factors of a well-established blood group system and absent when agglutinogens having the factors are absent, the specificity appears to belong in that particular system. Family studies will generally definitely establish such a relationship.

blood grouping; blood typing Division of all humans and animals into classes based on the reactions of their red blood cells with specific antisera and with the blood serum of one another. For example, in the A-B-O system there are four principal groups. Some authors use the term **blood groups** when referring to the A-B-O system and **blood types** when referring to other system such as group O, type Rh$_1$rh, type M, etc.

C-D-E notations System of identifying the blood group phenotypes in the Rh-Hr system, as advanced by British workers. One of the differences between this nomenclature and that of Wiener is that the Rh-Hr nomenclature is based on the **multiple allele gene theory** derived through population genetics and family studies, whereas the C-D-E notations are based on the **linked gene theory.** In the C-D-E system, C stands for rh′, D for Rh$_o$, E for rh″, c for hr′, d for (nonexistent) Hr$_o$, and e for hr″. At the time Fisher advanced this system, he assumed that when C is absent c is always present, or when E is absent e is always present, which has subsequently proved to be incorrect. Some workers use the small letters to indicate **presence** of a factor, others to denote **absence** of the antithetical factor. Table 8-1 is a comparison of three nomenclatures—the Rh-Hr of Wiener, the C-D-E of the British workers, and the numerals of Rosenfield.

cell panels Collection of vials containing red blood cells with as many as possible of the known blood group factors. When serum is tested to detect antibodies that react with red cells, all known antigens must be involved. It is virtually impossible to maintain a complete set of red cells, each with different specific factors, unless these panels of cells are used. They may be purchased or prepared in the laboratory; each vial of cells must have carefully tested and standardized agglutinogens. Each supplier gives a special name to the panels, which are laboratory reagents, for instance, **mixed antigen cells, panel cells,** and so on.

cell survival test Testing blood of the recipient in a transfusion for the presence of transfused red cells that display blood group specificities different from those of the recipient's own red cells, as **N** in a type M patient. The test is used as part of the posttransfusion work-up.

chi-square test See **statistical test.**

chromatin That portion of the nucleus of a cell which stains readily and which is made up of chromosomes containing DNA (deoxyribonucleic acid). The DNA is responsible for genetic information.

chromosomes Rodlike structures of chromatin within cell nuclei that carry the genes, which are the hereditary units, in linear order. Human cells contain twenty-three pairs of chromosomes, or forty-six chromosomes. The chromosomes become duplicated before the cell divides, one member of the resulting pairs of chromosomes going to each nucleus of the two daughter cells. Twenty-two of the pairs of chromosomes are **autosomal,** the twenty-third pair being the **sex chromosomes.** Chromosomes have been **mapped,** or **karyotyped,** and fall naturally into groups (Fig. 4-2). The Y chromosome is exclusive to males; the X occurs in males (XY) as well as in females (XX). See **gene.**

coating antibody Small IgG, 7S antibody that coats the erythrocytes when they are in saline medium but does not cause them to agglutinate unless an antiglobulin serum or high-protein medium is applied. See **blocking antibody** and **univalent (7S) antibody.**

coding of blood group reactions Scheme for systematizing all blood grouping reactions such as the binary coding system advocated by Wiener (p. 315). Computerizing all reactions in the laboratory is simply a matter of time. A number of schemes for coding blood groups or their reactions have been advanced, but the one suggested by Wiener is recommended because it is ideal for use in digital computers.

cold agglutinin Antibody that reacts at low, usually refrigerator, temperatures. The reaction usually disappears when the temperature is elevated above that at which the antibody reacted. Many of the autoagglutinins are cold-reacting antibodies.

combining site See **antigenic determinant.**

compatible bloods Bloods that mix with one another in vitro without any detectable reaction by any known laboratory method. When red cells of one person can be mixed with the serum of a second individual without a reaction, these cells are **compatible** with that serum. When the serum of this first person, whose cells were found compatible with the other serum, cannot be mixed with the cells of the second individual without a reaction, the serum is **incompatible** with the cells. The cells of group A, for example, are compatible with the serum of group AB, but the serum of group A is incompatible with the cells of group AB. Similarly, the cells of group O are compatible with the sera of all the A-B-O groups, but the serum of group O causes clumping of cells of groups A, B, and AB. Stating that the cells of group O are compatible, etc. refers only to the A-B-O system, and there are exceptions even within this system.

complement A complex substance with multiple discrete components, occurring naturally in blood plasma of various species of animals and in man and necessary in serologic hemolytic reactions, as well as in complement-fixation reactions. Its components are designated as C'1, C'2, C'3, C'4, and so on, with the numbers after the prime sign referring to the order of discovery of the component. Complement is active in fresh serum, but its activity gradually diminishes as the serum ages. It can be rendered inactive or destroyed by heating at 56° C for 15 minutes, in which case the serum is said to be **inactivated.** Complement reacts with hemolysin or isohemolysin to lyse, or dissolve, red cells having an antigen specific for that hemolysin. Some blood grouping tests require the presence of complement for activity of the antibody. Complement is most active at 37° C.

complete (**bivalent, IgM, large molecule, 19S, saline agglutinating**) **antibody** Antibody that reacts with red cells to cause them to clump when the cells are suspended in saline media. It is also reactive in a high-protein medium, but this medium is not essential. It is usually of the IgM, or 19S, antibody type and does not traverse the intact placenta. The term is seldom used today.

conglutination Specific clumping of cells caused by the combined action of IgG antibodies and conglutinin.

conglutinin Colloidal aggregate of serum proteins, formerly called X protein. When cells have been sensitized by their specific IgG antibody—that is, when they are coated with antibody—the conglutinin is adsorbed by the cells and causes them to stick together. Conglutinin does not act on nonsensitized cells. It is rela-

tively thermostable. It is sensitive to dilution with crystalline solutions and dissociates into its constituent molecules under such dilution. It appears to be related to complement. It should not be confused with antiglobulin.

conglutinin substitutes Some surface colloids such as acacia, gelatin, dextran, and PVP, which can be substituted for plasma in the conglutination test. They have cohesive and adhesive properties that enable them to act in a conglutination test, but they have the disadvantage of causing nonsensitized cells to clump weakly.

contingency table; 2 × 2 table Statistical method of testing association (or independence) between two genetic factors.

Coombs serum Antiglobulin serum produced in rabbits immunized with human globulin.

Coombs test Antiglobulin test, which may be either direct or indirect. See **antiglobulin.**

counterelectrophoresis Immunologic method of detecting the presence of specific antigen or antibody in a body substance by the combined use of diffusion, electrophoresis, and electroosmosis in agarose medium.

cross matching Compatibility test in which the serum of the patient is mixed with the cells of the donor and the cells of the patient are mixed with the serum of the donor to find out whether the cells remain free, that is, unclumped and not hemolyzed. Its purpose is to determine if a prospective donor is acceptable for a specific recipient. The tests are performed after blood grouping tests have shown that the patient and prospective donors belong to the same A-B-O blood group and Rh-Hr type.

cross-reaction Reaction of one antibody with two or more antigens.

crossing over Translocation of genes, genetic material, or portions of a chromosome that occurs at certain times during meiosis, leading to an exchange of chromosome parts by members of homologous chromosomes.

degrees of freedom Classes or categories in a statistical test, the frequencies of which may be assigned arbitrarily without changing the total number of items involved in the test.

diploid Cells bearing the regular number of chromosomes, twice the number in **haploid** cells.

discoplasm Cytoplasm of red blood cells.

DNA Deoxyribonucleic acid.

dominant; dominant characteristic Term in genetics indicating that a certain characteristic will develop in a subject who carries the corresponding determinant gene, whether in homozygous or heterozygous condition. A dominant gene is expressed in terms of its antigenic product when present either in single dose (one dominant and one recessive) or in double dose (two dominants) such as DR and DD, respectively.

donor One who gives blood in a transfusion or who donates his blood for the purpose of preparing typing sera or panel cells. Blood is given for panel cells when it contains a specific antibody or antigen useful for testing purposes.

dosage effect See **gene dosage effect.**

electrophoresis Movement of particles or molecules in an induced electric field, proportional to the amount of charge on the particles and the intensity of the electrical field.

eluate Product of elution.

elution Process by which red cells are made to release the antibody that has coated them or caused them to agglutinate.

enzyme-treated cells Red cells that have been mixed with a solution of a proteolytic enzyme like trypsin, papain, bromelin, or ficin, which alters the membrane or surface to aid in producing a reaction by an antibody. Some of the blood group antibodies will not react in the presence of enzyme-treated cells, and this nonreaction is one method by which the blood group systems are identified.

erythroblastosis fetalis; EBF; hemolytic disease of the newborn; icterus gravis neonatorum Condition characterized by abnormal destruction and regeneration of erythrocytes, with intravascular hemolysis or clumping, or both, and pathologic changes in the fetus or newborn infant resulting from the action of antibodies on its blood cells. The 7S antibodies are formed in the mother's circulation in response to stimulation by fetal red cells that have entered her bloodstream. The fetal cells are usually but not always of a different blood group such as an Rh-positive fetus and an Rh-negative mother. The mother's antibodies pass through the placenta and coat the infant's cells. In the presence of certain globulins the coated cells either hemolyze or clump; severe jaundice ensues with increase in bile pigment, nuclear jaundice, and death or serious damage to the infant or fetus. Erythroblastosis fetalis may also be due to incompatibilities other than Rh.

extrinsic attribute Attribute of agglutinogen or antigen substances, which would be technically nonexistent if there were no antisera with which it could be demonstrated. There are seemingly unlimited numbers of these attributes. For example, agglutinogen A has the extrinsic attributes (specificities, or factors) **A** and **C**, and agglutinogen B has both **B** and **C**, etc.; the extrinsic attribute **C** is shared by both agglutinogens. See **blood group factor.**

Fab; Fc Fragments of immunoglobulin split by papain. The Fc fragment (fragment, **c**rystalline) is the heavy chain of the immunoglobulin. The Fab fragment (fragment, **a**ntigen **b**inding) is the light chain of the immunoglobulin.

factor; blood group factor See **blood group factor** and **specificity.**

Freund's adjuvant Emulsion of certain mycobacteria used in immunologic studies with laboratory animals. The immune response to antigens by the animals, especially soluble antigens, is enhanced and prolonged when using antigens emulsified in the adjuvant. (For more complete information, consult the Difco Manual Supplementary Literature, May, 1972.)

gamma globulins See **immunoglobulins.**

gene Unit of inheritance carried supposedly in a linear order along the chromosome. There is a pair of genes for each characteristic of an organism. Genes and genotypes are designated by *italics.* See **alleles; allelic genes.**

gene deletion Loss of genetic material from a chromosome. Although it is possible that a small portion of a chromosome carrying a gene could be lost by accident at some cell division in the past, the so-called deletions may actually be special mutant allelic genes.

gene dosage effect When the antigen, which is an expression of the genes, in a homozygous individual is more reactive than in a heterozygous individual. A person who is heterozygous for a certain blood group characteristic may have red cells that react with less avidity than do those from a homozygous individual. An example would be the reactions with anti-N of type N, genotype *NN*, as opposed to type MN, genotype *MN*.

genotype Constitutional makeup of an individual in terms of his genes as determined by heredity. Genotypes are determined primarily by family studies after serologic blood grouping tests have been made. In some cases the genotype is obvious, as in group AB, in which the gene for antigen A has necessarily been derived from one parent and the gene for antigen B from another. The same is true of group O, for which only one genotype, *OO*, is possible. Genotypes are transmitted through the germ cells by means of the chromosomes, but there is evidence, in rare exceptional cases, of cytoplasmic inheritance. Each of the twenty-three pairs of chromosomes in the human contains numerous genes arranged in linear order, and every individual has a pair of each kind of gene for each characteristic—one derived from the maternal parent and the other from the paternal parent.

group-specific substance See Witebsky substance.

HAA Hepatitis-associated antigen.

haploid Cells bearing a single set of chromosomes, half the number of diploid cells. This is the normal complement of gametes (ova and spermatozoa).

hapten A term introduced by Landsteiner for substances that lack antigenicity but are capable of reacting specifically with immune sera in vitro. Polysaccharide antigenic determinants are haptens. They have a molecular weight of less than 4000.

HBAg Australia antigen. Hepatitis B antigen.

hemizygous Term applied when a gene is present only once in the genotype and not in the form of a pair of alleles, as for genes in the sex chromosomes, for example, genotype *XY* of males.

hemolysis Breaking down of the red cells with release of hemoglobin, often called simply dissolving, lysis, or disintegration of the red blood cells. It can be caused by physical means such as heat, electricity, or osmotic pressure when erythrocytes are placed in water. It can also be caused by chemical means such as detergents that lyse red cells or by serologic means like action of an antibody (**hemolysin**) on the cells that have the corresponding antigen, plus a third substance, **complement**. Some of the blood grouping antibodies are hemolytic; that is, when red cells are tested by freshly drawn serum containing that antibody and complement, the cells will dissolve instead of clumping, for example, anti-**A**, anti-**B**, anti-**Lewis**, anti-**Vel**.

hemolytic transfusion reaction Adverse reaction to a blood transfusion of incompatible blood cells in which the donor cells are destroyed in vivo.

heteroagglutination Clumping of cells of an animal or human by antibodies present in the serum of a member of a different species—an **interspecies** reaction—as opposed to isoagglutination.

heteroagglutinin Agglutinin that clumps red cells derived from a member of a different species.

heteroligating antibodies Antibodies that supposedly contain two different combining groups, said by Wiener to be nonexistent.

heterospecific pregnancy Pregnancy in which the mother's serum contains anti-**A** or anti-**B** antibodies that are incompatible with the red cells of her fetus, as in the case of a group O mother with a group A or group B fetus.

heterozygous Genetically impure, with a genotype consisting of two different allelic genes; for example, group A genotypes may be homozygous, *AA,* or heterozygous, *AO.* Inheritance of one dominant and one recessive characteristic, as in heterozygosity, results in expression of the dominant characteristic, but the unexpressed recessive gene can be transmitted to the offspring, where it can reveal itself if homozygous, as in group O.

homograft; homotransplant Transplantation of organs or tissues from man to man or from animal to animal of the same species. An **autograft** is a graft, or piece of tissue, removed from one part of the body and transferred to another part of the body of the same individual.

homologous blood Blood of an individual other than the subject under examination, belonging to the same blood group and usually referring to the A-B-O system.

homologous serum jaundice; hepatitis; serum hepatitis Hepatitis transferred through transfusion of whole blood, plasma, serum, thrombin, or fibrinogen. The danger of transmission of the viral cause of the disease is greatest, apparently, in pooled plasma transfusions and may cause death in as many as one in 600 transfusions. Many of the precautions taken in blood banks are for prevention of this disease.

homozygous When both alleles of a characteristic are alike. Homozygous individuals are referred to as **genetically pure.** See **heterozygous.**

Hr factors Blood group factors reciprocal to the Rh factors. They react with the various anti-Hr sera. They are important in determining phenotypes and probable genotypes in the Rh-Hr system and in some cases of intragroup transfusion reactions and erythroblastosis fetalis.

Hr sensitization Production of antibodies against Hr factors. If the exact Hr factor is not specified, it may be assumed that **hr'** is the specificity causing the production of antibodies, since it is the most antigenic of all the Hr factors.

Hr testing Examination of blood for Hr antigen on red cells, using Hr antisera.

human-type blood groups Blood groups of nonhuman primates determined by testing simian red cells and secretions with reagents used for blood grouping of human cells.

Ig See **immunoglobulins.**

immunization; immunized individual; sensitization; isoimmunization; isosensitization Production of antibodies against an antigenic stimulus. An immunized individual therefore is a person or an animal that has produced such antibodies either because of injection of the antigen or because of its presence through some process like transfusion or pregnancy. Sensitization also refers to production of antibodies in response to an antigenic stimulus. It is not to be confused with the expression "sensitized cells," which means cells that have been coated with antibody. Isosensitization is production of antibodies by one member of a species against an antigen in a different member of the same species, particularly against a **type-specific antigen** like anti-Rh in an Rh-negative person. Isoimmunization and isosensitization are often used interchangeably, but the term sensitization generally has the connotation of producing clinical problems, as in Rh sensitization, whereas immunization implies protective immunity, as in measles immunization.

immunogenetics Study of heredity in connection with the blood groups or the study of heredity of blood group factors by family studies or methods of population genetics.

immunogenicity See **antigenicity.**

immunoglobulins Proteins concerned with antibody formation. Electrophoretically they appear in the γ_2 to γ_1 band. Immunoglobulins are described on p. 23ff. When suitably modified as a result of the immune response, they act like antibodies. They are designated as IgG, IgM, IgA, IgD, and IgE, as well as 7S, 19S, 11S, etc.

immunohematology Branch of the study of blood that deals with antigens and antibodies and their clinical implications such as for blood transfusion, in particular, blood group serology, autoantibody formation, autosensitization, and autohemolytic anemias.

in vitro Literally, "in glass," or in the test tube. A reaction occurring outside the human or animal body; a laboratory reaction.

in vivo Within the living body or organism.

inactivation of serum Heating a serum to 56° C to render complement inactive or to destroy it.

incomplete (blocking, IgG, 7S, univalent) antibody Small molecule antibody that requires a third substance before it will combine with its specific antigen to cause a visible reaction. It *coats* red cells in saline media rather than causes them to agglutinate. When the appropriate antiglobulin serum or conglutinin, etc. is added, the coated cells clump. The term is seldom used today. See **antibody.**

independence of blood group specificities Occurrence of two or more specificities inherited by independent genes (genes located on different chromosomes or on different portions of one and the same chromosome).

inhibition of antibody Suppression of an expected serologic reaction. For example, a strong anti-P_1 was found in two patients with hydatid disease. Hydatid cyst fluid from sheep's livers, if it contains scolices, inhibits anti-P_1 sera but not anti-$P(Tj^a)$, which is inhibited only weakly if at all. Anti-I has also been inhibited by hydatid cyst fluid containing scolices. Saliva may inhibit anti-A, anti-B, or anti-H antibodies if it comes from a secretor of the appropriate blood group, as will semen, vaginal fluid, gastric fluid, dried red blood cells, and so on. The ability to inhibit antibody is the basis of the inhibition and absorption test for individual identification of stains of dried blood and body fluids.

intrinsic attribute See **antigenic determinant.**

irregular antibody Antibody not found as a regular occurrence, like anti-A and anti-B, but often formed artificially either by transfusion or pregnancy. Anti-Rh antibodies formed in individuals lacking the Rh factor is an example. Anti-P can be a naturally occurring, irregular agglutinin, or it can be artificially produced. The same is true of anti-M and anti-N.

iso- Prefix applied most frequently in blood grouping to human agglutinogens and agglutinins of the A-B-O blood group system. It refers to **intraspecies** reactions. Isosensitization, for example, means formation of antibodies by an animal or human in response to an antigen present in another member of the same species. Anti-**Rh** antibodies, formed in Rh-negative individuals injected with Rh-positive blood, are isoantibodies. Isoimmunization, preferably designated as isosensitization, occurs in pregnancies as well as in transfusions.

isoagglutination Reaction between an antibody and an antigen of different individuals of the same species such as clumping of cells of a group A person by serum of a group B person. It is an **intraspecies** reaction as opposed to **heteroagglutination,** which is an **interspecies** reaction.

isoagglutinin Antibody that causes clumping of red cells of another individual of the same species.

isoagglutinogen Antigen (agglutinogen) that reacts with agglutinins of a different member of the same species.

isoantibody; alloantibody Antibody that acts on red cells of other individuals of the same species but not on the individual's own red cells.

isoimmunization; isosensitization; alloimmunization Formation of antibodies by a member of a species in response to stimulation by an antigen from another member of the same species.

kernicterus; nuclear jaundice Severe form of icterus of the newborn in which degenerative lesions are found in the lenticular nucleus, subthalamus, and Ammon's horn. Damage to the brain cells is due to abnormally high levels of serum bilirubin.

lectin Plant agglutinins, or extracts of seeds, that cause agglutination of human and animal red cells. The most useful are anti-A_1 made from *Dolichos biflorus,* anti-H from *Ulex europeus,* and anti-N from *Vicia graminea,* and the leaves of the Korean *Vicia unijuga* (p. 296). The term lectin is reserved for those plant agglutinins that show group specificity. Other plant agglutinins are called **phytagglutinins.**

linkage; gene linkage; linked genes Two gene loci within measurable distance of one another on the same chromosome; the nearer they are to one another, the closer is the linkage. Two alleles with closely linked loci may pass through many generations together, until they are separated by **crossing over.** Linked genes tend to be inherited together.

locus (pl., **loci**) Site, or position, of a gene or its alleles on a chromosome.

lyophilization Freeze drying under vacuum.

lysis Disruption, dissolving, or dissolution of red blood cells.

meiosis Cell division with formation of gametes wherein the number of chromosomes is reduced from diploid to haploid (half the number).

mitosis Cell division with a series of changes in the nucleus and cytoplasm, in which the chromatin is modified into two sets of chromosomes that split longitudinally, one set going to each pole before the cell divides to form two daughter cells.

mixed antigen cells; multiple antigen cells See **cell panels.**

modifying genes Genes that can be detected only by their effect on the expression of other genes.

mosaicism; chimerism Refers to the presence in one individual of more than one kind of blood; for example, a person may have both A and B agglutinogens, which are present in different cells. This mixture of blood apparently takes place in utero by exchange of marrow cells from one fraternal twin to another or possibly from primary accident of gametogenesis.

mutation Change that takes place in the chromosomes resulting in production of a distinctive new characteristic that is then passed on to subsequent generations. The alteration takes place most often at the level of the gene.

NANA *N*-Acetylneuraminic acid (**sialic acid**).

nonsecretor See **secretor.**

null types Blood types that lack all demonstrable antigens, such as groups O, Rh$_{null}$, Lu(a-b-), Fy(a-b-), among others. See Table 11-1. They are usually discovered by accidental immunization. Most often they are inherited by autosomal recessives that are independent of the genes of the blood group system itself. One is known to be inherited by a dominant suppressor gene, and one probably depends on a gene on the sex chromosome X.

organ rejection When an organ or other tissue is transplanted from one person or animal to another or from an animal to a person or vice versa, and the tissues of the animal receiving the transplant react to cause destruction of the transplant. It is believed that this is a result of an immunologic reaction. Rejection of organs or tissues transplanted from one human to another may be due to a form of isoantibody production.

panagglutination; bacteriogenic agglutination; Huebener-Thomsen phenomenon Condition in which a serum causes agglutination of all cells, often even cells from the individual from whom the serum was derived. It is frequently a result of bacterial action and does not usually occur when blood and sera are fresh and sterile.

panmixia A system of mating characterized by random choice of mating partners, as opposed to nonrandom mating.

passive immunization Administration of specific antibodies to enhance immunity in an individual or to neutralize incompatible red cells circulating in an individual's blood. An example is anti-Rh antibodies (RhoGAM), given to prevent sensitization of a pregnant woman due to Rh incompatibility.

phenotype Characteristic of individuals of a species determined by direct observation, measurement, or chemical or serologic testing. It may be partly or wholly genetically determined, or it may be entirely determined by environmental influences. In the blood groups, phenotypes are an expression of the antigens on the red cells, produced by genes, but not all the genetic factors are necessarily represented. For example, phenotype Rh$_1$rh shows that genes R^1 and r are probably present, but family studies show that people of this phenotype could also be of genotypes R^1R^0 or R^0r'. In the Rh-Hr phenotypes, represented by a double symbol, reactions with anti-Rh sera are indicated by the left-hand portion of the symbol and reactions with anti-Hr sera by the right-hand portion. See Tables 8-3 and 8-9.

plasma Liquid portion of the blood in the blood vessels. When blood is removed from the body and mixed with an anticoagulant to keep it from clotting, the supernatant fluid after the blood cells settle is called plasma. It contains fibrinogen along with other proteins but not blood cells.

plasmapheresis Procedure in which blood is withdrawn from an individual, the red blood cells and plasma separated from one another, and the packed cells then returned to the circulation of the individual. Large quantities of plasma can thus be obtained from a single donor without reducing his red blood cell count.

population genetics Method of calculating gene frequencies in different groups of people or animals, using certain mathematical formulas. The mechanism of inheritance of an individual characteristic can be determined by such studies. The distribution within a population of certain blood group characteristics or agglutinogens and their allelic genes can also be determined in this manner.

probability (statistical) The relative frequency of the occurrence of an event as measured by the ratio of the number of cases or alternatives favorable to the event, to the total number of cases or alternatives.

popositus; proband First studied member of a family or one whose unusual blood type initiated a study of the blood of related members of the pedigree. In other words, it is the member of a family through whom the family came to be investigated.

proteolytic enzyme Organic substance, secreted by living cells, that catalyzes the digestion of protein. These are used in blood grouping to act on the red cell surface to render the cells more easily agglutinated, especially when mixed with small molecular antibodies. The enzymes most frequently used are trypsin, papain, bromelin, and ficin.

protocol Refers to a record of the reactions observed in the laboratory. (Its connotation in blood grouping is different from that in general parlance.)

prozone Phenomenon observed at times in titrations of antibodies in which the antibody apparently reacts more strongly when the serum is diluted than when undiluted.

pseudoagglutination False appearance of agglutination due to cause other than antigen-antibody reactions. Rouleaux formation of the erythrocytes is an example.

RDE Receptor-destroying enzymes.

recessive characteristic Mendelian characteristic transmitted by heredity, which is expressed only in homozygotes. When the recessive characteristic is present with a dominant gene, the recessive is not expressed, but when an individual is homozygous for a recessive gene, that individual develops as a recessive.

recipient Individual who receives blood (or plasma, serum, etc.) in a transfusion.

Rh antibodies; rhesus antibodies Antibodies formed as a result of a stimulus by any of the Rh specificities in an individual who lacks such factors.

Rh antisera Laboratory testing sera for identification of any of the Rh specificities. The antisera most widely and routinely used are anti-Rh_o, anti-rh′, and anti-rh″. Anti-rh^w is used routinely in some blood banks. Each antiserum detects its specific factor; thus anti-Rh_o detects specificity Rh_o, anti-rh′ detects rh′, anti-rh″ detects rh″, and anti-rh^w detects rh^w. By combining the information obtained in using these four antisera alone, twelve types can be identified, as in Table 8-3.

Rh conglutination test Test for anti-Rh IgG, 7S antibodies, also known as **indirect test for univalent Rh antibodies.** It is more sensitive than the blocking test for detecting such antibodies.

Rh factors; rhesus factors Serologic specificities on the red cell surface that are responsible for the reactions with Rh antisera. The most commonly tested for Rh factors are Rh_o, rh′, rh″, and rh^w. There are also variants of these.

Rh genes Series of allelic genes that determine the various Rh agglutinogens and Rh blood types. The most important so far identified are r, $r′$, $r^{′w}$, $r″$, r^y, R^o, R^1, R^{1w}, R^2, and R^Z, determining, respectively, agglutinogens rh, rh′, rh′^{w}, rh″, rh^y, Rh_o, Rh_1, Rh_1^w, Rh_2, and Rh_z. Genes are designated by the use of *italics,* and the "h" is dropped from the symbol so that genes and agglutinogens and blood specificities, or factors, will not be confused with one another. For example, gene R^1 determines the agglutinogen Rh_1 having specificities Rh_o and rh′; R^2 deter-

mines the agglutinogen Rh_2 having specificities Rh_o and rh″. Among Caucasoids, genes R^1, R^2, and r are those most commonly found; genes R^o, $r′$, and $r″$ are relatively rare; and R^Z and r^y are extremely rare. Gene R^o is found most commonly in Negroids, and the rare gene R^Z is found most often in East Asians (Mongolians), to a frequency of 3% to 5%.

Rh genes; rare allelic genes According to Wiener, genes r^v, r^G, R^{oV}, R^{od}, $\mathfrak{R}^o$, $\bar{R}^o$, $\hat{R}{}^o$, R^{1ab}, R^{2ab}, $\bar{\bar{R}}^o$, $\bar{\bar{R}}^w$, $\bar{r}$, etc. may additionally be postulated. See Tables 8-3 and 8-11 for other Rh-Hr genes.

Rh sensitization; Rh immunization Formation of antibodies against an Rh specificity in response to a transfusion or pregnancy. Clinically, two widely spaced transfusions of Rh-positive blood in Rh-negative persons are more likely to lead to Rh sensitization than are multiple transfusions covering only a short space of time. Those who have been sensitized to the Rh factor remain so for life, although the titer of antibodies becomes gradually weaker. A small injection of Rh-positive blood into such individuals will stimulate a pronounced and sustained rise in antibody titer (**anamnestic reaction**).

Rh testing Classifying blood by testing with anti-Rh_o serum alone, thus dividing all individuals into two groups—Rh positive and Rh negative.

Rh typing Classifying blood into one of the eight standard Rh types, using anti-Rh_o, anti-rh′, and anti-rh″ sera. Further classification is possible by using other Rh-Hr antisera in addition to these.

Rh variants Agglutinogens that give weak or **intermediate reactions** with one or more of the Rh-Hr antisera. The most important variants of Rh_o factors are $\mathfrak{R}h_o$, $\mathfrak{R}h_1$, $\mathfrak{R}h_2$, and $\mathfrak{R}h_z$. Such variants are more commonly found among Negroids than among Caucasians. The agglutinogens $\mathfrak{R}h_o$, $\mathfrak{R}h_1$, and $\mathfrak{R}h_2$ are believed to be inherited by the corresponding allelic genes, $\mathfrak{R}^o$, $\mathfrak{R}^1$, and $\mathfrak{R}^2$. For other variants, see p. 116ff.

Rh_o factor (specificity); standard Rh factor Original Rh factor corresponding to the rhesus factor of Landsteiner and Wiener. It is present in 85% of Caucasoids, 95% of Negroids, and almost 100% of Asiatics. It is the most antigenic of the Rh factors; this fact is indicated by the use of the capital "R" in the symbol. More than 90% of cases of erythroblastosis fetalis and intragroup hemolytic transfusion reactions are due to this factor.

Rh_o genotypes Since no anti-Hr_o serum has ever been found or produced, the genotypes of type Rh_o individuals cannot usually be determined directly by serologic methods alone. When tests are limited to Rh_o, three genotypes in the Rh system are possible, based on the theory that the Rh_o specificity is inherited as a simple mendelian dominant by means of a pair of allelic genes, *Rh* and *rh*. These genotypes are *RhRh*, *Rhrh*, and *rhrh*. Rh-negative people are always homozygous. The genotypes listed here are useful in helping to predict the presence or absence of the Rh factor in the offspring of a mating of an Rh-positive and an Rh-negative individual, but this oversimplifies the subject.

Rh₀ phenotypes Two phenotypes, Rh positive and Rh negative, which can be distinguished by using anti-**Rh₀** serum alone.

Rh-Hr types; Rh-Hr phenotypes Different types of blood demonstrable by testing the red cells with both anti-Rh and anti-Hr sera. The left-hand side of the symbol represents the results using Rh antisera, the right-hand side results with Hr antisera.

rouleaux formation of red cells When red cells are suspended, especially in certain high molecular colloids, and appear stacked on top of one another, like a roll of coins that has been pushed over. This appearance may stimulate agglutination and could be incorrectly reported as a positive laboratory result. Rouleaux formation may occur in patients having a rapid sedimentation rate, as in multiple myeloma. It is a form of pseudoagglutination. As a general rule, *rouleaux may be broken up by addition of saline.* See **pseudoagglutination.**

saline Salt solution. In blood grouping, it is physiologic sodium chloride solution, 0.85% sodium chloride in water.

saline antibody 19S, IgM antibody that reacts when the opposing cells are suspended in saline without antiglobulin serum or enzymes.

screening tests Tests made initially to separate specimens into categories, for example, testing to determine whether the blood is Rh positive or Rh negative. This eliminates performance of unnecessary laboratory tests. If the blood is Rh negative, only such tests will then be performed as should be made on Rh-negative blood. If the blood is Rh positive, further tests can be made to determine the exact Rh type, the phenotype, and the probable genotype. Screening tests are done in all branches of the laboratory, not only in blood grouping.

secretor; nonsecretor Persons who secrete the blood group substances, especially A-B-H, conditional to inheritance of the secretor gene *Se*. Blood group antigens are not confined to the red blood cells but can appear throughout the body, especially in the saliva, seminal or vaginal fluid, and gastric contents, of these individuals. Others who do not have the soluble substance in their body fluids are called **nonsecretors** and are homozygous for the *se* gene, genotype *sese*.

segregation Separation of allele pairs from one another and distribution to separate germ cells at meiosis. Segregation is observable only in het-

erozygous genotypes that have two different alleles.

sensitivity test A test of serum for irregular antibodies, such as anti-Rh and others.

sensitized cells Blood cells that have antibodies specifically attached to their surfaces but are not agglutinated or hemolyzed. Red cells may be artificially sensitized in the laboratory, or they may become coated in vivo as a result of sensitization by incompatible pregnancy or transfusion or by autoantibodies.

sensitization Formation of antibodies against a specific antigen. See **immunization** and **isoimmunization; isosensitization.**

seroanthropology Study of blood group distributions in various human populations.

seroprimatology Study of blood group distributions in various simian species, races, and populations.

serum (pl., sera) Fluid that collects from clotted blood. When fibrinogen is removed from plasma, the resulting fluid is serum.

serum grouping; reverse grouping Testing serum for the presence of anti-**A** and anti-**B** agglutinins as part of the A-B-O blood grouping procedure.

sex chromosome Chromosome, either X or Y, that determines sex. The male is XY, and female XX under normal circumstances.

sex-linked traits or characteristics Traits determined by genes located on sex chromosomes.

simian-type blood groups Blood groups of nonhuman primates determined by testing simian red cells with reagents produced by isoimmunization or cross-immunization of nonhuman primates.

somatic chromosomes; autosomal chromosomes; autosomes Nonsex chromosomes.

specific reaction Ability of an antibody to react only with cells having the antigen that corresponds to the antibody and with no other antigens. There is actually no 1:1 correspondence between antibody and agglutinogen, but instead between antibody and blood factor (serologic specificity).

specificity; serologic specificity See **blood group factor.**

statistical test Set of mathematical calculations that determine the probability of the occurrence of a phenomenon by chance only.

subtyping Further division of the various blood groups, or types, into their specific subdivisions; for example, group A can be further divided into subtypes A_1, A_2, $A_{1.2}$, A_3, A_4, etc., depending on the antisera used and on the kinds of reactions. Type rh′ can be subdivided into rh′ʷ as well as rh′, and so on. Also called **subgrouping.**

superfecundation Impregnation, by successive acts of coitus, of two or more ova liberated at the same ovulation. If it occurs at all, it is a very rare phenomenon.

suppressor genes Genes that can influence the effect of other genes on the same or different chromosomes and actually suppress or prevent expression of the other genes. An example is the Bombay blood type, which is due to homozygosity for a rare suppressor gene.

Svedberg coefficient; sedimentation constants Rate at which immunoglobulin components sediment. Immunoglobulins (Ig) are separated into a number of components according to their molecular weight as determined by means of ultracentrifugation, that is, centrifugation at a speed of over 50,000 rpm. The most rapidly sedimenting component is the M fraction, the second is G, and the slowest is the A fraction. The **Svedberg unit (S)** expresses the sedimentation coefficient per unit time in seconds. See Table 2-1 for sedimentation constants of the various immunoglobulins.

thermal amplitude Temperature range of activity of an antibody.

titer; titre Means by which the concentration of an antibody in a serum is measured. The serum is diluted serially and mixed with appropriate red cells. The highest dilution at which a reaction occurs is the end point of the titration. The titer is expressed in units and is the reciprocal of the highest dilution giving a distinct reaction. For example, if the highest dilution at which a reaction occurs is 1:16, the titer is 16 units.

titration Laboratory test by which certain reagents are tested for concentration. In blood grouping, titration refers to determination of the highest dilution of an antiserum demonstrably reactive for its corresponding antigen.

transfusion reaction Untoward manifestations of agglutination or hemolysis, or both, of red cells after infusion of blood of one individual into the bloodstream of another. Most such transfusion reactions are due to injecting blood containing an antigen to which the recipient has an antibody. Some reactions occur for reasons other than incompatibility of bloods, such as overaged or overheated blood, pyrogens in solutions, or allergens. These are due to nonspecific agents.

univalent (IgG, 7S) antibody Antibody of the small molecule type that readily passes through an intact placenta. It coats specific cells in saline media without causing them to agglutinate or hemolyze, and requires the presence of a third substance to complete the agglutination or hemolytic reaction. **Incomplete antibody.** The term preferred today is IgG, 7S antibody.

universal donor; universal recipient Now outdated concepts of use of certain blood in blood transfusion that can lead to dangerous reactions. It was formerly believed that group O blood (universal donor) could be safely transfused to individuals of any of the four A-B-O blood groups because group O cells do not have A or B agglutinogens and are therefore not agglutinable by the anti-A in blood group B or the anti-B in blood group A. A universal recipient was a group AB person, whose serum lacks the anti-A and anti-B antibodies and therefore will not clump incoming cells of any of the four blood groups. In certain emergencies, group O whole blood is still given to an A, B, or AB recipient.

warm agglutinin Antibody that reacts best in vitro at 37° C (body temperature).

washing cells Process of removing all traces of protein or other substances from cells, as well as from the medium in which such cells are suspended. It is accomplished by suspending the cells in saline, centrifuging, removing the supernate, and resuspending the cells in fresh saline, then repeating the process a number of times. Water cannot be used because it lyses red cells.

Witebsky substance, group-specific substances A and B Carbohydrate-like compounds displaying group A or group B specificity, extracted from horse saliva and from preparations of pepsin and peptone (A substance), or from stomach juice (B substance). Group-specific substances are added to blood used for transfusion to inhibit, or suppress, undesirable effects of anti-A or anti-B isoagglutinins present in the transfused blood; to stimulate formation of immune anti-A and anti-B agglutinins in voluntary human donors in the production of high-titered blood grouping reagents; and in tests to detect factor C of the A-B-O blood groups (Table 18-9).

zeta potential Potential at the boundary of shear, or the surface charge of erythrocytes. Such proteolytic enzymes as trypsin, papain, bromelin, and ficin reduce the net surface charge, or density, of the red cells and thus enhance agglutination by altering the so-called zeta potential. Bovine albumin and some of the synthetic polymers reduce the zeta potential by raising the dielectric constant of the reaction medium. In saline suspension, red cells carry a net negative charge that keeps them apart in stable suspension. This surface charge can be brought below a "critical potential" by multivalent cations. At this point the red cells will agglutinate.

Index